Stockley
Pocket C

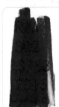

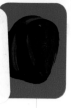

D0723687

interactions Pocket
companion 2015

DEC 03 2015

Stockley's Drug Interactions Pocket Companion 2015

Editor
Claire L Preston, BPharm, PGDipMedMan, MRPharmS

Editorial Staff
Elaina E Crehan, MChem
Samuel Driver, BSc
Chloë SAJ Hatwal, BSc, MRes
Stephanie L Jones, MPharm, MRPharmS
Sonia Z Khan, MPharm, PGCertPharmPrac
Rebecca E Luckhurst, BSc
Deirdre M McGuirk, BComm, MPharm, MRPharmS
Harpreet K Sandhu, MPharm, MRPharmS
Sandra Sutton, BPharm, MSc Med, Cert ProjMngt

Based on data produced by the Stockley Editorial Team
Ian A Baxter BSc, PhD, MRPharmS
Mildred Davis, BA, BSc, PhD, MRPharmS
Claire Jones, BPharm, MRPharmS, DipPresSci
Rebekah Raymond, BSc, DipPharmPrac
Julia Sawyer, BPharm, DipPharmPrac

Expert Contributor
C Rhoda Lee, BPharm, PhD, MRPharmS

PhP
Pharmaceutical Press

Published by Pharmaceutical Press

1 Lambeth High Street, London SE1 7JN, UK

© Royal Pharmaceutical Society of Great Britain 2015

(PP) is a trade mark of Pharmaceutical Press

Pharmaceutical Press is the publishing division of the Royal
Pharmaceutical Society

First published 2014

Typeset by Data Standards Ltd, Frome, Somerset
Printed in Italy by Rotolito Lombarda S.p.A.

ISBN 978 0 85711 167 8
ePDF 978 0 85711 199 9
ePub 978 0 85711 200 2

A catalogue record for this book is available from the British Library

Contents

Preface

What is *Stockley's Drug Interactions Pocket Companion*?

Stockley's Drug Interactions is a reference work that provides concise, accurate, and clinically relevant information to healthcare professionals. Monographs are based on published sources including clinical studies, case reports, and systematic reviews, and are fully referenced. *Stockley's Drug Interactions Pocket Companion* has summarised this comprehensive work to create a small and conveniently-sized quick-reference text.

  Stockley's Drug Interactions Pocket Companion provides the busy healthcare professional with quick and easy access to clinically relevant, evaluated and evidence-based information about drug interactions. As with the full reference work this publication attempts to answer the following questions:

- Are the drugs or substances in question known to interact or is the interaction only theoretical and speculative?
- If they do interact, how serious is it?
- Has it been described many times or only once
- Are all patients affected or only a few?
- Is it best to avoid some drug combinations altogether or can the interaction be accommodated in some way?
- What alternative and safer drugs can be used instead?

Coverage

Stockley's Drug Interactions Pocket Companion 2014 contains over 2200 interaction monographs pertaining to specific drugs or drug groups. Each monograph in *Stockley's Drug Interactions* was assessed by practising clinical pharmacists for its suitability for inclusion in the *Pocket Companion*. Broadly speaking interactions involving anaesthesia, the specialist use of multiple antiretrovirals, the specialist use of multiple antineoplastics or intravenous antineoplastics, and non-interactions were omitted. However, exceptions were made, particularly where there has been controversy over whether or not a drug interacts.

Monographs

Following the familiar format of the Stockley products, the information in this publication is organised into a brief summary of the evidence for the interaction and a description of how best to manage it. The information is based on the most recent quarterly update of *Stockley's Drug Interactions* at the time of going to press. This data is fully referenced and available at www.medicinescomplete.com. These references have not been included in the *Pocket Companion* to keep size to a minimum. Anyone interested in seeing our sources can consult *MedicinesComplete*, or the full reference work of *Stockley's Drug Interactions*.

Ratings

Each monograph has been assigned a rating symbol to offer guidance to the user on the clinical significance of the interaction. These ratings are the same as those used in *Stockley's Interaction Alerts*. The Alerts are rated using three separate categories:

- Action – This describes whether or not any action needs to be taken to accommodate the interaction. This category ranges from 'avoid' to 'no action needed'.
- Severity – This describes the likely effect of an unmanaged interaction on the patient. This category ranges from 'severe' to 'nothing expected'.
- Evidence – This describes the weight of evidence behind the interaction. This category ranges from 'extensive' to 'theoretical'.

These ratings are combined to produce one of four symbols:

❌ For interactions that have a life-threatening outcome, or where concurrent use is contraindicated by the manufacturers.

⚠ For interactions where concurrent use may result in a significant hazard to the patient and so dose adjustment or close monitoring is needed.

❓ For interactions where there is some doubt about the outcome of concurrent use, and therefore it may be necessary to give patients some guidance about possible adverse effects, and/or consider some monitoring.

✔ For interactions that are not considered to be of clinical significance, or where no interaction occurs.

We put a lot of thought in to the original design of these symbols, and have deliberately avoided a numerical or colour coding system as we did not want to imply any relationship between the symbols or colours. Instead we chose internationally recognisable symbols, which in testing were intuitively understood by our target audience of healthcare professionals.

Structure

Stockley's Drug Interactions Pocket Companion is structured alphabetically for ease of use, with International Nonproprietary Names (INNs) to identify drug names. Cross references to US Approved Names (USANs) are also included where drug names differ significantly. Consequently an interaction between aspirin and beta blockers will appear under A, and an interaction between beta blockers and digoxin will appear under B. We have only used drug groups where they are considered to be widely recognised, hence beta blockers is used, but alpha agonists is not. The drug groups we have used are as follows:

ACE inhibitors	Endothelin receptor	NSAIDs
Alpha blockers	antagonists	Opioids
Amfetamines	Ergot derivatives	Penicillins
Aminoglycosides	Fibrates	Phosphodiesterase
Angiotensin II	H$_2$-receptor	type-5 inhibitors
receptor antagonists	antagonists	Proton pump
Antimuscarinics	HRT	inhibitors
Antidiabetics	HIV-protease	Quinolones
Antihistamines	inhibitors	Salbutamol (Albuterol)
Antimuscarinics	5-HT$_3$-receptor	and related
Antipsychotics	antagonists	bronchodilators
Azoles	Inotropes and	SSRIs
Benzodiazepines	Vasopressors	Statins
Beta blockers	Low-molecular-weight	Sulfonamides
Bisphosphonates	heparins	Tetracyclines
Calcium-channel	Macrolides	Tricyclics
blockers	MAO-B inhibitors	Triptans
Cephalosporins	MAOIs	Vaccines
Contraceptives	Nasal decongestants	Warfarin and related
Corticosteroids	Nitrates	oral anticoagulants
Diuretics	NNRTIs	
Dopamine agonists	NRTIs	

Acknowledgements

Aside from the editorial staff many other people have contributed to this publication and the Editors gratefully acknowledge the assistance and guidance they have provided. In particular, we would like to express our gratitude to David Granger and Karl Parsons for their support in producing the final dataset, particularly the indexing, and to Linda Paulus who has handled the various aspects of the production of this book. Thanks are also due to Ivan Stockley and Alina Lourie for their support with this project.

Individual users of this product continue to take the time to provide us with feedback on the contents and structure of the data, and for that we are grateful. These comments are always useful to us in developing the products to better meet the needs of end-users.

Contact details

We are always very pleased to receive feedback from those using our products. Anyone wishing to comment can contact us at the following e-mail address: stockley@rpharms.com.

Abbreviations

ACE	angiotensin-converting enzyme
ALT	alanine aminotransferase
AST	aspartate aminotransferase
AUC	area under the time–concentration curve
BPH	benign prostatic hyperplasia
bpm	beats per minute
CNS	central nervous system
CSF	cerebrospinal fluid
CSM	Committee on Safety of Medicines (UK) (now subsumed within the Commission on Human Medicines)
DMARD	disease modifying antirheumatic drug
ECG	electrocardiogram
e.g.	*exempli gratia* (for example)
FFPRHC	The UK Faculty of Family Planning and Reproductive Health Care
HIV	human immunodeficiency virus
HRT	hormone replacement therapy
i.e.	*id est* (that is)
INR	international normalised ratio
IUD	intra-uterine device
LFT	liver function test
MAO	monoamine oxidase
MAO-A	monoamine oxidase, type A
MAO-B	monoamine oxidase, type B
MAOI	monoamine oxidase inhibitor
mg	milligram(s)
MHRA	Medicines and Healthcare products Regulatory Agency (UK)
mL	millilitre(s)
mmHg	millimetre(s) of mercury
mol	mole
NNRTI	non-nucleoside reverse transcriptase inhibitor
NRTI	nucleoside reverse transcriptase inhibitor
NSAID	non-steroidal anti-inflammatory drug
pH	the negative logarithm of the hydrogen ion concentration
PPI	proton pump inhibitor
RNA	ribonucleic acid
SSRI	selective serotonin reuptake inhibitor
TSH	thyroid-stimulating hormone
UK	United Kingdom
US	United States of America
WHO	World Health Organization

About the Editor

Claire L. Preston studied pharmacy at the University of Nottingham, graduating in 1998. She completed her pre-registration year in Ashford, Kent before working as a community pharmacist for several years. She then became a medicines management pharmacist at a Primary Care Trust in Kent where she undertook her Clinical Diploma. Claire started at the Pharmaceutical Press in 2007 as a Staff Editor on the *British National Formulary* and later became an Assistant Editor. Claire has been the Lead Editor for Drug Interactions for the Pharmaceutical Press since March 2012.

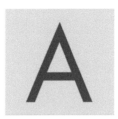

ACE inhibitors

Most ACE inhibitor interactions are pharmacodynamic, that is, interactions that result in an alteration in drug effects rather than drug disposition, so in most cases interactions of individual drugs will be applicable to the group as a whole. The ACE inhibitors do not appear to undergo interactions via cytochrome P450 isoenzymes.

ACE inhibitors + Aliskiren

The concurrent use of ACE inhibitors and aliskiren increases the risk of hyperkalaemia. Additive hypotension is likely to occur, which can be clinically beneficial, see also antihypertensives, page 97.

> Monitor potassium concentrations with concurrent use, particularly in patients at high risk of hyperkalaemia (such as those with reduced renal function and/or diabetes). Note that, in December 2011, the European Medicines Agency stated that aliskiren-containing medicines should not be given to diabetic patients in combination with ACE inhibitors.

ACE inhibitors + Allopurinol

A case of hypersensitivity has been attributed to the concurrent use of captopril and allopurinol. Other ACE inhibitors may interact similarly. Anaphylaxis and myocardial infarction occurred in one man taking enalapril with allopurinol. The combination of ACE inhibitors and allopurinol might increase the risk of leucopenia and serious infection.

> Patients taking both drugs should be very closely monitored for any signs of hypersensitivity (e.g. skin reactions) or low white cell count (sore throat, fever), especially if they have renal impairment. White blood cell counts should be monitored periodically: some manufacturers suggest checking before starting allopurinol, then every 2 weeks during the first 3 months of treatment, and periodically thereafter.

ACE inhibitors + Alpha blockers

The first-dose hypotensive effect seen with alpha blockers (particularly alfuzosin,

A

prazosin, and terazosin) is likely to be potentiated by ACE inhibitors. It is unclear whether there are real differences between the alpha blockers in their propensity to cause this first-dose effect. Note that the acute hypotensive reaction appears to be short-lived. In one small study tamsulosin did not have any clinically relevant effects on blood pressure that was already well controlled by enalapril.

When starting an alpha blocker it is often recommended that those already taking an antihypertensive should have their dose reduced to a maintenance level, while initiating the alpha blocker at a low dose, with the first dose taken just before going to bed. Patients should also be warned about the possibility of postural hypotension and how to manage it (i.e. lay down, raise the legs, and, when recovered, get up slowly). Similarly, when adding an antihypertensive to an alpha blocker, it might be prudent to decrease the dose of the alpha blocker and re-titrate as necessary.

ACE inhibitors + Antacids

Fosinopril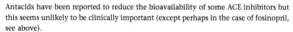

The bioavailability of fosinopril is moderately reduced by an aluminium/magnesium hydroxide-containing antacid.

The manufacturers suggest separating fosinopril administration from that of antacids by at least 2 hours.

Other ACE inhibitors

Antacids have been reported to reduce the bioavailability of some ACE inhibitors but this seems unlikely to be clinically important (except perhaps in the case of fosinopril, see above).

The manufacturers of some ACE inhibitors warn that antacids may reduce their bioavailability, but there seems to be no evidence of a clinically significant interaction in practice.

ACE inhibitors + Antidiabetics

The concurrent use of ACE inhibitors and antidiabetics normally appears to be uneventful. However, hypoglycaemia, marked in some instances, has occurred in a small number of diabetics taking insulin or sulfonylureas with captopril, enalapril, lisinopril, or perindopril. This has been attributed, but not proven, to be due to an interaction. Sitagliptin appears to alter the hypotensive effects of enalapril.

It would be advisable to warn all patients taking insulin or oral antidiabetics who are just starting any ACE inhibitors that excessive hypoglycaemia has been seen very occasionally and unpredictably. It might be prudent to temporarily increase the frequency of blood glucose monitoring. Any problem seems easily resolved by reducing the sulfonylurea dose. The risk of an interaction appears low, and the use of ACE inhibitors in diabetes is considered beneficial. The reported effect of sitagliptin on the blood pressure-lowering effects of ACE inhibitors requires further study, until more is known it would seem prudent to bear the possibility of an interaction in mind should any otherwise unexplained changes in blood pressure occur on concurrent use.

ACE inhibitors + **Aspirin** ❓

The antihypertensive efficacy of captopril and enalapril may be reduced by high-dose aspirin in about 50% of patients. Low-dose aspirin (less than or equal to 100 mg daily) appears to have little effect. It is unclear whether aspirin attenuates the benefits of ACE inhibitors in heart failure. The likelihood of an interaction may depend on disease state and its severity.

> For hypertension, no action is needed if antiplatelet dose aspirin is used. Suspect an interaction with analgesic dose aspirin if the ACE inhibitor seems less effective, or blood pressure control is erratic. Increase the ACE inhibitor dose or consider an alternative analgesic, but note that NSAIDs interact in the same way as high-dose aspirin. For heart failure it is generally advised that concurrent use is best avoided, unless a specific indication (e.g. coronary heart disease, stroke) exists.

ACE inhibitors + **Azathioprine** ⚠

Anaemia has been seen in kidney transplant patients given azathioprine with enalapril or captopril. Leucopenia occasionally occurs when captopril is given with azathioprine. Azathioprine is rapidly and extensively metabolised to mercaptopurine. Mercaptopurine is therefore expected to share the interactions of azathioprine.

> The manufacturer of captopril recommends that it should be used with extreme caution in patients taking immunosuppressants, especially if there is renal impairment. They advise that differential white blood cell counts should be checked before starting captopril, then every 2 weeks in the first 3 months of captopril use, and periodically thereafter, although this is most likely to already be occurring or planned because of the azathioprine. Any effect seems likely to be a group interaction, and it would therefore seem prudent to consider monitoring with any ACE inhibitor.

ACE inhibitors + **Ciclosporin (Cyclosporine)** ⚠

Acute renal failure has developed in kidney transplant patients taking ciclosporin with enalapril. Oliguria was seen in another patient taking ciclosporin with captopril. There is a possible increased risk of hyperkalaemia when ACE inhibitors are given with ciclosporin, as both drugs can increase potassium concentrations. It is anticipated that all ACE inhibitors will interact similarly.

> The incidence of renal failure appears to be low, nevertheless care and good monitoring are needed if ACE inhibitors and ciclosporin are used concurrently. Monitor potassium concentrations more closely in the initial weeks of concurrent use, bearing in mind that an increase in potassium concentrations might be due to worsening renal function as well as the use of these drugs.

ACE inhibitors + **Clonidine**

ACE inhibitors may potentiate the antihypertensive effects of clonidine, and this can be clinically useful. However, limited evidence suggests that the effects of captopril may be delayed when patients are switched from clonidine. Note that sudden withdrawal of clonidine may cause rebound hypertension.

> The general importance of this interaction is unknown, but be aware that it may occur.

A

ACE inhibitors + **Contraceptives**

Drospirenone, which is given as the progestogen component of oral combined hormonal contraceptives, might increase the risk of hyperkalaemia when given with other drugs that can cause hyperkalaemia such as ACE inhibitors. However, two studies found no evidence of an increased risk of hyperkalaemia on the concurrent use of with enalapril and drospirenone (given as *HRT*). Oral combined hormonal contraceptives are associated with increased blood pressure and might antagonise the efficacy of antihypertensive drugs, see Antihypertensives + Contraceptives, page 98.

> The risk of hyperkalaemia appears to be low, especially if renal function is normal. In the US, it is recommended that consideration be given to monitoring potassium concentrations during the first cycle in women [with normal renal function] who regularly take an ACE inhibitor, whereas the UK manufacturer recommends that the potassium concentration is measured during the first cycle or month of treatment in women with mild or moderate renal impairment only. For women with severe renal impairment, the UK manufacturer contraindicates the use of drospirenone-containing contraceptives, whereas, in the US, its use in renal impairment [to any degree] is contraindicated. In patients at higher risk of developing hyperkalaemia (e.g. in renal impairment) it is generally recommended that potassium concentrations are measured during the first cycle of treatment with drospirenone.

ACE inhibitors + **Co-trimoxazole**

Two reports describe serious hyperkalaemia, apparently caused by the concurrent use of trimethoprim (given as co-trimoxazole) and enalapril or quinapril, in association with renal impairment. In elderly patients taking an ACE inhibitor, the use of co-trimoxazole appears to increase the risk of hospitalisation for hyperkalaemia.

> Trimethoprim or ACE inhibitors alone can cause hyperkalaemia, particularly with other factors such as renal impairment. Monitor plasma potassium concentrations if this combination is used in those with renal impairment. Note that co-trimoxazole is a combination preparation containing trimethoprim, and might therefore interact similarly. It has been suggested that trimethoprim should probably be avoided in elderly patients, with or without chronic renal impairment, taking ACE inhibitors and patients with AIDS taking an ACE inhibitor for associated nephropathy should probably discontinue their ACE inhibitor during treatment with high-dose co-trimoxazole.

ACE inhibitors + **Digoxin** ✅

No clinically significant interaction has been seen between digoxin and most ACE inhibitors. Some studies have found that serum digoxin levels rise by about 20% or more if captopril is used, but others have found no significant changes. It has been suggested that any interaction is likely to occur only in those patients who have pre-existing renal impairment.

> No action usually needed. In patients with renal impairment given digoxin and captopril it may be prudent to be alert for increased digoxin effects (e.g. bradycardia).

ACE inhibitors + **Diuretics**

Loop diuretics and Thiazides 🔃

The use of ACE inhibitors with loop or thiazide diuretics is normally safe and effective, but first-dose hypotension (dizziness, fainting) can occur, particularly if the dose of diuretic is high (greater than furosemide 80 mg daily or equivalent) and often in association with predisposing conditions (heart failure, renovascular hypertension, haemodialysis, high levels of renin and angiotensin, low-sodium diet, dehydration, diarrhoea or vomiting, etc.). In addition, renal impairment, and even acute renal failure, have been reported, and diuretic-induced hypokalaemia can still occur when ACE inhibitors are used with potassium-depleting diuretics.

> First-dose hypotension is well established. In patients taking high-dose diuretics, ACE inhibitors should be initiated under close supervision. Consider temporarily stopping the diuretic or reducing its dose at least 24 hours before the ACE inhibitor is added. If this is not clinically appropriate the response to the first dose of the ACE inhibitor should be monitored for at least 2 hours, or until blood pressure has stabilised. ACE inhibitors should be started with a very low dose, even in patients at low risk (e.g. those with uncomplicated essential hypertension taking low-dose thiazides). All patients should be warned about what can happen, and advised to lie down if dizziness, lightheadedness or faintness occurs. Any marked hypotension is normally transient, but if problems persist it might be necessary to temporarily reduce the diuretic dose. Taking the first dose of the ACE inhibitor just before bedtime is also preferable. Severe reactions (e.g. renal impairment or hypokalaemia) are rare, and routine monitoring of the ACE inhibitor should suffice. However, if increases in urea and creatinine occur, a dose reduction and/or discontinuation of the diuretic and/or ACE inhibitor may be required.

Potassium-sparing diuretics ⚠️

The use of ACE inhibitors with potassium-sparing diuretics, such as amiloride, eplerenone, spironolactone, and triamterene, can result in hyperkalaemia, particularly in the presence of other risk factors (e.g. advanced age, diabetes, doses of spironolactone greater than 25 mg daily, and renal impairment).

> The concurrent use of ACE inhibitors and amiloride or triamterene is normally not advised, but if both drugs are appropriate potassium concentrations should be closely monitored. The presence of a loop or thiazide diuretic might not necessarily prevent hyperkalaemia. The combination of an ACE inhibitor and spironolactone or eplerenone is beneficial in some indications, but close monitoring of serum potassium concentrations and renal function is needed, especially with any changes in treatment or in the patient's clinical condition. It has been suggested that spironolactone should not be given with ACE inhibitors in those with a glomerular filtration rate of less than 30 mL/minute.

ACE inhibitors + **Epoetin** 🔃

Epoetin can cause hypertension and thereby reduce the effects of ACE inhibitors, and an additive hyperkalaemic effect is theoretically possible. ACE inhibitors appear to reduce the efficacy of epoetin, but any interaction could take many months to develop.

> Blood pressure and electrolytes, particularly potassium, should be routinely monitored in those given epoetin. An increase in the ACE inhibitor dose appears

to overcome any epoetin-induced increase in blood pressure; however, if blood pressure increases cannot be controlled or potassium concentrations increase, consider temporarily witholding the epoetin. Note that the UK and US manufacturers contraindicate epoetin in uncontrolled hypertension. The effect of ACE inhibitors on epoetin resistance is not established; it seems more likely to occur with concurrent use of high-dose ACE inhibitors and low-dose epoetin. As the epoetin dose is governed by response, no immediate intervention is necessary. If epoetin resistance occurs, consider increasing the epoetin dose.

ACE inhibitors + **Everolimus** 🔺

Angioedema has been reported in patients taking everolimus with ACE inhibitors.

Be alert to possibility of an increased risk of angioedema. Higher doses of both drugs might pose a greater risk.

ACE inhibitors + **Food** ✅

Food reduces the absorption of imidapril and moexipril, and reduces the conversion of perindopril to its active metabolite, perindoprilat.

The manufacturer recommends that perindopril is taken in the morning before a meal. The manufacturer recommends that imidapril is taken at the same time each day, about 15 minutes before a meal. Food has little or no clinically important effect on the absorption of captopril, cilazapril, enalapril, fosinopril, lisinopril, moexipril, quinapril, ramipril, spirapril, and trandolapril.

ACE inhibitors + **Gold** 🔺

Peripheral vasodilatation (facial flushing, nausea, dizziness, and occasionally, hypotension) has occurred when some patients given gold with ACE inhibitors. Isolated cases of loss of consciousness, cardiovascular collapse and cerebrovascular accident have been reported. In some patients the reaction occurred soon after the start of the ACE inhibitor, while in others there appeared to be a lag time of several months or more.

The general importance of this interaction is unclear. It has been recommended that patients taking ACE inhibitors who require gold compounds should, if possible, be given aurothioglucose. If this is not available, a 50% reduction in the sodium aurothiomalate dose is recommended with the patient in the recumbent position, and under observation for 20 minutes following the next few injections.

ACE inhibitors + **Heparin** 🔺

An extensive review of the literature found that heparin (both unfractionated and low-molecular-weight heparins) and heparinoids inhibit the secretion of aldosterone, which can cause hyperkalaemia. This effect may be additive with the hyperkalaemic effects of the ACE inhibitors.

The CSM in the UK suggests that potassium should be measured in all patients with risk factors (e.g. renal impairment, diabetes mellitus, pre-existing acidosis and those taking potassium-sparing drugs) before starting heparin, and monitored regularly thereafter (at least every 4 days has been suggested) particularly in patients receiving heparin for more than 7 days.

ACE inhibitors + **Herbal medicines or Dietary supplements**

A patient taking lisinopril developed marked hypotension and became faint after taking garlic capsules.

This seems to be the first and only report of this reaction, so its general importance is small. However, bear it in mind in case of an unexpected response to treatment.

ACE inhibitors + **HRT**

Drospirenone, which is given as the progestogen component in some HRT formulations, might increase the risk of hyperkalaemia when given with other drugs that can cause hyperkalaemia such as ACE inhibitors. However, two studies found no evidence of an increased risk of hyperkalaemia on the concurrent use of enalapril and drospirenone. The UK manufacturer of drospirenone-containing HRT notes that the increase in potassium levels may be more pronounced in diabetic women.

The risk of hyperkalaemia appears to be low, especially if renal function is normal. In the US, it is recommended that consideration be given to monitoring potassium levels during the first cycle in women [with normal renal function] who regularly take an ACE inhibitor, whereas the UK manufacturer recommends that the potassium level is measured during the first cycle or month of treatment only in women with mild or moderate renal impairment. In patients at higher risk of developing hyperkalaemia (e.g. in renal impairment) it is generally recommended that potassium levels are measured during the first cycle of treatment with drospirenone.

ACE inhibitors + **Lithium**

ACE inhibitors can increase lithium concentrations, and in some individuals 2- to 4-fold increases have occurred. Cases of lithium toxicity have been reported in patients given captopril, enalapril, or lisinopril (and possibly imidapril or perindopril). One analysis found an increased relative risk of 7.6 for lithium toxicity requiring hospitalisation in elderly patients newly started on an ACE inhibitor. Risk factors for this interaction seem to be poor renal function, heart failure, volume depletion, and increased age.

Adverse effects from concurrent use appear rare. Nevertheless, monitor for symptoms of lithium toxicity and consider monitoring lithium concentrations more frequently to avoid a potentially severe adverse interaction. As the onset of the interaction can be delayed, it has been advised that lithium concentrations should be monitored every week or every two weeks for several weeks. Patients taking lithium should be aware of the symptoms of lithium toxicity, see lithium, page 468 and told to immediately report them should they occur. This should be reinforced when they are given ACE inhibitors.

ACE inhibitors + **Low-molecular-weight heparins**

An extensive review of the literature found that heparin (both unfractionated and low-molecular-weight heparins) and heparinoids inhibit the secretion of aldosterone, which can cause hyperkalaemia. This effect may be additive with the hyperkalaemic effects of the ACE inhibitors.

The CSM in the UK suggests that potassium should be measured in all patients with risk factors (e.g. renal impairment, diabetes mellitus, pre-existing acidosis and those taking potassium-sparing drugs) before starting a low-molecular-weight heparin, and monitored regularly thereafter (at least every 4 days has been suggested) particularly in patients receiving a low-molecular-weight heparin for more than 7 days.

ACE inhibitors + **NSAIDs**

There is evidence that most NSAIDs (including the coxibs) can increase blood pressure in patients taking antihypertensives, including ACE inhibitors, although some studies have not found the increase to be clinically relevant. Indometacin appears to have the most substantial effect. The concurrent use of a NSAID and an ACE inhibitor might increase the risk of renal impairment, and rarely, hyperkalaemia.

Only some patients are affected. Consider increasing the frequency of blood pressure monitoring if an NSAID is started. Monitor renal function and electrolytes periodically.

ACE inhibitors + **Potassium**

ACE inhibitors can raise potassium levels. Hyperkalaemia is therefore possible if potassium supplements or potassium-containing salt substitutes are given, particularly in those patients where other risk factors are present, such as decreased renal function.

Monitor potassium levels, adjusting supplementation as necessary.

ACE inhibitors + **Probenecid**

Probenecid decreases the renal clearance of captopril and enalapril.

In general, these changes do not appear to result in a significant clinical effect, although it may be prudent to bear the possibility in mind in the case of any unexpected reductions in blood pressure in patients taking enalapril with probenecid. There is no information regarding other ACE inhibitors, but they would not be expected to interact any differently.

ACE inhibitors + **Procainamide**

The concurrent use of ACE inhibitors and procainamide possibly increases the risk of leucopenia, particularly in patients with renal impairment.

It is recommended that white cell counts are monitored before concurrent use, every 2 weeks during the first 3 months of concurrent use, and then periodically thereafter.

ACE inhibitors + **Rifampicin (Rifampin)**

An isolated report describes an increase in blood pressure in one hypertensive patient, which was attributed to an interaction between enalapril and rifampicin. Rifampicin might reduce the plasma concentrations of the active metabolites of imidapril and spirapril.

> The general importance of these interactions is unknown (although they are expected to be minor), but bear them in mind in case of any unexpected elevations in blood pressure. The manufacturers of imidapril state that rifampicin might reduce its antihypertensive efficacy, but this awaits clinical assessment.

ACE inhibitors + **Sirolimus**

Oedema of the tongue, face, lips, neck and chest has been reported in patients taking sirolimus with enalapril or ramipril who had previously taken these ACE inhibitors without any adverse effects.

> Caution should be used when either starting an ACE inhibitor in a patient already taking sirolimus or when starting sirolimus in a patient taking an ACE inhibitor. Higher doses of both drugs may pose a greater risk.

ACE inhibitors + **Tacrolimus**

Tacrolimus may cause nephrotoxicity and hyperkalaemia, which may be additive with the effects of the ACE inhibitors.

> Consider the possible contribution of ACE inhibitors if nephrotoxicity or hyperkalaemia occur in a patient also taking tacrolimus.

ACE inhibitors + **Tetracyclines**

The absorption of oral tetracycline (and therefore probably most tetracyclines) is moderately reduced by the magnesium carbonate excipient in some quinapril formulations (e.g. *Accupro*). On this basis, the manufacturer of another quinapril preparation (*Quinil*), which contains magnesium oxide, predicts that it will interact similarly.

> The manufacturers recommend avoiding concurrent use. One possible way to accommodate this interaction (as with the interaction between tetracyclines and antacids) is to separate the doses as much as possible (2 to 3 hours should be sufficient).

ACE inhibitors + **Trimethoprim**

Two reports describe serious hyperkalaemia, apparently caused by the concurrent use of trimethoprim (given as co-trimoxazole) and enalapril or quinapril, in association with renal impairment. In elderly patients taking an ACE inhibitor, the use of co-trimoxazole appears to increase the risk of hospitalisation for hyperkalaemia.

> Trimethoprim or ACE inhibitors alone can cause hyperkalaemia, particularly with other factors such as renal impairment. Monitor plasma potassium concentrations if this combination is used in those with renal impairment. It has been suggested

A

that trimethoprim should probably be avoided in elderly patients, with or without chronic renal impairment, taking ACE inhibitors and that patients with AIDS taking an ACE inhibitor for associated nephropathy should probably discontinue the ACE inhibitor during the use of high-dose co-trimoxazole.

Acetazolamide

Note that although hypokalaemia may occur with acetazolamide it is said to be transient and rarely clinically significant.

Acetazolamide + Aspirin

Metabolic acidosis can occur in those taking high-dose salicylates if they are given carbonic anhydrase inhibitors (e.g. acetazolamide).

> Carbonic anhydrase inhibitors should probably be avoided in those taking high-dose salicylates. If concurrent use is essential, the patient should be closely monitored for any evidence of toxicity (confusion, lethargy, hyperventilation, tinnitus) as the interaction may develop slowly and insidiously. In this context NSAIDs or paracetamol (acetaminophen) may be safer alternatives. It is not known whether eye drops interact similarly; there appear to be no reports of an interaction. No clinically relevant interaction would be expected with aspirin used in antiplatelet doses.

Acetazolamide + Carbamazepine

Increases in carbamazepine concentrations resulting in toxicity have been reported in a very small number of patients given acetazolamide.

> The general importance of this interaction is unknown, but it may be prudent to monitor for indicators of carbamazepine toxicity (nausea, vomiting, ataxia, drowsiness) and take levels if necessary.

Acetazolamide + Ciclosporin (Cyclosporine)

There is some limited evidence that oral acetazolamide can cause a large and rapid increase ciclosporin concentrations (up to 6-fold in 72 hours), possibly accompanied by renal toxicity.

> Ciclosporin concentrations and/or effects (e.g. on renal function) should be monitored as a matter of routine, but it might be prudent to increase monitoring if acetazolamide is started or stopped. Adjust the dose of ciclosporin as necessary.

Acetazolamide + Lithium

There is some evidence to suggest that the excretion of lithium can be increased by the short-term use of acetazolamide. However lithium *toxicity* occurred in one patient taking both drugs for a month.

> Lithium concentrations might be decreased by concurrent use. It would therefore

be prudent to be aware of this possibility, monitoring lithium concentrations if an interaction is suspected.

Acetazolamide + Mexiletine

Large changes in urinary pH caused by the concurrent use of alkalinising drugs (such as acetazolamide) can, in some patients, have a marked effect on the plasma concentrations of mexiletine.

The effect does not appear to be predictable. There appear to be no reports of adverse interactions but if concurrent use is necessary, it should be closely monitored. Mexiletine is no longer widely available, but the UK manufacturer previously recommended that concurrent use should be avoided.

Acetazolamide + Opioids

Theoretically, urinary alkalinisers such as acetazolamide may increase the effects of methadone.

The clinical significance of this interaction is unclear, but bear it in mind in case of an unexpected response to methadone.

Acetazolamide + Phenobarbital

Severe osteomalacia and rickets have been seen in a few patients taking phenobarbital or primidone with acetazolamide. A marked reduction in primidone levels with a loss in seizure control has also been described in a very small number of patients.

The general importance of this interaction is unknown. Concurrent use should be monitored for signs or symptoms of low levels of vitamin D or osteomalacia and for reduced primidone efficacy. Stop acetazolamide if possible should osteomalacia occur.

Acetazolamide + Phenytoin

Severe osteomalacia and rickets have been seen in a few patients taking phenytoin with acetazolamide. Rises in phenytoin levels have also been described in a very small number of patients. Fosphenytoin, a prodrug of phenytoin, may interact similarly.

The clinical importance of this interaction is unknown. Concurrent use should be monitored for signs or symptoms of low levels of vitamin D, osteomalacia or phenytoin toxicity. Stop acetazolamide if possible should osteomalacia occur. Indicators of phenytoin toxicity include blurred vision, nystagmus, ataxia or drowsiness.

Acetazolamide + Quinidine

Large rises in urinary pH due to the concurrent use of acetazolamide could cause the retention of quinidine, which could lead to quinidine toxicity. Also note that hypokalaemia, which may rarely be caused by acetazolamide, can increase the toxicity of QT-prolonging drugs such as quinidine.

Monitor the effects if acetazolamide is started or stopped and adjust the quinidine dose as necessary. Also consider monitoring potassium to ensure it is within the accepted range.

Aciclovir

Valaciclovir is a prodrug of aciclovir and therefore has the potential to interact similarly.

Aciclovir + Ciclosporin (Cyclosporine)

Aciclovir does not normally seem to affect ciclosporin concentrations or worsen renal function on concurrent use, but cases of nephrotoxicity and increased ciclosporin concentrations have been reported. Valaciclovir, a prodrug of aciclovir, is expected to interact similarly.

The handful of cases where problems have arisen clearly indicate that renal function should be closely monitored if both drugs are given. The manufacturers recommend that renal function is closely monitored if valaciclovir, or aciclovir infusion, are given with ciclosporin.

Aciclovir + H₂-receptor antagonists

Single-dose studies have found that cimetidine increases the exposure to valaciclovir and its metabolite, aciclovir, but this is thought unlikely to be clinically important.

No action is generally needed. However, the UK manufacturer of valaciclovir recommend caution if high-dose valaciclovir is used. A similar interaction seems possible with aciclovir.

Aciclovir + HIV-protease inhibitors

The concurrent use of aciclovir and indinavir might increase the risk of indinavir-associated renal complications.

The clinical relevance of this effect is unclear: bear it in mind the possibility of additive drug-induced crystalluria if both drugs are given. This would also apply to the aciclovir prodrug, valaciclovir. This adverse effect is particularly associated with indinavir, and not the other HIV-protease inhibitors.

Aciclovir + Mycophenolate ❓

No clinically significant pharmacokinetic interaction appears to occur between aciclovir and mycophenolate. However, the manufacturers state that in renal impairment there may be competition for tubular secretion and increased concentrations of both drugs may occur. This is also possible with valaciclovir. A case report describes neutropenia in a patient taking valaciclovir with mycophenolate.

No action is needed, but increased monitoring may be prudent in patients with reduced renal function. Neutropenia is a rare adverse effect of valaciclovir alone. Nevertheless, bear the possibility of an interaction in mind should neutropenia occur if mycophenolate is also given.

Aciclovir + NRTIs ⚠

Tenofovir alone can cause renal failure and this might be additive with other drugs that are nephrotoxic: the US manufacturer names aciclovir and valaciclovir.

Avoid concurrent use. If this is not possible, the UK & US manufacturers of tenofovir advise that renal function should be monitored at least weekly.

Aciclovir + Probenecid

Probenecid reduces the renal excretion of, and therefore increases the exposure to, aciclovir and valaciclovir.

Dose alterations are unlikely to be needed due to the wide therapeutic range of aciclovir and valaciclovir. However, the UK manufacturer of valaciclovir states that caution is warranted if high-dose valaciclovir is given. Note that a clinically relevant interaction is more likely in those with reduced renal function.

Aciclovir + Theophylline

Preliminary evidence suggests that aciclovir can reduce the clearance of theophylline (and therefore possibly aminophylline) by about 30%.

Evidence appears to be limited. Be alert for an increase in the adverse effects of theophylline (nausea, headache, tremor) if aciclovir is added, and consider monitoring theophylline concentrations.

Aciclovir + Tizanidine ⚠

Aciclovir is predicted to increase the exposure to tizanidine, increasing its hypotensive and sedative effects.

The UK and US manufacturers suggest that concurrent use should be avoided. Until more is known be alert for adverse effects such as bradycardia, hypotension, and drowsiness.

Adenosine

Adenosine + Dipyridamole ⚠

Dipyridamole greatly reduces the bolus dose of adenosine necessary to convert supraventricular tachycardia to sinus rhythm. Profound bradycardia occurred in a patient taking dipyridamole when an adenosine infusion was given for myocardial stress testing.

The UK manufacturers advise the avoidance of adenosine in patients taking dipyridamole for supraventricular tachycardia, and contraindicate the use of dipyridamole with adenosine for myocardial perfusion imaging. Patients will need much less adenosine to treat arrhythmias while taking dipyridamole. It has been suggested that the initial dose of adenosine should be reduced 2-fold or 4-fold. If adenosine is considered necessary for myocardial imaging in a patient taking dipyridamole, the dipyridamole should be stopped 24 hours before imaging, or the dose of adenosine should be greatly reduced. This could be insufficient for extended-release dipyridamole preparations, and in this case it has been suggested that the dipyridamole will need to be stopped several days before the test.

Adenosine + Theophylline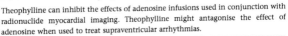

Theophylline can inhibit the effects of adenosine infusions used in conjunction with radionuclide myocardial imaging. Theophylline might antagonise the effect of adenosine when used to treat supraventricular arrhythmias.

Theophylline, aminophylline, and other xanthines should be avoided for 24 hours before using an adenosine infusion for radionuclide myocardial imaging. Adenosine bolus injections for the termination of paroxysmal supraventricular tachycardia might still be effective in patients taking xanthines. The usual dose schedule should be followed. However, note that adenosine has induced bronchospasm and it has been suggested that adenosine should be avoided in patients with bronchoconstriction or bronchospasm, and used cautiously in those with obstructive pulmonary disease not associated with bronchospasm. The UK manufacturers contraindicate the use of adenosine in chronic obstructive lung disease with evidence of bronchospasm and warn that adenosine might aggravate or precipitate bronchospasm. The UK manufacturers of adenosine also state that theophylline, aminophylline, and other xanthines should be avoided for 24 hours before administration of adenosine, and that xanthine-containing drinks should be avoided for at least 12 hours before administration. Xanthines, such as intravenous aminophylline, can be used to terminate any persistent adverse effects of adenosine infusions given for myocardial imaging.

Albendazole

Albendazole + Carbamazepine ⚠

Carbamazepine lowers the plasma concentrations of albendazole.

For systemic infections it might be necessary to increase the albendazole dose. Monitor the outcome of concurrent use. This interaction is of no importance in the treatment of intestinal worm infections.

Albendazole + Food ⚠

Giving albendazole with a meal (especially fatty meals) causes a large increases the concentrations of its active metabolite.

Albendazole absorption is poor, and if it is being used for systemic infections, it is advisable to take it with a meal.

Albendazole + HIV-protease inhibitors

Ritonavir reduces the exposure to albendazole and to its active metabolite, albendazole sulfoxide.

> It might be necessary to increase the albendazole dose when treating systemic worm infections in patients also taking ritonavir. Monitor the outcome of concurrent use. The interaction is of no importance when albendazole is used for intestinal worm infections.

Albendazole + Phenobarbital

Phenobarbital (and therefore probably primidone) lowers the plasma concentrations of albendazole.

> For systemic infections it might be necessary to increase the albendazole dose. Monitor the outcome of concurrent use. This interaction is of no importance in the treatment of intestinal worm infections.

Albendazole + Phenytoin

Phenytoin lowers the plasma concentrations of albendazole. Fosphenytoin, a prodrug of phenytoin, would be expected to interact similarly.

> For systemic infections it might be necessary to increase the albendazole dose. Monitor the outcome of concurrent use. This interaction is of no importance in the treatment of intestinal worm infections.

Alcohol

Probably the most common drug interaction of all occurs if alcohol is drunk by those taking other drugs that have CNS depressant activity, the result being even further CNS depression. Blood-alcohol concentrations well within the legal driving limit can, in the presence of other CNS depressants, be equivalent to blood-alcohol concentrations at or above the legal limit in terms of worsened driving and other skills. A less common interaction that can occur between alcohol and some drugs, chemicals, and fungi is the flushing reaction. This is exploited in the case of disulfiram (*Antabuse*) as an alcohol deterrent. However, it can occur unexpectedly with some other drugs and can be both unpleasant and possibly frightening, but it is not usually dangerous. See also antihypertensives, page 97, for general comments about hypertension and alcohol consumption.

Alcohol + Alpha blockers

Alpha blockers can enhance the hypotensive effect of alcohol in subjects susceptible to the alcohol flush syndrome. The plasma concentrations of both indoramin and alcohol might be increased by concurrent use, which could lead to increased drowsiness.

> The general significance of the hypotensive effects are unclear, but it would be

prudent to warn susceptible patients when they start treatment. The degree of impairment caused by drinking alcohol whilst taking indoramin will depend on the individual patient. However, warn all patients of the potential effects, especially on driving or undertaking other skilled tasks. See also antihypertensives, page 97, for general comments about hypertension and alcohol consumption.

Alcohol + Amfetamines

Dexamfetamine, and related drugs such as ecstasy, can reduce the deleterious effects of alcohol (such as sedation), but some impairment still occurs making it unsafe to drive or undertake other skilled tasks. Tests with metamfetamine suggest that it increases the feeling of intoxication caused by alcohol. Alcohol might increase the cardiac adverse effects of amfetamines The concurrent use of alcohol and ecstasy results in very small changes in the pharmacokinetics of both drugs.

> The effects of this interaction are not clear, but as some psychomotor impairment occurs, warn all patients of the potential effects, and counsel against driving or undertaking other skilled tasks. Information about an increase in cardiac toxicity with the combination of amfetamines and alcohol is limited, and no general conclusions can be drawn.

Alcohol + Antidiabetics

Diabetics managed with insulin, oral antidiabetics, or diet alone need not abstain from alcohol, but they should drink only in moderation and accompanied by food. However, alcohol makes the signs of hypoglycaemia less clear, and delayed hypoglycaemia can occur. The CNS depressant effects of alcohol in association with hypoglycaemia can make driving or the operation of dangerous machinery much more hazardous. Metformin does not carry the same risk of lactic acidosis seen with phenformin and it is suggested by the British Diabetic Association that one or two drinks a day are unlikely to be harmful to those taking metformin. A flushing reaction is common in patients taking chlorpropamide who drink alcohol, but is rare with other sulfonylureas.

> Diabetics are advised not to exceed 2 drinks (for women) or 3 drinks (for men) daily and limit the intake of drinks with high-carbohydrate content (e.g. sweet sherries, liqueurs, low alcohol wines). Diabetics should not drink on an empty stomach and they should know that the warning signs of hypoglycaemia may possibly be obscured by the effects of the alcohol and that the hypoglycaemic effects of alcohol may occur several hours after drinking. Driving or handling dangerous machinery should be avoided because the CNS depressant effects of alcohol in association with hypoglycaemia can be particularly hazardous. The chlorpropamide-alcohol interaction (flushing reaction) is very well documented, but of minimal importance. It is a nuisance and possibly socially embarrassing but normally requires no treatment. Patients should be warned.

Alcohol + Antihistamines

Some antihistamines cause drowsiness, which can be increased by alcohol. The detrimental effects of alcohol on driving skills are considerably increased by the use of the more sedative antihistamines (e.g. chlorphenamine, diphenhydramine, hydroxyzine) and appear to be minimal or absent with the non-sedating antihistamines (e.g.

cetirizine, loratadine). Note that some of the more sedative antihistamines are common ingredients of cough, cold, and influenza remedies.

> The degree of impairment will depend on the individual patient. However, warn all patients taking sedating antihistamines of the potential effects, especially on driving or undertaking other skilled tasks. The incidence of sedation varies with the non-sedating antihistamine and depends on the individual patient. Therefore patients should be advised to be alert to the possibility of drowsiness if they have not taken the drug before. Any drowsiness would be apparent after the first few doses.

Alcohol + Antipsychotics ❓

The detrimental effects of alcohol on the skills related to driving are greatly increased by chlorpromazine, increased by flupentixol, sulpiride, and thioridazine, and possibly increased by olanzapine, prochlorperazine and quetiapine. Any interaction with amisulpride, haloperidol, or tiapride seems to be mild; nevertheless, all antipsychotic drugs that cause drowsiness have the potential to enhance the effects of alcohol. The postural hypotension seen with antipsychotics is likely to be worsened by alcohol. There is some evidence that drinking can precipitate extrapyramidal adverse effects in patients taking antipsychotics.

> The degree of sedation will depend on the antipsychotic given and the individual patient. However, warn all patients of the potential effects, and counsel against driving or undertaking other skilled tasks. It has been suggested that patients should routinely be advised to abstain from alcohol during antipsychotic treatment in order to avoid potentiating extrapyramidal adverse effects, although note that cases of a problem seem rare. Patients should also be warned about postural hypotension and counselled on how to manage it (i.e. lay down, raise the legs, and on recovering to get up slowly).

Alcohol + Apomorphine ❓

Apomorphine can increase the effects of alcohol, and the hypotensive adverse effects of apomorphine might be increased by alcohol.

> Warn patients they may feel dizzy if they drink alcohol when taking apomorphine, and to sit or lie down if this occurs. One US manufacturer of subcutaneous apomorphine advises avoiding alcohol.

Alcohol + Aspirin ✅

A small increase in the gastrointestinal blood loss caused by aspirin occurs if individuals also drink alcohol, but any increased damage to the lining of the stomach is small and appears usually to be of minimal importance in most healthy individuals taking moderate doses of aspirin and drinking moderate amounts of alcohol. However, people who consume at least 3 or more alcoholic drinks daily and who regularly take more than 325 mg of aspirin have been shown to have a high risk of bleeding. Chronic and/or gross overuse of aspirin and alcohol can result in gastric ulceration. Other salicylates would be expected to have similar effects to aspirin.

> This interaction is only likely to be of clinical relevance where high doses of aspirin or other oral salicylates are given to heavy drinkers.

Alcohol + **Azoles**

A few cases of disulfiram-like reactions (nausea, vomiting, facial flushing) have been seen in patients who drank alcohol while taking ketoconazole.

> The incidence of this reaction appears to be very low and its importance is probably small. Reactions of this kind are usually more unpleasant than serious and normally require no treatment. Nevertheless, the UK manufacturer of ketoconazole advises avoiding alcohol.

Alcohol + **Benzodiazepines**

Benzodiazepine and related anxiolytics and hypnotics increase the CNS depressant effects of alcohol to some extent. Alcohol modestly affects the pharmacokinetics of some benzodiazepines, and can increase aggression or amnesia, and/or reduce their anxiolytic effects.

> The deterioration in psychomotor skills (as a result of the increased CNS depression that might occur) will depend on the individual patient, the particular drug in question, its dose and the amounts of alcohol taken. The risk is heightened because the patient might be unaware of being affected. Some benzodiazepines used at night for sedation are still present in appreciable amounts the next day and therefore could continue to interact. Anyone taking any of these drugs should be warned that their usual response to alcohol can be greater than expected, and their ability to drive a car, or carry out any other tasks requiring alertness, might be impaired.

Alcohol + **Beta blockers**

The effects of atenolol and metoprolol do not appear to be changed by alcohol. Some preliminary evidence suggests that the detrimental effects of alcohol and atenolol (with chlortalidone) or propranolol are additive on the performance of some psychomotor tests. There is some evidence that alcohol modestly reduces the haemodynamic effects of propranolol and that the blood pressure-lowering effects of sotalol appear to be increased by alcohol.

> The clinical importance of these minor effects is undetermined, but they seem unlikely to be of great importance. See also antihypertensives, page 97, for general comments about antihypertensives and alcohol consumption.

Alcohol + **Bupropion**

The concurrent use of bupropion and alcohol does not appear to affect the pharmacokinetics of either drug; however, adverse CNS effects or reduced alcohol tolerance have been reported on concurrent use. The risk of seizures with bupropion might be increased with both the excessive use and abrupt withdrawal of alcohol.

> The UK and US manufacturers of bupropion recommend that the consumption of alcohol should be minimised or avoided. Additionally, they contraindicate its use during abrupt withdrawal from alcohol, and advise caution with its use in alcohol abuse.

Alcohol + **Buspirone** 🛈

The use of buspirone with alcohol can cause drowsiness and weakness, although it does not appear to impair the performance of a number of psychomotor tests.

> The degree of impairment will depend on the individual patient. However, warn all patients of the potential effects, and counsel against driving or undertaking other skilled tasks. The UK manufacturer notes that there is no information on higher therapeutic doses of buspirone given with alcohol, and they suggest that it would be prudent to avoid alcohol while taking buspirone.

Alcohol + **Calcium-channel blockers**

Felodipine, Diltiazem, or Nifedipine 🛈

Alcohol might increase the exposure to felodipine and nifedipine. This resulted in an increase in heart rate in patients taking felodipine but no effects were noted in patients taking nifedipine. The UK manufacturers of one prolonged-release diltiazem preparation (*Adizem*) warns that alcohol might increase the rate of diltiazem release.

> Information about these interactions is limited. Their clinical significance is uncertain, but probably small. Note that the UK manufacturer of the prolonged-release diltiazem preparation (*Adizem*) states that alcohol should not be taken at the same time as this preparation. See also antihypertensives, page 97, for general comments about antihypertensives and alcohol consumption.

Verapamil 🛈

Blood alcohol concentrations were slightly raised, and remained elevated for five times longer than normal, in patients taking verapamil.

> Information about this interaction is limited and unconfirmed. The increased blood alcohol concentration could be enough to increase legal blood concentrations to illegal concentrations if driving. Moreover, the intoxicant effects of alcohol might persist for a much longer period of time. Warn patients of these potential effects, and counsel against driving or undertaking other skilled tasks. See also antihypertensives, page 97, for general comments about antihypertensives and alcohol consumption.

Alcohol + **Carbamazepine** 🛈

Moderate social drinking does not appear to affect carbamazepine plasma concentrations. Heavy drinking might increase the metabolism of carbamazepine, and this might be further increased in alcoholics who abstain from drinking alcohol.

> The degree of impairment will depend on the individual. However, warn all patients of the potential effects, especially on driving or undertaking other skilled tasks. Most people with epilepsy can have 1 or 2 units of alcohol without increasing the chances of having a seizure. The risk of seizures might be increased in heavy drinkers on tapering or stopping alcohol.

Alcohol + Cephalosporins

Disulfiram-like reactions have been seen in patients taking cefamandole, cefmenoxime, cefoperazone, and possibly cefonicid after drinking alcohol or following an injection of alcohol. This is not a general reaction of the cephalosporins, but is confined to those with particular chemical structures. Due to their structure ceforanide, cefotiam, and cefpiramide also present a risk. Other cephalosporins are not expected to interact.

> The reaction appears normally to be more embarrassing or unpleasant and frightening than serious, with the symptoms subsiding spontaneously after a few hours. Treatment is not usually needed, although two elderly patients needed treatment for hypotension. Patients taking the interacting cephalosporins should be advised to avoid alcohol during treatment and for up to 3 days (7 days in the presence of renal or hepatic impairment) after the course of cephalosporin is completed.

Alcohol + Ciclosporin (Cyclosporine)

An isolated report describes an increase in serum ciclosporin concentrations in a patient after an episode of binge drinking, but a subsequent study found that moderate single doses of alcohol in other patients had no such effect. Red wine (350 mL) appears to decrease ciclosporin bioavailability.

> It seems that alcohol in moderation will not affect ciclosporin concentrations, although greater care might be advised with red wine. However, the study findings do not imply that an interaction would occur with an occasional single glass of red wine taken with a meal and separate from ciclosporin dosing. Note that patients might be advised to avoid alcohol if they are taking ciclosporin after transplantation.

Alcohol + Contraceptives

Alcohol clearance might be reduced in women taking combined hormonal contraceptives.

> No action is needed in those taking contraceptives.

Alcohol + Dapoxetine

No pharmacokinetic interaction appears to occur between dapoxetine and alcohol. However, concurrent use is predicted to increase alcohol-related adverse reactions, such as dizziness, drowsiness, slow reflexes, or altered judgement, and might increase the risk of syncope.

> The manufacturer advises that patients taking dapoxetine should avoid drinking alcohol.

Alcohol + Disulfiram ✕

Drinking alcohol while taking disulfiram will result in flushing and fullness of the face and neck, tachycardia, breathlessness, giddiness, hypotension, nausea, and vomiting.

This is called the disulfiram reaction. A mild flushing reaction of the skin can occur in particularly sensitive individuals if alcohol is applied to the skin or if alcohol vapour is inhaled. Note that some products (e.g. *Norvir oral solution*) are formulated with alcohol and, although the volume of alcohol taken with the dose is likely to be small, might still provoke this reaction.

This interaction is exploited therapeutically to deter alcoholics from drinking. Patients should also be warned about the exposure to alcohol from some unexpected sources such as foods, cosmetics, medicinal remedies, and solvents. Disulfiram is eliminated slowly from the body and therefore exposure to alcohol can produce unpleasant symptoms up to 14 days after taking the last dose of disulfiram.

Alcohol + Duloxetine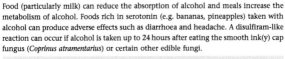

No important psychomotor interaction normally appears to occur between duloxetine and alcohol. However, additive effects (e.g. drowsiness) are considered possible.

The degree of impairment will depend on the individual patient. However, warn all patients of the potential effects, and counsel against driving or undertaking other skilled tasks. Note that the US manufacturer states that duloxetine should ordinarily not be prescribed for patients with substantial alcohol use as severe liver injury may result.

Alcohol + Food

Food (particularly milk) can reduce the absorption of alcohol and meals increase the metabolism of alcohol. Foods rich in serotonin (e.g. bananas, pineapples) taken with alcohol can produce adverse effects such as diarrhoea and headache. A disulfiram-like reaction can occur if alcohol is taken up to 24 hours after eating the smooth ink(y) cap fungus (*Coprinus atramentarius*) or certain other edible fungi.

No action is generally needed, although whether the interaction with food leading to reduced alcohol absorption can be regarded as advantageous or undesirable is a moot point. The intensity of the disulfiram-like reaction depends upon the quantity of fungus and alcohol consumed, and the time interval between them. However, reports of this reaction in the medical literature are few and far between. Treatment does not normally appear to be necessary.

Alcohol + Furazolidone

A disulfiram-like reaction might occur in patients taking furazolidone if they drink alcohol. One report suggests that about 1 in 5 patients might be affected.

Reactions of this kind appear to be more unpleasant and possibly frightening than serious, and normally need no treatment. Nevertheless, patients should be warned about what could happen if they drink alcohol.

Alcohol + Griseofulvin

An isolated case report describes a very severe disulfiram-like reaction when a man taking griseofulvin drank a can of beer. Other isolated reports describe flushing and

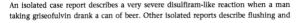

tachycardia, or increased alcohol effects, when patients taking griseofulvin consumed alcohol.

> The documentation is extremely sparse, which would seem to suggest that adverse interactions between alcohol and griseofulvin are uncommon. Concurrent use need not be avoided, but it might be prudent to warn all patients of the potential effects (e.g. flushing and tachycardia).

Alcohol + H$_2$-receptor antagonists

Although some studies have found that blood alcohol concentrations can be increased to some extent, and possibly remain elevated for longer than usual, in patients taking H$_2$-receptor antagonists, other studies report that no clinically relevant interaction occurs. Hypoglycaemia, which can occur following alcohol intake, might be enhanced by H$_2$-receptor antagonists.

> Extensive reviews of the data have concluded that the interaction is not, in general, clinically relevant. There are insufficient grounds to justify any general warning regarding alcohol and H$_2$-receptor antagonists, but note that many of the conditions for which H$_2$-receptor antagonists are used may be made worse by alcohol, so restriction of alcohol intake might be prudent.

Alcohol + Herbal medicines or Dietary supplements

Ginseng

Panax ginseng (Asian ginseng) increases the clearance of alcohol and lowers blood alcohol concentrations.

> The available data suggests that the concurrent use of alcohol and *Panax ginseng* is unlikely to be detrimental.

Kava ⚠

There is some evidence that kava might worsen the CNS depressant effects of alcohol. The concurrent use of alcohol has been suggested as a possible contributing factor in some cases of kava hepatotoxicity.

> The effects of this interaction are not clear, but as some psychomotor impairment occurs warn all patients of the potential effects, and counsel against driving or undertaking other skilled tasks. The use of kava is restricted in the UK because of reports of idiosyncratic hepatotoxicity.

Liv 52 ❓

Liv 52, an Ayurvedic herbal remedy, appears to reduce the hangover symptoms after drinking alcohol. However it also increases the blood alcohol concentration of moderate drinkers (by about 30%) for the first few hours after drinking.

> These increases might be enough to raise the blood alcohol from legal to illegal concentrations when driving. Moderate drinkers should be warned.

Alcohol + HRT ✓

Acute ingestion of alcohol increases the concentrations of circulating estradiol in women using oral HRT. A smaller increase occurs with transdermal HRT. In addition, regular alcohol intake (as low as 1 to 2 drinks per day) appears to modestly increase the risk of some types of breast cancer in women receiving HRT. Estradiol does not affect blood alcohol concentrations.

It has been suggested that women taking HRT should limit their alcohol intake (about one drink or less per day has been proposed), but more study is needed to confirm any interaction and its importance.

Alcohol + Hyoscine (Scopolamine) ❓

Although additive CNS effects are possible, a study found no adverse interaction appears to occur if patients using transdermal hyoscine (*Scopoderm TTS*) drink alcohol. Hyoscine butylbromide might delay peak serum alcohol concentrations, but the clinical relevance of this is unclear.

In general, the manufacturers of several hyoscine hydrobromide preparations suggest that alcohol should be avoided, although note that hyoscine butylbromide and hyoscine methobromide do not readily pass the blood-brain barrier, and would not be expected to cause additive adverse effects with alcohol.

Alcohol + Isoniazid ❓

Isoniazid slightly increases the hazards of driving after drinking alcohol. Isoniazid-induced hepatitis might also possibly be increased, and the effects of isoniazid are possibly reduced in some heavy drinkers.

There appear to be some extra risks for patients taking isoniazid who drink, but the effect does not appear to be large. Patients should nevertheless be warned about the potential effects, especially on driving or undertaking other skilled tasks. The clinical significance of the other effects are unclear, but the UK manufacturer advises care if giving isoniazid to patients with chronic alcoholism.

Alcohol + Leflunomide ⚠

The UK manufacturers state that the concurrent use of alcohol and leflunomide has the potential to cause additive hepatotoxic effects. However, one study suggested that self-reported alcohol consumption had no significant influence on ALT levels.

The manufacturers recommend that alcohol should be avoided by patients taking leflunomide, whereas the British Society for Rheumatology guidelines make a practical recommendation, suggesting that alcohol intake should be limited to 4 to 8 units a week.

Alcohol + Levamisole ❓

A disulfiram-like reaction has been reported when levamisole was given with alcohol.

Reactions of this kind normally seems to be more unpleasant and possibly frightening than serious. Symptoms usually resolve in a few hours, and it usually requires no treatment. However, it would seem prudent to warn patients of the possibility.

Alcohol + Lithium ❓

Some limited evidence suggests that the use of lithium with alcohol might impair the performance of skills related to driving, without affecting blood-alcohol concentrations.

Information is limited, but patients should be warned of the potential psychomotor adverse effects, and counselled against driving or undertaking other skilled tasks. The degree of impairment will depend on the individual.

Alcohol + Macrolides ❓

Alcohol can cause a small reduction in the absorption of erythromycin ethylsuccinate. There is some evidence that intravenous erythromycin can raise blood alcohol concentrations.

The extent to which this reduced absorption might alter the antibacterial effects of erythromycin is uncertain, but it seems likely to be small. The extent and the practical importance of the increased blood alcohol concentrations (e.g. on driving ability) is unknown.

Alcohol + MAOIs ✖

Patients taking non-selective MAOIs can suffer a serious hypertensive reaction if they drink some beers, lagers, or wines, including low-alcohol drinks, but apparently not spirits; however, this is a reaction to the tyramine content rather than the alcohol. The hypotensive adverse effects of the MAOIs can be exaggerated in a few patients by alcohol and they might experience dizziness and faintness after drinking relatively modest amounts.

Avoid tyramine-rich drinks and counsel patients on the possible response to alcohol. Patients taking MAOIs should also be warned of the possibility of orthostatic hypotension and fainting if they drink alcohol. They should be advised not to stand up too quickly, and to remain sitting or lying if they experience dizziness or faintness.

Alcohol + Maprotiline ❓

Maprotiline can cause drowsiness (particularly during the first few days of treatment) which is worsened by alcohol. Giving alcohol with mianserin impairs performance in psychomotor tests.

Patients should be warned that their usual response to alcohol may be greater than expected, and their ability to drive a car, or carry out any other skilled tasks, might be impaired.

Alcohol + Methotrexate

There is some inconclusive evidence to suggest that the consumption of alcohol might increase the risk of methotrexate-induced hepatic cirrhosis and fibrosis.

One UK manufacturer of methotrexate advises the avoidance of drugs, including alcohol, which have hepatotoxic potential, and a US manufacturer contraindicates the use of methotrexate in patients with alcoholism or alcoholic liver disease.

Alcohol + Methylphenidate

Alcohol can increase methylphenidate exposure and exacerbate some of its CNS effects.

The UK manufacturer recommends that alcohol should be avoided in those taking methylphenidate. In addition, methylphenidate should be given cautiously to patients with a history of drug dependence or alcoholism because of its potential for abuse.

Alcohol + Metoclopramide

There is some evidence to suggest that metoclopramide can increase the rate of absorption of alcohol, increase maximum blood alcohol concentrations, and possibly increase alcohol-related sedation.

The degree of impairment will depend on the individual. However, warn all patients of the potential adverse effects, and counsel against driving or undertaking other skilled tasks. Note that metoclopramide alone can sometimes cause drowsiness.

Alcohol + Metronidazole

A disulfiram-like reaction has occurred in a number of patients taking oral metronidazole who drank alcohol. There is one report of its occurrence when metronidazole was applied as a vaginal insert, and another when metronidazole was given intravenously. The interaction has been reported in one case with ornidazole, and is alleged to occur with all other 5-nitroimidazoles (e.g. tinidazole).

This interaction has been extensively studied but it remains slightly controversial because the incidence has been reported as between 0 and 100%. Because of its unpredictability all patients given metronidazole should be warned what may happen if they drink alcohol. Alcohol should be avoided for 24 to 48 hours (72 hours for extended-release preparations) after metronidazole is stopped, and for 72 hours after tinidazole is stopped. The reaction, when it occurs, normally seems to be more unpleasant and possibly frightening than serious, and usually requires no treatment, although one possible fatality has been reported.

Alcohol + Mianserin

Mianserin can cause drowsiness (particularly during the first few days of treatment) which is worsened by alcohol. Giving alcohol with mianserin impairs performance in psychomotor tests.

The degree of impairment will depend on the individual patient. Patients should be warned that their usual response to alcohol may be greater than expected, and their ability to drive or carry out any other skilled tasks, might be impaired.

Alcohol + Mirtazapine ⚠

The sedative effects of mirtazapine might be increased by alcohol.

The UK and US manufacturers advise against concurrent use. Patients should be warned that their usual response to alcohol may be greater than expected, and their ability to drive, or undertake other skilled tasks, might be impaired.

Alcohol + Nicotinic acid (Niacin) ⚠

One patient taking nicotinic acid experienced delirium and metabolic acidosis after drinking about 1 litre of wine.

The manufacturers suggest avoiding concurrent use as adverse effects (flushing and pruritus), and possibly liver toxicity, might be increased.

Alcohol + Nilutamide ⚠

Several studies have described alcohol intolerance (facial flushing, malaise, hypotension) in patients taking nilutamide.

It is recommended that patients who experience this reaction should avoid drinking alcohol. Flutamide and bicalutamide have not been reported to produce these effects when patients drink alcohol, so in some cases they might be considered as an alternative to nilutamide.

Alcohol + Nitrates ❓

Patients who take glyceryl trinitrate (nitroglycerin) and drink alcohol might feel faint and dizzy because of an increased susceptibility to postural hypotension. Consider also, antihypertensives, page 97.

The consumption of alcohol should not stop patients from using glyceryl trinitrate (nitroglycerin), but they should be warned of the possible effects and told to sit or lie down if they feel faint and dizzy, until symptoms abate.

Alcohol + NSAIDs

Indometacin and Phenylbutazone ⚠

The skills related to driving are impaired by indometacin and phenylbutazone. Additive sedation occurs if patients drink while taking phenylbutazone, but this does not appear to occur with indometacin. See also *Miscellaneous NSAIDs*, below.

The degree of impairment will depend on the individual patient. However, warn all patients of the potential effects, and counsel against driving or undertaking other skilled tasks.

Miscellaneous NSAIDs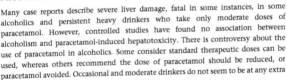

Alcohol might increase the risk of gastrointestinal haemorrhage associated with NSAIDs, and a few isolated reports attribute acute renal failure to the acute excessive consumption of alcohol in patients taking NSAIDs.

Serious problems seem rare. Concurrent use need not be avoided with moderate alcohol intake but be aware that there are some risks and these are increased in heavy drinkers.

Alcohol + Opioids

The opioid analgesics can enhance the CNS depressant effects of alcohol, which has been fatal in some cases. The CNS depressant effects of alcohol are modestly increased by normal therapeutic doses of dextropropoxyphene (propoxyphene), but in deliberate suicidal overdose the CNS depressant effects appear to be additive, and can be fatal. A single case report describes a fatality due to the combined CNS depressant effects of hydromorphone and alcohol. Alcohol has been associated with rapid release of hydromorphone and morphine from extended-release preparations, which could result in potentially fatal doses.

The degree of impairment and/or sedation will depend on the individual patient, the opioid dose used, and the amount of alcohol consumed. However, warn all patients of the potential effects, and with larger doses counsel against driving or undertaking other skilled tasks.

Alcohol + Paracetamol (Acetaminophen)

Many case reports describe severe liver damage, fatal in some instances, in some alcoholics and persistent heavy drinkers who take only moderate doses of paracetamol. However, controlled studies have found no association between alcoholism and paracetamol-induced hepatotoxicity. There is controversy about the use of paracetamol in alcoholics. Some consider standard therapeutic doses can be used, whereas others recommend the dose of paracetamol should be reduced, or paracetamol avoided. Occasional and moderate drinkers do not seem to be at any extra risk.

There seems to be no way of identifying those alcoholics at risk. The combination need not be avoided, but caution patients against long-term regular use without close monitoring.

Alcohol + Perampanel

The effects of perampanel on CNS depression might be synergistic with those of alcohol.

The degree of impairment will depend on the individual patient. However, warn all patients of the potential effects, and counsel against driving or undertaking other skilled tasks.

A

Alcohol + Phenobarbital ❓

Moderate social drinking does not appear to cause a clinically relevant alteration in phenobarbital serum concentrations, and does not appear to cause changes in the control of epilepsy. Alcohol and the barbiturates are CNS depressants, which together can have additive and possibly even synergistic effects. Activities requiring alertness and good co-ordination can be made more difficult and more hazardous. Alcohol might also continue to interact the next day if the barbiturate has hangover effects.

The degree of impairment will depend on the individual patient. Patients should be warned that their usual response to alcohol may be greater than expected, and their ability to drive a car, or carry out any other tasks requiring alertness, might be impaired. Most people with epilepsy can have 1 or 2 units of alcohol without increasing the chances of having a seizure.

Alcohol + Phenytoin ❓

Chronic heavy drinking reduces serum phenytoin concentrations. Acute alcohol intake can possibly increase phenytoin concentrations, but moderate social drinking appears to have little clinical effect in those taking phenytoin. Fosphenytoin, a prodrug of phenytoin, might interact similarly.

Monitor heavy drinkers for decreased phenytoin effects, as they might need above-average doses of phenytoin to maintain adequate serum concentrations. However, be aware that patients with liver impairment usually need lower doses of phenytoin, so the picture can be more complicated.

Alcohol + Pimecrolimus ❓

Alcohol intolerance (moderate to severe facial flushing) and application site erythema have been reported rarely with pimecrolimus cream.

Patients should be warned of the possibility of a flushing reaction with alcohol, although the incidence of this reaction seems to be rare.

Alcohol + Pregabalin ❓

No clinically relevant pharmacokinetic interaction occurs between pregabalin and alcohol, and concurrent use does not appear to have a clinically important effect on respiration. However, the manufacturers suggest that pregabalin may potentiate the effects of alcohol.

The degree of impairment will depend on the individual patient. Patients should be warned that their usual response to alcohol may be greater than expected, and their ability to drive a car, or carry out any other tasks requiring alertness, may be impaired.

Alcohol + Retinoids ❓

The consumption of alcohol can increase the serum concentrations of etretinate in patients taking acitretin.

The clinical relevance of this interaction is unknown. However, it might have

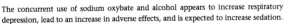
some bearing on the length of the period after acitretin therapy during which women are advised not to conceive.

Alcohol + Sodium oxybate

The concurrent use of sodium oxybate and alcohol appears to increase respiratory depression, lead to an increase in adverse effects, and is expected to increase sedation.

Patients should be warned not to drink alcoholic beverages while taking sodium oxybate.

Alcohol + SSRIs

Fluoxetine, paroxetine and sertraline have no clinically relevant pharmacokinetic interaction with alcohol, but some modest increase in sedation might possibly occur with fluvoxamine or paroxetine. No pharmacodynamic interaction is expected to occur between escitalopram or citalopram and alcohol.

Although no interaction has clearly been demonstrated, most manufacturers of SSRIs suggest that concurrent use with alcohol is not advisable. This is presumably because both drugs act on the CNS and also because of the risk of alcohol abuse in depressed patients.

Alcohol + Tacrolimus

Alcohol can cause facial flushing or skin erythema in patients using tacrolimus ointment. This reaction appears to be fairly common and has also occurred with medicines formulated with alcohol.

Patients should be warned of the possibility of a flushing reaction with alcohol and that alcohol might need to be avoided if flushing occurs.

Alcohol + Tetracyclines ✅

Doxycycline serum concentrations might fall below minimum therapeutic concentrations in alcoholic patients, but tetracycline is not affected. There is nothing to suggest that moderate amounts of alcohol have a clinically relevant effect on the serum concentrations of any tetracycline in non-alcoholic subjects.

One possible solution is to give alcoholic subjects double the dose of doxycycline. Alternatively tetracycline might be a suitable non-interacting alternative.

Alcohol + Tizanidine ❓

Sedation occurs in up to 50% of patients taking tizanidine; these effects may be additive with alcohol. Additive hypotensive effects also considered possible, see antihypertensives, page 97. Alcohol modestly increases tizanidine levels, which may enhance these effects.

The degree of impairment will depend on the individual patient. However, warn all patients of the potential adverse effects, and counsel against driving or undertaking other skilled tasks, and to sit or lie down if they become dizzy or faint.

A

Alcohol + Trazodone ❓

Trazodone impairs performance in some psychomotor tests, and further impairment can occur with alcohol.

> The degree of impairment will depend on the individual patient. However, warn all patients of the potential effects, and counsel against driving or undertaking other skilled tasks.

Alcohol + Tricyclics ❓

Psychomotor skills can be impaired by amitriptyline, and to a lesser extent by doxepin and imipramine, particularly during the first few days of treatment. This impairment can be increased by alcohol. Amoxapine, clomipramine, desipramine, and nortriptyline appear to interact with alcohol only minimally. Specific information about other tricyclic antidepressants appears to be lacking. However, the toxicity of some tricyclics might be increased by alcohol, and in alcoholics with liver disease.

> Although an interaction has not been clearly demonstrated with all tricyclics, some caution is warranted as they all have some sedative effects. The degree of impairment will depend on the individual patient. However, warn all patients of the potential effects, and counsel against driving or undertaking other skilled tasks. In addition some prescribers may feel it appropriate to offer further precautionary advice, because during the first 1 to 2 weeks of treatment many tricyclics (without alcohol) can temporarily impair the skills related to driving, although the effects of the interaction diminish during continued treatment.

Alcohol + Venlafaxine ❓

No important psychomotor interaction normally appears to occur between alcohol and venlafaxine. However, additive CNS effects (such as drowsiness) are considered possible.

> The UK and US manufacturers state that patients should be advised to avoid alcohol while taking venlafaxine. Nevertheless, it might be prudent to warn all patients of the potential effects, and counsel against driving or undertaking other skilled tasks. The degree of impairment will depend on the individual patient.

Alcohol + Warfarin and related oral anticoagulants ✓

The effects of anticoagulants such as warfarin are unlikely to be changed in those with normal liver function who drink small or moderate amounts of alcohol: one large study showed no relationship between raised INR and alcohol consumption. However, heavy drinkers or patients with some liver disease may show considerable fluctuations in their prothrombin times when they drink alcohol. Some sources also say that the indanedione phenindione may interact with alcohol, but there seems no direct evidence available to support this prediction.

> Patients should be counselled about appropriate alcohol consumption when they start anticoagulant therapy.

Aliskiren

Aliskiren + Amiodarone

Ketoconazole modestly increases the exposure to aliskiren. The UK manufacturer of aliskiren predicts that amiodarone will interact similarly.

Monitor concurrent use for aliskiren adverse effects such as diarrhoea, dyspepsia, and hypotension. Adjust the aliskiren dose as necessary. Note that doses twice the usual recommended dose of aliskiren have been safely used in clinical studies.

Aliskiren + Angiotensin II receptor antagonists

The concurrent use of aliskiren and angiotensin II receptor antagonists may increase the risk of hyperkalaemia. Additive blood pressure-lowering effects are likely to occur, which may be clinically beneficial, see also antihypertensives, page 97.

Monitor potassium concentrations on concurrent use, particularly in patients at high risk of hyperkalaemia (such as those with reduced renal function and/or diabetes). Note that, in December 2011, the European Medicines Agency stated that aliskiren should not be given to diabetic patients in combination with angiotensin II receptor antagonists.

Aliskiren + Azoles

Itraconazole

Itraconazole markedly increases the exposure to aliskiren by about 6–fold and decreases the plasma renin activity in response to aliskiren.

The manufacturers contraindicate concurrent use.

Ketoconazole

Ketoconazole modestly increases the exposure to aliskiren.

Monitor concurrent use for aliskiren adverse effects such as diarrhoea, dyspepsia, and hypotension. Adjust the aliskiren dose as necessary. Note that doses twice the usual recommended dose of aliskiren have been safely used in clinical studies.

Aliskiren + Calcium-channel blockers

Verapamil

Verapamil doubled the exposure to aliskiren in one study. Aliskiren does not affect verapamil pharmacokinetics.

It has been suggested that no initial aliskiren dose adjustment is required with verapamil; however, it would be prudent to monitor concurrent use for aliskiren adverse effects, such as diarrhoea or dyspepsia, and to ensure that the blood pressure-lowering effects of aliskiren do not become excessive.

Other calcium-channel blockers

The use of aliskiren with calcium-channel blockers is expected to result in additive blood pressure-lowering effects.

> This is likely to be a desirable interaction. No action is needed unless the reduction in blood pressure becomes excessive.

Aliskiren + Ciclosporin (Cyclosporine)

Ciclosporin markedly increases the exposure to aliskiren.

> The UK and US manufacturers of aliskiren contraindicate concurrent use. If both drugs are considered essential the dose of aliskiren will need to be reduced; concurrent use should be closely monitored for aliskiren adverse effects such as diarrhoea, dyspepsia, and hypotension.

Aliskiren + Diuretics

Loop diuretics

Aliskiren reduces the plasma levels of furosemide by about 50%. Additive hypotensive effects are likely when aliskiren is given with any diuretic, see antihypertensives, page 97.

> The effects of furosemide may be reduced. Monitor blood pressure and/or disease control, and adjust the doses/treatment accordingly.

Potassium-sparing diuretics

Based on experience with the use of other substances that affect the renin-angiotensin system, the concurrent use of potassium-sparing diuretics and aliskiren may lead to increases in serum potassium. Additive hypotensive effects are likely when aliskiren is given with any diuretic, see antihypertensives, page 97.

> Monitor potassium levels and adjust treatment as necessary.

Aliskiren + Food

A high-fat meal moderately reduces the exposure to aliskiren.

> The UK manufacturer advises taking aliskiren with a light meal, preferably at the same time each day.

Aliskiren + Grapefruit juice ⊗

Grapefruit juice appears to greatly reduce the exposure to aliskiren, which might reduce the effects of aliskiren on blood pressure. Apple juice and orange juice have a similar effect on the exposure to aliskiren.

> Patients should be advised to avoid drinking these fruit juices while taking aliskiren.

Aliskiren + **Herbal medicines or Dietary supplements**

Rifampicin reduces the exposure to aliskiren and reduces its effects on plasma renin activity. The manufacturers of aliskiren predict that St John's wort might interact similarly.

Monitor concurrent use for a reduced effect on blood pressure and increase the dose of aliskiren if necessary.

Aliskiren + **Macrolides**

Ketoconazole moderately increases the exposure to aliskiren. The UK manufacturer of aliskiren predicts that some macrolides (clarithromycin, erythromycin, and telithromycin) will interact similarly.

Monitor concurrent use for aliskiren adverse effects such as diarrhoea, dyspepsia, and hypotension. Adjust the aliskiren dose as necessary. Note that doses twice the usual recommended dose of aliskiren have been safely used in clinical studies.

Aliskiren + **NSAIDs**

NSAIDs might reduce the antihypertensive effects of aliskiren. In dehydrated or elderly patients with pre-existing renal impairment, the concurrent use of aliskiren and NSAIDs may result in a further deterioration of renal function and possible renal failure.

Monitor the outcome of concurrent use, and consider monitoring renal function.

Aliskiren + **Quinidine**

Ciclosporin, a potent inhibitor of P-glycoprotein, markedly increases the exposure to aliskiren. Quinidine is predicted to interact similarly.

The UK manufacturer of aliskiren contraindicates concurrent use.

Aliskiren + **Rifampicin (Rifampin)**

Rifampicin reduces the exposure to aliskiren. Plasma renin activity was 61% greater during rifampicin use, suggesting that rifampicin reduces the effects of aliskiren on renin activity.

Monitor concurrent use for a reduced effect on blood pressure and increase the dose of aliskiren if necessary.

Aliskiren + **Statins**

Atorvastatin increases the exposure to aliskiren.

Monitor concurrent use for aliskiren adverse effects such as diarrhoea, dyspepsia, and hypotension. Adjust the aliskiren dose as necessary. Note that doses twice the usual recommended dose of aliskiren have been safely used in clinical studies.

Allopurinol

Allopurinol + Antidiabetics

Allopurinol adversely affected glycaemic control in a patient with type 2 diabetes receiving insulin. Marked hypoglycaemia and coma occurred in one patient taking gliclazide and allopurinol. Allopurinol causes an increase in the half-life of chlorpropamide, and a minor decrease in the half-life of tolbutamide.

> More study is needed to find out whether any of these interactions has general clinical importance, but it seems unlikely.

Allopurinol + Azathioprine

The haematological effects of azathioprine and mercaptopurine are markedly increased by the concurrent use of allopurinol.

> The dose of azathioprine or mercaptopurine should be reduced by two-thirds to three-quarters to minimise the risk of toxicity. Despite taking these precautions toxicity may still be seen and very close haematological monitoring is advisable if concurrent use is necessary.

Allopurinol + Capecitabine

The activity of capecitabine is predicted to be decreased by allopurinol.

> The UK manufacturers of capecitabine say that allopurinol should be avoided.

Allopurinol + Carbamazepine

There is some evidence to suggest that high-dose allopurinol (15 mg/kg or 600 mg daily) can gradually raise serum carbamazepine levels by about one-third. It appears that allopurinol 300 mg daily has no effect on carbamazepine levels.

> This interaction may take weeks or months to develop. Warn patients taking high-dose allopurinol to monitor for indicators of carbamazepine toxicity, which include nausea, vomiting, ataxia and drowsiness. Monitor carbamazepine levels as necessary.

Allopurinol + Ciclosporin (Cyclosporine)

Isolated case reports describe large increases in ciclosporin concentrations in patients given allopurinol (100 or 200 mg). However, two clinical studies found a trend towards lower ciclosporin concentrations with low-dose allopurinol (e.g. 25 mg).

> This interaction is unconfirmed and of uncertain clinical significance. There is insufficient evidence to recommend increased monitoring, but be aware of the potential for an interaction in case of an unexpected response to treatment.

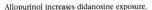

Allopurinol + Diuretics ❓

The thiazide diuretics may increase the incidence of hypersensitivity reactions (rash, vasculitis, hepatitis, eosinophilia, progressive renal impairment) in patients taking allopurinol, especially in the presence of renal impairment.

> The clinical significance of this interaction is unclear but some caution is warranted, particularly if the patient has renal impairment. Remember that thiazides can cause hyperuricaemia.

Allopurinol + NRTIs ✖

Allopurinol increases didanosine exposure.

> The UK manufacturer of didanosine contraindicates concurrent use, and advises that patients requiring allopurinol should be changed from didanosine to an alternative antiretroviral regimen.

Allopurinol + Penicillins ❓

The incidence of skin rashes among those taking either ampicillin or amoxicillin is increased by allopurinol.

> There would seem to be no strong reason for avoiding concurrent use, but prescribers should recognise that the development of a rash is by no means unusual. Whether this also occurs with penicillins other than ampicillin or amoxicillin is uncertain, but it does not seem to have been reported.

Allopurinol + Phenytoin ❓

A case report describes phenytoin toxicity in a boy given allopurinol. Another study found raised phenytoin levels in 2 of 18 patients given allopurinol.

> Although information is limited, it appears that allopurinol may raise phenytoin levels in some patients. It would therefore be prudent to monitor for phenytoin toxicity when allopurinol, particularly in high doses, is added. Indicators of phenytoin toxicity include blurred vision, nystagmus, ataxia or drowsiness.

Allopurinol + Probenecid ⚠

Probenecid appears to increase the renal excretion of the active metabolite of allopurinol, while allopurinol is thought to inhibit the metabolism of probenecid. Theoretically, the concurrent use of allopurinol and probenecid could lead to uric acid precipitation in the kidneys.

> The clinical significance of these interactions appears to be minimal. Nevertheless, the UK manufacturer of allopurinol recommends any reduction in efficacy should be assessed in each case. For allopurinol injection, the US manufacturer recommends a high urinary output of at least 2 litres daily, and the maintenance of neutral or slightly alkaline urine, to help prevent renal precipitation of urates.

A

Allopurinol + Pyrazinamide ⚠

Allopurinol is expected to increase the levels of pyrazinoic acid (an active metabolite of pyrazinamide), and increase its hyperuricaemic effect.

Allopurinol is unlikely to be an effective treatment for pyrazinamide-induced hyperuricaemia, and may exacerbate the situation. Note that pyrazinamide should be used with caution or is contraindicated in patients with a history of gout. If hyperuricaemia accompanied by gouty arthritis (without liver dysfunction) occurs, pyrazinamide should be stopped.

Allopurinol + Theophylline ❓

Allopurinol might slightly increase the exposure to theophylline, but not all studies have found this effect. It seems likely that aminophylline might interact similarly.

Be alert for symptoms of theophylline adverse effects (such as headache, nausea, tremor), particularly in situations where its metabolism might already be reduced (other drugs or diseases). If adverse effects occur, monitor theophylline concentrations, and adjust the dose of theophylline or aminophylline accordingly.

Allopurinol + Warfarin and related oral anticoagulants ⚠

Most patients taking coumarins with allopurinol do not develop an adverse interaction, but excessive hypoprothrombinaemia and bleeding can occur quite unpredictably in a few individuals. The interaction has only been reported with warfarin and phenprocoumon, but it would be prudent to apply the same precautions with any coumarin.

An interaction between allopurinol and the coumarins is not established; however, bear it in mind when using both drugs. Consider increasing the frequency of INR monitoring during the initial stages of concurrent use.

Alpha blockers

Alpha blockers + Angiotensin II receptor antagonists ❓

The first-dose hypotensive effect seen with alpha blockers (particularly alfuzosin, prazosin, and terazosin) is likely to be potentiated by angiotensin II receptor antagonists. It is unclear whether there are real differences between the alpha blockers in their propensity to cause this first-dose effect. Note that the acute hypotensive reaction appears to be short-lived.

When starting an alpha blocker it is often recommended that those already taking an antihypertensive should have their dose reduced to a maintenance level, while initiating the alpha blocker at a low dose, with the first dose taken just before going to bed. Patients should also be warned about the possibility of postural

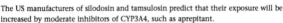
hypotension and how to manage it (i.e. lay down, raise the legs, and, when recovered, get up slowly). Similarly, when adding an antihypertensive to an alpha blocker, it might be prudent to decrease the dose of the alpha blocker and re-titrate as necessary.

Alpha blockers + Aprepitant

The US manufacturers of silodosin and tamsulosin predict that their exposure will be increased by moderate inhibitors of CYP3A4, such as aprepitant.

> The US manufacturers of silodosin and tamsulosin advise caution on concurrent use with moderate inhibitors of CYP3A4, such aprepitant, particularly at tamsulosin doses higher than 400 micrograms; be aware that the effects of these alpha blockers (dizziness, headache, postural hypotension) might be increased.

Alpha blockers + Azoles

Alfuzosin, Silodosin, and Tamsulosin

Ketoconazole, a potent inhibitor of CYP3A4, moderately increases the exposure to alfuzosin, silodosin, and tamsulosin. Itraconazole is predicted to interact with these alpha blockers similarly.

> The US manufacturers of these alpha blockers contraindicate the concurrent use of potent inhibitors of CYP3A4, such as ketoconazole, itraconazole and voriconazole. However, if concurrent use is essential, it would seem prudent to use the minimum dose of the alpha blocker and titrate as necessary, monitoring for adverse effects, particularly first-dose hypotension. The risks are likely to be greater in patients also taking other antihypertensives. The US manufacturers of silodosin and tamsulosin also advise caution on concurrent use with moderate inhibitors of CYP3A4, such as fluconazole and posaconazole, particularly at tamsulosin doses higher than 400 micrograms daily; be aware that the effects of these alpha blockers (dizziness, headache, postural hypotension) might be increased.

Doxazosin

Doxazosin is primarily metabolised by CYP3A4. The US manufacturer therefore predicts that potent inhibitors of CYP3A4, such as ketoconazole, itraconazole, and voriconazole might inhibit the metabolism of doxazosin.

> The clinical relevance of this prediction is unclear as other pathways are involved in doxazosin metabolism, but until more is known some caution seems prudent. If concurrent use is undertaken be aware that the adverse effects of doxazosin (e.g. dizziness, headache, postural hypotension) might be increased.

Alpha blockers + Beta blockers

The risk of first-dose hypotension with prazosin (resulting in dizziness or even fainting) is higher if the patient is already taking a beta blocker. This is likely to be true of other alpha blockers, particularly alfuzosin and terazosin, although it is unclear whether there are real differences between the alpha blockers in their propensity to cause this first dose effect. Alpha blockers and beta blockers can be given together for additional lowering of blood pressure in patients with hypertension, and studies with patients taking beta blockers suggest that silodosin or tamsulosin can be used concurrently without adverse effect on blood pressure.

It is recommended that those already taking beta blockers should have the dose reduced to a maintenance dose and begin with a low-dose of an alpha blocker, with the first dose taken just before going to bed. They should also be warned about the possibility of postural hypotension and how to manage it (i.e. lay down, raise the legs, and get up slowly when recovered). Similarly, when adding a beta blocker to an alpha blocker, it might be prudent to decrease the dose of the alpha blocker and re-titrate as necessary to achieve adequate blood pressure control.

Alpha blockers + Bupropion ❓

Bupropion (a potent CYP2D6 inhibitor) is predicted to slightly increase tamsulosin exposure.

The US manufacturers of tamsulosin advise caution on concurrent use, particularly at tamsulosin doses higher than 400 micrograms daily. Be aware that the effects of tamsulosin (dizziness, headache, postural hypotension) might be increased.

Alpha blockers + Calcium-channel blockers

Diltiazem and Verapamil ⚠️

Verapamil might increase the exposure to prazosin and terazosin, and might also increase the adverse effects related to tamsulosin. The concurrent use of diltiazem and alfuzosin can increase the concentrations of prazosin and terazosin. The US manu-facturers of silodosin and tamsulosin predict that diltiazem and verapamil might inhibit the metabolism of these alpha blockers (particularly at tamsulosin doses higher than 400 micrograms), leading to an increase in exposure and effects.

It seems likely that any pharmacokinetic interaction between the alpha blockers and the calcium-channel blockers will be accounted for by the dose titration that is recommended when starting concurrent use, see under Other calcium-channel blockers, below.

Other calcium-channel blockers ❓

Blood pressure might decrease sharply when calcium-channel blockers are first given to patients already taking alpha blockers (particularly alfuzosin, prazosin, bunazosin, and terazosin), and *vice versa*. Alpha blockers and calcium-channel blockers can be combined for additional blood pressure-lowering in patients with hypertension.

It is recommended that patients already taking calcium-channel blockers should have the dose reduced and start with a low-dose of alpha blocker, with the first dose taken just before going to bed. Caution should also be exercised when calcium-channel blockers are added to established alpha blocker therapy. Patients should also be warned about the possibility of postural hypotension and how to manage it (i.e. lay down, raise the legs, and get up slowly when recovered).

Alpha blockers + Ciclosporin (Cyclosporine)

Prazosin

Preliminary studies show that prazosin causes a small reduction in the glomerular filtration rate of kidney transplant patients taking ciclosporin.

There would seem to be no strong reasons for totally avoiding prazosin in patients taking ciclosporin, but the authors of the report point out that the fall in glomerular filtration rate makes prazosin a less attractive antihypertensive.

Silodosin

Ciclosporin is predicted to increase silodosin exposure by inhibiting P-glycoprotein.

Concurrent use is not recommended; however, if both drugs are given it would seem prudent to be alert for any evidence of silodosin adverse effects (e.g. dizziness, diarrhoea and orthostatic hypotension). If these become troublesome consider reducing the dose of silodosin or withdrawing the drug as necessary.

Alpha blockers + Cinacalcet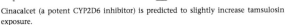

Cinacalcet (a potent CYP2D6 inhibitor) is predicted to slightly increase tamsulosin exposure.

The US manufacturers of tamsulosin advise caution on concurrent use, particularly at tamsulosin doses higher than 400 micrograms daily. Be aware that the effects of tamsulosin (dizziness, headache, postural hypotension) might be increased.

Alpha blockers + Clonidine

There is evidence that prazosin can reduce the antihypertensive effects of clonidine, whereas some other evidence suggests that this does not occur.

No action needed unless hypotension becomes excessive. If the combination of prazosin and clonidine is less effective than expected consider an interaction as the cause.

Alpha blockers + Cobicistat

Cobicistat, a very potent inhibitor of CYP3A4, is predicted to moderately increase the exposure to alfuzosin, silodosin, and tamsulosin. *In vitro* studies suggest that the metabolism of doxazosin might also be inhibited by potent CYP3A4 inhibitors.

The US manufacturers of alfuzosin, silodosin and tamsulosin contraindicate the concurrent use of potent inhibitors of CYP3A4. However, if concurrent use is essential, it would seem prudent to use the minimum dose of the alpha blocker and titrate as necessary, monitoring for adverse effects, particularly first-dose hypotension. The risks are likely to be greater in patients also taking other antihypertensives.

Alpha blockers + **Dapoxetine** ❓

The concurrent use of tamsulosin and dapoxetine does not appear to affect the pharmacokinetics of either drug. Nevertheless, the Swedish manufacturer of dapoxetine predicts that concurrent use with an alpha blocker might have additive effects on blood pressure.

> Tamsulosin is less likely to cause orthostatic hypotension than other alpha blockers, however caution is still required. Bear the possibility of an interaction in mind should excessive blood pressure-lowering effects occur.

Alpha blockers + **Digoxin** ❓

A 60% rise in digoxin levels occurred over 3 days in one study when prazosin was also given. Another study found the opposite effect. Clinical experience suggests that any interaction is rare.

> No action is usually need when prazosin is given with digoxin, although consider an interaction if adverse effects, such as bradycardia, or evidence of a reduction in effect, occur. Alfuzosin, doxazosin, silodosin, tamsulosin and terazosin appear not to interact with digoxin.

Alpha blockers + **Diuretics** ❓

As would be expected, the use of an alpha blocker with a diuretic might result in an additive hypotensive effect, but aside from first-dose hypotension, this usually seems to be a beneficial interaction in patients with hypertension. The effects in patients with congestive heart failure might be more severe.

> As postural hypotension is a possibility, warn patients to lie down if symptoms such as dizziness, fatigue, or sweating develop, and to remain lying down until they abate completely. An alpha blocker dose reduction and then re-titration might be necessary in some patients. In particular, patients with congestive heart failure, who have had large doses of diuretics, should start prazosin treatment at the lowest dose, with the initial dose given at bedtime.

Alpha blockers + **Duloxetine**

Duloxetine (a moderate CYP2D6 inhibitor) is predicted to slightly increase tamsulosin exposure.

> The US manufacturers of tamsulosin advise caution on concurrent use, particularly at tamsulosin doses higher than 400 micrograms daily. Be aware that the effects of tamsulosin (dizziness, headache, postural hypotension) might be increased.

Alpha blockers + **H₂-receptor antagonists**

No clinically important interaction occurs between cimetidine and alfuzosin, doxazosin, or tamsulosin.

> No action needed. However, note that because tamsulosin concentrations are slightly increased, the US manufacturers state that caution should be used on concurrent use with cimetidine, particularly with tamsulosin doses greater than 400 micrograms. In practice this probably means being aware that an increase in

the adverse effects of tamsulosin (e.g. dizziness, headache, postural hypotension) might occur as a result of this interaction. Other H_2–receptor antagonists would not be expected to interact this way.

Alpha blockers + HIV-protease inhibitors

The HIV-protease inhibitors boosted with ritonavir (all very potent inhibitors of CYP3A4), and saquinavir or ritonavir alone, are predicted to moderately increase the exposure to alfuzosin, silodosin, and tamsulosin. *In vitro* studies suggest that the metabolism of doxazosin might also be inhibited by these HIV-protease inhibitors.

The US manufacturers contraindicate the use of alfuzosin, silodosin or tamsulosin with potent inhibitors of CYP3A4, such as the HIV-protease inhibitors boosted with ritonavir, saquinavir, or ritonavir. However, if concurrent use is essential, it would seem prudent to use the minimum dose of the alpha blocker and titrate as necessary, monitoring for adverse effects, particularly first-dose hypotension. The risks are likely to be greater in patients also taking other antihypertensives.

Alpha blockers + Macrolides

Clarithromycin and telithromycin (both potent inhibitors of CYP3A4) are predicted to moderately increase the exposure to alfuzosin, silodosin, and tamsulosin. *In vitro* studies suggest that the metabolism of doxazosin might also be inhibited by these macrolides. The US manufacturers of silodosin and tamsulosin predict that their exposure will be increased by erythromycin (a moderate inhibitor of CYP3A4).

The US manufacturers of alfuzosin, silodosin and tamsulosin contraindicate the concurrent use of potent inhibitors of CYP3A4, such as clarithromycin and telithromycin. However, if concurrent use is essential, it would seem prudent to use the minimum dose of the alpha blocker and titrate as necessary, monitoring for adverse effects, particularly first-dose hypotension. The risks are likely to be greater in patients also taking other antihypertensives. The US manufacturers of silodosin and tamsulosin also advise caution on concurrent use with moderate inhibitors of CYP3A4, such as erythromycin, particularly at tamsulosin doses higher than 400 micrograms daily; be aware that the effects of these alpha blockers (dizziness, headache, postural hypotension) might be increased.

Alpha blockers + MAOIs

Indoramin

It has been predicted that the concurrent use of indoramin and MAOIs might lead to hypertension. However, the pharmacology of these drugs suggests just the opposite, namely that hypotension is the more likely outcome.

The UK manufacturer of indoramin contraindicates concurrent use.

Other alpha blockers ❓

Both the MAOIs and the alpha blockers have hypotensive effects, which might be additive.

No action needed, but be aware that hypotension is a possibility if any alpha blocker is given with an MAOI.

Alpha blockers + NSAIDs ❓

Indometacin reduces the blood pressure-lowering effects of prazosin in some individuals. However, indometacin does not appear to interact adversely with other alpha blockers.

If indometacin is added to established treatment with prazosin, be alert for a reduced antihypertensive response. It is not known exactly what happens in patients taking both drugs long-term, but note that with other interactions between antihypertensives and NSAIDs the effects seem to be modest.

Alpha blockers + Opioids ❓

Dextropropoxyphene (propoxyphene), a moderate CYP2D6 inhibitor, is predicted to slightly increase tamsulosin exposure.

The US manufacturers of tamsulosin advise caution on concurrent use, particularly at tamsulosin doses higher than 400 micrograms daily. Be aware that the effects of tamsulosin (dizziness, headache, postural hypotension) might be increased.

Alpha blockers + Phosphodiesterase type-5 inhibitors ⚠️

Postural hypotension might occur with higher doses of avanafil, sildenafil, tadalafil, or vardenafil given at the same time as doxazosin or terazosin. It seems likely that this effect will occur with most alpha blockers, although it is seen less frequently with modified-release alfuzosin and tamsulosin, and possibly silodosin.

Patients should be stable on an alpha blocker before a phosphodiesterase type-5 inhibitor is started, and the lowest starting dose of the phosphodiesterase inhibitor (e.g. sildenafil 25 mg) should be considered. If an alpha blocker is required in a patient already taking a phosphodiesterase type-5 inhibitor, additional caution is required and the alpha blocker should be started at the lowest dose. Patients should be advised what to do if they develop postural hypotension (i.e. lay down, raise the legs and, when recovered, get up slowly). However the UK manufacturer of tadalafil does not recommend concomitant use with doxazosin, and the US manufacturer does not recommend concurrent use with alpha blockers for treating benign prostatic hyperplasia.

Alpha blockers + Propafenone ❓

Propafenone (a moderate CYP2D6 inhibitor) is predicted to slightly increase tamsulosin exposure.

The US manufacturers of tamsulosin advise caution on concurrent use, particularly at tamsulosin doses higher than 400 micrograms daily. Be aware that the effects of tamsulosin (dizziness, headache, postural hypotension) might be increased.

Alpha blockers + SSRIs ❓

Paroxetine slightly increases tamsulosin exposure. Other potent inhibitors of CYP2D6 (such as fluoxetine) are expected to interact similarly.

The slight increase in tamsulosin exposure by paroxetine is unlikely to be clinically important. The US manufacturer advises caution, particularly at tamsulosin doses higher than 400 micrograms daily. Be aware that the effects of tamsulosin (dizziness, headache, postural hypotension) might be increased.

Alpha blockers + Terbinafine [?]

Terbinafine (a potent CYP2D6 inhibitor) is predicted to slightly increase tamsulosin exposure.

The US manufacturer of tamsulosin advises caution on concurrent use, particularly at tamsulosin doses higher than 400 micrograms daily. Be aware that the effects of tamsulosin (dizziness, headache, postural hypotension) might be increased.

Amantadine

Amantadine + Bupropion [!]

The manufacturer of bupropion states that limited clinical data suggests a higher incidence of undesirable effects (nausea, vomiting, excitement, restlessness, postural tremor) in patients also given amantadine.

Patients taking amantadine should be given small initial doses of bupropion, which are increased gradually. Good monitoring is advisable.

Amantadine + Dopamine agonists [?]

The manufacturers of pramipexole predict that its clearance will be reduced by amantadine.

The clinical significance of this is uncertain, and there appear to be no reports of any adverse interactions. The manufacturers suggest a reduction of the pramipexole dose should be considered in patients taking amantadine.

Amfetamines

Amfetamines + Antipsychotics [?]

The manufacturers of amfetamine, dexamfetamine and lisdexamfetamine note that haloperidol may inhibit the central stimulant effects of the amfetamines.

The amfetamines may be less effective in those taking haloperidol. Be alert for this effect on concurrent use.

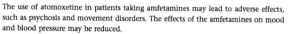

A

Amfetamines + **Atomoxetine**

The use of atomoxetine in patients taking amfetamines may lead to adverse effects, such as psychosis and movement disorders. The effects of the amfetamines on mood and blood pressure may be reduced.

> If both drugs are given, be aware that adverse CNS effects may develop, and consider reducing the doses or stopping one of the drugs should this occur.

Amfetamines + **Beta blockers**

It has been suggested that the effects of the beta blockers (e.g. their blood pressure-lowering effects) might be inhibited by amfetamines. Others suggest that concurrent use might result in severe hypertension and antagonism of the effects of amfetamines. The UK manufacturer of dexamfetamine also warns that the concurrent use of beta blockers might result in severe hypertension and, in addition, states that adrenoceptor blocking drugs, such as propranolol might antagonise the effects of dexamfetamine (a sympathomimetic).

> It would seem prudent to monitor blood pressure if amfetamines are given to patients taking beta blockers, and consider the contribution of the amfetamine if a patient taking an amfetamine and an antihypertensive has inadequate blood pressure control.

Amfetamines + **Furazolidone**

The pressor responses to dexamfetamine in 4 hypertensive patients were increased 2- to 3-fold after 6 days of furazolidone use, and after 13 days they had increased by about 10-fold. Furazolidone has MAO-inhibitory activity, after 5 to 10 days of use, which is about equivalent to that of the non-selective MAOIs.

> The concurrent use of furazolidone with amfetamines might be expected to result in a potentially serious rise in blood pressure and should therefore be avoided.

Amfetamines + **Guanethidine**

When hypertensive patients taking guanethidine were given single doses of dexamfetamine or metamfetamine, the hypotensive effects of the guanethidine were completely abolished, and in some instances the blood pressures rose higher than before treatment with the guanethidine. Other amfetamines would be expected to interact similarly.

> Concurrent use should be avoided.

Amfetamines + **HIV-protease inhibitors**

An HIV-positive man taking ritonavir and saquinavir died after also taking metamfetamine and amyl nitrate. Toxicology reported extremely high metamfetamine concentrations, which were attributed to an interaction with ritonavir. Evidence is limited, but ritonavir and tipranavir are expected to raise the concentrations of the amfetamines (by inhibiting CYP2D6). Haemolytic anaemia has also been reported in a patient taking metamfetamine with indinavir.

> Patients should be made aware of the additional potential risks of using

amfetamines with ritonavir and tipranavir (deaths have occurred). Some recommend that patients taking ritonavir should avoid amfetamines. It would seem prudent to reduce the amfetamine dose.

Amfetamines + Inotropes and Vasopressors

The manufacturers of amfetamine, dexamfetamine and lisdexamfetamine state that amfetamines enhance the adrenergic effects of noradrenaline (norepinephrine). This may result in increased vasoconstriction, and could enhance the pressor effects of noradrenaline. Other inotropes and vasopressors with adrenergic actions may be similarly affected, but this does not appear to be specifically mentioned.

As the effects of these inotropes and vasopressors on blood pressure are likely to be closely monitored, any interaction should be picked up by routine monitoring.

Amfetamines + MAOIs

The concurrent use of amfetamines and non-selective MAOIs can result in a potentially fatal hypertensive crisis and/or serotonin syndrome, page 580.

Concurrent use is contraindicated. It would seem prudent to also avoid the use of an amfetamine for 14 days after an MAOI has been taken.

Amfetamines + Moclobemide

The concurrent use of an amfetamine and an MAOI can result in a potentially fatal hypertensive crisis and/or serotonin syndrome. Moclobemide may interact with the amfetamines similarly.

It may be prudent to avoid the concurrent use of moclobemide and an amfetamine.

Amfetamines + SSRIs

There may be an increased risk of serotonin syndrome and neurotoxic reactions if amfetamines or related drugs are given with SSRIs. Fluoxetine and paroxetine may inhibit the metabolism of the amfetamines; toxicity has been reported.

Be alert for evidence of amfetamine adverse effects if fluoxetine and paroxetine are also given. The general significance of the case reports describing serotonin syndrome, page 580 and neurotoxicity is unknown, but bear it in mind in case of an unexpected response to treatment.

Amfetamines + Tricyclics

The UK and US manufacturers state that amfetamines might increase the effects of tricyclics, and that some tricyclics might potentiate cardiac adverse effects and increase the concentration of dexamfetamine in the brain.

The clinical relevance of these warnings is unclear. It might be prudent to consider the risks of combining an amfetamine with a tricyclic in patients with pre-existing cardiovascular disorders.

Amfetamines + Venlafaxine

An isolated case of serotonin syndrome, page 580, has been attributed to the concurrent use of dexamfetamine and venlafaxine.

> The clinical significance of this interaction is unknown, but bear it in mind in case of an unexpected response to treatment.

Aminoglycosides

The aminoglycosides are known to be nephrotoxic and many of their interactions occur as a result of this effect. Due to the number of known interactions with other nephrotoxic drugs (for examples see amphotericin B, below, and ciclosporin, page 47), many manufacturers of other drugs with nephrotoxic effects advise caution on their concurrent use. It is advisable to monitor renal function in patients taking aminoglycosides, and it may be prudent to increase the frequency of this monitoring in patients taking other nephrotoxic drugs.

Aminoglycosides + Amphotericin B

A number of patients developed nephrotoxicity, which was attributed to amphotericin B. Raised gentamicin or amikacin levels, without significant changes in creatinine, were seen in children also given amphotericin B.

> Aminoglycosides are nephrotoxic and it is generally recommended that they should be avoided with other nephrotoxic drugs (such as amphotericin B, particularly the conventional formulation). However, if concurrent use is essential it may be prudent to increase the renal function and drug level monitoring that is advised during the use of an aminoglycoside.

Aminoglycosides + Bisphosphonates

Severe hypocalcaemia has been reported in three patients given sodium clodronate when they were also given netilmicin or amikacin. Theoretically, additive calcium lowering effects could occur with any bisphosphonate and aminoglycoside combination. Note that some manufacturers predict that the concurrent use of drugs that cause nephrotoxicity (such as the aminoglycosides) may lead to an increase in bisphosphonate levels.

> If bisphosphonates are given with aminoglycosides, caution and close monitoring of calcium and magnesium levels has been advised. The renal loss of calcium and magnesium can continue for weeks after aminoglycosides are stopped, and bisphosphonates can also persist in bone for weeks. This means that the interaction is potentially possible whether the drugs are given concurrently or sequentially.

Aminoglycosides + Ciclosporin (Cyclosporine)

Nephrotoxicity is increased in some patients by the concurrent use of ciclosporin and amikacin, gentamicin, or tobramycin. This interaction would be expected with all systemic aminoglycosides.

In general the concurrent use of two drugs with nephrotoxic potential should be avoided; however, the concurrent use of ciclosporin and aminoglycosides is clinically valuable. It would be prudent to increase the monitoring of renal function on concurrent use.

Aminoglycosides + Digoxin

Digoxin levels have been reported to be increased (more than doubled) by the concurrent use of gentamicin in patients with congestive cardiac failure and diabetes.

This interaction seems rare. Patients should be monitored for signs of digoxin toxicity if gentamicin is given, especially those with diabetes or impaired renal function. Initially, checking pulse rate is probably adequate. There seems to be no information about other parenteral aminoglycosides. Consider also neomycin, page 330.

Aminoglycosides + Diuretics

Etacrynic acid

The concurrent use of aminoglycosides and etacrynic acid should be avoided because their damaging actions on the ear can be additive. The intravenous use of etacrynic acid and renal impairment are additional causative factors. Even sequential use may not be safe, and the effects may be irreversible.

Avoid concurrent use. Other loop diuretics appear to be safer.

Other loop diuretics

Although some patients have developed nephrotoxicity and/or ototoxicity while taking furosemide and an aminoglycoside, it has not been established that this was as a result of an interaction. It has been suggested that any interaction may be more likely to occur if high-dose infusions of furosemide are used.

As there is some uncertainty about the safety of concurrent use, increased monitoring (e.g. of renal function) would seem appropriate, particularly if high doses of furosemide are given. The same precautions would seem to be appropriate with other loop diuretics (although see *Etacrynic acid*, above).

Aminoglycosides + Mycophenolate

A selective bowel decontamination regimen of tobramycin and nystatin (with cefuroxime) modestly reduced mycophenolate bioavailability.

Until further information is available, it would seem prudent to monitor the outcome of concurrent use, and for a short period after stopping the antibacterial, to ensure that mycophenolate remains effective.

Aminoglycosides + NRTIs

Cidofovir or tenofovir alone can cause renal failure and this might be additive with other drugs that are nephrotoxic: the manufacturers name the aminoglycosides.

Concurrent use of cidofovir and an aminoglycoside is contraindicated; the UK and US manufacturers advise stopping potentially nephrotoxic drugs at least 7 days before starting cidofovir. The concurrent use of tenofovir with an aminoglycoside should also be avoided.; If this is not possible, monitoring of renal function should be increased: the UK and US manufacturers of tenofovir suggest at least weekly monitoring on concurrent use.

Aminoglycosides + NSAIDs

Some reports claim that gentamicin and amikacin levels may be raised by indometacin, and that amikacin levels may be raised by ibuprofen lysine, when given to premature babies to treat patent ductus arteriosus, whereas others have not found an interaction.

Concurrent use should be closely monitored (e.g. renal function, aminoglycoside levels) because of the toxicity that is associated with raised aminoglycoside levels. It has been suggested that the aminoglycoside dose should be reduced before giving indometacin. It has also been suggested that the dose interval of amikacin should be increased by at least 6 to 8 hours if ibuprofen lysine is also given during the first days of life. Other aminoglycosides possibly behave similarly. This interaction does not seem to have been studied in adults.

Aminoglycosides + Penicillins

A reduction in aminoglycoside levels can occur if aminoglycosides and penicillins are given together to patients with severe renal impairment. Carbenicillin, piperacillin and ticarcillin have been implicated with both gentamicin and tobramycin. No interaction of importance appears to occur either with intravenous aminoglycoside and penicillins in those with normal renal function.

In patients with renal impairment it has been recommended that the penicillin dose should be adjusted according to renal function, and the levels of both antibacterials closely monitored. However, note that antibacterial inactivation can continue in the assay sample, and rapid assay is probably necessary. There would seem to be no reason for avoiding concurrent use in patients with normal renal function because no significant *in vivo* inactivation appears to occur. Moreover there is good clinical evidence that concurrent use is valuable, especially in the treatment of *Pseudomonas* infections. Consider also neomycin, page 512.

Aminoglycosides + Proton pump inhibitors

Proton pump inhibitors can cause hypomagnesaemia, which might be additive with the magnesium-lowering effects of the aminoglycosides.

Hypomagnesaemia can develop after more than one year of concurrent use, so consider monitoring magnesium concentrations before and annually during proton pump inhibitor use, or in response to symptoms of hypomagnesaemia (e.g. muscle twitching or cramps, tremors, vomiting, tiredness, or loss of appetite). In those patients who develop hypomagnesaemia, oral and parenteral magnesium supplements might not be as effective as anticipated. Stopping the proton pump inhibitor (where possible) might be necessary.

Aminoglycosides + Tacrolimus

The aminoglycosides are known to be nephrotoxic and many of their interactions occur as a result of this effect. Due to the number of known interactions with other nephrotoxic drugs (for examples see amphotericin B, page 46, and ciclosporin, page 47), many manufacturers of other drugs with nephrotoxic effects, including tacrolimus, advise caution on their concurrent use.

It is advisable to monitor renal function in patients taking aminoglycosides, and it may be prudent to increase the frequency of this monitoring in patients taking other nephrotoxic drugs.

Aminoglycosides + Vancomycin

The nephrotoxicity of the aminoglycosides appears to be potentiated by vancomycin.

Concurrent use is therapeutically useful, but the risk of increased nephrotoxicity should be borne in mind. Therapeutic drug monitoring and regular assessment of renal function is warranted.

Amiodarone

Note that amiodarone has a long half-life (25 to 100 days) so that interactions may occur for some time after amiodarone has been withdrawn.

Amiodarone + Beta blockers

Hypotension, bradycardia, ventricular fibrillation, and asystole have been seen in a few patients given amiodarone with propranolol, metoprolol, or sotalol (for sotalol, see also drugs that prolong the QT interval, page 352). Amiodarone increases metoprolol concentrations, and might increase the concentrations of other beta blockers metabolised by CYP2D6, which might contribute to both the beneficial and adverse effects reported. However, analysis of clinical studies suggests that the combination of amiodarone and beta blockers can be beneficial.

The concurrent use of beta blockers and amiodarone is not uncommon and can be therapeutically useful. However, it should be undertaken with caution and an appreciation of the potential adverse effects, especially with sotalol. Monitor for bradycardia, adjusting the doses or stopping one drug if the heart rate becomes too slow.

Amiodarone + Calcium-channel blockers

Increased cardiac depressant effects (potentiation of negative chronotropic properties and conduction slowing effects) would be expected if amiodarone is given with diltiazem or verapamil. One case of sinus arrest and serious hypotension has been reported in a woman taking diltiazem with amiodarone.

> It is advised that amiodarone should be avoided or used with caution with diltiazem or verapamil because cardiodepression may occur. Note that diltiazem has been used for rate control in patients developing postoperative atrial fibrillation despite the use of prophylactic amiodarone. There do not appear to be any reports of adverse effects attributed to the use of amiodarone with the dihydropyridine class of calcium-channel blockers (e.g. nifedipine), which typically have little or no negative inotropic activity at usual doses.

Amiodarone + Chloroquine

Some UK manufacturers of amiodarone and chloroquine suggest that concurrent use may increase the risk of torsade de pointes. Chloroquine may cause arrhythmias and ECG changes when used alone, particularly in high doses and for prolonged periods; however, chloroquine is not generally considered a high risk for causing cardiovascular toxicity, especially when given at the correct dose and administered appropriately.

> Some (but not all) UK manufacturers of amiodarone and chloroquine contra-indicate concurrent use, whereas the US manufacturers do not include any warnings about this theoretical interaction.

Amiodarone + Ciclosporin (Cyclosporine)

Ciclosporin serum concentrations can be increased by amiodarone and nephrotoxicity has occurred as a result. Increased amiodarone concentrations and pulmonary toxicity have been reported in patients stopping amiodarone and starting ciclosporin.

> Concurrent use need not be avoided but close monitoring of ciclosporin serum concentrations and renal function is needed, and ciclosporin dose reductions might be required to minimise potential nephrotoxicity. Remember to re-adjust the ciclosporin dose if amiodarone is stopped, bearing in mind that it might take weeks before amiodarone is totally cleared from the body. The general significance of the increase in amiodarone concentrations and the occurrence of pulmonary toxicity is unclear, but bear these reports in mind in case of unexpected effects.

Amiodarone + Cobicistat

The US manufacturer of elvitegravir boosted with cobicistat (in a fixed-dose combination also including emtricitabine and tenofovir) predicts that cobicistat will increase amiodarone concentrations.

> Monitor for amiodarone adverse effects (bradycardia, taste disturbances, tremor, ECG changes) and adjust the amiodarone dose if necessary.

Amiodarone + Colestyramine and related drugs

Colestyramine appears to reduce amiodarone levels by about 50%.

> Because amiodarone undergoes some enterohepatic recirculation, separating the doses may only minimise the interaction. Monitor for decreased amiodarone

effects if colestyramine is started, and adjust the amiodarone dose as necessary, or consider an alternative to colestyramine.

Amiodarone + Co-trimoxazole

Some UK manufacturers of amiodarone state that co-trimoxazole (trimethoprim with sulfamethoxazole) prolongs the QT interval and increases the risk of torsade de pointes; however co-trimoxazole is not generally associated with causing significant QT interval prolongation and torsade de pointes.

One UK manufacturer contraindicates concurrent use. However, the US manufacturers and other UK manufacturers make no mention of any possible interaction.

Amiodarone + Dabigatran

Amiodarone, a P-glycoprotein inhibitor, increases the exposure to dabigatran.

For thromboembolism prophylaxis, reduce the dabigatran dose to 150 mg daily and take both drugs at the same time. No dabigatran dose adjustment is necessary for stroke prophylaxis. Monitor for bleeding and anaemia and discontinue dabigatran if severe bleeding occurs. Any interaction might persist for several weeks after stopping amiodarone.

Amiodarone + Digoxin

Digoxin levels can be approximately doubled by amiodarone. Some individuals may show even greater increases. Digitalis toxicity is likely to occur if the dose of digoxin is not reduced appropriately.

The interaction occurs in most patients and is clearly evident after a few days but may take 4 weeks to fully develop. Reduce the digoxin dose by between one-third to one-half initially and monitor digoxin levels. Further adjustment of the digoxin dose may be needed after a week or two, and possibly a month or more depending on digoxin levels. Particular care is needed in children, who may show much larger rises in digoxin levels.

Amiodarone + Disopyramide

The QT interval prolonging effects are increased when disopyramide and amiodarone are used together (see drugs that prolong the QT interval, page 352, for a general discussion of QT prolongation).

The UK manufacturer contraindicates concurrent use. If concurrent use is essential, the dose of disopyramide should be reduced by 30 to 50% several days after starting amiodarone. The continued need for disopyramide should be monitored, and withdrawal attempted if possible. If disopyramide is added to amiodarone, the initial dose of disopyramide should be about half of the usual recommended dose. Close monitoring is essential.

Amiodarone + Diuretics

Mild to moderate inhibitors of CYP3A4 (such as amiodarone) may increase the AUC of eplerenone up to threefold, which increases the risk of hyperkalaemia.

> It is generally recommended that the dose of eplerenone should not exceed 25 mg daily in patients taking amiodarone.

Amiodarone + Donepezil

The risk of adverse effects, including bradycardia, may be increased if a centrally-acting anticholinesterase is given with amiodarone.

> Be alert for bradycardia if amiodarone is given with donepezil.

Amiodarone + Flecainide

Serum flecainide concentrations are increased by amiodarone. An isolated report describes torsade de pointes in a patient taking amiodarone with flecainide.

> Reduce the flecainide dose by one-third to one-half if amiodarone is added and monitor for flecainide adverse effects (dizziness, nausea, and tremor). The interaction could take 2 weeks or more to develop fully and can persist for some weeks after amiodarone is withdrawn.

Amiodarone + Galantamine

The risk of adverse effects, including bradycardia, may be increased if a centrally-acting anticholinesterase is given with amiodarone.

> Be alert for bradycardia if amiodarone is given with galantamine.

Amiodarone + Grapefruit juice

Grapefruit juice appears to completely inhibit the metabolism of amiodarone to its major active metabolite, increases the AUC of amiodarone by 50% and increases its peak level by 84%, which may lead to toxicity. However, the effect of amiodarone on the PR and QTc intervals is apparently *decreased*, possibly due to reduced levels of the active metabolite.

> Further study is needed. In the meantime, it may be prudent to suggest to patients that they avoid grapefruit juice.

Amiodarone + H₂-receptor antagonists

Cimetidine possibly causes a modest rise in amiodarone levels in some patients.

> Information seems to be limited to one study but this interaction may be clinically important in some patients. Be alert for amiodarone adverse effects (e.g. bradycardia, taste disturbances, tremor, nausea).

Amiodarone + HIV-protease inhibitors

A rise in amiodarone levels of about 50% has been seen in a patient given indinavir.

Other HIV-protease inhibitors would be expected to interact similarly. Saquinavir has QT-prolonging effects, which might be additive with those of other drugs with such effects, such as amiodarone, see drugs that prolong the QT interval, page 352.

The concurrent use of amiodarone with a HIV-protease inhibitor is generally contraindicated. However, in the UK the exception is atazanavir boosted with ritonavir, and in the US, caution and increased monitoring, including taking amiodarone levels, is recommended with amprenavir, atazanavir, darunavir boosted with ritonavir, fosamprenavir, and lopinavir boosted with ritonavir.

Amiodarone + Levothyroxine

Patients taking levothyroxine for hypothyroidism might develop elevated thyroid-stimulating hormone concentrations or overt hypothyroidism when also given amiodarone.

The UK manufacturer of amiodarone contraindicates its use in patients with current, or a history of, thyroid dysfunction. Close monitoring of thyroid function is required if amiodarone is given with levothyroxine. Note that levothyroxine has been given to correct hypothyroidism induced by amiodarone.

Amiodarone + Lidocaine

Isolated reports describe a seizure in a man given intravenous lidocaine about 2 days after he started to take amiodarone, and sinoatrial arrest in another man with sick sinus syndrome who was given both drugs. There is conflicting evidence as to whether or not amiodarone affects the pharmacokinetics of intravenous lidocaine.

Careful monitoring is required if both drugs are used. The manufacturers of topical lidocaine also advise caution, especially if large amounts of lidocaine are applied.

Amiodarone + Lithium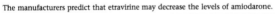

Hypothyroidism developed very rapidly in 2 patients taking amiodarone when lithium was started.

Note that lithium has been tried for the treatment of amiodarone-induced hyperthyroidism, and regular monitoring of thyroid status is recommended throughout amiodarone treatment. Lithium has rarely been associated with QT prolongation, and consequently the UK manufacturer of amiodarone contra-indicates its concurrent use (see drugs that prolong the QT interval, page 352, for a general discussion of QT prolongation).

Amiodarone + NNRTIs

The manufacturers predict that etravirine may decrease the levels of amiodarone.

The manufacturers recommend caution on concurrent use and state that amiodarone levels should be monitored, if this is possible.

Amiodarone + Phenytoin

Phenytoin levels can be raised by amiodarone, markedly so in some individuals (4-fold rise reported) and phenytoin toxicity may occur. Amiodarone levels are reduced by phenytoin.

Monitor phenytoin levels and for phenytoin adverse effects (e.g. blurred vision, nystagmus, ataxia or drowsiness), and adjust the phenytoin dose if necessary. A 25 to 30% reduction in the phenytoin dose has been recommended for those taking 2 to 4 mg/kg daily, but it should be remembered that small alterations in phenytoin dose may result in a large change in phenytoin levels, as phenytoin kinetics are non-linear. The clinical significance of the effects on amiodarone are unclear.

Amiodarone + Procainamide ✕

The QT interval prolonging effects are increased when procainamide and amiodarone are used together (see drugs that prolong the QT interval, page 352, for a general discussion of QT prolongation). Amiodarone increases the levels of procainamide and its metabolite by 60% and 30%, respectively.

Concurrent use should generally be avoided due to the QT prolonging effects of the combination. If the two drugs are considered essential, the ECG should be closely monitored and the dose of procainamide may need to be reduced by 20 to 50%. Levels should be monitored where possible, and patients observed closely for adverse effects.

Amiodarone + Quinidine ✕

The QT interval prolonging effects of quinidine and amiodarone are increased when they are used together, and torsade de pointes has occurred (see drugs that prolong the QT interval, page 352, for a general discussion of QT prolongation). Quinidine levels can be increased by about 30% by amiodarone, although larger increases have been reported in some individuals.

Concurrent use is generally contraindicated due to the QT prolonging effects of the combination. If the two drugs are considered essential, the dose of quinidine may need to be reduced by 30 to 50%. Levels should be monitored where possible. The QT interval on the ECG should also be monitored and patients observed closely for quinidine-related adverse effects.

Amiodarone + Rivastigmine ❓

The risk of adverse effects, including bradycardia, may be increased if a centrally-acting anticholinesterase is given with amiodarone.

Be alert for bradycardia if amiodarone is given with rivastigmine.

Amiodarone + Statins ⚠

Amiodarone increases exposure to simvastatin, and there is some evidence of a higher incidence of myopathy when amiodarone is given with high doses of simvastatin. Furthermore, cases of myopathy and rhabdomyolysis have been reported in patients taking amiodarone and simvastatin. Lovastatin, and possibly to a lesser extent atorvastatin, might interact similarly.

The dose of simvastatin should not exceed 20 mg daily in patients taking amiodarone, unless the clinical benefit is likely to outweigh the increased risk of myopathy and rhabdomyolysis. The US manufacturer of lovastatin suggests a maximum dose of 40 mg daily in the presence of amiodarone. For atorvastatin, the UK manufacturer advises that a lower dose of atorvastatin should be considered, with close monitoring at the start of treatment or if the dose of amiodarone is changed. In all cases, patients taking these statins with amiodarone should be warned to report promptly any unexplained muscle aches, tenderness, cramps, stiffness, or weakness. However, note that the UK manufacturer of amiodarone actually recommends that when a statin is required with amiodarone, one that is not metabolised by CYP3A4 (that is, none of these three statins) should be used.

Amiodarone + Tacrine

The risk of adverse effects, including bradycardia, may be increased if a centrally-acting anticholinesterase is given with amiodarone.

Be alert for bradycardia if amiodarone is given with tacrine.

Amiodarone + Warfarin and related oral anticoagulants

The anticoagulant effects of warfarin, phenprocoumon and acenocoumarol are increased by amiodarone in most patients and bleeding may occur. The extent of the interaction appears to be dependent on the dose of amiodarone, with higher doses having a greater effect. The interaction starts within a few days and is usually maximal by 2 to 7 weeks.

The dose of warfarin and phenprocoumon should be reduced by one- to two-thirds if amiodarone is added, and the dose of acenocoumarol should be reduced by between about 30 and 50%. However, these suggested reductions are only broad generalisations and individual patients may need more or less. Monitor the INR (or prothrombin times) on concurrent use at least weekly until a new steady-state has been achieved, and for several weeks after amiodarone is stopped. Some sources state that the metabolism of the indanedione phenindione is inhibited by amiodarone, but this appears to be an extrapolation from the known interaction with warfarin. There seems to be no clinical evidence available to support this prediction.

Amphotericin B

See also drugs that prolong the QT interval, page 352, as QT-prolongation can be exacerbated by hypokalaemia, which is a common adverse effect of amphotericin B. The renal toxicity of amphotericin B may be associated with sodium depletion.

Amphotericin B + Azoles

The effects of amphotericin B and the azoles would be expected to be antagonistic, and

A

there is some clinical evidence that supports this suggestion. Concurrent use might increase the incidence of hepatotoxicity.

Despite extensive *in vitro* and *animal* data, it is not entirely clear whether or not azoles inhibit the efficacy of amphotericin B. Until more is known concurrent use should be limited to specific cases and the outcome should be well monitored for both a reduced antifungal response and an increase in adverse effects, such as increasing LFTs.

Amphotericin B + Ciclosporin (Cyclosporine)

The risk of nephrotoxicity appears to be increased if ciclosporin is given with amphotericin B. Limited evidence suggests that liposomal amphotericin B (*AmBisome*) does not increase nephrotoxicity or hepatotoxicity when given to infants taking ciclosporin. Ciclosporin blood concentrations might be increased or decreased by amphotericin B.

It has been suggested that if amphotericin must be given, withholding ciclosporin until the serum concentration is less than about 150 nanograms/mL might be a means of decreasing renal toxicity without losing the immunosuppressive effect. The reports supporting a lack of significant nephrotoxicity all used liposomal amphotericin B, which would seem to suggest that, in patients taking ciclosporin, these formulations are advisable. Monitor both ciclosporin concentration and renal function carefully on concurrent use.

Amphotericin B + Corticosteroids

Amphotericin B and corticosteroids can cause potassium loss and salt and water retention, which can have adverse effects on cardiac function.

Monitor electrolytes (especially potassium, which should be closely monitored in any patient taking amphotericin B) and fluid balance if amphotericin B is given with corticosteroids. The elderly would seem to be particularly at risk. Note that the renal toxicity of amphotericin B might be associated with sodium depletion. Note that one UK manufacturer of a non-lipid formulation of amphotericin B advises that corticosteroids should not be used concurrently unless they are necessary to control drug reactions.

Amphotericin B + Digoxin

Amphotericin B causes potassium loss which could lead to the development of digitalis toxicity.

Potassium levels should be monitored when amphotericin B is given, but extra care is needed in those taking digoxin. Supplement potassium or prevent its loss as appropriate.

Amphotericin B + Diuretics

Amphotericin B can cause hypokalaemia. Loop diuretics or thiazide and related diuretics increase the risk of hypokalaemia when given with amphotericin.

Potassium should be monitored closely on concurrent use, with levels adjusted accordingly.

Amphotericin B + Flucytosine

For some fungal infections the combination of flucytosine with amphotericin B can be more effective than flucytosine alone, but increased flucytosine toxicity might also occur.

> For some systemic fungal infections concurrent use is specifically recommended. Nevertheless, flucytosine concentrations and renal function should be very closely monitored when the drugs are given.

Amphotericin B + Ganciclovir

Ganciclovir or valganciclovir toxicity might be enhanced when they are given with, immediately before, or after, other drugs that inhibit the replication of rapidly dividing cells (e.g. bone marrow, gastrointestinal mucosa), or are nephrotoxic, such as amphotericin B.

> The UK and US manufacturers of ganciclovir advise that concurrent use should only be undertaken if the benefits outweigh the risks. Monitor renal function and toxicity on concurrent use. Similar precautions would seem prudent with valganciclovir.

Amphotericin B + NRTIs

Cidofovir or tenofovir alone can cause renal failure and this might be additive with other drugs that are nephrotoxic: the UK and US manufacturers name amphotericin B.

> Concurrent use of cidofovir and amphotericin B is contraindicated: the UK and US manufacturers advise stopping potentially nephrotoxic drugs at least 7 days before starting cidofovir. The concurrent use of tenofovir with amphotericin B should also be avoided. If this is not possible, monitoring of renal function should be increased: the UK and US manufacturers of tenofovir suggest at least weekly monitoring on concurrent use.

Amphotericin B + Pentamidine

There is evidence that acute renal failure and electrolyte disturbances (e.g. hypomagnesaemia) might develop in patients given amphotericin B if they are also given parenteral pentamidine: both drugs are known to be nephrotoxic. See also drugs that prolong the QT interval, page 352.

> Close monitoring of renal function and electrolytes should be routine when either drug is used and it is essential that this recommendation is adhered to if both drugs are given: daily monitoring is recommended with parenteral pentamidine. It might be prudent to use liposomal amphotericin B rather than conventional amphotericin B to reduce the risk of renal impairment. No interaction seems to occur when pentamidine is given by inhalation, probably because the serum concentrations achieved are low.

A

Amphotericin B + **Proton pump inhibitors**

Proton pump inhibitors can cause hypomagnesaemia, which might be additive with the magnesium-lowering effects of amphotericin B.

> Hypomagnesaemia can develop after more than one year of concurrent use, so consider monitoring magnesium concentrations before and annually during proton pump inhibitor use, or in response to symptoms of hypomagnesaemia (e.g. muscle twitching or cramps, tremors, vomiting, tiredness, or loss of appetite). In those patients who develop hypomagnesaemia, oral and parenteral magnesium supplements might not be as effective as anticipated. Stopping the proton pump inhibitor (where possible) might be necessary.

Amphotericin B + **Salbutamol (Albuterol) and related bronchodilators**

Beta$_2$ agonists, such as salbutamol and terbutaline, can cause hypokalaemia. This can be increased by other potassium-depleting drugs such as amphotericin B. In severe cases the risk of serious cardiac arrhythmias could be increased.

> The CSM in the UK advises monitoring potassium in severe asthma, because of the probability of multiple potassium-depleting drugs being used, and because some conditions predispose these patients to hypokalaemia (e.g. hypoxia). Consider monitoring based on the severity of the patient's condition, and the number of potassium-depleting drugs used.

Amphotericin B + **Tacrolimus**

Both amphotericin B and tacrolimus may cause renal failure and this may be additive on concurrent use: cases of nephrotoxicity have been reported.

> Renal function should be monitored when either drug is used alone, but it may be prudent to increase the frequency of this monitoring if both drugs are given.

Amphotericin B + **Vancomycin**

The risk of nephrotoxicity with vancomycin may possibly be increased if it is given with other drugs with similar nephrotoxic effects, such as amphotericin B.

> There seems to be no direct evidence to support the existence of an interaction, and some evidence suggesting that no interaction occurs. Even so, the general warning issued by the manufacturers to monitor carefully is a reasonable precaution, given the known adverse effects of these drugs.

Anastrozole

Anastrozole + **HRT** ✕

HRT would be expected to diminish the effects of anastrozole.

> Oestrogen-containing HRT is generally considered contraindicated in patients

with current or a history of breast cancer: concurrent use is contraindicated by the manufacturers of anastrozole. If it is essential, use the lowest HRT dose for the shortest duration: the patient should be fully aware of the potential risks.

Anastrozole + Tibolone

Tibolone appears to increase the risk of recurrent breast cancer in women taking an aromatase inhibitor (such as anastrozole).

Concurrent use is not recommended.

Angiotensin II receptor antagonists

Most angiotensin II receptor antagonist interactions are pharmacodynamic, that is, interactions that result in an alteration in drug effects rather than drug disposition, so in most cases interactions of individual drugs will be applicable to the group as a whole.

Angiotensin II receptor antagonists + Antidiabetics

No clinically relevant pharmacokinetic interactions occur between glibenclamide (glyburide) and candesartan, telmisartan or valsartan, or between tolbutamide and irbesartan. Losartan and possibly eprosartan may reduce awareness of hypoglycaemic symptoms.

The symptoms of hypoglycaemia may be reduced by losartan and possibly other angiotensin II receptor antagonists. Further study is needed to establish this interaction, but note that this is similar to the effect of ACE inhibitors, page 2.

Angiotensin II receptor antagonists + Aspirin

Low-dose aspirin does not appear to affect the antihypertensive efficacy of losartan and would therefore not be expected to alter the effects of other angiotensin II receptor antagonists. High-dose aspirin does not appear to have been studied.

No action needed if low-dose aspirin is used. Suspect an interaction with high-dose aspirin if the angiotensin II receptor antagonist seems less effective or blood pressure control is erratic. Consider an alternative analgesic, but note that NSAIDs may also affect blood pressure control.

Angiotensin II receptor antagonists + Azoles

Fluconazole decreases the metabolism of irbesartan and reduces the conversion of losartan to its active metabolite, although no significant changes in the hypotensive effect of losartan were noted.

No clinically significant interaction appears to occur between the angiotensin II receptor antagonists and the azoles; however, bear the pharmacokinetic interaction between losartan and fluconazole in mind in case of any unexplained reduction in the antihypertensive effects of losartan.

Angiotensin II receptor antagonists + Ciclosporin (Cyclosporine) ⚠

Studies have found no significant changes in renal function in patients taking ciclosporin with candesartan, losartan, and valsartan. There is a possible increased risk of hyperkalaemia if angiotensin II receptor antagonists are given with ciclosporin, as both drugs might raise potassium concentrations.

> Although renal failure has not been reported on concurrent use, note that cases have occurred with ACE inhibitors, page 3. Monitor potassium concentrations more closely in the initial weeks of concurrent use, bearing in mind that an increase in potassium concentrations might be due to worsening renal function as well as the use of these drugs.

Angiotensin II receptor antagonists + Contraceptives ❓

Drospirenone, which is given as the progestogen component of oral combined hormonal contraceptives, might increase the risk of hyperkalaemia when given with other drugs that can cause hyperkalaemia such as angiotensin II receptor antagonists. Oral combined hormonal contraceptives are associated with increased blood pressure and might antagonise the efficacy of antihypertensive drugs, see Antihypertensives + Contraceptives, page 98.

> The risk of hyperkalaemia appears to be low, especially if renal function is normal. In the US, it is recommended that consideration be given to monitoring potassium concentrations during the first cycle in women [with normal renal function] who regularly take an angiotensin II receptor antagonist, whereas the UK manufacturer recommends that the potassium concentration is measured during the first cycle or month of treatment in women with mild or moderate renal impairment only. For women with severe renal impairment, the UK manufacturer contraindicates the use of drospirenone-containing contraceptives, whereas, in the US, its use in renal impairment [to any degree] is contraindicated. In patients at higher risk of developing hyperkalaemia (e.g. in renal impairment) it is generally recommended that potassium concentrations are measured during the first cycle of treatment with drospirenone. .

Angiotensin II receptor antagonists + Co-trimoxazole ⚠

In elderly patients taking an angiotensin II receptor antagonist, the use of co-trimoxazole appears to increase the risk of hospitalisation for hyperkalaemia.

> Trimethoprim or angiotensin II receptor antagonists alone can cause hyperkalaemia, particularly with other factors such as renal impairment. Note that co-trimoxazole is a combination preparation containing trimethoprim, and might therefore interact similarly. Monitor plasma potassium concentrations if this combination is used in those with renal impairment. It has been suggested that trimethoprim should probably be avoided in elderly patients, with or without chronic renal impairment, taking angiotensin II receptor antagonists.

Angiotensin II receptor antagonists + **Digoxin**

Telmisartan may increase digoxin trough and peak levels by 13% and 50%, respectively.

> The small increase in the trough levels suggests that the dose of digoxin need not automatically be reduced when telmisartan is started, but consideration should be given to monitoring for digoxin adverse effects such as bradycardia, taking digoxin levels if necessary. Candesartan, eprosartan, irbesartan, losartan, olmesartan, and valsartan appear not to affect digoxin levels.

Angiotensin II receptor antagonists + **Diuretics**

Loop diuretics

Symptomatic hypotension may occur if an angiotensin II receptor antagonist is started in patients taking high-dose diuretics. Potassium levels may be either increased, decreased or not affected.

> Concurrent use is generally well tolerated and may be clinically beneficial. Monitor blood pressure and potassium levels initially. In patients with heart failure or those who are volume or sodium depleted, it has been recommended that the dose of diuretic or angiotensin II receptor antagonist be reduced to begin with, to avoid hypotension.

Potassium-sparing diuretics

There is an increased risk of hyperkalaemia if angiotensin II receptor antagonists are given with potassium-sparing diuretics (such as amiloride, triamterene or the aldosterone antagonists eplerenone, spironolactone), particularly if other risk factors (such as advanced age, dose of spironolactone greater than 25 mg, reduced renal function and type II diabetes) are also present.

> The concurrent use of amiloride or triamterene and an angiotensin II receptor antagonist is not usually recommended and should be avoided in patients with moderate or severe renal impairment, whereas the concurrent use of an angiotensin II receptor antagonists with an aldosterone antagonist such as spironolactone may be useful in heart failure. If any of these potassium-sparing diuretics is given with an angiotensin II receptor antagonist increased monitoring of potassium levels is required.

Thiazide diuretics

Symptomatic hypotension may occur if an angiotensin II receptor antagonist is started in a patient taking high-dose diuretics. Potassium levels may be either increased, decreased or not affected by the concurrent use of these drugs. No clinically relevant pharmacokinetic interactions appear to occur between candesartan, eprosartan, irbesartan, losartan, olmesartan, telmisartan or valsartan, and hydrochlorothiazide, although the bioavailability of hydrochlorothiazide may be modestly reduced.

> Concurrent use is generally well tolerated and may be clinically beneficial. Monitor blood pressure and potassium levels initially. In patients with heart failure or those who are volume or sodium depleted, it has been recommended that the dose of diuretic or angiotensin II receptor antagonist be reduced to avoid hypotension.

A

Angiotensin II receptor antagonists + Epoetin

Epoetin can cause hypertension and thereby reduce the effects of angiotensin II receptor antagonists. An additive hyperkalaemic effect is theoretically possible. In one study, patients taking losartan needed higher epoetin doses to achieve similar haemoglobin concentrations to those in patients not taking losartan.

Blood pressure and electrolytes, particularly potassium, should be routinely monitored in patients given epoetin. If blood pressure increases cannot be controlled, or potassium concentrations increase, consider temporarily withholding the epoetin. Note that the UK and US manufacturers contraindicate epoetin in uncontrolled hypertension. The clinical relevance of the effect of losartan on epoetin efficacy is unclear; however, as the epoetin dose is titrated to effect, no immediate intervention is necessary.

Angiotensin II receptor antagonists + Food

Food decreases eprosartan levels and slightly reduces the exposure to valsartan. Food appears to have a negligible or no effect on the bioavailability of candesartan, irbesartan, losartan, olmesartan, or telmisartan.

None of these changes is likely to be clinically important. The UK manufacturer recommends that eprosartan is given with food, but the US manufacturer suggests that eprosartan can be taken with or without food.

Angiotensin II receptor antagonists + Heparin

An extensive review of the literature found that heparin (both unfractionated and low-molecular-weight heparins) and heparinoids inhibit the secretion of aldosterone, which can cause hyperkalaemia. This may be additive with the hyperkalaemic effects of angiotensin II receptor antagonists.

The CSM in the UK suggests that potassium should be measured in all patients with risk factors (renal impairment, diabetes mellitus, pre-existing acidosis and those taking potassium-sparing drugs) before starting heparin, and monitored regularly thereafter (at least every 4 days has been suggested).

Angiotensin II receptor antagonists + HRT

Drospirenone, which is given as the progestogen component in some HRT formulations, might increase the risk of hyperkalaemia when given with other drugs that can cause hyperkalaemia such as the angiotensin II receptor antagonists. The UK manufacturer of drospirenone-containing HRT notes that the increase in potassium levels may be more pronounced in diabetic women.

The risk of hyperkalaemia appears to be low, especially if renal function is normal. In the US, it is recommended that consideration be given to monitoring potassium levels during the first cycle in women [with normal renal function] who regularly take an angiotensin II receptor antagonist, whereas the UK manufacturer recommends that the potassium level is measured during the first cycle or month of treatment only in women with mild or moderate renal impairment. In patients at higher risk of developing hyperkalaemia (e.g. in renal impairment) it is generally recommended that potassium levels are measured during the first cycle of treatment with drospirenone.

Angiotensin II receptor antagonists + Lithium

Case reports describe lithium toxicity in patients given candesartan, losartan, valsartan and possibly irbesartan. Other angiotensin II receptor antagonists would be expected to interact similarly. The risk of lithium toxicity would be expected to increase when risk factors such as advanced age, renal impairment, heart failure and volume depletion are also present.

Even though the interaction appears rare, patients should have their lithium levels monitored to avoid a potentially severe adverse interaction. The development of the interaction may be delayed (up to 7 weeks seen) so that weekly monitoring of lithium levels for several weeks has been advised. Patients taking lithium should be aware of the symptoms of lithium toxicity, page 468 and told to immediately report them should they occur. This should be reinforced when they are given angiotensin II receptor antagonists. Note that some manufacturers do not recommend concurrent use.

Angiotensin II receptor antagonists + Low-molecular-weight heparins

An extensive review of the literature found that heparin (both unfractionated and low-molecular-weight heparins) and heparinoids inhibit the secretion of aldosterone, which can cause hyperkalaemia. This may be additive with the hyperkalaemic effects of angiotensin II receptor antagonists.

The CSM in the UK suggests that potassium should be measured in all patients with risk factors (renal impairment, diabetes mellitus, pre-existing acidosis and those taking potassium-sparing drugs) before starting a low-molecular-weight heparin and monitored regularly thereafter (at least every 4 days has been suggested).

Angiotensin II receptor antagonists + Mycophenolate

Telmisartan appears to decrease mycophenolic acid exposure.

Consider periodic monitoring of mycophenolic acid concentrations and consider an interaction if mycophenolic exposure declines.

Angiotensin II receptor antagonists + NSAIDs ❓

Indometacin may attenuate the antihypertensive effect of losartan, valsartan, or other angiotensin II receptor antagonists, although only some patients are affected. Other NSAIDs may interact similarly. No clinically relevant pharmacokinetic interactions occur between telmisartan and ibuprofen or between valsartan and indometacin. The combination of an NSAID and angiotensin II receptor antagonist can increase the risk of renal impairment and hyperkalaemia.

Patients taking angiotensin II receptor antagonists who require indometacin and probably other NSAIDs should be monitored for alterations in blood pressure control. Poor renal perfusion may increase the risk of renal failure if angiotensin II receptor antagonists are given with NSAIDs and so regular hydration of the patient and monitoring of renal function is recommended.

Angiotensin II receptor antagonists + Potassium

There is an increased risk of hyperkalaemia if angiotensin II receptor antagonists are given with potassium supplements or potassium-containing salt substitutes, particularly in those patients where other risk factors (such as advanced age, reduced renal function, and type II diabetes) are present.

If concurrent use is necessary, monitor potassium levels, adjusting supplementation as necessary.

Angiotensin II receptor antagonists + Rifampicin (Rifampin)

Rifampicin reduces the levels of the active metabolite of losartan and therefore diminishes its blood pressure-lowering effects. In theory, irbesartan and possibly candesartan may also be affected.

This interaction is by no means established, but monitor the effects of concurrent use on blood pressure. Consider raising the losartan dose or using an alternative to losartan if problems occur.

Angiotensin II receptor antagonists + Tacrolimus

Candesartan and losartan do not affect the pharmacokinetics of tacrolimus. Concurrent use with angiotensin II receptor antagonists may increase the risk of developing hyperkalaemia and/or nephrotoxicity in those taking tacrolimus.

Consider the possible contribution of angiotensin II receptor antagonists should hyperkalaemia and/or nephrotoxicity occur.

Angiotensin II receptor antagonists + Trimethoprim

In elderly patients taking an angiotensin II receptor antagonist, the use of co-trimoxazole appears to increase the risk of hospitalisation for hyperkalaemia.

Trimethoprim or angiotensin II receptor antagonists alone can cause hyperkalaemia, particularly with other factors such as renal impairment. Monitor plasma potassium concentrations if this combination is used in those with renal impairment. It has been suggested that trimethoprim should probably be avoided in elderly patients, with or without chronic renal impairment, taking angiotensin II receptor antagonists.

Antacids

Antacids + Antihistamines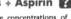

An aluminium/magnesium hydroxide-containing antacid reduced the AUC of fexofenadine by about 40% in one study.

Although the clinical significance of this effect has not been assessed it is recommended that administration is separated by 2 hours.

Antacids + Antipsychotics

Antacids containing aluminium/magnesium hydroxide or magnesium trisilicate can reduce the urinary excretion of chlorpromazine by up to 45%. Similarly, an aluminium/magnesium hydroxide antacid reduced the absorption of sulpiride. Anecdotal evidence suggests a possible interaction between haloperidol and aluminium hydroxide-containing antacids. *In vitro* studies suggest that this interaction may possibly also occur with other antacids and phenothiazines.

The clinical importance of these interactions are not established, but it would seem reasonable to separating the doses of chlorpromazine or sulpiride and aluminium/magnesium hydroxide antacids by 2 to 3 hours to minimise any interaction. Similarly, consider separating the doses if an interaction between haloperidol and antacids is suspected.

Antacids + Aspirin

The salicylate concentrations of patients taking large doses of aspirin or other salicylates as anti-inflammatory drugs can be reduced to subtherapeutic levels by aluminium/magnesium hydroxide or sodium bicarbonate antacids.

Care should be taken to monitor salicylate levels if any antacid is started or stopped in patients where the control of salicylate levels is critical. Probably of little importance with small or one-off doses of aspirin. Note that antacids may also increase the rate of absorption of aspirin given as enteric-coated tablets.

Antacids + Azoles

The absorption of ketoconazole and itraconazole capsules is moderately to markedly reduced by antacids.

Advise patients to take antacids not less than 2 to 3 hours before or after ketoconazole and at least one hour before or 2 hours after itraconazole capsules. Monitor the effects to confirm that these azoles are effective. The absorption of fluconazole, itraconazole solution and posaconazole does not appear to be affected by antacids to a clinically relevant extent, so these azoles may be suitable alternatives. However, the UK manufacturer of posaconazole still considers that its absorption might be affected by drugs that affect gastric acidity, including antacids.

Antacids + **Bisphosphonates**

The oral absorption of bisphosphonates is significantly reduced by aluminium/magnesium hydroxide and other antacids containing metallic tri- and divalent ions.

Bisphosphonates should be prevented from coming into contact with antacids (containing aluminium, bismuth, calcium, magnesium). Recommendations on the timing of administration of bisphosphonates in relation to food and other drugs varies. Alendronate should be taken (after an overnight fast) at least 30 minutes before antacids, clodronate should probably be taken at least 1 hour before or after antacids, ibandronate should be taken (after at least a 6 hour fast) at least 30 minutes to 1 hour before antacids, risedronate should be taken at least 30 minutes before the first dose of antacid in the morning and at least 2 hours from any further doses of antacids during the rest of the day, and etidronate and tiludronate should be taken at least 2 hours apart from antacids.

Antacids + **Cephalosporins**

Cefpodoxime

Aluminium/magnesium hydroxide has been shown to reduce the bioavailability of cefpodoxime proxetil by about 40%. Sodium bicarbonate and aluminium hydroxide alone seem to have similar effects.

It has been recommended that cefpodoxime is given at least 2 hours apart from antacids.

Other cephalosporins

Aluminium/magnesium hydroxide reduced the AUC of a modified-release preparation of cefaclor by 18%, but this reduction is small and considered unlikely to be clinically important.

No action needed.

Antacids + **Chloroquine**

In a small study magnesium trisilicate reduced the exposure to chloroquine by about 20%. Related *in vitro* studies found that the absorption of chloroquine was also decreased by magnesium trisilicate, calcium carbonate and gerdiga. Gerdiga is a clay-based antacid containing hydrated silicates, and various carbonates and bicarbonates. Hydroxychloroquine is predicted to interact like chloroquine.

The clinical significance of this reduction is unclear, but one way to minimise any possible effect on chloroquine absorption is to separate the doses from the antacids by at least 2 to 3 hours. One UK manufacturer recommends that the chloroquine dose should be separated from antacids by at least 4 hours. The UK manufacturer of hydroxychloroquine recommends that it is given 4 hours before or after antacids.

Antacids + **Corticosteroids**

The absorption of prednisone can be reduced by up to 40% by large (60 mL) doses of aluminium/magnesium hydroxide antacids; small doses (20 or 30 mL) of antacid do not appear to interact. Prednisolone probably behaves similarly. Dexamethasone absorption is reduced by about 75% by magnesium trisilicate.

> Some manufacturers of dexamethasone suggest that the doses of antacid should be separated as far as possible from the dexamethasone. In other similar antacid interactions 2 to 3 hours is usually sufficient. The manufacturers of deflazacort also issue a similar warning. It would seem prudent to follow this advice for large doses of antacid and any corticosteroid. Concurrent use should be monitored to confirm that the therapeutic response is adequate.

Antacids + **Digoxin**

Antacids

Although some studies suggest that antacids can reduce the bioavailability of digoxin, there is other evidence suggesting that no clinically relevant interaction occurs.

> A clinically relevant interaction seems unlikely, although it may be worth bearing in mind if, on rare occasions, a patient seems to experience an interaction. In this situation, consider separating the dosing by 2 to 3 hours, as this minimises other absorption interactions with antacids.

Calcium 🔺

The effects of digitalis glycosides might be increased by rises in blood calcium levels, and in two cases the concurrent use of intravenous calcium and digoxin resulted in fatal arrhythmias. This seems to be the only direct clinical evidence of a serious adverse interaction, although there is plenty of less direct evidence that an interaction is possible.

> Intravenous calcium should be avoided in patients taking digoxin. If that is not possible, it has been suggested that it should be given slowly or only in small amounts in order to avoid transient high serum calcium levels.

Antacids + **Dipyridamole** ❓

The effective disintegration, dissolution and eventual absorption of dipyridamole in tablet or suspension form depends upon having a low pH in the stomach. Drugs that raise the gastric pH (such as the antacids) are expected to reduce the bioavailability of immediate-release formulations of dipyridamole.

> The clinical significance of this possible interaction is unknown. Consider separating the dosing of immediate-release dipyridamole tablets or suspension and antacids by 2 to 3 hours, as this minimises other absorption interactions with antacids. Note that modified-release preparations of dipyridamole (that are buffered) do not appear to be affected, and might therefore be a suitable alternative.

Antacids + **Diuretics** 🔺

Hypercalcaemia and possibly metabolic alkalosis can develop in patients given large amounts of calcium (with or without high doses of vitamin D) if they are also given thiazide diuretics, which can reduce the urinary excretion of calcium.

> Consider monitoring calcium levels in those given a thiazide and a calcium supplement or large amounts of calcium antacids regularly. Patients taking thiazides should be warned about the ingestion of very large amounts of calcium carbonate (readily available without prescription). This interaction is unlikely to be of importance in patients taking occasional calcium e.g. in antacids.

Antacids + Elvitegravir

Aluminium and magnesium-containing antacids appear to reduce elvitegravir exposure

> Separate administration by at least 2 hours.

Antacids + Enteral feeds

Aluminium-containing antacids can interact with high-protein liquid enteral feeds (in enteral or nasogastric tubes) within the oesophagus to produce an obstructive plug (a bezoar).

> It has been suggested that if an antacid is needed, it should be given some time after the nutrients, and the tube should be vigorously flushed beforehand.

Antacids + Ethambutol

Both aluminium hydroxide and aluminium/magnesium hydroxide can cause a small reduction in the absorption of ethambutol (e.g. AUC decreased by 10%) in some patients.

> The reduction in absorption is generally small and variable, and it seems doubtful if it will have a significant effect on the treatment of tuberculosis. However, the US manufacturer suggests that aluminium hydroxide-containing antacids should not be taken until 4 hours after a dose of ethambutol.

Antacids + Fibrates

Antacids (aluminium hydroxide, aluminium magnesium silica hydrate) slightly to moderately reduce gemfibrozil exposure.

> It has been suggested that gemfibrozil should be given 1 to 2 hours before antacids.

Antacids + Gabapentin

An aluminium/magnesium hydroxide antacid given with or 2 hours after gabapentin reduced its bioavailability by about 20%. When the antacid was given 2 hours before gabapentin, the bioavailability was reduced by about 10%.

> These small changes are unlikely to be of clinical importance. However, the

manufacturer recommends that gabapentin is taken about 2 hours after aluminium/magnesium-containing antacids.

Antacids + HIV-protease inhibitors

Drugs that increase gastric pH (such as the H_2-receptor antagonists) reduce atazanavir exposure: and antacids would be expected to interact similarly. Tipranavir exposure is slightly decreased by antacids (containing aluminium/magnesium hydroxide).

The UK and US manufacturers of atazanavir recommend that it should be given 2 hours before, or one hour after, buffered medicinal products. This would include didanosine-buffered tablets and antacids. The UK manufacturer of tipranavir recommends that it should not be given within 2 hours of antacids.

Antacids + Iron

Calcium

Calcium carbonate and calcium acetate (doses from 500 mg to 3 g) may cause a modest reduction in the absorption of iron from ferrous sulfate. Smaller doses of calcium (e.g. in multivitamin supplements) appear unlikely to have a clinically significant effect. All iron compounds would be expected to be similarly affected.

Monitor the response to iron in patients taking large doses of calcium. It may be prudent to separate the administration of iron preparations and calcium as much as possible to avoid admixture in the gut. Bear it in mind in case of a reduced response to iron.

Iron

The absorption of iron and the expected haematological response can be reduced by the concurrent use of antacids (sodium bicarbonate, calcium carbonate, aluminium/magnesium hydroxide, magnesium trisilicate). However, information is limited and difficult to assess.

As a general precaution, separate the administration of iron compounds and antacids as much as possible to avoid admixture in the gut. Note that separating the dosing by 2 to 3 hours minimises other absorption interactions with antacids.

Antacids + Isoniazid

The absorption of isoniazid is modestly reduced by aluminium hydroxide (about 25%), less so by magaldrate, and not affected by aluminium/magnesium hydroxide tablets or didanosine chewable tablets (formulated with an antacid buffer).

The clinical importance of the modest reductions in isoniazid levels is uncertain, but it is likely to be small.

Antacids + Levodopa

Antacids do not appear to interact significantly with immediate-release levodopa, but

A

they may reduce the bioavailability of modified-release preparations of levodopa (e.g. *Madopar CR*).

Concurrent use need not be avoided with standard preparations. With modified-release preparations it would seem advisable to separate administration (2 to 3 hours is usually enough in other similar situations). The outcome should be monitored.

Antacids + **Levothyroxine**

A few reports describe reduced levothyroxine effects in patients given aluminium/magnesium-containing antacids. The efficacy of levothyroxine can also be reduced by the concurrent use of calcium carbonate, whereas limited evidence suggests that calcium acetate might not interact.

The general importance of the interaction with aluminium/magnesium-containing antacids is not known. If an interaction is suspected, monitor thyroid function and adjust the levothyroxine dose accordingly in any patient given antacids. Separating dosing might minimise this interaction. With calcium carbonate, the mean reduction in the absorption of levothyroxine is quite small, but some individuals can experience a clinically important effect. The cautious approach would be to advise all patients to separate the doses by at least 4 hours.

Antacids + **Lithium**

The ingestion of marked amounts of sodium can prevent the establishment or maintenance of adequate lithium levels. Conversely, dietary salt restriction can cause lithium levels to rise to toxic concentrations if the lithium dose is not reduced appropriately.

Warn patients not to take non-prescription antacids or urinary alkalinisers without first seeking informed advice. Sodium bicarbonate comes in various guises and disguises e.g. *Alka-Seltzer* (55.8%), *Andrews Salts* (22.6%), *Eno* (46.4%), *Jaap's Health Salts* (21.3%), or *Peptac* (28.8%). Substantial amounts of sodium also occur in some urinary alkalinising agents (e.g. *Citralka*, *Citravescent*). An antacid containing aluminium/magnesium hydroxide with simeticone has been found to have no effect on the bioavailability of lithium carbonate, and so antacids of this type may be suitable alternatives.

Antacids + **Macrolides**

Aluminium/magnesium hydroxide antacids may reduce the peak levels of azithromycin but the overall absorption was unchanged.

It is suggested that azithromycin should not be given at the same time as antacids, but should be taken at least 1 hour before or 2 hours after.

Antacids + **Mexiletine** ✕

Large changes in urinary pH caused by the concurrent use of alkalinising drugs such as sodium bicarbonate can, in some patients, have a marked effect on mexiletine concentrations.

The effect does not appear to be predictable. Mexiletine is no longer widely

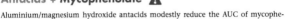
available, but the UK manufacturer previously recommended that concurrent use should be avoided.

Antacids + Mycophenolate ⚠

Aluminium/magnesium hydroxide antacids modestly reduce the AUC of mycophenolate.

The US manufacturer says that aluminium/magnesium antacids can be used in patients taking mycophenolate, but that they should not be given simultaneously. With many other antacid interactions, a 2 to 3 hour separation is usually sufficient to avoid an interaction. One UK manufacturer advises against long-term use of antacids with mycophenolate. It would seem prudent to check that the immunosuppressant effects of mycophenolate remain adequate.

Antacids + NNRTIs ⚠

When delavirdine was given 10 minutes after an antacid (type and dose not stated) delavirdine exposure was moderately decreased. Rilpivirine is predicted to be similarly affected.

The manufacturer of delavirdine recommends separating administration by at least one hour. The UK and US manufacturers of rilpivirine advise that aluminium-, magnesium-, or calcium-containing antacids are taken at least 2 hours before, or 4 hours, after rilpivirine.

Antacids + NSAIDs

Diflunisal ✓

Antacids containing aluminium with or without magnesium can reduce the absorption of diflunisal by up to 40%, but no important interaction occurs if food is taken at the same time. Magnesium hydroxide can increase the rate of diflunisal absorption, which may improve the onset of analgesia.

If diflunisal is taken with or after food as advised, it appears that this interaction should have little clinical relevance.

Other NSAIDs ✓

Studies have shown that antacids have no clinically significant effect on the pharmacokinetics of azapropazone, celecoxib, dexketoprofen, diclofenac, etodolac, etoricoxib, ibuprofen, indometacin, flurbiprofen, ketoprofen, ketorolac, lornoxicam, mefenamic acid, meloxicam, metamizole, nabumetone, piroxicam, sulindac, tenoxicam, tolfenamic acid, or tolmetin. The rate of absorption of some of these NSAIDs is moderately affected by antacids, which may affect the onset of analgesia. However, if NSAIDs are taken after food, as recommended, these effects are unlikely to be clinically significant.

No action needed.

A

Antacids + Penicillamine ⚠

The absorption of penicillamine can be reduced by 30 to 40% by antacids containing aluminium/magnesium hydroxide.

For maximal absorption separate administration. A separation of 2 to 3 hours is usually sufficient with other similar interactions. Note that sodium bicarbonate does not appear to interact to a clinically significant extent.

Antacids + Phenytoin ❓

Some, but not all studies have shown that antacids (containing aluminium, calcium or magnesium) do not usually interact to a clinically relevant extent with phenytoin. However, in some instances antacids have reduced phenytoin serum levels and this may have been responsible for loss of seizure control in some patients.

A clinically relevant interaction does not appear to occur in most patients. However, if there is any sign that phenytoin levels are being reduced, separating the doses by 2 to 3 hours may minimise the effects. In this situation monitor concurrent use to ensure phenytoin remains effective.

Antacids + Proguanil ⚠

The bioavailability of proguanil is moderately reduced by magnesium trisilicate. Other antacids, such as those containing aluminium, might interact similarly.

The clinical significance of this reduction is unclear, but one way to minimise any possible effect is to separate the doses by at least 2 to 3 hours.

Antacids + Proton pump inhibitors ⚠

Aluminium/magnesium-containing antacids may cause a slight 13% reduction in the bioavailability of lansoprazole, but no interaction was seen when the lansoprazole was given one hour after the antacid.

This interaction is not expected to be clinically significant. However the UK manufacturers recommend separating administration by one hour, although this seems overly cautious.

Antacids + Quinidine ⚠

Large rises in urinary pH due to the concurrent use of some antacids (such as sodium bicarbonate) can cause the retention of quinidine, which could lead to toxicity, but there seems to be only one case on record of an adverse interaction (with aluminium/magnesium hydroxide).

It is difficult to predict which antacids, if any, are likely to interact (although note that aluminium hydroxide alone does not appear to interact). Monitor the effects if drugs that can markedly change urinary pH are started or stopped. Adjust the quinidine dose as necessary.

Antacids + **Quinolones**

The levels of many of the quinolones can be reduced by aluminium/magnesium antacids. Calcium compounds interact to a lesser extent, and bismuth compounds only minimally.

As a very broad rule-of-thumb, the quinolones should be taken at least 2 hours before and not less than 4 to 6 hours after aluminium/magnesium antacids. The only obvious exception is fleroxacin, which appears to interact minimally. The interaction with calcium compounds is variable, and some quinolones may not interact (levofloxacin, lomefloxacin, moxifloxacin or ofloxacin), but in the absence of direct information a 2-hour separation errs on the side of caution. The interaction with bismuth is minimal and no action is likely to be needed. The H_2-receptor antagonists and the proton pump inhibitors do not interact and may therefore be suitable alternatives.

Antacids + **Raltegravir**

Aluminium and magnesium-containing antacids are predicted to reduce raltegravir exposure.

Until more is known, separate administration by at least 2 hours.

Antacids + **Rifampicin (Rifampin)**

The absorption of rifampicin can be reduced up to about one-third by antacids.

If antacids are given it would be prudent to be alert for any evidence that rifampicin is less effective than expected. The US manufacturers advise giving rifampicin one hour before antacids.

Antacids + **Riociguat**

Co-administration of aluminium and magnesium containing antacids reduces riociguat exposure.

The UK manufacturer recommends taking antacids 2 hours before, or 1 hour after riociguat. The US manufacturer however, recommends separating administration by at least 1 hour.

Antacids + **Statins**

Rosuvastatin

The bioavailability of rosuvastatin is moderately reduced by aluminium/magnesium-containing antacids. The effect is reduced if the antacid is given 2 hours after rosuvastatin.

Separate the doses of rosuvastatin and antacids by at least 2 hours.

Other statins

Aluminium/magnesium hydroxide antacids cause a slight reduction in the bioavailability of atorvastatin and pravastatin, but this does not appear to reduce their lipid-lowering efficacy.

No action needed.

Antacids + Strontium

Aluminium/magnesium hydroxide slightly reduces the absorption of strontium ranelate (AUC decreased by 20 to 25%) if given with or 2 hours before strontium, but not when given 2 hours after strontium. Calcium reduces the bioavailability of strontium ranelate by about 60 to 70%.

Antacids should be taken 2 hours after strontium ranelate. However, because it is also recommended that strontium is taken at bedtime, the manufacturers say that if this dosing interval is impractical, concurrent intake is acceptable. For calcium preparations administration should be separated by 2 hours.

Antacids + Tetracyclines

The levels and therefore the therapeutic effectiveness of the tetracyclines can be markedly reduced or even abolished by antacids containing aluminium, bismuth, calcium or magnesium. Other antacids, such as sodium bicarbonate, may also reduce the bioavailability of some tetracyclines. Even intravenous doxycycline levels can be reduced by antacids. Note that interactions with antacids within formulations may also occur, such as didanosine tablets.

As a general rule aluminium, bismuth, calcium or magnesium-containing antacids should not be given at the same time as the tetracyclines. If they must be used, patients should be advised to separate the doses by 2 to 3 hours or more, to prevent their admixture in the gut. This also applies to quinapril formulations containing substantial quantities of magnesium (such as *Accupro*), although the interaction is less pronounced, and buffered didanosine tablets formulated with antacids. H_2-receptor antagonists do not interact, and they may therefore be a suitable alternative.

Antacids + Ursodeoxycholic acid (Ursodiol)

Some antacids (including aluminium-containing antacids) have been shown to adsorb bile acids *in vitro* and some UK and US manufacturers of ursodeoxycholic acid suggest therefore predict that antacids might reduce ursodeoxycholic acid absorption.

Simultaneous concurrent use should be avoided. If concurrent use is necessary, separating administration by at least 2 hours is recommended.

Antacids + Zinc

Calcium (either as the carbonate or the citrate) reduces the AUC of zinc by up to 80%.

The clinical importance of this interaction is unknown, but it would seem prudent to separate the administration of zinc and calcium. Note that separating the doses by 2 to 3 hours minimises other absorption interactions with antacids.

Antidiabetics

Antidiabetics + **Antidiabetics**

Pioglitazone and Rosiglitazone

Pioglitazone and rosiglitazone can cause fluid retention and peripheral oedema, which can worsen or cause heart failure. There is evidence that the incidence of these effects is higher when pioglitazone or rosiglitazone are combined with insulin, sulfonylureas or saxagliptin. In addition, there might be an increased risk of myocardial ischaemia when rosiglitazone is used with insulin. The incidence of hypoglycaemia might also be increased on concurrent use.

In October 2007 the European Medicines Agency concluded that the combination of rosiglitazone and insulin should only be used in exceptional cases and under close supervision. In the UK and US concurrent use is contraindicated or not advised. If both drugs are given, close monitoring is warranted If oedema occurs in a patient taking a thiazolidinedione it has been recommended that the possible causes be assessed, and that if symptoms and signs suggest congestive heart failure, a dose change and temporary or permanent discontinuance of the thiazolidinedione should be considered. The UK manufacturer advises that when rosiglitazone is used with a sulfonylurea, the dose of rosiglitazone should be increased to 8 mg daily only with caution, assessing the risk of fluid retention. Bear in mind the possibility of an increased risk of peripheral oedema if saxagliptin is added to thiazolidinedione therapy.

Other antidiabetics

The UK and US manufacturers of exenatide state that the concurrent use of exenatide and acarbose, insulin, miglitol, repaglinide, or nateglinide has not been studied and therefore cannot be recommended. However, one UK manufacturer states that exenatide can be used as adjunctive therapy to basal insulin. The UK manufacturer of liraglutide advises against concurrent use with insulin as this combination has not been studied.

If both drugs are given, monitor for adverse effects (such as hypoglycaemia) and diabetic control more closely.

Antidiabetics + **Antihistamines**

The concurrent use of biguanides (e.g. metformin) and ketotifen appears to be well tolerated, but a fall in the number of platelets has been seen in one study in patients taking the combination.

The general importance of this report is uncertain. The manufacturers contra-indicate concurrent use until the effect is explained.

Antidiabetics + **Antimalarials**

Hydroxychloroquine can reduce insulin requirements, which has resulted in hypoglycaemia in diabetics managed with insulin. Hydroxychloroquine has also improved glycaemic control in patients taking glibenclamide (glyburide). Similarly, hypoglycaemia has occurred in a patient taking chloroquine and insulin, and quinine reduces blood glucose concentrations in patients taking gliclazide.

It appears that hydroxychloroquine and chloroquine can cause a modest reduction in blood glucose concentrations, which is additive with antidiabetic treatment. Mefloquine and quinine have also been reported to reduce blood glucose concentrations, although some evidence is complicated by the use of quinine in malaria, as malaria can also cause hypoglycaemia. The interactions are not well established, however bear the possibility of an interaction in mind should any unexpected change in diabetic control occur, and adjust the dose of the antidiabetic drug as necessary.

Antidiabetics + Antipsychotics

Chlorpromazine can increase blood glucose concentrations, particularly in daily doses of 100 mg or more (incidence of hyperglycaemia is about 25%). Smaller chlorpromazine doses of 50 to 70 mg daily do not appear to cause hyperglycaemia. Other classical antipsychotics can also affect diabetic control (haloperidol, zuclopenthixol, and a number of phenothiazines have been implicated) and the atypical antipsychotics, clozapine, olanzapine, and risperidone, are also associated with an increased risk of glucose intolerance. One epidemiological study found evidence of an association between antipsychotic drug use and worsening of metabolic control, and another found an increased risk of hospitalisation for hyperglycaemia, especially in the first month of use of the antipsychotic.

Increases in the dose requirements of the antidiabetic drug should be anticipated during concurrent use. It would seem prudent to increase monitoring of glycaemic control, particularly when starting or stopping any classical or atypical antipsychotic in a patient with diabetes.

Antidiabetics + Aprepitant

Aprepitant reduces the AUC of tolbutamide by about 25%. Fosaprepitant is a prodrug of aprepitant and would be expected to interact similarly.

As the clinical relevance of this reduction in tolbutamide has not been assessed the manufacturer advises caution, but changes of this magnitude are rarely clinically significant.

Antidiabetics + Aspirin

Analgesic doses of aspirin and other salicylates can lower blood glucose levels, but small analgesic doses do not normally have an adverse effect on patients taking antidiabetics. Large doses of salicylates may have a more significant effect.

It may be prudent to increase monitoring of blood glucose levels during the initial use of large doses of aspirin or salicylates, and adjust the antidiabetic dose accordingly. Small antiplatelet doses of aspirin are unlikely to cause a problem.

Antidiabetics + **Azoles**

Fluconazole

Fluconazole normally appears not to affect the diabetic control of most patients taking sulfonylureas, but isolated reports describe hypoglycaemic coma and aggressive behaviour following concurrent use. There is some evidence that the blood-glucose-lowering effects of both glipizide and glibenclamide (glyburide) might be moderately increased by fluconazole. Fluconazole can also cause a moderate increase in the plasma concentration of glimepiride. The plasma concentration of nateglinide is increased by fluconazole, but this does not potentiate the blood-glucose lowering effects of low-dose nateglinide.

> There is no reason to avoid the concurrent use of fluconazole and these sulfonylureas, but warn patients to report any signs of hypoglycaemia. A greater blood-glucose lowering effect might possibly occur with higher doses of nateglinide in clinical practice. Monitor the outcome of concurrent use on blood glucose concentrations and adjust the antidiabetic treatment accordingly.

Itraconazole

Itraconazole causes modest increases in the plasma concentrations of repaglinide and nateglinide, but in one study this did not affect the control of blood glucose concentrations. Ketoconazole, a potent CYP3A4 inhibitor, increases the exposure to saxagliptin. Itraconazole is predicted to interact similarly.

> Consider monitoring blood glucose concentrations on concurrent use. The US manufacturer of saxagliptin recommends that the dose of saxagliptin should be limited to 2.5 mg daily.

Ketoconazole

Ketoconazole increases the blood glucose-lowering effects of tolbutamide in healthy subjects, and modestly increases the exposure to pioglitazone, rosiglitazone and saxagliptin.

> It might be prudent to increase the frequency of blood glucose monitoring if any of these antidiabetics is given with ketoconazole. Adjust the antidiabetic medication accordingly. Note that the US manufacturer recommends that the dose of saxagliptin should be limited to 2.5 mg daily.

Miconazole

Hypoglycaemia has been seen in a few diabetics taking tolbutamide, glibenclamide (glyburide), or gliclazide when they were given oral miconazole. Nateglinide is predicted to be similarly affected.

> Concurrent use of oral miconazole should be monitored and the dose of the sulfonylurea or nateglinide reduced if necessary. Warn patients to report any unexpected changes in blood glucose concentrations. Miconazole oral gel (which may be sufficiently absorbed to potentially have systemic effects) might interact similarly. Note that intravaginal miconazole and miconazole topical creams are probably unlikely to interact, because absorption by these routes is minimal.

Posaconazole

The concurrent use of posaconazole and glipizide did not affect the pharmacokinetics

A

of either drug, but posaconazole slightly enhanced the blood glucose-lowering effects of glipizide in healthy subjects.

> The clinical significance of this interaction is unclear, but bear it in mind in case of an unexpected change in diabetic control. It may be prudent to warn patients to report any unexpected changes in blood glucose concentrations.

Voriconazole

The manufacturers of voriconazole predict that it may increase the plasma concentrations of the sulfonylureas, and a case report describes this effect in a patient given voriconazole and glimepiride.

> Until more is known careful monitoring of blood glucose is advisable during concurrent use.

Antidiabetics + Beta blockers ❓

In diabetics using insulin, the normal increase in blood glucose in response to hypoglycaemia might be impaired by propranolol, but serious and severe hypoglycaemia (sometimes accompanied by an increase in blood pressure) seems rare. Other beta blockers normally interact to a lesser extent or not at all. The blood glucose-lowering effects of sulfonylureas might possibly be reduced by beta blockers. Be aware that in the presence of beta blockers some of the familiar warning signs of hypoglycaemia might not occur.

> Monitor the effects of concurrent use well, avoid the non-selective beta blockers where possible, and check for any evidence that the dose of the antidiabetic needs some adjustment. Warn all patients that some of the normal premonitory signs of a hypoglycaemic attack might not appear, in particular tachycardia and tremor, whereas hunger, irritability and nausea might be unaffected, and sweating can even be increased.

Antidiabetics + Calcium-channel blockers ❓

Diltiazem moderately increases the exposure to saxagliptin. Verapamil would be expected to interact similarly. Calcium-channel blockers are known to have effects on insulin secretion and glucose regulation, but significant disturbances in the control of diabetes appear to be rare.

> Consider monitoring blood glucose concentrations more closely on concurrent use, and reduce the dose of saxagliptin if necessary. No particular precautions normally seem to be necessary with other antidiabetics, but bear the potential for interaction in mind if the control of diabetes seems unusually difficult.

Antidiabetics + Carbamazepine

Linagliptin or Repaglinide ⚠

Carbamazepine is predicted to reduce the exposure to linagliptin and repaglinide.

> Consider giving an alternative to carbamazepine. If concurrent use is necessary,

increase blood glucose concentration monitoring, and adjust the antidiabetic treatment accordingly.

Saxagliptin

Carbamazepine is predicted to reduce saxagliptin, exposure.

The US manufacturer considers that no dose adjustment of saxagliptin is needed as dipeptidylpeptidase-4 inhibitory activity was unaffected. However, as it cannot be ruled out that carbamazepine might reduce the blood-glucose lowering effect of saxagliptin, the UK manufacturer advises caution. Bear this interaction in mind should any reduced saxagliptin effects occur.

Antidiabetics + Chloramphenicol

The blood glucose-lowering effects of tolbutamide and chlorpropamide can be increased by chloramphenicol and acute hypoglycaemia can occur. Other sulfonylureas are often predicted to interact similarly, but there does not seem to be any direct evidence of this.

An increased blood glucose-lowering effect should be expected if both drugs are given but few patients experience a severe effect. Monitor concurrent use carefully and reduce the dose of the sulfonylurea as necessary. No interaction would be expected with topical chloramphenicol because the systemic absorption is likely to be small.

Antidiabetics + Ciclosporin (Cyclosporine)

Some preliminary evidence suggests that glibenclamide (glyburide) can increase serum ciclosporin concentrations. Glipizide approximately doubled ciclosporin concentrations in 2 patients, but one study found no interaction. Ciclosporin increased repaglinide bioavailability in one study. Repaglinide had no effect on ciclosporin concentrations in another study.

The interactions between ciclosporin and glibenclamide or glipizide are unconfirmed, and of uncertain clinical significance. There is insufficient evidence to generally recommend increased monitoring, but be aware of the potential for an interaction with the sulfonylureas if ciclosporin concentrations are unexpectedly increased. Data for an interaction between repaglinide and ciclosporin is inconclusive. The possibility of an increased blood-glucose lowering effect should be borne in mind if ciclosporin is added to established repaglinide therapy, and patients should be advised to report any adverse effects, particularly an increase in the number of hypoglycaemic events. In patients already stable on ciclosporin, start repaglinide at a low dose and titrate upwards as necessary. Note that ciclosporin can cause hyperglycaemia, and therefore interfere with diabetic control. However, the effect is rare, and does not justify an increase in monitoring all patients.

Antidiabetics + Clonidine

Clonidine may possibly suppress the signs and symptoms of hypoglycaemia in diabetics. Marked hyperglycaemia occurred in a child using insulin when clonidine was given. However, the effect of clonidine on carbohydrate metabolism appears to be variable, as other reports have described both increases and decreases in blood glucose levels. Clonidine premedication may decrease or increase the hyperglycaemic response to surgery.

> The general importance of this interaction is unclear. It would seem prudent to warn all patients that some of the normal premonitory signs of hypoglycaemia may not appear. Suspect an interaction if disturbances in the control of diabetes occur in patients given clonidine. Monitor blood glucose levels closely if clonidine is used as a premedication before surgery.

Antidiabetics + Colestyramine and related drugs

Acarbose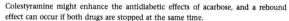

Colestyramine might enhance the antidiabetic effects of acarbose, and a rebound effect can occur if both drugs are stopped at the same time.

> The clinical importance of the effects of colestyramine on acarbose in diabetics is uncertain, but some care seems appropriate. It would seem prudent to increase blood-glucose monitoring if concurrent use is started or stopped and adjust the antidiabetic treatment accordingly.

Chlorpropamide or Tolbutamide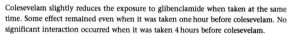

The concurrent use of chlorpropamide (with phenformin) or tolbutamide inhibited the normal hypocholesterolaemic effects of colestipol in 12 diabetic patients.

> Colestipol might not be suitable for lowering blood cholesterol in diabetics taking chlorpropamide or tolbutamide, but more study is needed.

Glibenclamide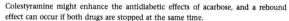

Colesevelam slightly reduces the exposure to glibenclamide when taken at the same time. Some effect remained even when it was taken one hour before colesevelam. No significant interaction occurred when it was taken 4 hours before colesevelam.

> The manufacturers recommend that glibenclamide is taken at least 4 hours before colesevelam.

Glipizide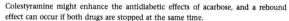

The absorption of glipizide might be reduced by about 30% if it is taken at the same time as colestyramine.

> It has been suggested that glipizide should be taken 1 to 2 hours before colestyramine, but this might only be partially effective because glipizide might undergo some enterohepatic recirculation.

Antidiabetics + Contraceptives

Some women may require small increases or decreases in their dose of antidiabetic while taking hormonal contraceptives, but it is unusual for the control of diabetes to be seriously disturbed.

> Routine monitoring should be adequate to detect any interaction as the effects

seem to be gradual. However, note that occasionally severe disturbances in control do occur. Irrespective of diabetic control, hormonal contraceptives should be used with caution in patients with diabetes because of the increased risk of arterial disease: the lowest-strength combined oral contraceptive preparations (20 micrograms of oestrogen) is advised and this might minimise the adverse effect on diabetic control. The choice of progestogen might also be important, with levonorgestrel appearing to have the most detrimental effect on blood glucose control.

Antidiabetics + **Corticosteroids**

Corticosteroids with glucocorticoid (hyperglycaemic) activity oppose the blood glucose-lowering effects of the antidiabetics. Significant hyperglycaemia has been seen with systemic corticosteroids, and in cases with high-dose inhaled corticosteroids or high-potency topical corticosteroids.

It would seem prudent to increase blood glucose monitoring when a corticosteroid is started and adjust the antidiabetic treatment accordingly. Routine monitoring of local corticosteroids appears over-cautious, but be aware that isolated cases of hyperglycaemia have been reported.

Antidiabetics + **Co-trimoxazole**

Occasionally and unpredictably acute hypoglycaemia has occurred in patients given various sulfonylureas and co-trimoxazole, although pharmacokinetic studies have not established an interaction. Note that co-trimoxazole alone may rarely cause hypoglycaemia. See also trimethoprim, page 92, for its effects on repaglinide and rosiglitazone.

Information is limited and serious adverse effects appear to be rare. Nevertheless, the cautious approach would be to increase blood glucose monitoring in diabetics taking co-trimoxazole and warn the patient that increased blood glucose-lowering effects, sometimes excessive, are a possibility.

Antidiabetics + **Digoxin**

Acarbose

Some but not all studies have found that digoxin plasma levels can be markedly reduced by acarbose.

Just why there is an inconsistency between these reports is not understood but it would clearly be prudent to consider monitoring digoxin levels for any evidence of a reduced effect.

Sitagliptin

Sitagliptin slightly increases digoxin exposure.

The very slight rise in digoxin exposure is unlikely to be clinically relevant, and no digoxin dose adjustment is needed when sitagliptin is started. However, the UK manufacturer recommends that patients at risk of digoxin toxicity should be monitored for this when sitagliptin is used, which is a cautious approach.

Antidiabetics + **Disopyramide**

Disopyramide occasionally and unpredictably causes hypoglycaemia, which may be severe. Isolated reports describe severe hypoglycaemia when disopyramide was given to diabetic patients taking gliclazide, or metformin and/or insulin.

Patients at particular risk of hypoglycaemia are the elderly, the malnourished, and diabetics. Impaired renal function or cardiac function might also be predisposing factors. It has been suggested that blood glucose concentrations should be closely monitored and the disopyramide stopped if problems arise.

Antidiabetics + **Diuretics**

Loop diuretics

The control of diabetes is not usually significantly disturbed by etacrynic acid, furosemide, or torasemide, although there are a few reports showing that etacrynic acid and furosemide can sometimes raise blood glucose levels.

No action needed.

Thiazide diuretics

By raising blood glucose levels, the thiazide and related diuretics can reduce the effects of the antidiabetics and impair the control of diabetes. However, this effect appears to be dose-related, and is less frequent at the low doses now commonly used for hypertension. Hyponatraemia has rarely been reported with chlorpropamide combined with a thiazide and potassium-sparing diuretic.

This interaction is of only moderate practical importance. Guidelines on the treatment of hypertension in diabetes (2009) recommend the use of thiazides. However, if higher doses are used, increased monitoring of diabetic control would seem prudent. The full effects may take many months to develop in some patients.

Antidiabetics + **Endothelin receptor antagonists**

There appears to be an increased risk of liver toxicity if bosentan is used with glibenclamide (glyburide). Glibenclamide (glyburide) modestly reduces the plasma levels of bosentan, and bosentan reduces the plasma levels of glibenclamide (glyburide).

The manufacturers suggest the combination should be avoided.

Antidiabetics + **Fibrates**

Sulfonylureas or Insulin

TA number of reports describe hypoglycaemia and/or an enhancement of the effects of insulin and sulfonylureas in patients given fibrates.

There would seem to be no good reason for avoiding concurrent use, but be aware that the dose of the antidiabetic may need adjustment. Patients should be warned that excessive hypoglycaemia occurs occasionally and unpredictably.

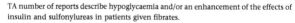

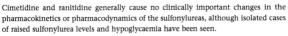

Nateglinide

Only a modest pharmacokinetic interaction occurs between gemfibrozil and nateglinide.

> The manufacturer of nateglinide recommends particular caution, but this seems a very wary approach. Consider increasing the frequency of blood glucose monitoring until treatment is stabilised.

Pioglitazone or Rosiglitazone

Gemfibrozil causes large increases in the AUCs of pioglitazone and rosiglitazone.

> The clinical relevance of this interaction has not been assessed. Until further experience is gained, caution is warranted. Consider an increased frequency of blood glucose monitoring if gemfibrozil is started or stopped, adjusting the pioglitazone or rosiglitazone dose as necessary.

Repaglinide

Gemfibrozil markedly increases the levels and blood glucose-lowering effects of repaglinide and cases of serious hypoglycaemia have been reported.

> On the basis of studies and reports of serious hypoglycaemic episodes with gemfibrozil and repaglinide, the European Medicines Agency contraindicate concurrent use.

Antidiabetics + H₂-receptor antagonists

Metformin

Cimetidine appears to reduce the clearance of metformin, and may have contributed to a case of metformin-associated lactic acidosis.

> The dose of metformin may need to be reduced if cimetidine is used, bearing in mind the possibility of lactic acidosis if levels become too high.

Miglitol ▲

Miglitol decreases the AUC of ranitidine by 60%.

> The clinical significance of this effect is unknown. It may be prudent to monitor for ranitidine efficacy.

Sulfonylureas ?

Cimetidine and ranitidine generally cause no clinically important changes in the pharmacokinetics or pharmacodynamics of the sulfonylureas, although isolated cases of raised sulfonylurea levels and hypoglycaemia have been seen.

> The evidence suggests that most diabetics do not experience any marked changes in their diabetic control if they are given cimetidine or ranitidine. However, consider the possibility of an interaction if any unexplained loss of diabetic control occurs.

Antidiabetics + **Herbal medicines or Dietary supplements**

Glucosamine +/- Chondroitin

In a controlled study glucosamine with chondroitin had no effect on the glycaemic control of patients taking oral antidiabetics, but one report notes that unexpected increases in blood glucose concentrations have occurred.

> It might be prudent to increase monitoring of blood glucose if glucosamine supplements are taken. Also, if glucose control unexpectedly deteriorates, bear in mind the possibility of self-medication with supplements such as glucosamine.

Karela (Momordica charantia)

The blood glucose-lowering effects of antidiabetics can be increased by karela.

> Karela is used to flavour foods such as curries, and also used as a herbal medicine for the treatment of diabetes mellitus. Health professionals should therefore be aware that patients may possibly be using karela as well as more orthodox drugs to control their diabetes. Irregular consumption of karela as part of the diet could possibly contribute to unexplained fluctuations in diabetic control.

St John's wort (Hypericum perforatum)

St John's wort modestly decreases the exposure to rosiglitazone by about 25%. Pioglitazone might be similarly affected.

> The clinical relevance of the modest reduction in rosiglitazone exposure has not been assessed, but an interaction with rosiglitazone or pioglitazone seems unlikely to be important. However, note that the UK manufacturer of pioglitazone advises caution on concurrent use.

Antidiabetics + **HIV-protease inhibitors**

The US manufacturer of saxagliptin predicts that atazanavir, indinavir, nelfinavir, ritonavir, and saquinavir will increase the exposure to saxagliptin.

> The US manufacturer of saxagliptin recommends that the dose of saxagliptin should be limited to 2.5 mg daily with most of these HIV-protease inhibitors, although no dose adjustment is necessary with amprenavir and fosamprenavir. It would seem prudent to increase the monitoring of blood glucose concentrations with any HIV-protease inhibitor, and adjust treatment accordingly.

Antidiabetics + **HRT**

Some women may require small increases or decreases in their dose of antidiabetic while taking HRT, but it is unusual for the control of diabetes to be seriously disturbed.

> Routine monitoring should be adequate to detect any interaction as the effects seem to be gradual. However, note that occasionally severe disturbances in control do occur. Menopausal HRT should be used with caution in diabetics because of the increased risk of arterial disease.

Antidiabetics + Isoniazid

Isoniazid is known to be associated with hyperglycaemia and some reports suggest that isoniazid might affect the control of diabetes with insulin and tolbutamide.

> Strictly speaking this seems to be a drug-disease interaction. Given the effects of isoniazid on blood glucose, it would be prudent for diabetics given isoniazid to be monitored for changes in the control of the diabetes. Monitoring and appropriate dose adjustments of the antidiabetic should be considered where necessary.

Antidiabetics + Lanreotide

Lanreotide can affect blood glucose concentrations in diabetic patients.

> Blood glucose concentrations should be checked in diabetic patients to determine whether antidiabetic treatment needs to be adjusted.

Antidiabetics + Leflunomide

The active metabolite of leflunomide (A771726) has been shown by *in vitro* studies to be an inhibitor of CYP2C9, which is concerned with the metabolism of tolbutamide. The manufacturers advise caution if leflunomide is given with tolbutamide as increased tolbutamide levels may result.

> It may be prudent to monitor blood glucose levels on concurrent use.

Antidiabetics + Macrolides

Sulfonylureas

Isolated cases of hypoglycaemia have been described in patients taking glibenclamide (glyburide) or glipizide with clarithromycin or erythromycin. In a pharmacokinetic study, clarithromycin slightly increased glibenclamide concentrations. The same effect might occur with tolbutamide.

> It might be prudent to increase monitoring of blood glucose concentration, and adjust the dose of the antidiabetic as necessary.

Repaglinide

Clarithromycin and telithromycin appear to increase the exposure to repaglinide and might enhance its blood glucose-lowering effects: a case of hypoglycaemia has been reported with clarithromycin. Erythromycin might interact similarly.

> It might be prudent to increase blood glucose monitoring on concurrent use and adjust the dose of repaglinide if necessary.

Saxagliptin

Clarithromycin and telithromycin are predicted to increase saxagliptin exposure. Erythromycin might also interact, although to a lesser extent.

> The US manufacturer recommends that the dose of saxagliptin should be limited to 2.5 mg daily with clarithromycin or telithromycin. It would seem prudent to

increase monitoring of blood glucose concentrations and adjust treatment accordingly. No initial saxagliptin dose adjustment is recommended with erythromycin; however, consider monitoring blood glucose concentrations more closely and reduce the dose if clinically indicated.

Antidiabetics + MAOIs

The blood glucose-lowering effects of insulin and the oral antidiabetics can be increased by MAOIs. This may improve the control of blood glucose levels in most diabetics, but in a few it may cause undesirable hypoglycaemia.

It may be prudent to increase blood glucose monitoring on concurrent use.

Antidiabetics + Neomycin

Neomycin alone can reduce postprandial blood glucose levels, and may enhance the reduction in postprandial glucose levels associated with acarbose. Neomycin also appears to increase the unpleasant gastrointestinal adverse effects (flatulence, cramps and diarrhoea) of acarbose.

The manufacturers suggest that if these adverse effects are severe the dose of acarbose should be reduced.

Antidiabetics + Nicotinic acid (Niacin)

Nicotinic acid causes deterioration in glucose tolerance, which might be dose-related, and can result in the need for dose adjustment of a patient's antidiabetic drugs. Nevertheless, its beneficial effects on lipids might outweigh its effects on glucose tolerance in some diabetic patients.

Diabetic control should be closely monitored, recognising that some adjustment of the antidiabetic drugs might be needed.

Antidiabetics + NNRTIs

Rilpivirine is predicted to reduce metformin exposure by inhibiting its renal excretion.

Monitor concurrent use for metformin adverse effects (anorexia, abdominal pain) and adjust the metformin dose if necessary.

Antidiabetics + NSAIDs

Antidiabetics with Azapropazone or Phenylbutazone

Although in general NSAIDs do not appear to interact with antidiabetics (see below) azapropazone and particularly phenylbutazone seem to cause a consistent lowering of blood glucose levels (probably by inhibiting the metabolism of the sulphonylureas), which has resulted in severe hypoglycaemia in a number of cases.

Concurrent use with phenylbutazone should be well monitored and a reduction in the dosage of the sulphonylurea may be necessary to avoid excessive hypoglycaemia. The manufacturers of azapropazone say that the concurrent use of sulphonylureas is not recommended.

Pioglitazone or Rosiglitazone with NSAIDs

The risk of fluid retention with pioglitazone or rosiglitazone is increased by NSAIDs, and this may exacerbate or precipitate heart failure and/or oedema, particularly in those with limited cardiac reserve.

Caution is appropriate, and patients should be monitored for signs of fluid retention and heart failure (e.g. shortness of breath or swollen ankles). Patients who develop these symptoms should seek a medical review.

Antidiabetics, general with NSAIDs

No adverse interaction normally occurs between most NSAIDs and antidiabetics, although in some isolated cases hypoglycaemia has occurred.

No action needed, but be aware that NSAIDs may rarely and unpredictably cause hypoglycaemia.

Antidiabetics + Octreotide

Octreotide decreases insulin resistance which might affect diabetic control. Octreotide appears to have no benefits in those with intact insulin reserves (type 2 diabetes) and it might reduce sulfonylurea-induced hypoglycaemia.

If octreotide is used with insulin, anticipate the need to reduce the insulin dose (studies suggest by up to 50%). Octreotide might affect insulin secretion, and therefore glucose tolerance, and so it would be prudent to monitor the effects of giving octreotide with any of the oral antidiabetics.

Antidiabetics + Orlistat

Acarbose

The manufacturers of orlistat recommend avoiding the concurrent use of acarbose because of a lack of interaction studies.

Avoid concurrent use.

Other antidiabetics

Orlistat improved glycaemic control, which resulted in the need to reduce the dose of glibenclamide (glyburide) or glipizide in almost half of the patients in one study. In other studies, orlistat reduced the dose requirement for metformin and insulin.

Monitor the outcome of concurrent use on blood sugar levels and adjust the antidiabetic treatment accordingly.

A

Antidiabetics + **Pancreatic enzymes**

The manufacturers of acarbose and miglitol reasonably suggest that digestive enzyme preparations (such as amylase, pancreatin) would be expected to reduce the effects of these antidiabetics.

The manufacturers advise avoiding concurrent use.

Antidiabetics + **Pasireotide**

Pasireotide can affect blood glucose concentrations in pre-diabetic and diabetic patients.

Blood glucose concentrations should be checked in diabetic patients to determine whether doses of antidiabetic drugs need to be adjusted.

Antidiabetics + **Phenobarbital**

Linagliptin or Repaglinide

Phenobarbital (and therefore probably primidone, which is metabolised to phenobarbital), are predicted to decrease the exposure to linagliptin and repaglinide.

Consider giving an alternative, non-interacting alternative to phenobarbital or primidone. If concurrent use is necessary, it would seem prudent to increase blood glucose concentration monitoring, and adjust the antidiabetic treatment accordingly.

Saxagliptin

Phenobarbital and primidone (which is metabolised to phenobarbital), are predicted to reduce saxagliptin exposure.

The US manufacturer considers that no dose adjustment of saxagliptin is needed as overall dipeptidylpeptidase-4 inhibitory activity was unaffected. However, as it cannot be ruled out that enzyme inducers might reduce the blood-glucose lowering effect of saxagliptin the UK manufacturer advises caution. Bear this interaction in mind should any reduced saxagliptin effects occur.

Antidiabetics + **Phenytoin**

Repaglinide and Linagliptin

Phenytoin (and therefore probably its prodrug, fosphenytoin), are predicted to reduce the exposure to linagliptin or repaglinide.

Consider giving an alternative, non-interacting drug to phenytoin, if possible. If concurrent use is necessary, increase blood glucose concentration monitoring to ensure that the antidiabetic drug is still effective, and adjust the antidiabetic treatment accordingly.

Saxagliptin

Phenytoin and therefore probably its prodrug, fosphenytoin, are predicted to increase the exposure to saxagliptin.

The US manufacturer considers that no dose adjustment of saxagliptin is needed as overall dipeptidylpeptidase-4 inhibitory activity was unaffected. However, as it cannot be ruled out that enzyme inducers might reduce the blood-glucose lowering effect of saxagliptin the UK manufacturer advises caution. Bear this interaction in mind should any reduced saxagliptin effects occur.

Other antidiabetics

Large and toxic doses of phenytoin have been observed to cause hyperglycaemia, but normal therapeutic doses do not usually affect the control of diabetes. Two isolated cases of phenytoin toxicity have been attributed to the use of tolbutamide.

No interaction of clinical importance normally occurs and so no special precautions would seem to be necessary, but bear it in mind in the case of an unexpected response to treatment. Indicators of phenytoin toxicity include blurred vision, nystagmus, ataxia, or drowsiness.

Antidiabetics + Probenecid

The clearance of chlorpropamide is prolonged by probenecid, but the clinical importance of this is uncertain.

Monitor the effect of concurrent use on blood glucose levels and adjust the chlorpropamide dose if necessary. Tolbutamide appears not to interact with probenecid, and so may be a suitable alternative.

Antidiabetics + Quinolones

A number of reports describe severe hypoglycaemia (and, rarely, hyperglycaemia) in patients with diabetes taking gatifloxacin with various antidiabetics, including some sulfonylureas, insulin, metformin, pioglitazone, repaglinide, rosiglitazone, and voglibose. Isolated cases describe hypoglycaemia in patients with diabetes taking glibenclamide (glyburide) with ciprofloxacin, levofloxacin, or norfloxacin, and fatalities have occurred.

Studies have shown that systemic gatifloxacin can cause hypoglycaemia and hyperglycaemia with at least a 10-fold higher incidence than other quinolones. The use of systemic gatifloxacin in patients with diabetes has been contra-indicated, however gatifloxacin eye drops are not expected to interact. Studies using ciprofloxacin and levofloxacin with glibenclamide (glyburide) suggest plasma glucose concentrations are not usually affected to a clinically relevant extent. Therefore in general these interactions seem unlikely to be clinically significant with most quinolones; however, it might be prudent to consider increasing the frequency of blood glucose monitoring in the elderly, who appear more at risk of hypoglycaemia.

Antidiabetics + **Rifabutin**

The manufacturers and the CSM in the UK warn that rifabutin may possibly reduce the effects of oral antidiabetics, although this is likely to be to at lesser extent than rifampicin. For information on the effects *rifampicin* has on antidiabetics, see Antidiabetics + Rifampicin (Rifampin), page 90.

Monitor the outcome of concurrent use on blood glucose levels and adjust the antidiabetic treatment accordingly. In many cases an increase in the dose of the antidiabetic may possibly be needed. Note that the US manufacturer considers that no dose adjustment of saxagliptin is needed with *rifampicin (rifampin)*, and therefore an initial dose adjustment seems unlikely to be needed with rifabutin.

Antidiabetics + **Rifampicin (Rifampin)**

Rifampicin reduces the exposure and blood glucose-lowering effects of tolbutamide, gliclazide, chlorpropamide (single case) and glibenclamide (glyburide), and to a lesser extent glimepiride, glipizide and glymidine. Rifampicin also reduces the exposure and effects of repaglinide, and possibly nateglinide, pioglitazone, and rosiglitazone. Rifampicin moderately reduces the exposure to saxagliptin, without affecting the exposure to its active metabolite, and slightly reduces the exposure to linagliptin.

Monitor the outcome of concurrent use on blood glucose concentrations and adjust the antidiabetic treatment accordingly. In many cases an increase in the dose of the antidiabetic seems likely to be needed. The US manufacturer states that no dose adjustment of saxagliptin is needed as overall efficacy was unaffected. The US manufacturer of linagliptin states that an alternative antidiabetic should be used, if possible.

Antidiabetics + **SSRIs**

In various clinical studies in patients with diabetes, the SSRIs have generally caused minor improvements in glycaemic control. However, isolated cases of severe hypoglycaemia, hyperglycaemia, and hypoglycaemia unawareness have been reported.

It might be prudent to consider increasing the frequency of blood glucose monitoring if an SSRI is started or stopped, adjusting the antidiabetic drugs as necessary.

Antidiabetics + **Statins**

Glibenclamide

Fluvastatin may raise glibenclamide levels, but this possibly only occurs with doses above 40 mg daily. Blood glucose levels were not affected by concurrent use.

The UK manufacturers of fluvastatin suggest that concurrent use should be avoided because of the risk of hypoglycaemia. The US manufacturers advise close monitoring, which should continue if the fluvastatin dose is increased to 40 mg twice daily. This seems prudent.

Other antidiabetics

One study reported an increased incidence of adverse effects when repaglinide was given with simvastatin, and there is a possibility of increased liver and muscle effects when pioglitazone or rosiglitazone are used with atorvastatin.

As yet there is insufficient evidence to recommend special precautions when the statins are used with any antidiabetic drug. No clinically relevant adverse interactions appear to have been reported between statins and sulfonylureas. The use of statins in patients with diabetes is known to be beneficial for both primary and secondary prevention of cardiovascular events.

Antidiabetics + **Sulfinpyrazone**

Sulfinpyrazone reduces the clearance of tolbutamide by about 40%.

There appear to be no reports of a clinically relevant interaction with these or any other sulfonylureas; however what is known suggests that increased blood glucose-lowering effects, and possibly hypoglycaemia, could occur. It would therefore seem prudent to consider monitoring blood-glucose levels, and warn patients that hypoglycaemia may occur.

Antidiabetics + **Sulfonamides**

The blood glucose-lowering effects of some of the sulfonylureas are increased by some, but not all, sulfonamides. The sulfonamides now available appear less likely to interact. Nevertheless, occasionally and unpredictably acute hypoglycaemia has occurred.

Information is limited and serious adverse effects appear to be rare. Nevertheless, the cautious approach would be to increase the frequency of blood glucose monitoring and warn the patient that increased blood glucose-lowering effects, sometimes excessive, are a possibility.

Antidiabetics + **Testosterone**

Testosterone can enhance the blood glucose-lowering effects of insulin, and might also improve glycaemic control in those taking oral antidiabetics.

It would seem prudent to increase monitoring of blood glucose if testosterone is started and adjust the antidiabetic dose accordingly. A reduction in patients' dose requirements of insulin (of about one-third) might be expected.

Antidiabetics + **Tibolone**

Tibolone may slightly impair glucose tolerance and therefore possibly reduce the effects of antidiabetics. Strictly speaking this is a drug-disease interaction.

The manufacturers of tibolone state that patients with diabetes should be closely supervised. It would therefore seem prudent to increase the frequency of blood glucose monitoring if tibolone is started or stopped.

Antidiabetics + Tricyclics ❓

Interactions between antidiabetics and tricyclic antidepressants appear to be rare, but isolated cases of hypoglycaemia have occurred in patients given insulin or a sulfonylurea with a tricyclic.

These isolated cases seem unlikely to be of general importance.

Antidiabetics + Trimethoprim

Repaglinide ⚠

In one study trimethoprim increased the AUC of single-dose repaglinide by about 60% without changing its blood-glucose lowering effects.

The UK manufacturers advise that concurrent use should be avoided as the effect of larger doses of both drugs are unknown. However, the US manufacturers suggest that repaglinide dose adjustments may be necessary. If both drugs are used it would seem prudent to increase the frequency of blood glucose monitoring until the effects are known.

Rosiglitazone ❓

Trimethoprim appears to modestly increase the AUC of rosiglitazone and pioglitazone.

This interaction is not expected to be clinically significant, but, until more experience is gained, some caution is warranted.

Sulfonylureas ✔

Trimethoprim does not appear to significantly affect the pharmacokinetics of tolbutamide. Consider also co-trimoxazole, page 81, which may interact.

No action needed.

Antidiabetics + Warfarin and related oral anticoagulants

Exenatide ❓

A controlled study found that exenatide had no effect on the pharmacokinetics and only slightly raised the INR (by 12%). However, the manufacturer states that cases of raised INRs have been reported with concurrent use, and predict that other coumarins will interact similarly.

A clinically significant interaction seems unlikely. However, the manufacturer advises that the INR should be closely monitored when exenatide is started, stopped, or the dose altered.

Liraglutide ❓

Liraglutide is not expected to alter the absorption of warfarin. In addition, liraglutide does not affect cytochrome P450, by which warfarin is principally metabolised. No interaction would therefore be expected. However, the UK manufacturer states that a clinically relevant interaction with active substances with narrow therapeutic index such as warfarin cannot be excluded.

> The UK manufacturer recommends that more frequent monitoring of the INR is recommended if patients taking warfarin are given liraglutide. As there is little clinical experience with liraglutide, this might be prudent.

Other antidiabetics

Although isolated cases of interactions (raised prothrombin times, bleeding or hypoglycaemia) have been seen in patients taking anticoagulants and acarbose, metformin or sulfonylureas, in general no important interaction appears to occur. A decrease in prothrombin time has also been seen with acarbose or metformin.

> The isolated cases of bleeding are not expected to represent a general interaction.

Antihistamines

No specific interaction studies have been performed with antihistamine eye drops. However, interactions are not anticipated since very little drug is expected to reach the systemic circulation. Note also that the sedative antihistamines may cause additive sedation with any other CNS depressant drug.

Antihistamines + Azoles

Ebastine

Ketoconazole very markedly increases ebastine concentrations. Itraconazole is expected to interact similarly.

> Although the risk of an interaction seems small, because of the potential for life-threatening torsade de pointes arrhythmia, the manufacturer of ebastine advises against the use of itraconazole or ketoconazole.

Loratadine

Ketoconazole moderately increases loratadine exposure. In one study, this was associated with a small increase in the QT interval, but there was no obvious alteration in the adverse event profile.

> No special precautions appear to have been recommended for the use of loratadine with ketoconazole.

Mizolastine

Ketoconazole increases mizolastine concentrations, which caused a small increase in the QT interval in one study.

> The UK manufacturer of mizolastine contraindicates its concurrent use with systemic imidazole antifungals (e.g. ketoconazole, miconazole), and use with other CYP3A4 inhibitors is cautioned, which would include all other azoles. However, note that itraconazole, a triazole, would be expected to interact to the same extent as ketoconazole.

A

Other antihistamines ❓

Desloratadine, emedastine, and rupatadine concentrations are increased by ketoconazole, and fexofenadine concentrations are increased by both itraconazole and ketoconazole, but no adverse cardiac events have been seen.

Because there is no data on an interaction between acrivastine and ketoconazole, the UK manufacturer advises caution. As no change in QT interval or in adverse events occurred, the combination of ketoconazole or itraconazole with fexofenadine, desloratadine, or emedastine is assumed to be safe in terms of cardiac effects. The UK manufacturer of rupatadine advises that it is used with caution with ketoconazole and other azoles. No special precautions appear to have been recommended for the use of loratadine with azoles. Azelastine, cetirizine (and therefore probably its isomer levocetirizine), and levocabastine do not appear to interact with the azole antifungals and might therefore be suitable alternatives.

Antihistamines + **Benzodiazepines** ❓

An enhanced sedative effect would be expected if known sedative antihistamines are given with benzodiazepines.

Warn all patients taking sedating antihistamines of the potential effects, and counsel against driving or undertaking other skilled tasks. The degree of impairment will depend on the individual patient.

Antihistamines + **Betahistine** ❓

A single report describes the re-emergence of labyrinthine symptoms in a patient taking betahistine with terfenadine. This interaction had been predicted on theoretical grounds because betahistine is an analogue of histamine. Betahistine may therefore oppose the effects of all antihistamines.

Although the general relevance of this isolated case report is unclear, the use of antihistamines should be carefully considered in patients taking betahistine.

Antihistamines + **Grapefruit juice**

Rupatadine ⚠

Grapefruit juice increases the exposure to rupatadine 3.5-fold.

The manufacturer advises that grapefruit juice should not be taken at the same time as rupatadine.

Other antihistamines ❓

Grapefruit juice has been found to reduce the AUC of fexofenadine by up to 67%, which may reduce its efficacy.

The general importance of reduction in fexofenadine levels is unclear, but bear it in mind in case of a lack of response to treatment. Note that the manufacturer of acrivastine advises caution with grapefruit juice but notes that there are no data to demonstrate an interaction.

Antihistamines + H$_2$-receptor antagonists

Cimetidine moderately raises hydroxyzine levels and considerably raises loratadine levels, but this is not thought to be of clinical significance. The manufacturer of mizolastine predicts that cimetidine may raise mizolastine levels.

No action is generally needed. Note that the manufacturer of mizolastine recommends caution because raised mizolastine levels may prolong the QT interval.

Antihistamines + Herbal medicines or Dietary supplements

Some studies have found that St John's wort increased the clearance of fexofenadine up to 2-fold, whereas another study found no clinically relevant effect.

If fexofenadine is less effective in a patient taking regular St John's wort, consider this interaction as a possible cause.

Antihistamines + HIV-protease inhibitors

Loratadine

The UK manufacturer states that ritonavir, including ritonavir given to boost other HIV-protease inhibitors, is expected to increase the plasma concentrations of loratadine.

They advise that patients should be alert for loratadine adverse effects (e.g. fatigue, nausea, headache) if they are also given ritonavir.

Mizolastine

The manufacturers of mizolastine predict that drugs that are potent inhibitors of CYP3A4 (such as the HIV-protease inhibitors) will increase mizolastine concentrations.

The manufacturer of mizolastine advises caution on concurrent use. However, note that they contraindicate the use of the azoles, page 93, which would not be expected to interact to the same extent as the HIV-protease inhibitors. Note that the UK manufacturer of saquinavir contraindicates the concurrent use of mizolastine because of a possible risk of QT prolongation.

Other antihistamines

Ritonavir modestly increases cetirizine concentrations. Ritonavir, indinavir (alone or boosted by ritonavir) and lopinavir boosted with ritonavir increase fexofenadine exposure.

These interactions are not expected to be clinically significant. No action needed.

A

Antihistamines + **Macrolides**

Ebastine or Mizolastine ✖

Erythromycin causes a large increase in ebastine concentrations, which resulted in a modest prolongation of the QT interval in one study. Erythromycin also increases mizolastine concentrations, although this has no effect on the QT interval.

> The manufacturer of ebastine advises against the concurrent use of erythromycin, clarithromycin, and josamycin. The manufacturer of mizolastine contraindicates the concurrent use of the macrolides.

Other antihistamines ❓

Erythromycin increases fexofenadine and rupatadine concentrations, although this has no effect on the QT interval. Azithromycin has also been reported to increase fexofenadine concentrations, but this also had no effect on the QT interval, or on adverse events. One study found that the combination of erythromycin and loratadine caused a very slight increase in the QT interval.

> The manufacturer of rupatadine advises caution on the concurrent use of erythromycin and other CYP3A4 inhibitors, which would be expected to include clarithromycin and telithromycin. The situation with erythromycin and loratadine is unclear; however, no special precautions appear to have been recommended. Because there are no data on acrivastine with erythromycin, the manufacturer advises caution. Azelastine, cetirizine (and probably levocetirizine), desloratadine, and levocabastine might be suitable non-interacting alternatives for some patients. As the use of fexofenadine with erythromycin did not result in significant adverse cardiac effects, concurrent use with erythromycin is considered safe.

Antihistamines + **MAOIs**

Antihistamines, general ❓

The alleged interaction between MAOIs and most antihistamines appears to be based on a single animal study, and is probably more theoretical than real. The exceptions seem to be cyproheptadine and promethazine (see below).

> In general, there would appear to be no good reason to avoid the concurrent use of sedating or non-sedating antihistamines with an MAOI. However, the UK manufacturers of some of the sedating antihistamines (alimemazine, chlorphenamine, diphenhydramine) state that MAOIs may intensify the antimuscarinic effect of antihistamines, and many contraindicate or advise caution on concurrent use, both with and for 14 days after stopping an MAOI. The US manufacturers of isocarboxazid and tranylcypromine contraindicate all antihistamines.

Cyproheptadine ❓

Isolated reports describe delayed hallucinations in a patient taking phenelzine and cyproheptadine, and the rapid re-emergence of depression when cyproheptadine was given to two other patients taking brofaromine or phenelzine.

> It would be prudent to monitor for a reduction in efficacy or an adverse response if cyproheptadine is given with any MAOI or RIMA. The manufacturer of cyproheptadine contraindicates concurrent use with MAOIs, however, there appears to be no reason why cyproheptadine cannot be used to treat serotonin syndrome occurring in a patient taking an MAOI.

Promethazine

Promethazine is a phenothiazine antihistamine. Rarely, cases of neuroleptic malignant syndrome or extrapyramidal symptoms have been seen when phenothiazines have been given with MAOIs.

> The UK manufacturer contraindicates the use of promethazine, both with and for 14 days after stopping treatment with an MAOI.

Antihistamines + Rifampicin (Rifampin)

Rifampicin increases the oral clearance of fexofenadine, more than 5-fold in some cases, but the clinical significance of this is unclear.

> Until more is known it would seem prudent to monitor the efficacy of fexofenadine if it is given with rifampicin.

Antihistamines + Ulipristal

Ulipristal does not alter the pharmacokinetics of fexofenadine when given 1.5 hours before.

> The UK manufacturer of *low-dose* ulipristal suggests that as ulipristal appears to inhibit P-glycoprotein *in vitro*, the administration of ulipristal and P glycoprotein substrates such as fexofenadine, should be separated by at least 1.5 hours.

Antihypertensives

The hypotensive effect of antihypertensives can be enhanced by other antihypertensives, as would be expected. Although first-dose hypotension' (dizziness, light-headedness, fainting) can occur with some combinations (e.g. see ACE inhibitors, page 1 and alpha blockers, page 37), the additive effects are usually clinically useful. Perhaps of more concern is the use of antihypertensives with drugs that have hypotension as an adverse effect, where the effects might not be anticipated or deliberately sought. The situation with alcohol is slightly more complex. Chronic moderate to heavy drinking raises blood pressure and reduces, to some extent, the effectiveness of antihypertensive drugs. A few patients taking antihypertensives might experience postural hypotension, dizziness, and fainting shortly after having an alcoholic drink. See also alpha blockers, page 15, beta blockers, page 18, and calcium-channel blockers, page 19, for more specific information on these individual groups. Patients with hypertension who are moderate to heavy drinkers should be encouraged to reduce their intake of alcohol. It might then become possible to reduce the dose of the antihypertensive. It should be noted that epidemiological studies show that regular light to moderate alcohol consumption is associated with a *lower* risk of cardiovascular disease. Drugs where hypotension is the main effect include:

- ACE inhibitors
- Aliskiren
- Alpha blockers
- Angiotensin II receptor antagonists
- Beta blockers
- Calcium-channel blockers
- Clonidine
- Diazoxide
- Diuretics

- Guanethidine
- Hydralazine
- Methyldopa
- Minoxidil
- Moxonidine
- Nitrates
- Nitroprusside

Drugs where hypotension is a significant adverse effect include:

- Alcohol
- Aldesleukin
- Alprostadil
- Antipsychotics
- Dopamine agonists (e.g. apomorphine, bromocriptine, pergolide)
- Drospirenone
- Levodopa
- MAOIs
- Moxisylyte
- Nicorandil
- Tizanidine

Antihypertensives + Contraceptives

Oral combined hormonal contraceptives might increase blood pressure and antagon-ise the efficacy of antihypertensives. The risks appear to be modest with newer contraceptives than with historically used higher-dose contraceptives. The UK Faculty of Sexual and Reproductive Healthcare (FSRH) consider that the use of a combined hormonal contraceptive (tablet, transdermal patch, or vaginal ring) is not usually recommended in women with adequately controlled hypertension with no other risk factors for cardiovascular disease, unless other more appropriate methods are not available or acceptable. In these women, there is no restriction on the use of oral progestogen-only contraceptives or progestogen-only implants, and the benefits of the use of depot medroxyprogesterone acetate or norethisterone enantate are considered to usually outweigh the theoretical risks. Additive hypotension might also occur when drospirenone, an analogue of spironolactone is given with antihypertensives, see Antihypertensives, page 97.

> It is generally advised that combined hormonal contraceptives are not used in women with hypertension with no other risk factors for cardiovascular disease, and that they should be avoided in women with hypertension and other risk factors for cardiovascular disease. Progestogen-only contraceptives are usually the preferred hormonal method of contraception in women with hypertension. If combined hormonal contraceptives are used in women taking antihypertensives, blood pressure should be monitored more frequently.

Antimuscarinics

Remember that other drugs, (e.g. clozapine, nefopam, tricyclic antidepressants) have antimuscarinic adverse effects, and therefore may interact similarly.

Antimuscarinics + Antimuscarinics

Additive antimuscarinic effects can develop if two or more drugs with antimuscarinic effects are used together. The easily recognised and common peripheral antimuscarinic effects are blurred vision, dry mouth, constipation, difficulty in urination, reduced sweating and tachycardia. Central effects include confusion, disorientation, visual hallucinations, agitation, irritability, delirium, memory problems, belligerence and even aggressiveness. Problems are most likely to arise in patients with particular physical conditions such as glaucoma, prostatic hypertrophy or constipation, in whom antimuscarinic drugs should be used with caution, if at all. It has been pointed out that the antimuscarinic adverse effects can mimic the effects of normal ageing. Consider also antipsychotics, below.

Concurrent use need not be avoided but some caution is warranted, especially in the disease states mentioned.

Antimuscarinics + **Antipsychotics** ❓

Antipsychotics and antimuscarinics are often given together advantageously and uneventfully, but occasionally serious and even life-threatening interactions occur. These include heat stroke in hot and humid conditions, severe constipation and paralytic ileus, and atropine-like psychoses. Antimuscarinics used to counteract the extrapyramidal adverse effects of antipsychotics may also reduce or abolish their therapeutic effects. See also antimuscarinics, page 98, as many antipsychotics also have antimuscarinic adverse effects.

These drugs have been widely used together with apparent advantage and often without problems. However, be aware that low-grade antimuscarinic toxicity can easily go undetected, particularly in the elderly. Also note that serious problems can sometimes develop, particularly if high doses are used. Consider:

- warning patients (particularly those on high doses) to minimise outdoor exposure and/or exercise in hot and humid climates.
- being alert for severe constipation and for the development of complete gut stasis, which can be fatal.
- that the symptoms of central antimuscarinic psychosis can be confused with the basic psychotic symptoms of the patient.
- withdrawal of one or more of the drugs, or a dose reduction and/or appropriate symptomatic treatment if any of these interactions occur.
- that the concurrent use of antimuscarinics to control the extrapyramidal adverse effects of neuroleptics is necessary, and be aware that the therapeutic effects may possibly be reduced as a result.

Some antipsychotics and antimuscarinics prolong the QT interval. For interactions resulting from additive effects on the QT interval see drugs that prolong the QT interval, page 352. Remember that many drugs have antimuscarinic adverse effects (e.g. tricyclics, page 117).

Antimuscarinics + **Donepezil** ⚠

The effects of donepezil are expected to oppose the actions of drugs with antimuscarinic effects, and in turn to be opposed by antimuscarinics. However, two cases describe confusional states resulting from the concurrent use of anticholinesterases and drugs with antimuscarinic effects, which is the opposite effect to that expected.

Whether this interaction is of real practical importance awaits confirmation, but it would seem prudent to monitor concurrent use for an increase in adverse effects.

A

Antimuscarinics + **Galantamine**

The effects of galantamine are expected to oppose the actions of drugs with antimuscarinic effects, and in turn to be opposed by antimuscarinics. However, two cases describe confusional states resulting from the concurrent use of other anticholinesterases and drugs with antimuscarinic effects, which is the opposite effect to that expected.

Whether this interaction is of real practical importance awaits confirmation, but it may be prudent to monitor concurrent use for an increase in adverse effects.

Antimuscarinics + **Levodopa**

Antimuscarinics may modestly reduce the rate and possibly the extent of levodopa absorption. One case describes levodopa toxicity, which occurred after the withdrawal of an antimuscarinic.

Concurrent use is of established benefit. The presence of a dopa-decarboxylase inhibitor would be expected to minimise the effects of any interaction, however reduced levodopa absorption has still been reported with this combination. There is certainly no need to avoid concurrent use, but it would be prudent to be alert for any evidence of a reduced levodopa response if antimuscarinics are added, or for levodopa toxicity if they are withdrawn.

Antimuscarinics + **MAOIs**

No adverse interactions between the MAOIs and antimuscarinics appear to have been reported. However, some manufacturers of non-selective MAOIs and antimuscarinics advise caution because of the theoretical possibility that concurrent use may lead to increased antimuscarinic effects.

Bear this possible interaction in mind on concurrent use.

Antimuscarinics + **Nitrates**

Drugs with antimuscarinic effects, such as the tricyclic antidepressants and disopyramide, depress salivation and many patients complain of having a dry mouth. In theory sublingual glyceryl trinitrate (nitroglycerin) tablets will dissolve less readily under the tongue in these patients, thereby reducing their absorption and effects.

A possible alternative is to use a glyceryl trinitrate (nitroglycerin) spray in patients who suffer from dry mouth.

Antimuscarinics + **Rivastigmine**

The effects of rivastigmine are expected to oppose the actions of drugs with antimuscarinic effects, and in turn to be opposed by antimuscarinics. However, in practice two cases describe confusional states resulting from the concurrent use of anticholinesterases and drugs with antimuscarinic effects, which is the opposite effect to that expected.

Whether this interaction is of real practical importance awaits confirmation, but it may be prudent to monitor concurrent use for an increase in adverse effects.

Antimuscarinics + SSRIs

Several patients have developed delirium when given fluoxetine, paroxetine or sertraline with benzatropine, in the presence of an antipsychotic (usually perphenazine or haloperidol). Concurrent use in other patients has been uneventful. Paroxetine may increase the levels of procyclidine.

> The general clinical importance of this interaction is uncertain, but be alert for evidence of confusion and possible delirium in patients given SSRIs with benzatropine, particularly if they are also taking other drugs with antimuscarinic actions. If antimuscarinic effects are seen in patients taking paroxetine and procyclidine, the dose of procyclidine should be reduced.

Antimuscarinics + Tacrine

The effects of tacrine are expected to oppose the actions of drugs with antimuscarinic effects, and in turn to be opposed by antimuscarinics. However, in practice two cases describe confusional states resulting from the concurrent use of anticholinesterases and drugs with antimuscarinic effects, which is the opposite effect to that expected.

> Whether this interaction is of real practical importance awaits confirmation, but it may be prudent to monitor concurrent use for an increase in adverse effects.

Antipsychotics

Antipsychotics + Antipsychotics

Quetiapine

Limited evidence suggest that thioridazine slightly reduces quetiapine concentrations. A case report describes a seizure in a patient taking olanzapine and quetiapine.

> Concurrent use need not be avoided. Until more is known, monitor concurrent use of thioridazine with quetiapine for efficacy, being alert for the need to raise the quetiapine dose. The case highlights the importance of considering seizure potential when prescribing multiple antipsychotic medications. For the risk of additive QT prolongation, see under Other antipsychotics, below

Other antipsychotics

Additive QT-prolonging effects are likely with some antipsychotic combinations.

> For more information on the effects of using multiple drugs with QT-prolonging effects, see drugs that prolong the QT interval, page 352.

Antipsychotics + Apomorphine

Centrally-acting dopamine antagonists (such as the antipsychotics, including prochlorperazine used at an antiemetic dose) may antagonise the effects of apomorphine. However, note that clozapine may be used to reduce the symptoms of neuropsychiatric complications of Parkinson's disease. Additive hypotensive effects are also possible, see antihypertensives, page 97.

> Concurrent use should be avoided, or monitored closely to ensure apomorphine

remains effective. Note that prochlorperazine has been used safely in patients taking apomorphine for erectile dysfunction.

Antipsychotics + **Aprepitant** ❌

Aprepitant can increase the exposure to CYP3A4 substrates, such as pimozide, in the short term, then reduce their exposure within 2 weeks. An increase in the concentration of pimozide, might result in the potentially fatal torsade de pointes, (see Drugs that prolong the QT interval, page 352). Fosaprepitant, a prodrug of aprepitant, would be expected to interact similarly.

> Concurrent use is contraindicated. Caution is needed in the 2 weeks after aprepitant is stopped because it is also a mild *inducer* of CYP3A4 and the induction is transient. Therefore, it might *induce* the metabolism of pimozide leading to *reduced* pimozide concentrations.

Antipsychotics + **Azoles**

Pimozide and Sertindole ❌

The azoles are predicted to raise the concentrations of pimozide and sertindole, which could lead to potentially fatal torsade de pointes.

> The concurrent use of azoles with pimozide or sertindole is contraindicated. Note that miconazole oral gel might be swallowed in sufficient amounts to cause a systemic effect, and the manufacturer also contraindicates its use with sertindole.

Quetiapine ⚠

Quetiapine exposure is markedly increased by ketoconazole. Other azoles, page 143 are predicted to interact similarly, although probably to a greater or lesser extent.

> The UK manufacturer contraindicates concurrent use, whereas the US manufacturer advises that lower quetiapine doses might be needed. If both drugs are given monitor for quetiapine adverse effects (such as somnolence, dry mouth, tachycardia) and adjust the quetiapine dose accordingly.

Other antipsychotics ⚠

The concentrations of some antipsychotics might be raised by the azoles:

- Aripiprazole exposure is slightly increased by itraconazole and ketoconazole by about 20 to 40%.
- Haloperidol concentrations are raised by 30% or more by itraconazole, but there was wide variation between subjects. Adverse neurological effects were seen in some subjects. Other azoles that inhibit CYP3A4, such as ketoconazole, would be expected interact, see azoles, page 143.
- Risperidone concentrations and those of its active metabolite, 9-hydroxyrisperidone, were increased by about 80% by itraconazole in one study. Azoles that are potent inhibitors of CYP3A4, such as ketoconazole and voriconazole, would be expected interact similarly, see azoles, page 143.

> Monitor for signs of adverse antipsychotic effects (such as sedation, agitation, movement disorders) if these azoles are given, and consider reducing the antipsychotic dose, in particular quetiapine. The manufacturers of aripiprazole

suggest halving its dose if itraconazole or ketoconazole are given. The US manufacturers further recommend a 75% reduction in the aripiprazole dose when both a CYP3A4 inhibitor (such as itraconazole or ketoconazole) and a CYP2D6 inhibitor (such as quinidine, page 114) are given together.

Antipsychotics + **Benzodiazepines**

Antipsychotics, general 🔺

Additive CNS depressant effects would be expected when antipsychotics are given with benzodiazepines or related drugs (such as zopiclone or zolpidem). Concurrent use has resulted in excessive sedation, severe hypotension, respiratory depression and, in rare cases, unconfirmed neuroleptic malignant syndrome. Rarely, fatal hypotension and respiratory arrest have been reported when clozapine was given with benzodiazepines. Note that the parenteral use of these drugs is frequent in the more severe cases.

> Be aware of these potential adverse effects, but note that concurrent use is common and most often uneventful. The US manufacturer recommends that if an intravenous benzodiazepine is required in addition to parenteral aripiprazole, the patient should be monitored for excessive sedation and orthostatic hypotension.

Olanzapine 🔺

Excessive sedation and hypotension might occur if parenteral benzodiazepines are given with intramuscular olanzapine: fatalities have been reported.

> Concurrent use is not recommended. If both drugs are needed, parenteral benzodiazepines should not be given until at least one hour after intramuscular olanzapine. If a parenteral benzodiazepine has already been given, intramuscular olanzapine should be given with care and the patient should be closely monitored for sedation and cardiorespiratory depression.

Antipsychotics + **Beta blockers**

Sotalol ✖

Additive QT-prolonging effects are likely with a number of the antipsychotics, see drugs that prolong the QT interval, page 352.

> Concurrent use should generally be avoided.

Beta blockers, general 🔺

The concurrent use of chlorpromazine and propranolol can result in a marked rise in the levels of both drugs. Propranolol also markedly increases thioridazine levels. Additive hypotensive effects are also possible, see antihypertensives, page 97.

> Monitor the outcome of concurrent use, adjusting the doses of both drugs as necessary.

A

Antipsychotics + Bupropion ⚠

Bupropion is predicted to inhibit the metabolism of haloperidol, risperidone, and thioridazine.

> The manufacturers recommend that if any of these drugs are added to treatment with bupropion, they should be given in doses at the lower end of the range. If bupropion is added to existing treatment, decreased doses of the antipsychotics should be considered. However, there appear to be no reports of problems with the concurrent use of any of these drugs. Note that both bupropion and antipsychotics can lower the seizure threshold, and a maximum dose of 150 mg of bupropion should be considered for patients prescribed other drugs that may lower the convulsive threshold.

Antipsychotics + Buspirone ❓

Two studies found that buspirone can cause a rise in haloperidol levels, while another found that no interaction occurred.

> There would seem to be no reason for avoiding concurrent use. However, be aware that some patients seem to experience large rises in haloperidol levels, so consider this interaction if the adverse effects of haloperidol (e.g. sedation, agitation, movement disorders) become troublesome.

Antipsychotics + Calcium-channel blockers

Aripiprazole or Droperidol ⚠

Diltiazem is predicted to increase aripiprazole and droperidol levels. Verapamil would be expected to interact similarly.

> Patients should be closely monitored for signs of aripiprazole or droperidol toxicity (such as sedation, hypotension, dizziness). An initial dose reduction of aripiprazole is probably not required, but if adverse effects develop, consider adjusting the dose.

Risperidone ❓

The UK manufacturer briefly notes that verapamil increases the plasma concentrations of risperidone.

> Bear the possibility of an interaction in mind should risperidone adverse effects (e.g. agitation, insomnia, headache) occur.

Sertindole ⚠

Diltiazem and verapamil reduce the clearance of sertindole by about 20%.

> The manufacturers of sertindole contraindicate concurrent use because raised sertindole levels can prolong the QT interval, see Drugs that prolong the QT interval, page 352.

Antipsychotics, general ❓

In general, the hypotensive adverse effects of phenothiazines would be expected to be additive with the blood pressure-lowering effects of the calcium-channel blockers, see antihypertensives, page 97.

> Bear the possibility of hypotension in mind on concurrent use. Warn patients to take time in getting up to minimise orthostatic hypotension.

Antipsychotics + **Carbamazepine** ?

Clozapine, haloperidol and risperidone plasma concentrations can be roughly halved by carbamazepine. Plasma concentrations of aripiprazole, bromperidol, fluphenazine, olanzapine, paliperidone, quetiapine, sertindole, tiotixene, and possibly chlorpromazine, flupentixol and zuclopenthixol, are also reduced by carbamazepine. An increase in the concentrations of carbamazepine or its epoxide metabolite (which is thought to cause some of the adverse effects of carbamazepine) has been reported in patients given loxapine, haloperidol, quetiapine, risperidone, or chlorpromazine with amoxapine. Toxicity has occurred. Isolated cases of neuroleptic malignant syndrome have occurred in patients taking antipsychotics with carbamazepine. The combination of clozapine and carbamazepine is predicted to increase agranulocytosis and one case of fatal pancytopenia has been reported.

> Monitor carbamazepine concentrations if loxapine, haloperidol, quetiapine, risperidone, or chlorpromazine are given. Also monitor concurrent use to ensure that the antipsychotics remain effective (especially risperidone, clozapine, olanzapine, sertindole and haloperidol), and consider a dose increase if needed. The manufacturers recommend using double the dose of aripiprazole in patients taking carbamazepine. The UK manufacturer advises that carbamazepine should only be given with quetiapine if the benefits outweigh the risks: they suggest that consideration should be given to changing to a drug with no enzyme-inducing effects and name valproate. The manufacturers of sertindole state that the daily dose of sertindole might need to be increased towards the upper end of the maximum dose range to accommodate this interaction. Note that the induction effects of carbamazepine on paliperidone concentrations become maximal after 2 to 3 weeks. The manufacturers advise that clozapine should not be given with carbamazepine: if both drugs are necessary, full blood counts should be closely monitored, as should clozapine efficacy (increase the clozapine dose as required). The general significance of the raised concentrations of the carbamazepine epoxide metabolite is unclear but the possibility of an interaction should be considered in patients who develop neurotoxic adverse effects. It is also important to consider the seizure potential when prescribing antipsychotic medications.

Antipsychotics + **Cilostazol**

The UK manufacturer predicts that cilostazol will increase the exposure to drugs that are metabolised by CYP3A4, and they name pimozide.

> If cilostazol does increase pimozide exposure, it seems likely that the QT interval will be prolonged and therefore it might be prudent to avoid concurrent use where possible. See drugs that prolong the QT interval, page 352 for further information.

A

Antipsychotics + **Cobicistat**

Perphenazine, risperidone or thioridazine

The US manufacturer of elvitegravir with cobicistat (in a fixed-dose combination also including emtricitabine and tenofovir) predicts that it might increase the plasma concentrations of antipsychotics and they name perphenazine, risperidone, and thioridazine.

> Monitor for adverse effects of these antipsychotics on concurrent use, and reduce the dose if necessary.

Pimozide

The US manufacturer of elvitegravir with cobicistat (in a fixed-dose combination also including emtricitabine and tenofovir) predicts that it might increase the plasma concentrations of pimozide, which might increase the risk of cardiac toxicity (e.g. QT prolongation).

> Concurrent use is contraindicated.

Antipsychotics + **Corticosteroids**

CYP3A4 inducers such as *carbamazepine* reduce quetiapine exposure. The US manufacturer predicts that the corticosteroids will interact similarly.

> The corticosteroid do not usually interact with other drugs by inducing CYP3A4, and there appear to be no published reports of an interaction. Nevertheless, until more is known, consider the possibility of an interaction if quetiapine efficacy appears reduced in patients also given corticosteroids. Note that quetiapine and drugs that can cause hypokalaemia (such as corticosteroids) have been associated with QT prolongation, see Drugs that prolong the QT interval, page 352 for more information.

Antipsychotics + **Dapoxetine**

The Swedish manufacturer of dapoxetine predicts that it might increase thioridazine exposure (by inhibiting CYP2D6), which might increase the risk of cardiac adverse effects such as QT prolongation and torsade de pointes, see drugs that prolong the QT interval, page 352. However, limited data suggests that dapoxetine does not have a clinically relevant inhibitory effect on CYP2D6.

> A clinically relevant pharmacokinetic interaction seems unlikely. Nevertheless, the Swedish manufacturer of dapoxetine contraindicates concurrent use, during and for 14 days after stopping thioridazine, and further recommends that thioridazine should not be given for at least 7 days after stopping dapoxetine.

Antipsychotics + **Darifenacin**

Darifenacin increases the levels of CYP2D6 substrates such as the *tricyclics* (imipramine AUC increased by 70%). The manufacturers therefore advise caution with other CYP2D6 substrates, and specifically name thioridazine.

> If the combination is used it would be prudent to closely monitor for thioridazine adverse effects, and consider the possibility of ventricular arrhythmias.

Antipsychotics + **Desmopressin**

Drugs that can cause water retention or hyponatraemia (e.g. chlorpromazine) may have an additive effect with desmopressin: water overload and/or hyponatraemia may occur.

The increased risk may be small, with severe complications being rare; however, it would be prudent to exercise caution on concurrent use, with more frequent monitoring of serum sodium.

Antipsychotics + **Dopamine agonists**

Centrally-acting dopamine antagonists (such as the antipsychotics, including prochlorperazine used at an antiemetic dose) are expected to oppose the effects of the dopamine agonists.

Concurrent use should be avoided, or monitored closely to ensure that the dopamine agonist remains effective. Additive hypotensive effects are possible, see antihypertensives, page 97.

Antipsychotics + **Diuretics**

In controlled studies in elderly patients with dementia, the concurrent use of furosemide with risperidone appeared to be associated with a higher incidence of mortality than risperidone or furosemide alone.

The UK manufacturer recommends caution on concurrent use, considering the risks and benefits: dehydration was an overall risk factor for mortality and should therefore be carefully avoided in elderly patients with dementia.

Antipsychotics + **Duloxetine**

Duloxetine is predicted to inhibit the metabolism of thioridazine and risperidone.

In the US concurrent use of duloxetine and thioridazine is contraindicated. If the combination is used it would be prudent to closely monitor for thioridazine or risperidone adverse effects (such as sedation, hypotension, dizziness). With thioridazine, consider the possibility of ventricular arrhythmias.

Antipsychotics + **Food**

Paliperidone ❓

Paliperidone exposure is increased by a high-fat, high-calorie meal by about 50 to 60%.

The UK manufacturer states that paliperidone should be consistently taken either on an empty stomach or with breakfast, whereas the US manufacturer advises that paliperidone can be taken without regard to food, which was the protocol in the clinical efficacy studies of paliperidone.

A

Ziprasidone

Food increases the absorption of ziprasidone. The fat content of meals appears to have little effect on the outcome.

> The US manufacturer recommends that oral ziprasidone is always taken with food.

Antipsychotics + Grapefruit juice

The manufacturers predict that grapefruit juice will, like other CYP3A4 inhibitors, raise pimozide levels. This may lead to potentially life-threatening torsade de pointes. Grapefruit juice is also predicted to increase quetiapine levels.

> The concurrent intake of grapefruit juice is contraindicated with pimozide and is not recommended with quetiapine.

Antipsychotics + Guanethidine

Large doses of chlorpromazine may reduce or even abolish the antihypertensive effects of guanethidine. However, in some patients the hypotensive effect of chlorpromazine may predominate. The antihypertensive effects of guanethidine can also be reduced by haloperidol and thiothixene. Note also, that the antipsychotics can cause postural hypotension, therefore additive hypotensive effects are possible with combined use, see antihypertensives, page 97.

> Increases or decreases in blood pressure may occur as a result of concurrent use. Monitor blood pressure adjusting the guanethidine dose as necessary.

Antipsychotics + H$_2$-receptor antagonists

Chlorpromazine, Clozapine or Droperidol

One study found that chlorpromazine concentrations are reduced by cimetidine, whereas a single case report describes clozapine toxicity when cimetidine was also taken. The manufacturers predict that cimetidine will inhibit the metabolism of droperidol.

> The general significance of these interactions is unclear, but it would seem prudent to monitor concurrent use for both excessive antipsychotic adverse effects (such as drowsiness, hypotension) and/or loss of efficacy. Consider monitoring clozapine concentrations.

Sertindole

Cimetidine is predicted to increase sertindole levels (by inhibiting CYP3A4), which might result in potentially fatal torsade de pointes, see Drugs that prolong the QT interval, page 352.

> The manufacturers contraindicate concurrent use.

Antipsychotics + **Herbal medicines or Dietary supplements**

Evening primrose oil

Although seizures have occurred in a few patients with schizophrenia taking phenothiazines with evening primrose oil, no adverse effects were seen in others, and there appears to be no firm evidence that evening primrose oil should be avoided by epileptic patients.

No action needed; it seems likely that the phenothiazine rather than the evening primrose oil caused this adverse reaction.

St John's wort (Hypericum perforatum)

The manufacturers of aripiprazole and paliperidone predict that St John's wort will reduce the level of these drugs.

The manufacturers recommend using double the dose of aripiprazole, then titrating to effect, in patients taking potent CYP3A4 inducers. The manufacturer of paliperidone advise monitoring paliperidone effects and adjusting the dose of paliperidone if necessary.

Antipsychotics + **HIV-protease inhibitors**

Aripiprazole

Aripiprazole is metabolised by CYP3A4, which is strongly inhibited by the HIV-protease inhibitors. Increased aripiprazole concentrations are therefore expected.

Caution and monitoring are recommended. The manufacturers suggest that the dose of aripiprazole should be halved.

Clozapine

Clozapine concentrations are predicted to be raised by ritonavir, resulting in serious haematological toxicity.

Concurrent use is contraindicated.

Haloperidol

The manufacturer predicts that ritonavir will increase haloperidol concentrations.

Monitor for haloperidol adverse effects (e.g. sedation, agitation, movement disorders) and consider a haloperidol dose reduction, if necessary. Note that concurrent use with saquinavir is predicted to increase the risk of QT prolongation, see Drugs that prolong the QT interval, page 352 for further information.

Olanzapine

Olanzapine concentrations are roughly halved by ritonavir.

If concurrent use is necessary monitor olanzapine efficacy and increase the dose if necessary. Note that concurrent use with saquinavir might increase the risk of QT

A

prolongation, see Drugs that prolong the QT interval, page 352 for further information.

Pimozide or Sertindole ⊗

Pimozide and sertindole are metabolised by CYP3A4, which is inhibited by the HIV-protease inhibitors. Raised pimozide or sertindole concentrations, which increase the risk of potentially fatal arrhythmias, would be expected.

Concurrent use is contraindicated. Note that concurrent use with saquinavir is predicted to increase the risk of QT prolongation, see Drugs that prolong the QT interval, page 352 for further information.

Quetiapine ⚠

Quetiapine exposure is markedly increased by *ketoconazole*, a potent inhibitor of CYP3A4. HIV-protease inhibitors are also inhibitors of CYP3A4 and are therefore predicted to interact similarly.

The UK manufacturer contraindicates concurrent use, whereas the US manufacturer advises that lower quetiapine doses might be needed. If concurrent use is necessary, monitor for signs of quetiapine adverse effects (e.g. dizziness, anxiety, orthostatic hypotension), and expect the need to reduce the quetiapine dose. Note that concurrent use with saquinavir might increase the risk of QT prolongation, see Drugs that prolong the QT interval, page 352 for further information.

Risperidone ⚠

Neuroleptic malignant syndrome, ataxia and severe lethargy leading to coma, and extrapyramidal adverse effects have been seen in patients given risperidone with indinavir and ritonavir.

If risperidone is given to any patient taking ritonavir (including ritonavir given as a pharmacokinetic enhancer) be alert for risperidone adverse effects (e.g. agitation, insomnia, headache, extrapyramidal effects). If these become troublesome consider decreasing the risperidone dose. Note that additive QT prolongation might occur on the concurrent use of risperidone and saquinavir boosted with ritonavir, see drugs that prolong the QT interval, page 352 for further information.

Thioridazine ⚠

Antiretroviral doses of ritonavir (300 mg twice daily or more) are predicted to increase thioridazine concentrations.

The manufacturer of ritonavir recommends monitoring for thioridazine adverse effects during concurrent use. Note that concurrent use with saquinavir is predicted to increase the risk of QT prolongation, see drugs that prolong the QT interval, page 352 for further information.

Antipsychotics + Levodopa ⚠

Centrally-acting dopamine antagonists (such as the antipsychotics, including prochlorperazine used at an antiemetic dose) may antagonise the effects of levodopa. The antipsychotic effects and extrapyramidal adverse effects of these drugs can be opposed by levodopa. Of the atypical antipsychotics, risperidone, and olanzapine cause deterioration in motor function in Parkinson's disease. Ziprasidone and

Antipsychotics + **Rifabutin** ⚠

Rifabutin is predicted to reduce aripiprazole levels.

The manufacturers recommend using double the dose of aripiprazole then titrating to effect. Remember to re-adjust the dose if rifabutin is stopped.

Antipsychotics + **Rifampicin (Rifampin)** ⚠

Rifampicin decreases haloperidol, risperidone (and its active metabolite, hydroxyrisperidone) and sertindole concentrations and is also predicted to decrease aripiprazole, paliperidone and quetiapine concentrations. Case reports suggest that rifampicin reduces clozapine concentrations.

Monitor the concurrent use of these antipsychotics with rifampicin: clozapine concentrations should be closely monitored. Be alert for the need to increase the dose of any of these antipsychotics in the presence of rifampicin. The manufacturers of sertindole state that the daily dose of sertindole might need to be increased towards the upper end of the maximum dose range. The manufacturers recommend that the dose of aripiprazole should be doubled. Note that increasing the dose of clozapine might not be successful in managing this interaction; it may be prudent to consider the use of other drugs. The UK manufacturer advises that enzyme inducers (such as rifampicin) should only be given with quetiapine if the benefits outweigh the risks: they suggest that consideration should be given to changing to a drug with no enzyme-inducing effects and name valproate.

Antipsychotics + **SSRIs**

Pimozide ✗

Pimozide exposure is moderately increased by paroxetine, slightly increased by sertraline, and is predicted to be raised by fluoxetine and fluvoxamine which could increase the risk of QT prolongation and potentially fatal torsade de pointes arrhythmias, see drugs that prolong the QT interval, page 352. The use of SSRIs and pimozide has also led to extrapyramidal adverse effects, oculogyric crises and sedation in rare cases. QT prolongation has been reported with the concurrent use of pimozide and citalopram, and escitalopram is predicted to interact similarly.

The UK manufacturer of pimozide contraindicates its use with all SSRIs as a class and they specifically name sertraline, paroxetine, citalopram, and escitalopram, whereas the US manufacturer contraindicates only sertraline, and additionally advises avoiding fluvoxamine.

Thioridazine ✗

Thioridazine concentrations are increased by fluvoxamine (about 3-fold), and are predicted to be increased by fluoxetine or paroxetine.

The manufacturers of fluoxetine, fluvoxamine and paroxetine contraindicate the concurrent use of thioridazine as raised concentrations increase the risk of QT prolongation, see drugs that prolong the QT interval, page 352. The use of thioridazine is also contraindicated for 5 weeks after fluoxetine has been stopped. The UK manufacturer suggests that the dose of thioridazine might need to be reduced when it is given with citalopram or escitalopram; however, a clinically important pharmacokinetic interaction seems unlikely. Note that caution is

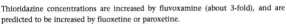

advised when thioridazine is taken with other drugs that can lower the seizure threshold such as the SSRIs.

Other antipsychotics ⚠

On the whole no significant adverse interactions appear to occur between most antipsychotics and the SSRIs. However, a number of case reports describe extrapyramidal adverse effects and serotonin syndrome following the use of fluoxetine or paroxetine with an antipsychotic. The concentrations of some antipsychotics are raised by SSRIs:

- Aripiprazole concentrations are raised by fluoxetine and paroxetine.
- Clozapine concentrations are raised by fluoxetine, paroxetine and sertraline: particularly large increases can occur with fluvoxamine. Toxicity has been seen in some patients. Studies suggest that citalopram generally does not interact, although one case report describes raised clozapine concentrations in a patient taking citalopram.
- Haloperidol concentrations are raised up to twofold by fluoxetine and by 20 to 60% by fluvoxamine. Sertraline caused a minor increase in haloperidol concentrations in one study, but not another. Escitalopram is predicted to increase haloperidol concentrations.Additive QT prolongation is predicted if citalopram, or possibly escitalopram, are given with haloperidol.
- Fluvoxamine moderately increases olanzapine exposure, increasing olanzapine adverse effects. Other SSRIs have negligible or no effect.
- Perphenazine exposure is markedly raised by paroxetine, and possibly raised by fluoxetine, which increased extrapyramidal adverse effects in a few cases.
- Quetiapine concentrations are possibly raised by fluvoxamine.
- Risperidone concentrations are moderately to markedly raised by fluoxetine and paroxetine, and slightly increased by fluvoxamine and sertraline.
- Sertindole concentrations are raised 2- to 3-fold by fluoxetine and paroxetine, which could increase the risk of QT prolongation.
- Zotepine concentrations are raised by fluoxetine by 10%; however, the concentrations of norzotepine are doubled.

Monitor the outcome of concurrent use and adjust the antipsychotic dose as necessary. Some have suggested that the antipsychotic dose should be re-evaluated before the SSRI is started. The manufacturers of sertindole suggest that low maintenance doses of sertindole are used and that ECG monitoring is necessary as sertindole can prolong the QT interval. A risperidone dose reduction by one-third has been suggested with fluoxetine. The manufacturers recommend halving the dose of aripiprazole with CYP2D6 inhibitors such as fluoxetine or paroxetine. In addition, the US manufacturer also recommends a 75% reduction in the aripiprazole dose when both a CYP2D6 inhibitor and a CYP3A4 inhibitor (such as ketoconazole, page 102) are given together. The manufacturers of olanzapine recommend that a lower starting dose, or a dose reduction, should be considered with fluvoxamine; a dose adjustment with SSRIs other than fluvoxamine is not expected to be necessary. A dose adjustment of risperidone with SSRIs other than fluoxetine or paroxetine is not expected to be necessary. Note that both groups of drugs lower the seizure threshold. Caution is advised when paliperidone or phenothiazines are taken with other drugs that might lower the seizure threshold, such as the SSRIs. Both citalopram and escitalopram cause QT prolongation, as do a number of the antipsychotics, see drugs that prolong the QT interval, page 352. It might be prudent to use an alternative SSRI which is not known to be associated with QT prolongation.

Antipsychotics + **Sucralfate** ⚠

Sucralfate can reduce the absorption of sulpiride by about 40%.

Separating dosing by 1 to 2 hours appears to minimise this interaction.

Antipsychotics + **Teduglutide** ❓

Teduglutide might increase the absorption of other drugs given concurrently, although evidence for this appears limited to an association with altered mental status in patients also taking benzodiazepines. The manufacturers state that the possibility of this effect should be considered, particularly for those drugs a narrow therapeutic range or where the dose is titrated against effect (they specifically name the phenothiazines), as dose adjustments might be required.

Until more is known, it would seem prudent to consider the possibility of an interaction if the adverse effects of these drugs increase in patients given teduglutide.

Antipsychotics + **Tricyclics** ❓

Studies and case reports have described increased tricyclic antidepressant levels with phenothiazines. There is currently evidence for this interaction between:

- chlorpromazine and imipramine
- flupentixol and imipramine or desipramine
- fluphenazine and imipramine
- haloperidol and desipramine
- levomepromazine and nortriptyline
- perphenazine and amitriptyline, imipramine, desipramine or nortriptyline
- thioridazine and desipramine, imipramine or nortriptyline

Further, antipsychotic levels may be raised or their clearance reduced by the tricyclics, and this has been seen with:

- amitriptyline, imipramine or nortriptyline and chlorpromazine

The concurrent use of antipsychotics and tricyclics has also resulted in extrapyramidal reactions and seizures (both groups of drugs lower the seizure threshold). Despite these reactions these drugs are widely used in combination, and a number of fixed-dose combinations have been marketed. Also note that additive QT-prolonging effects are possible with certain combinations, see drugs that prolong the QT interval, page 352.

Concurrent use is common. No action is generally needed but bear the interaction in mind in case of problems. Additive antimuscarinic adverse effects are also possible, see antimuscarinics, page 98.

Antipsychotics + **Valproate** ⚠

Valproate can apparently lower clozapine and olanzapine levels. Valproate may also *increase* clozapine levels. The combination of olanzapine and valproate appears to increase the risk of hepatic injury in children. Extended-release valproate semisodium (divalproex sodium) has been reported to increase the levels of paliperidone by 50%.

Bear in mind the potential for a change in the levels of clozapine and/or an increase in its adverse effects, and adjust the dose as necessary. With olanzapine, it has been suggested that liver enzymes should be monitored every 3 to 4 months for the first year of treatment, thereafter monitoring every 6 months if no adverse effects are detected. Consider a dose reduction of paliperidone if it is given with valproate semisodium (divalproex sodium).

Antipsychotics + Venlafaxine ⚠

Venlafaxine can almost double haloperidol levels. Adverse effects resulting from this interaction have been seen in practice.

Be aware that increased haloperidol adverse effects (e.g. sedation, agitation, movement disorders) may occur. It may be necessary to reduce the haloperidol dose.

Antipsychotics + Zileuton ⊗

Zileuton is predicted to increase pimozide exposure and increase the risk of QT-interval prolongation and the development of life-threatening arrhythmias.

The US manufacturer of pimozide contraindicates concurrent use.

Apixaban

Apixaban + Aspirin ⚠

The UK manufacturer of apixaban states that no pharmacokinetic or pharmacodynamic interaction occurs between apixaban and aspirin. Nevertheless, they predict that concurrent use might increase the risk of bleeding: significant bleeding was reported on concurrent use of apixaban with both aspirin and clopidogrel.

If concurrent use is necessary, monitor for signs of excessive bleeding.

Apixaban + Cilostazol ⚠

The UK manufacturer predicts that the effects of apixaban can be increased by drugs that affect platelet function, such as cilostazol.

If concurrent use is necessary, monitor for signs of excessive bleeding.

Apixaban + Clopidogrel ⚠

Phase I studies have reported that the concurrent use of apixaban and clopidogrel (with or without aspirin) does not affect bleeding time, platelet aggregation, or clotting tests; however, the UK manufacturer reports that concurrent use of apixaban with both aspirin and clopidogrel causes significant bleeding.

If concurrent use is necessary, monitor for signs of excessive bleeding.

Apixaban + **Dabigatran**

The concurrent use of apixaban with dabigatran might theoretically increase the risk of bleeding.

> The UK manufacturers of apixaban and dabigatran contraindicate concurrent use unless switching between anticoagulants; monitor for signs of excessive bleeding.

Apixaban + **Dipyridamole**

The UK manufacturer predicts that the effects of apixaban can be increased by drugs that affect platelet function, such as dipyridamole.

> If both drugs are necessary, monitor for signs of excessive bleeding.

Apixaban + **Heparin**

The UK manufacturer predicts that the effects of apixaban can be increased by other drugs that affect coagulation, such as heparin.

> The UK manufacturer of apixaban contraindicates concurrent use unless switching between anticoagulants; monitor for signs of excessive bleeding.

Apixaban + **Low-molecular-weight heparins**

The concurrent use of apixaban and enoxaparin has additive effects on anti-factor Xa activity, and therefore increases the risk of bleeding.

> The UK manufacturer of apixaban contraindicates concurrent use unless switching between anticoagulants; monitor for signs of excessive bleeding.

Apixaban + **NSAIDs**

The UK manufacturer predicts that the effects of apixaban can be increased by drugs that affect platelet function or increase the risks of bleeding, such as the NSAIDs.

> If both drugs are necessary, monitor for signs of excessive bleeding.

Apixaban + **Prasugrel**

The UK manufacturer predicts that the effects of apixaban can be increased by drugs that affect platelet function, such as prasugrel.

> If concurrent use is necessary, monitor for signs of excessive bleeding.

Apixaban + **Rivaroxaban**

The UK manufacturer predicts that the effects of apixaban can be increased by other drugs that affect coagulation, platelet function, or increase the risks of bleeding, such as rivaroxaban.

> The UK manufacturers of apixaban and rivaroxaban contraindicate concurrent

use unless switching between anticoagulants; if this is necessary, monitor for signs of excessive bleeding.

Apixaban + Sulfinpyrazone

The concurrent use of antiplatelet drugs with apixaban might theoretically increase the risk of bleeding.

The UK manufacturer of apixaban does not recommend concurrent use. If both drugs are essential, patients should be closely monitored for signs and symptoms of bleeding.

Apixaban + Ticagrelor

The UK manufacturer predicts that the effects of apixaban can be increased by drugs that affect platelet function, such as ticagrelor.

If both drugs are necessary, monitor for signs of excessive bleeding.

Apixaban + Ticlopidine

The UK manufacturer predicts that the effects of apixaban can be increased by drugs that affect platelet function, such as ticlopidine.

If concurrent use is necessary, monitor for signs of excessive bleeding.

Apixaban + Warfarin and related oral anticoagulants

The UK manufacturer predicts that the effects of apixaban can be increased by other drugs that affect coagulation, such as the oral anticoagulants.

The UK manufacturer of apixaban contraindicates concurrent use unless switching between anticoagulants; monitor for signs of excessive bleeding.

Apomorphine

Apomorphine + 5-HT₃-receptor antagonists

Extrapyramidal adverse effects, profound hypotension and loss of consciousness have been reported with the concurrent use of ondansetron and subcutaneous apomorphine (for Parkinson's disease). Other 5-HT₃-receptor antagonists may interact similarly.

The US manufacturer of subcutaneous apomorphine for Parkinson's disease contraindicates concurrent use of all 5-HT₃-receptor antagonists. However, the manufacturers of sublingual apomorphine used for erectile dysfunction state that it may be used safely with ondansetron.

Apomorphine + Metoclopramide

Metoclopramide is a centrally-acting dopamine antagonist and can oppose the effects of apomorphine, and also worsen Parkinson's disease.

Concurrent use should generally be avoided. Domperidone is the antiemetic of choice in Parkinson's disease, and may also be used safely in patients taking sublingual apomorphine for erectile dysfunction.

Aprepitant

Fosaprepitant is a prodrug of aprepitant, and therefore has the potential to interact similarly.

Aprepitant + Azoles

Ketoconazole increases the AUC of aprepitant 5-fold. The manufacturer predicts that itraconazole, posaconazole and voriconazole may interact similarly. Fosaprepitant, a prodrug of aprepitant, would be expected to interact similarly.

The manufacturers recommend caution when aprepitant is given with these azoles. The lowest dose of aprepitant may be appropriate. Counsel patients about aprepitant adverse effects (e.g. hiccups, fatigue, constipation, headache).

Aprepitant + Benzodiazepines

Aprepitant increases the exposure to oral midazolam after a few days of concurrent use. A few days after aprepitant treatment is stopped a transient slight reduction in midazolam plasma concentrations could occur. Aprepitant appears to have less effect on *intravenous* midazolam. Triazolam, and to a lesser extent alprazolam, are expected to be affected similarly. Fosaprepitant, a prodrug of aprepitant, has also been shown to increase oral midazolam exposure.

Aprepitant would be expected to increase the drowsiness and length of sedation and amnesia in patients given midazolam (and possibly alprazolam or triazolam). Consider reducing the dose of these benzodiazepines and monitor the outcome of concurrent use carefully. The effects of aprepitant on the plasma concentration of intravenously administered benzodiazepines are expected to be less than its effects on those administered orally.

Aprepitant + Calcium-channel blockers

The concurrent use of aprepitant and diltiazem increases the levels of both drugs by almost 2-fold, although this did not result in any significant cardiovascular effects. Fosaprepitant moderately raises diltiazem levels, and a small decrease in blood pressure was reported. It seems likely that verapamil will interact with both drugs in the same way as diltiazem.

Consider giving the lowest dose of aprepitant and be alert for aprepitant adverse effects such as hiccups, fatigue, constipation and headache. Also be aware of a potential decrease in blood pressure if either of these antiemetics is given to a patient taking diltiazem or verapamil.

Aprepitant + **Carbamazepine**

Rifampicin, a potent inducer of CYP3A4, reduces the exposure to aprepitant by 91%; reduced efficacy would be expected. Carbamazepine, another potent inducer of CYP3A4, is predicted to interact similarly, both with aprepitant, and its prodrug, fosaprepitant.

The UK manufacturer recommends that concurrent use should be avoided.

Aprepitant + **Ciclosporin (Cyclosporine)**

Aprepitant can increase the exposure to CYP3A4 substrates such as ciclosporin, in the short term then reduce their exposure within 2 weeks. Fosaprepitant, a prodrug of aprepitant, would be expected to interact similarly.

Ciclosporin concentrations and/or effects (e.g. on renal function) should be monitored as a matter of routine, but it may be prudent to increase monitoring if either drug is stopped, started, or the dose altered.

Aprepitant + **Colchicine**

Aprepitant and its pro-drug, fosaprepitant, are predicted to increase the exposure to colchicine.

The US manufacturer of colchicine recommends that the colchicine dose is reduced in patients taking moderate CYP3A4 inhibitors, such as aprepitant, or if they have stopped taking any of these drugs within 2 weeks of starting colchicine, see Ciclosporin (Cyclosporine) + Colchicine, page 251 for further details. The manufacturers also contraindicate the concurrent use of colchicine and P-glycoprotein inhibitors, such as aprepitant or fosaprepitant, in patients with renal or hepatic impairment.

Aprepitant + **Contraceptives**

Aprepitant reduces the levels of ethinylestradiol and norethisterone (given as an oral combined hormonal contraceptive). Greater effects were seen in another study when dexamethasone was also given with aprepitant. Contraceptive efficacy would be expected to be reduced. Fosaprepitant, a prodrug of aprepitant, would be expected to interact similarly. The contraceptive efficacy of oral progestogen-only contraceptives, the progestogen-only implant and emergency hormonal contraceptives (both progestogen-only and combined hormonal preparations) are also expected to be reduced.

The manufacturer recommends that alternative or additional contraceptive methods should be used during aprepitant therapy and for 2 months (UK advice) or one month (US advice) after the last dose of aprepitant. The same advice is given for fosaprepitant. In the UK, the Faculty of Sexual and Reproductive Healthcare (FSRH) include aprepitant in their list of enzyme inducing drugs in their 2011 guideline on hormonal contraception and drug interactions; see contraceptives, page 288, for details of this guidance.

Aprepitant + Corticosteroids

In the short-term, aprepitant increases the AUC of dexamethasone (by about 2.2-fold) and methylprednisolone (by up to 2.5-fold). Fosaprepitant, a prodrug of aprepitant, would be expected to interact similarly.

> The manufacturers recommend that the usual dose of dexamethasone should be reduced by about 50% when given with aprepitant (although note that the dose given in the manufacturer's dexamethasone/aprepitant antiemetic regimen accounts for the interaction).. They also recommend that the usual dose of intravenous methylprednisolone is reduced by 25%, and the usual oral dose by 50%, in the presence of aprepitant. However, the manufacturer also notes that during continuous treatment with methylprednisolone, levels would be expected to *decrease* over the following 2 weeks. The effect is expected to be greater if methylprednisolone is given orally rather than intravenously.

Aprepitant + Dapoxetine

Aprepitant, and therefore its prodrug fosaprepitant, are predicted to increase the exposure to dapoxetine. As dapoxetine is also metabolised by CYP2D6, CYP2D6 metaboliser status is predicted to also affect this interaction.

> The Swedish manufacturer of dapoxetine recommends a maximum dose of dapoxetine 30 mg on concurrent use with aprepitant. In patients known to be CYP2D6 extensive metabolisers (which is generally unlikely), the manufacturer advises a maximum dapoxetine dose of 60 mg.

Aprepitant + Darifenacin

Aprepitant is predicted to increase the exposure to darifenacin in the short-term, then reduce its exposure within 2 weeks. Fosaprepitant, a prodrug of aprepitant, is expected to interact similarly.

> Monitor for an increase in darifenacin adverse effects. Dose reductions might be needed. On longer-term use, monitor for darifenacin efficacy.

Aprepitant + Ergot derivatives

Aprepitant can increase the exposure to CYP3A4 substrates such as ergot derivatives, in the short-term, then reduce their exposure within 2 weeks. Ergotism could occur. Fosaprepitant, a prodrug of aprepitant, would be expected to interact similarly.

> The effect may persist for 2 weeks after aprepitant is stopped. Avoid the combination where possible. Concurrent use needs close monitoring (e.g. for cold extremities and other signs of ergot adverse effects).

Aprepitant + **Everolimus**

Aprepitant can increase the exposure to CYP3A4 substrates such as everolimus in the short-term, then reduce their exposure within 2 weeks. Fosaprepitant, a prodrug of aprepitant, would be expected to interact similarly.

> Everolimus concentrations and/or effects (e.g. on renal function) should be monitored as a matter of routine, but it would be prudent to increase monitoring if either drug is started, stopped, or the dose altered.

Aprepitant + **Fesoterodine**

Aprepitant is predicted to increase the exposure to fesoterodine in the short-term, then reduce its exposure within 2 weeks. Fosaprepitant, a prodrug of aprepitant, is predicted to interact similarly.

> Bear in mind the possibility of an interaction should an increase in adverse effects occur (e.g. dry mouth, dizziness, insomnia). On longer-term use, monitor for fesoterodine efficacy. Concurrent use should be avoided in patients with severe renal impairment, and a maximum fesoterodine dose of 4 mg daily given to those with mild to moderate renal impairment. Concurrent use should also be avoided in patients with moderate or severe hepatic impairment, and a maximum dose of fesoterodine 4 mg daily given to those with mild hepatic impairment.

Aprepitant + **Gestrinone**

The manufacturers warn that *rifampicin* (*rifampin*) might increase the metabolism of gestrinone and thereby reduce its effects. Other enzyme inducers, such as aprepitant and its prodrug, fosaprepitant, might interact similarly.

> The clinical significance of this warning is unclear and there appear to be no reports of an interaction in practice; however, be aware that gestrinone might be less effective if aprepitant or fosaprepitant are given concurrently.

Aprepitant + **Herbal medicines or Dietary supplements**

Rifampicin, a potent inducer of CYP3A4, reduces the exposure to aprepitant by 91%; reduced efficacy would be expected. St John's wort, another inducer of CYP3A4, is predicted to interact similarly, both with aprepitant, and its prodrug, fosaprepitant.

> The UK manufacturer recommends that concurrent use should be avoided.

Aprepitant + **HIV-protease inhibitors**

Ketoconazole increases the AUC of aprepitant 5-fold. The manufacturers suggest that potent inhibitors of CYP3A4 may interact similarly; the US manufacturer specifically names ritonavir and nelfinavir although other HIV-protease inhibitors could also interact in this way. Fosaprepitant, a prodrug of aprepitant, would be expected to interact with the HIV-protease inhibitors in the same way as aprepitant.

> The lowest dose of aprepitant may be appropriate. Counsel patients about adverse effects (e.g. hiccups, fatigue, constipation, headache).

Aprepitant + HRT

The hormones in HRT are similar to those used in hormonal contraceptives, page 122, and so may be affected by enzyme-inducing drugs, such as aprepitant, in the same way. Note that fosaprepitant, a prodrug of aprepitant, would also be expected to reduce HRT levels.

> The clinical significance of any interaction is unclear; however, consider the possibility of reduced HRT efficacy. This effect would be most likely noticed where HRT is prescribed for menopausal vasomotor symptoms, but might be difficult to detect where the indication is osteoporosis. The interaction is not relevant to HRT applied locally for menopausal vaginitis.

Aprepitant + Macrolides

Ketoconazole, a potent CYP3A4 inhibitor, increases the exposure to aprepitant 5-fold. The manufacturer predicts that clarithromycin and telithromycin will interact similarly. Fosaprepitant, a prodrug of aprepitant, would also be expected to interact with these macrolides in this way.

> The manufacturer recommends caution when aprepitant is used with any potent inhibitor of CYP3A4 (they name clarithromycin and telithromycin). The lowest dose of aprepitant may be appropriate. Counsel patients about adverse effects (e.g. hiccups, fatigue, constipation, headache). Other macrolides may also interact, although it seems unlikely that they all will, see macrolides, page 474.

Aprepitant + Opioids

Aprepitant can increase the exposure to CYP3A4 substrates (such as alfentanil and fentanyl) in the short-term, then reduce their exposure within 2 weeks. Fosaprepitant, a prodrug of aprepitant, would be expected to interact similarly.

> If concurrent use is considered necessary monitor for prolonged sedation and respiratory depression. Dose reductions may be needed. On longer-term use monitor for fentanyl or alfentanil efficacy.

Aprepitant + Oxybutynin

Aprepitant is predicted to increase the exposure to oxybutynin in the short-term, then reduce its exposure within 2 weeks. Further evidence suggests interactions between oxybutynin and CYP3A4 inhibitors are not clinically relevant, however manufacturers advise an increase in oxybutynin concentration cannot be ruled out. Fosaprepitant, a prodrug of aprepitant, is predicted to interact similarly.

> Monitor for an increase in oxybutynin adverse effects, such as dry mouth, constipation, and drowsiness, and reduce the dose if needed. On longer-term use, monitor for oxybutynin efficacy.

Aprepitant + Phenobarbital

Rifampicin, a potent inducer of CYP3A4, reduces the exposure to aprepitant (and probably its prodrug, fosaprepitant) by 91%; reduced efficacy would be expected. Phenobarbital (and therefore probably primidone), another potent inducer of CYP3A4, is predicted to interact similarly.

The UK manufacturer recommends that concurrent use should be avoided.

Aprepitant + **Phenytoin**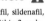

The manufacturers predict that phenytoin (and therefore probably its prodrug, fosphenytoin) may reduce the levels of aprepitant and therefore reduce its efficacy. Phenytoin levels may also be reduced by aprepitant. Fosaprepitant, a prodrug of aprepitant, would be expected to interact similarly.

Avoid concurrent use. If both drugs are given monitor aprepitant (and fosaprepitant) and phenytoin (and fosphenytoin) efficacy carefully.

Aprepitant + **Phosphodiesterase type-5 inhibitors**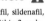

Aprepitant can increase the exposure to CYP3A4 substrates (e.g. avanafil, sildenafil, tadalafil, and vardenafil) in the short term then reduce their exposure within 2 weeks. Fosaprepitant, a prodrug of aprepitant, would be expected to interact similarly.

Monitor for an increase in phosphodiesterase type-5 inhibitor adverse effects (such as headache, flushing, and visual disturbances). Dose reductions might be needed. On longer-term use, monitor for phosphodiesterase type-5 inhibitor efficacy. The US manufacturer advises that a maximum avanafil dose of 50 mg every 24 hours should not be exceeded with moderate CYP3A4 inhibitors, such as aprepitant. The UK manufacturer however, advises a maximum dose of 100 mg once every 48 hours with moderate CYP3A4 inhibitors.

Aprepitant + **Quinidine**

Aprepitant can increase the exposure to CYP3A4 substrates such as quinidine, in the short term then reduce them within 2 weeks. Fosaprepitant, a prodrug of aprepitant, would be expected to interact similarly.

Monitor for adverse effects such as hypotension, tinnitus and diarrhoea. If these occur, take quinidine plasma concentrations, if possible. Reduce the quinidine dose as necessary.

Aprepitant + **Rifampicin (Rifampin)**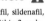

Rifampicin, an inducer of CYP3A4, reduces the exposure to aprepitant by 91%, and reduced efficacy would be expected. Fosaprepitant, a prodrug of aprepitant, would be expected to interact similarly.

The UK manufacturer recommends that concurrent use should be avoided.

Aprepitant + **Sirolimus**

Aprepitant is predicted to raise the levels of CYP3A4 substrates (such as sirolimus), then reduce them within 2 weeks. Fosaprepitant, a prodrug of aprepitant, would be expected to interact similarly.

> Sirolimus levels and/or effects (e.g. on renal function) should be monitored as a matter of routine, but it may be prudent to increase monitoring if either drug is stopped, started, or the dose altered.

Aprepitant + Solifenacin

Aprepitant is predicted to increase the exposure to solifenacin in the short-term, then reduce its exposure within 2 weeks. Fosaprepitant, a prodrug of aprepitant, is predicted to interact similarly.

> Monitor for an increase in solifenacin adverse effects. Dose reductions might be needed. On longer-term use, monitor for solifenacin efficacy.

Aprepitant + Tacrolimus

Aprepitant is predicted to raise the levels of CYP3A4 substrates (such as tacrolimus), then reduce them within 2 weeks. Fosaprepitant, a prodrug of aprepitant, would be expected to interact similarly.

> Tacrolimus levels and/or effects (e.g. on renal function) should be monitored as a matter of routine, but it may be prudent to increase monitoring if either drug is stopped, started, or the dose altered.

Aprepitant + Tolterodine

Aprepitant is predicted to increase the exposure to tolterodine in the short-term, then reduce its exposure within 2 weeks. Fosaprepitant, a prodrug of aprepitant is predicted to interact similarly.

> Monitor for an increase in tolterodine adverse effects. Dose reductions might be needed. On longer-term use, monitor for tolterodine efficacy.

Aprepitant + Ulipristal

Moderate inhibitors of CYP3A4, such as aprepitant, are predicted to moderately increase the exposure to ulipristal. Fosaprepitant, a prodrug of aprepitant, would be expected to interact in a similar way.

> The UK manufacturer of low-dose ulipristal for the symptomatic management of uterine fibroids does not recommend its concurrent use with moderate CYP3A4 inhibitors. If low-dose ulipristal is given with aprepitant or fosaprepitant, monitor for an increase in the adverse effects of ulipristal (for example nausea, abdominal pain, and breast tenderness) or any unexpected outcome occurring during concurrent use. The UK manufacturer of ulipristal for emergency contraception states that CYP3A4 inhibitors are unlikely to have any clinically relevant effects.

A

Aprepitant + **Warfarin and related oral anticoagulants** ⚠

Aprepitant modestly reduces warfarin levels and slightly decreases the INR in healthy subjects. Fosaprepitant, a prodrug of aprepitant, would be expected to interact similarly.

The manufacturer recommends that the INR should be monitored closely for 2 weeks, particularly 7 to 10 days after each 3-day course of aprepitant. They also recommend similar caution with acenocoumarol. Similar advice is given by the manufacturers of fosaprepitant.

Artemether

Co-artemether is a combination product containing artemether and lumefantrine, and its interactions are discussed under the individual constituents.

Artemether + **Azoles** ✅

Ketoconazole moderately increased the exposure to artemether in one study. However, this is within the range of inter-individual variability and no changes in ECG parameters or increases in adverse events were reported.

This increase is unlikely to be clinically relevant, and the UK manufacturer advises that no dose adjustment is necessary when artemether with lumefantrine is given with ketoconazole.

Artemether + **Food** ❓

Food, especially high-fat food, moderately increases the bioavailability of artemether.

As soon as patients can tolerate food, artemether should be taken with food to increase absorption. Patients who are unable to eat during treatment should be closely monitored as they might be at greater risk of treatment failure.

Artemether + **Grapefruit juice** ✅

Grapefruit juice increases the exposure to artemether.

Based on the evidence with ketoconazole, page 128, this increase is not expected to be clinically significant and no dose adjustment of artemether is required.

Aspirin

Aspirin + **Cilostazol** ⚠

The concurrent use of more than one antiplatelet drug might increase the risk of bleeding. However, the incidence of bleeding does not appear to be further increased if cilostazol is added to low-dose aspirin. In contrast, in patients taking clopidogrel and aspirin, the addition of cilostazol might increase the risk of bleeding.

> Combinations of antiplatelet drugs are commonly used and can be clinically beneficial; however, be aware of the increased risk of bleeding. Note that the European Medicines Agency contraindicate the use of cilostazol with two or more antiplatelet drugs or anticoagulants. The US manufacturer of cilostazol generally advises caution on the concurrent use of other antiplatelet drugs.

Aspirin + Clopidogrel

The clinical benefit of giving aspirin with clopidogrel is established for some indications; however, there is an increased risk of bleeding relative to either drug alone.

> Although combinations of antiplatelet drugs are commonly used, be aware of the increased risk of bleeding. The UK manufacturer advises a maximum dose of aspirin 100 mg daily with concurrent use of clopidogrel.

Aspirin + Contraceptives

Hormonal contraceptives lower aspirin levels. A few early reports suggest that the very occasional failure of copper IUDs to prevent pregnancy may have been due to an interaction with aspirin.

> The evidence is insufficient to justify general precautions. No action is needed.

Aspirin + Corticosteroids

Salicylate levels are reduced by corticosteroids, and therefore salicylate levels may rise, possibly to toxic concentrations, if the corticosteroid is withdrawn without salicylate dose adjustment. Concurrent use increases the risk of gastrointestinal bleeding and ulceration.

> Patients taking high-dose salicylates should be monitored to ensure that the levels remain adequate when corticosteroids are added and do not become excessive if they are withdrawn.

Aspirin + Dabigatran

The concurrent use of aspirin and high-dose dabigatran slightly increased the risk of major haemorrhage.

> The UK manufacturer of dabigatran does not recommend concurrent use with aspirin. If both drugs are essential, patients should be closely monitored for signs and symptoms of bleeding. It would be prudent to similarly monitor the concurrent use of antiplatelet doses of aspirin.

Aspirin + Dipyridamole

The concurrent use of more than one antiplatelet drug might increase the risk of bleeding. However, the addition of dipyridamole to low-dose aspirin does not appear to further increase the incidence of bleeding.

> The concurrent use of dipyridamole and aspirin can be clinically beneficial for some indications. However, it might be prudent to monitor concurrent use for an increase in bleeding particularly in patients who are at a high risk of bleeding.

Aspirin + Diuretics

Loop diuretics ❓

Aspirin may reduce the diuretic effect of bumetanide, furosemide, and piretanide, and the combination of aspirin and furosemide may increase the risk of acute renal failure and salicylate toxicity. The risk of ototoxicity with high doses of salicylates may theoretically be increased by loop diuretics.

> The clinical significance of this interaction is unclear. However, aspirin should be avoided in patients with recurrent hospital admissions for worsening heart failure. Salicylate toxicity may occur if furosemide is given concurrently in patients receiving high doses of salicylates. Be aware that renal impairment and ototoxicity are a possibility in patients receiving high dose of salicylates, and consider increasing monitoring for these effects.

Spironolactone ❓

Although studies in healthy subjects have found that the spironolactone-induced loss of sodium in the urine is reduced, a study in hypertensive patients showed that the blood pressure-lowering effects of spironolactone were not affected by analgesic dose aspirin.

> Concurrent use need not be avoided, but if the diuretic response to spironolactone is less than expected, consider this interaction as a cause.

Aspirin + Duloxetine ❓

The bleeding risk associated with antiplatelet drugs such as aspirin might be further increased by the concurrent use of an SSRI, although the data appears to be conflicting. SNRIs (e.g. duloxetine) are expected to interact similarly.

> The UK manufacturers of duloxetine advise caution on concurrent use in patients taking antiplatelet drugs (such as aspirin). Consider giving gastroprotective drugs to those at high risk of gastrointestinal bleeding (e.g. the elderly, those with a history of gastrointestinal bleeding, patients taking multiple antiplatelet drugs). Advise patients to report any signs of excessive bleeding.

Aspirin + Food ✅

Food delays the absorption of aspirin but does not affect the overall amount absorbed.

> Avoid food if rapid analgesia is needed. Otherwise aspirin is better taken with or after food to minimise gastric irritation.

Aspirin + **Gold**

A study in patients given analgesic doses of aspirin suggested that the concurrent use of gold can increase aspirin-induced hepatotoxicity.

> Other analgesics, such as fenoprofen, appear safer than aspirin (in analgesic doses) so it is probably wise to consider an alternative analgesic.

Aspirin + **Heparin**

Although the concurrent use of aspirin and heparin is indicated in specific situations (such as acute coronary syndromes), combined use slightly increases the risk of haemorrhage, and may contribute to the development of epidural or spinal haematoma after epidural anaesthesia.

> Unless specifically indicated, it may be prudent to avoid the combined use of aspirin with heparin because of the likely increased risk of bleeding. Patients should be monitored closely for signs of bleeding. Extreme caution is needed if combined use is considered appropriate in patients undergoing epidural anaesthesia.

Aspirin + **Herbal medicines or Dietary supplements**

Fish Oils

The concurrent use of aspirin and fish oils caused at least additive effects on bleeding time in healthy subjects, although clinical studies in patients taking aspirin alone, and with clopidogrel, found no evidence of an increase incidence of bleeding episodes. Bleeding is more likely with high-dose fish oils (more than 4 g daily).

> Bear the possibility of increased bleeding in mind on concurrent use. Note that a lower dose preparation (1 g daily) is also licensed to be used with other standard therapies, including antiplatelets, as adjuvant treatment after myocardial infarction.

Ginkgo biloba

Ginkgo biloba alone has been associated with platelet, bleeding, and clotting disorders, and there are isolated reports of clinically significant bleeding after its concurrent use with antiplatelet drugs such as aspirin. However, several studies have found no evidence of an increased risk of bleeding with concurrent use.

> The evidence is too slim to advise patients against taking aspirin with *Ginkgo biloba*, but some do recommend caution. This seems prudent as caution is generally recommended with concurrent use of more than one conventional antiplatelet drug. Patients should be told to seek professional advice if any bleeding problems arise.

Tamarindus indica

Tamarindus indica (tamarind) fruit extract markedly increased the absorption of aspirin and caused a 3-fold increase in its levels.

> The clinical relevance of this interaction is unknown, but large rises in the levels of analgesic dose aspirin may result in toxicity. Bear this in mind if analgesic doses of aspirin are taken with this fruit extract.

A

Aspirin + Kaolin

Kaolin-pectin causes a small reduction in the absorption of aspirin, which is not clinically relevant.

No action needed.

Aspirin + Low-molecular-weight heparins ⚠

Although the concurrent use of aspirin and a low-molecular-weight-heparin is indicated in specific situations (such as acute coronary syndromes), combined use slightly increases the risk of haemorrhage. Cases of retroperitoneal and spinal haematoma have been reported with concurrent use of low-molecular-weight heparins (e.g. enoxaparin) and aspirin.

Unless specifically indicated, it may be prudent to avoid the combined use of aspirin with a low-molecular-weight-heparin because of the likely increased risk of bleeding. Patients should be monitored closely for signs of bleeding. Extreme caution is needed if combined use is considered appropriate in patients undergoing epidural anaesthesia.

Aspirin + Methotrexate

Analgesic-dose aspirin slightly reduces the clearance of methotrexate. Concurrent use may increase the incidence of methotrexate toxicity (pancytopenia, pneumonitis).

Regular antiplatelet-dose aspirin in patients stabilised on methotrexate seems unlikely to cause a significant problem. With analgesic-dose aspirin the risks are likely to be lowest in those taking low-dose methotrexate for psoriasis or rheumatoid arthritis. Patients should be counselled regarding non-prescription aspirin use. Patients should be told to report any sign or symptom suggestive of infection, particularly sore throat (which might possibly indicate that white cell counts have fallen) or dyspnoea or cough (suggestive of pulmonary toxicity).

Aspirin + Metoclopramide

Although some studies have found that metoclopramide increases the rate of aspirin absorption, others have found no change, and the clinical efficacy of aspirin seems unaltered.

No action needed. This may be a beneficial interaction if a faster onset of analgesia is needed.

Aspirin + Mifepristone

Theoretically NSAIDs (including aspirin) might reduce the efficacy of mifepristone, and combined use is often not recommended. However, evidence from two studies with naproxen and diclofenac suggests no reduction in mifepristone efficacy.

Because of theoretical concerns of antagonistic effects, NSAID analgesics have been avoided in protocols for medical abortion. However, the limited available evidence suggests that this might not be necessary.

Aspirin + NSAIDs

Non-selective NSAIDs might antagonise the antiplatelet effects of aspirin and reduce its cardioprotective effects. Some NSAIDs (particularly coxibs and diclofenac) are also associated with an increased thrombotic/cardiovascular risk. Combined use of NSAIDs (including coxibs) and aspirin, even in low-dose, increases the risk of gastrointestinal bleeds.

> The need for any NSAID should be very carefully considered as NSAIDs (particularly coxibs and diclofenac, but also other non-selective NSAIDs) are associated with an increased thrombotic/cardiovascular risk, particularly when used at high doses and for long-term treatment. Therefore coxibs and diclofenac are contraindicated, and other NSAIDs should generally be avoided, in those with ischaemic heart disease, cerebrovascular disease, or peripheral artery disease. Diclofenac is also contraindicated in those with congestive heart failure. In addition, the European Society of Cardiology guidelines recommend that patients resistant to antiplatelet treatment should not be given either coxibs or non-selective NSAIDs with aspirin, and recommend that coxibs and NSAIDs should not be used after myocardial infarction. If antiplatelet dose aspirin is used with NSAIDs, gastroprotection (e.g. a proton pump inhibitor) should be considered, especially when other risk factors (e.g. corticosteroids) are present. There is no clinical rationale for the combined use of anti-inflammatory/analgesic doses of aspirin and NSAIDs, and such use should be avoided.

Aspirin + Phenytoin

Although it has been suggested that aspirin enhances the effects of phenytoin, there appears to be no good evidence to show that a clinically significant interaction occurs.

> No action needed.

Aspirin + Prasugrel

The concurrent use of aspirin and prasugrel might increase the risk of bleeding. The risk appears to vary with different combinations of antiplatelet drugs: one study found that the risk of bleeding with concurrent use of aspirin with prasugrel was greater than that seen with *clopidogrel*.

> Although combinations of antiplatelet drugs are commonly used and can be clinically beneficial, be aware of the increased risk of bleeding.

Aspirin + Probenecid

The uricosuric effects of high doses of aspirin or other salicylates and probenecid are mutually antagonistic. Low dose, enteric-coated aspirin appears not to interact.

> Regular dosing with substantial amounts of salicylates should be avoided, but small very occasional analgesic doses probably do not matter. Salicylate levels of 50 to 100 mg/L are necessary before this interaction occurs.

Aspirin + Quinidine

A patient and two healthy subjects given quinidine with aspirin (325 mg twice daily or

A

more) showed a 2- to 3-fold increase in bleeding times. The patient developed petechiae and gastrointestinal bleeding.

> This interaction appears to result from the additive effects of the two drugs. Be aware of the potential for this interaction if the combination is used. However, significant interactions seem rare.

Aspirin + Rivaroxaban ❓

Aspirin does not affect the pharmacokinetics of rivaroxaban, or cause a clinically relevant change in the anticoagulant effects of rivaroxaban. However, the bleeding time during concurrent use might be slightly prolonged. Note that aspirin increases the risk of bleeding, and concurrent use with rivaroxaban might possibly increase this risk.

> Advise patients to be aware of increased bruising or prolonged bleeding, and to seek medical advice if this occurs.

Aspirin + SSRIs ❓

The SSRIs might increase the risk of upper gastrointestinal bleeding and the risk appears to be further increased by the concurrent use of antiplatelet drugs including aspirin. The overall evidence for an increased risk of bleeding when giving an SSRI with antiplatelet-dose aspirin is conflicting, with some studies demonstrating an increased risk and others suggesting no additional antiplatelet effect occurs.

> In general, the manufacturers of the SSRIs advise caution on the concurrent use of drugs that affect platelet function, such as aspirin. If the combination of an SSRI and aspirin cannot be avoided, consider giving a gastroprotective drug (such as a proton pump inhibitor), especially to those at high risk of gastrointestinal bleeding (such as the elderly, those with a history of gastrointestinal bleeding, or patients taking multiple antiplatelet drugs). Advise patients to report any signs of excessive bleeding. Note that this advice would also apply to those patients taking analgesic-dose aspirin with an SSRI.

Aspirin + Sulfinpyrazone ⚠

The uricosuric effects of the salicylates, including analgesic-dose aspirin, and sulfinpyrazone are mutually antagonistic.

> Concurrent use for uricosuria should be avoided. Analgesic doses of aspirin as low as 700 mg can cause an appreciable fall in uric acid excretion. Regular dosing with substantial amounts of salicylates should be avoided, but small very occasional analgesic doses probably do not matter. Salicylate levels of 50 to 100 mg/L are necessary before this interaction occurs. Note that sulfinpyrazone can cause gastric bleeding and inhibit platelet aggregation which may be additive with aspirin.

Aspirin + Ticagrelor ❓

The concurrent use of ticagrelor and aspirin might increase the risk of bleeding, and the efficacy of ticagrelor might be reduced with doses of aspirin greater than 300 mg daily.

> Ticagrelor is specifically licensed for use with aspirin, but be aware of the increased

risk of bleeding. The UK manufacturer of ticagrelor states that an aspirin dose of 75 to 150 mg daily should be used, and, because of the potential for a decrease in the efficacy of ticagrelor, aspirin doses above 300 mg daily are not recommended. However, in the US, doses of aspirin above 100 mg daily are not recommended, and the US manufacturers state that a dose of aspirin of 75 to 100 mg daily should be used with ticagrelor.

Aspirin + Ticlopidine

Low-dose aspirin and ticlopidine have additive inhibitory effects on platelet aggregation and combined use increases the risk of bleeding relative to aspirin alone.

Although combinations of antiplatelet drugs can be clinically beneficial, be aware of the increased risk of bleeding. Note that US manufacturer states that the safety of concurrent use beyond 30 days has not been established.

Aspirin + Valproate

Sodium valproate toxicity developed in several patients given large and repeated doses of aspirin and one elderly patient given regular low-dose aspirin.

Any interaction seems rare. Bear the potential for an interaction in mind should any unexpected valproate adverse effects occur in patients taking aspirin, particularly in high doses, and consider advising patients to monitor for indicators of valproate toxicity (such as nausea, vomiting, dizziness, rash, ataxia).

Aspirin + Venlafaxine

The bleeding risk associated with antiplatelet drugs such as aspirin might be further increased by the concurrent use of an SSRI, although the data appears to be conflicting. SNRIs (e.g. venlafaxine) are expected to interact similarly.

The UK manufacturer of venlafaxine advises caution on concurrent use in patients taking antiplatelet drugs (such as aspirin). Consider giving gastroprotective drugs to those at high risk of gastrointestinal bleeding (e.g. the elderly, those with a history of gastrointestinal bleeding, patients taking multiple antiplatelet drugs). Advise patients to report any signs of excessive bleeding.

Aspirin + Vitamin C 🚫

Aspirin appears to reduce the absorption of vitamin C by about one-third.

The clinical importance of this interaction is unclear, however it has been suggested that normal physiological requirements of vitamin C (30 to 60 mg ascorbic acid daily) may need to be increased to 100 to 200 mg daily.

Aspirin + Warfarin and related oral anticoagulants ⚠

High doses of aspirin (4 g daily or more) can increase prothrombin times. It also damages the stomach wall, which increases the risks of bleeding. Low-dose aspirin (75 to 325 mg daily) increases the risk of bleeding when given with warfarin, although,

A

in most studies the absolute risks have been small. Increased warfarin effects have been seen when the salicylates methyl salicylate or trolamine salicylate, were used on the skin.

It is usual to avoid analgesic and anti-inflammatory doses of aspirin while taking any anticoagulant. Patients should be told that many non-prescription analgesic, antipyretic, cold and influenza preparations might contain substantial amounts of aspirin. Warn them that it might be listed as acetylsalicylic acid. Paracetamol (acetaminophen) is a safer analgesic substitute (but not entirely without problems). Low-dose aspirin is also associated with an increased risk of bleeding. However, in certain patient groups (for example, those with prosthetic heart valves at high risk of thromboembolism) the benefits might outweigh the risks. Consider adding a gastroprotective drug in those who are at risk of gastrointestinal bleeding. In addition, in the long-term, aspirin doses should be limited to no more than 81 mg daily in those taking oral anticoagulants. Any interaction with topical salicylates seems likely to be rare.

Aspirin + Zafirlukast

The plasma concentration of zafirlukast is modestly increased by analgesic-dose aspirin.

This interaction is not expected to be clinically relevant.

Atomoxetine

Atomoxetine + MAOIs

The manufacturer notes that other drugs that affect brain monoamine levels (like atomoxetine) have caused serious reactions (including symptoms of serotonin syndrome, page 580 and symptoms similar to neuroleptic malignant syndrome) when taken with MAOIs.

The manufacturer contraindicates the use of atomoxetine during and for 2 weeks after stopping an MAOI.

Atomoxetine + Mirtazapine

Atomoxetine is a sympathomimetic that acts as a noradrenaline (norepinephrine) reuptake inhibitor. The manufacturers therefore predict that it may have additive or synergistic pharmacological effects with other drugs that affect noradrenaline, such as mirtazapine.

The manufacturer recommends caution. Be aware that additive effects are possible and monitor e.g. somnolence or agitation, as appropriate.

Atomoxetine + Nasal decongestants

Atomoxetine is a sympathomimetic that acts as a noradrenaline (norepinephrine) reuptake inhibitor. The manufacturers therefore predict that it may have additive or synergistic pharmacological effects with other drugs that affect noradrenaline, such as pseudoephedrine.

> The manufacturer recommends caution. Be aware that additive effects are possible and monitor e.g. somnolence or agitation, as appropriate.

Atomoxetine + Quinidine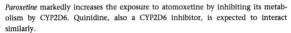

Paroxetine markedly increases the exposure to atomoxetine by inhibiting its metabolism by CYP2D6. Quinidine, also a CYP2D6 inhibitor, is expected to interact similarly.

> It would seem prudent to monitor for an increase in atomoxetine adverse effects (somnolence, agitation). The atomoxetine dose should be titrated slowly with the dose increased only if symptoms fail to improve and if the initial dose is well tolerated. The US manufacturer suggests a starting dose of atomoxetine 0.5 mg/kg daily (40 mg per day in those over 70 kg) and only increasing the dose to 1.2 mg/kg daily (or 80 mg per day) if symptoms do not improve after 4 weeks and the initial dose is well tolerated. The UK manufacturer states that the initial dose should be maintained for a minimum of 7 days before considering an increase. Note that both atomoxetine and quinidine have been associated with QT prolongation, see Drugs that prolong the QT interval, page 352 for more information.

Atomoxetine + Salbutamol (Albuterol) and related bronchodilators

Atomoxetine potentiated the increase in heart rate and blood pressure caused by salbutamol infusions in one study, but another study found no adverse interaction.

> The manufacturers recommend caution when atomoxetine is given to patients receiving intravenous, oral, or high-dose nebulised salbutamol or other beta$_2$ agonists. Monitor heart rate and blood pressure carefully in the initial stages of concurrent use. Note that atomoxetine and drugs that can cause hypokalaemia (such as salbutamol and related bronchodilators) have been associated with QT prolongation, see Drugs that prolong the QT interval, page 352 for more information.

Atomoxetine + SSRIs

Paroxetine markedly increases the exposure to atomoxetine, which might increase the incidence of adverse effects. Fluoxetine appears to interact similarly.

> It would seem prudent to monitor for an increase in adverse effects (somnolence, agitation). The atomoxetine dose should be started low and titrated slowly. The US manufacturer suggests a starting dose of atomoxetine 0.5 mg/kg daily (40 mg per day in those over 70 kg) and only increasing the dose to 1.2 mg/kg daily (or 80 mg per day) if symptoms do not improve after 4 weeks and the initial dose is well tolerated. The UK manufacturer states that the initial dose should be maintained for a minimum of 7 days before considering an increase. Note that atomoxetine and some SSRIs (escitalopram and citalopram) have been associated with QT prolongation, see Drugs that prolong the QT interval, page 352 for more information.

Atomoxetine + Terbinafine

Paroxetine markedly increases the exposure to atomoxetine by inhibiting its metabolism by CYP2D6. Terbinafine, also a CYP2D6 inhibitor, is expected to interact similarly.

It would seem prudent to monitor for an increase in adverse effects (somnolence, agitation). The atomoxetine dose should be started low and titrated slowly, with the dose increased only if symptoms fail to improve and if the initial dose is well tolerated. The US manufacturer suggests a starting dose of atomoxetine 0.5 mg/kg daily (40 mg per day in those over 70 kg) and only increasing the dose to 1.2 mg/kg daily (or 80 mg per day) if symptoms do not improve after 4 weeks and the initial dose is well tolerated. The UK manufacturer states that the initial dose should be maintained for a minimum of 7 days before considering an increase.

Atomoxetine + Tricyclics

Atomoxetine is a sympathomimetic that acts as a noradrenaline (norepinephrine) reuptake inhibitor. The manufacturers therefore predict that it may have additive or synergistic pharmacological effects with other drugs that affect noradrenaline, such as imipramine, and other tricyclics.

The manufacturer recommends caution. Be aware that additive effects are possible and monitor e.g. somnolence or agitation, as appropriate. Note that both atomoxetine and the tricyclics have been associated with QT prolongation, see Drugs that prolong the QT interval, page 352 for more information.

Atomoxetine + Venlafaxine

Atomoxetine is a sympathomimetic that acts as a noradrenaline (norepinephrine) reuptake inhibitor. The manufacturers therefore predict that it may have additive or synergistic pharmacological effects with other drugs that affect noradrenaline, such as venlafaxine.

The manufacturer recommends caution. Be aware that additive effects are possible and monitor e.g. somnolence or agitation, as appropriate.

Atovaquone

Atovaquone + Food

Fatty foods markedly increase the exposure to atovaquone tablets and suspension.

Atovaquone (with proguanil) tablets should be taken with food or a milky drink, and atovaquone suspension should be taken with food or with an enteral nutritional supplement with a high-fat content. Monitor patients who are unable to tolerate taking atovaquone with food for treatment failure: consider intravenous treatment in the case of pneumocystis pneumonia.

Atovaquone + HIV-protease inhibitors

Atovaquone causes a minor decrease in the minimum concentration of indinavir, and might increase saquinavir exposure. The UK and US manufacturers of ritonavir predict that it will decrease atovaquone concentrations, and this has been seen with both atazanavir and lopinavir boosted with ritonavir.

The UK manufacturer of atovaquone recommends caution because of the potential risk of indinavir treatment failure, although the effect on indinavir alone was small. However, indinavir is usually used with ritonavir as a pharmacological booster and with other antiretrovirals, which might modify the interaction. Some manufacturers recommend careful monitoring of atovaquone concentrations and/or therapeutic effects when it is used with HIV-protease inhibitors boosted with ritonavir as it is possible that both prophylaxis and treatment with atovaquone might be ineffective. A dose increase might be necessary. Note that other manufactures advise avoiding concurrent use.

Atovaquone + Metoclopramide

Preliminary evidence suggests that metoclopramide decreases the concentration of atovaquone.

The UK manufacturer of atovaquone suspension recommends caution on the concurrent use of metoclopramide, whereas the US manufacturer of atovaquone suspension does not mention metoclopramide. If an antiemetic is required in patients taking atovaquone with proguanil, the US manufacturer suggests that metoclopramide should be given only if other antiemetics are unavailable, whereas the UK manufacturer does not recommend concurrent use.

Atovaquone + NNRTIs

Atovaquone exposure appears to be moderately reduced by efavirenz.

The reduction in atovaquone exposure by efavirenz could result in reduced efficacy. It would therefore seem prudent to avoid concurrent use.

Atovaquone + NRTIs

Slight increases in zidovudine exposure have been seen with atovaquone in one study, whereas another study found no pharmacokinetic changes.

The increased zidovudine exposure is unlikely to increase its adverse effects during a short-course of atovaquone and no dose adjustments are required. Nevertheless, the UK manufacturer of atovaquone recommends regular monitoring for zidovudine-associated adverse effects, particularly if atovaquone suspension is used, as this achieves higher atovaquone concentrations. For longer courses of atovaquone, monitor concurrent use for zidovudine toxicity (such as bone marrow suppression).

Atovaquone + Rifabutin

In one study the concurrent use of atovaquone and rifabutin resulted in a slight decrease in the exposure to atovaquone.

It has been suggested that no atovaquone dose adjustment is needed. However, the

A

UK and US manufacturers of atovaquone still consider that rifabutin could result in subtherapeutic atovaquone concentrations and so the UK manufacturer advises against concurrent use.

Atovaquone + Rifampicin (Rifampin)

Rifampicin reduces the plasma concentration of atovaquone and atovaquone raises the plasma concentration of rifampicin.

Concurrent use should be avoided because of the likelihood of sub-therapeutic atovaquone concentrations.

Atovaquone + Tetracyclines

Tetracycline reduces the plasma concentration of atovaquone.

The manufacturers suggest that parasitaemia should be closely monitored in patients taking atovaquone (with proguanil) and tetracycline. In the UK, they also state that tetracycline should be given with caution to patients taking atovaquone suspension.

Azathioprine

Azathioprine is rapidly and extensively metabolised to mercaptopurine. Mercaptopurine is therefore expected to share the interactions of azathioprine.

Azathioprine + Balsalazide

The haematological toxicity of azathioprine and mercaptopurine may be increased by 5-aminosalicylates. Balsalazide may be less likely to interact although this requires confirmation.

Full blood counts should be monitored routinely if azathioprine or mercaptopurine is used; however, it may be prudent to increase the frequency of monitoring when starting this combination. If any abnormalities arise, consider this interaction as a possible cause.

Azathioprine + Co-trimoxazole

There is some evidence that the risk of haematological toxicity may be increased in renal transplant patients taking azathioprine if they are also given co-trimoxazole (which contains sulfamethoxazole with trimethoprim) or trimethoprim, particularly if both drugs are taken for extended periods. However, other evidence suggests that the drugs may be used together safely, and the combination is commonly used in practice. Azathioprine is rapidly and extensively metabolised to mercaptopurine. Mercaptopurine is therefore expected to interact similarly.

Full blood count should be monitored if azathioprine or mercaptopurine is used. If any abnormalities arise, consider this interaction as a possible cause.

Azathioprine + Febuxostat

The manufacturers of febuxostat predict that it will increase the levels of azathioprine. Azathioprine is rapidly and extensively metabolised to mercaptopurine. Mercaptopurine is therefore expected to interact similarly.

> Concurrent use is not recommended by the UK manufacturers and is contraindicated by the US manufacturers. If the concurrent use of febuxostat is considered essential, it would seem prudent to reduce the dose of azathioprine or mercaptopurine and monitor closely for haematological toxicity.

Azathioprine + Leflunomide

The manufacturers state that the concurrent use of leflunomide and azathioprine has not yet been studied but it would be expected to increase the risk of serious adverse reactions (haematological toxicity or hepatotoxicity). Azathioprine is rapidly and extensively metabolised to mercaptopurine. Mercaptopurine is therefore expected to interact similarly.

> The manufacturers advise avoiding concurrent use. As the active metabolite of leflunomide has a long half-life of 1 to 4 weeks, a washout with colestyramine or activated charcoal should be given if patients are to be switched to other DMARDs.

Azathioprine + Mesalazine (Mesalamine)

The haematological toxicity of azathioprine and mercaptopurine may be increased by mesalazine.

> Full blood counts should be monitored if azathioprine or mercaptopurine is used; however it may be prudent to increase the frequency of monitoring when starting this combination. If any abnormalities arise, consider this interaction as a possible cause.

Azathioprine + Mycophenolate

The manufacturers have recommended that mycophenolate should not be given with azathioprine because concurrent use has not been studied and both drugs have the potential to cause bone marrow suppression. Azathioprine is rapidly and extensively metabolised to mercaptopurine. Mercaptopurine is therefore expected to interact similarly.

> Avoid concurrent use.

Azathioprine + Olsalazine

The haematological toxicity of azathioprine and mercaptopurine may be increased by olsalazine.

> Full blood counts should be monitored if azathioprine or mercaptopurine is used; however, it may be prudent to increase the frequency of monitoring when starting this combination. If any abnormalities arise, consider this interaction as a possible cause.

A

Azathioprine + **Sulfasalazine**

The haematological toxicity of azathioprine and mercaptopurine may be increased by sulfasalazine.

> Full blood counts should be monitored if azathioprine or mercaptopurine is used; however, it may be prudent to increase the frequency of monitoring when starting this combination. If any abnormalities arise, consider this interaction as a possible cause.

Azathioprine + **Sulfonamides**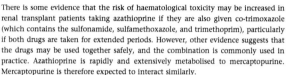

There is some evidence that the risk of haematological toxicity may be increased in renal transplant patients taking azathioprine if they are also given co-trimoxazole (which contains the sulfonamide, sulfamethoxazole, and trimethoprim), particularly if both drugs are taken for extended periods. However, other evidence suggests that the drugs may be used together safely, and the combination is commonly used in practice. Azathioprine is rapidly and extensively metabolised to mercaptopurine. Mercaptopurine is therefore expected to interact similarly.

> Full blood count should be monitored if azathioprine or mercaptopurine is used. If any abnormalities arise, consider this interaction as a possible cause.

Azathioprine + **Trimethoprim**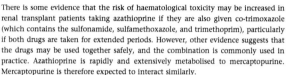

There is some evidence that the risk of haematological toxicity may be increased in renal transplant patients taking azathioprine if they are also given trimethoprim, particularly if both drugs are taken for extended periods. However, other evidence suggests that the drugs may be used together safely, and the combination of azathioprine or mercaptopurine and trimethoprim with sulfamethoxazole is commonly used in practice. Azathioprine is rapidly and extensively metabolised to mercaptopurine. Mercaptopurine is therefore expected to interact similarly.

> Full blood count should be monitored if azathioprine or mercaptopurine is used. If any abnormalities arise, consider this interaction as a possible cause.

Azathioprine + **Vaccines** ❌

The immune response of the body is suppressed by cytotoxic antineoplastics. The effectiveness of vaccines may be poor and generalised infection may occur in patients immunised with live vaccines. In one study the antibody response to pneumococcal vaccination was reduced by 60% in patients receiving antineoplastics, and suboptimal responses to influenza and measles vaccines have been reported.

> Live vaccines should not be given to patients who are receiving cytotoxics or other immunosuppressant antineoplastics. In the UK, it is recommended that live vaccines should not be given during or within at least 6 months of such treatment. Monitor the immune response to other types of vaccine. Consider whether vaccination can be carried out before or after azathioprine or mercaptopurine use.

Azathioprine + **Warfarin and related oral anticoagulants**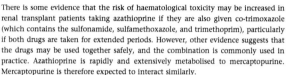

Azathioprine appears to increase warfarin requirements, and cases of bleeding have occurred when azathioprine is stopped. Dose increases of up to 4-fold have been needed. Mercaptopurine appears to interact similarly with acenocoumarol.

Monitor the anticoagulant effect closely if azathioprine or mercaptopurine is added or withdrawn and adjust the warfarin dose as necessary. Similar precautions would seem necessary with any coumarin.

Azoles

The azole antifungals are potent enzyme inhibitors, but they do not all affect the same isoenzymes. This explains their differing interaction profiles.

- Fluconazole is a potent inhibitor of CYP2C9 and CYP2C19, and generally only inhibits CYP3A4 at high doses (greater than 200 mg daily). Interactions are less likely with single doses used for genital candidiasis than with longer term use.
- Itraconazole and its major metabolite, hydroxy-itraconazole, are potent inhibitors of CYP3A4.
- Ketoconazole is a potent inhibitor of CYP3A4.
- Miconazole is a potent inhibitor of CYP2C9.
- Posaconazole is an inhibitor of CYP3A4.
- Voriconazole is an inhibitor of CYP2C9, CYP2C19 and CYP3A4, a moderate inhibitor of CYP2C19 and a weak inhibitor of CYP2C9.

A number of other azoles are only used topically in the form of skin creams or intravaginal preparations, and are not usually been associated with drug interactions, presumably because their systemic absorption is so low. However, note that isolated cases of an interaction have been reported with coumarins, page 174. Fluconazole, ketoconazole and voriconazole have been associated with prolongation of the QT interval, although generally not to a clinically relevant extent. However, they may also raise the levels of other drugs that prolong the QT interval, and these combinations are often contraindicated.

Azoles + Benzodiazepines

Midazolam and Triazolam

Itraconazole and ketoconazole markedly or very markedly increase the exposure to oral midazolam and triazolam, thereby increasing and prolonging their sedative and amnesic effects. Fluconazole moderately increases the exposure to oral midazolam and triazolam; intravenous midazolam is less affected. Posaconazole and voriconazole moderately to markedly increases both oral and intravenous midazolam exposure; triazolam might be similarly affected.

Most manufacturers contraindicate the concurrent use of oral midazolam or triazolam with itraconazole or ketoconazole. Similarly, the manufacturer of miconazole oral gel also contraindicates use with triazolam and oral midazolam. Expect increased and prolonged sedation. If concurrent use with an azole is necessary, consider reducing the dose of midazolam or triazolam. Dose adjustments of single bolus doses of intravenous midazolam might not be necessary (except with posaconazole); however, the dose of high-dose, long-term intravenous midazolam will need to be titrated to avoid long-lasting hypnotic effects. Patients should be warned about increased sedation and counselled against driving or undertaking other skilled tasks.

Other benzodiazepines

The effects of the benzodiazepines might be increased and prolonged by azole antifungals. Modest pharmacokinetic interactions have been seen between alprazolam and itraconazole or ketoconazole, and brotizolam and itraconazole. Fluconazole and voriconazole moderately increase the exposure to diazepam. Alprazolam and brotizolam should also be used with caution with oral miconazole. Posaconazole is expected to increase exposure to alprazolam. Ketoconazole or itraconazole slightly increase the exposure to the non-benzodiazepine hypnotics, zolpidem, eszopiclone, and zopiclone. Voriconazole slightly increases the exposure to zolpidem.

The deepness of sleep and its duration might be increased. Monitor the outcome of concurrent use and consider decreasing the benzodiazepine or zopiclone, eszopiclone, or zolpidem dose. Patients should be warned about increased sedation and counselled against driving or undertaking other skilled tasks. Note that while most manufacturers advise caution on concurrent use, a few manufacturers contraindicate the concurrent use of ketoconazole or itraconazole with alprazolam and brotizolam.

Azoles + Bicalutamide

The manufacturer of bicalutamide predicts that inhibitors of CYP3A4 may increase the levels of bicalutamide, which may increase the risk of adverse effects: they specifically name ketoconazole.

The manufacturer advises caution as bicalutamide adverse effects may be increased. However, as steady-state levels of bicalutamide are highly variable, any increase seems unlikely to be clinically relevant.

Azoles + Buspirone ⚠

Buspirone exposure is markedly increased by itraconazole (13-fold). Ketoconazole and voriconazole are likely to interact similarly, and posaconazole and fluconazole might also interact in this way, but to a lesser extent. The UK manufacturer also predicts that miconazole oral gel (which at high doses, might be sufficiently absorbed to potentially have systemic effects) will interact similarly.

The manufacturers recommend reducing the buspirone dose to 2.5 mg either daily or twice daily if itraconazole is used. Similar dose reductions would seem prudent with ketoconazole and voriconazole. Some caution is also needed with posaconazole and fluconazole. The manufacturer of miconazole oral gel also advises caution and suggests that buspirone dose reductions might be needed on concurrent use.

Azoles + Busulfan ⚠

Itraconazole reduces the clearance of busulfan by a modest 20%. There is some limited evidence that ketoconazole may increase the risk of hepatic veno-occlusive disease in those given high-dose busulfan. The manufacturer of miconazole oral gel (which may be sufficiently absorbed to potentially have systemic effects) predicts that it will also inhibit the metabolism of busulfan.

Although the rise in levels is only moderate, it would be prudent to monitor for busulfan toxicity. The manufacturer of miconazole oral gel suggests that dose reductions of busulfan may be necessary. Fluconazole appears not to interact, and so may be a useful alternative.

Azoles + Calcium-channel blockers

Lercanidipine

Ketoconazole markedly increases lercanidipine levels up to about 8-fold. Itraconazole, posaconazole and voriconazole are expected to interact similarly. Fluconazole is only likely to interact in doses of greater than 200 mg daily. At the maximum doses miconazole oral gel is sufficiently absorbed to potentially have systemic effects, and may also interact.

The concurrent use of lercanidipine with itraconazole or ketoconazole is contra-indicated. If other azoles are given with lercanidipine, be alert for the need to lower the lercanidipine dose and monitor for adverse effects, such as hypotension, headache, flushing, and oedema.

Other calcium-channel blockers

Itraconazole can raise felodipine levels up to 8-fold, which increases its adverse effects, in particular ankle and leg oedema. Ketoconazole can have a similar effect on nisoldipine levels. A few case reports suggest that isradipine and nifedipine can interact similarly with itraconazole, and that fluconazole can also interact with nifedipine. It is likely that all calcium-channel blockers will be affected in the same way, although probably to a greater or lesser extent. Posaconazole and voriconazole are expected to increase calcium-channel blocker levels. Fluconazole is only likely to interact in doses of greater than 200 mg daily. At the maximum doses miconazole oral gel is sufficiently absorbed to potentially have systemic effects, and may also interact.

Monitor the outcome of concurrent use, being prepared to reduce the dose of calcium-channel blocker as necessary. Monitor for calcium-channel blocker adverse effects, such as hypotension, headache, flushing, and oedema.

Azoles + Carbamazepine

Fluconazole or Miconazole

Carbamazepine toxicity has been caused by fluconazole and miconazole.

Evidence is limited. Nevertheless, monitor for signs of carbamazepine toxicity, which can present as nausea, vomiting, ataxia or drowsiness, and adjust the carbamazepine dose if necessary.

Other azoles

Carbamazepine, either alone or when given with phenobarbital or phenytoin, has been shown to markedly decrease itraconazole concentrations resulting in treatment failure. Carbamazepine is predicted to decrease posaconazole and voriconazole concentrations. Ketoconazole causes a small to moderate rise in serum carbamazepine concentrations; other azoles might interact similarly.

Concurrent use should be avoided unless the benefits are expected to outweigh the risks, although note that the use of voriconazole is specifically contraindicated. If concurrent use is necessary it seems likely that the antifungal dose will need to be increased. It would seem prudent to use other alternatives wherever possible or monitor efficacy very closely. Be alert for any evidence of increased carbamazepine adverse effects (e.g. nausea, vomiting, ataxia and drowsiness).

Azoles + Ciclosporin (Cyclosporine)

Ketoconazole

Ciclosporin concentrations increase rapidly and sharply with ketoconazole. Topical ketoconazole 2% cream has been reported to not interact with ciclosporin.

Monitor the concentrations and effects (e.g. on renal function) of ciclosporin more frequently if ketoconazole is started or stopped, adjusting the ciclosporin dose as necessary. Ciclosporin dose reductions of 70 to 80% might be required.

Posaconazole

Posaconazole can increase ciclosporin concentrations: ciclosporin toxicity has occurred. Ciclosporin is predicted to increase posaconazole concentrations.

The UK and US manufacturers suggest that the dose of ciclosporin should be reduced by about 25% when posaconazole is started, with careful monitoring of ciclosporin plasma concentrations and effects (e.g. on renal function) and further dose adjustment as needed, including when posaconazole is stopped.

Voriconazole

Voriconazole increases ciclosporin concentrations.

The dose of ciclosporin should be halved when initiating voriconazole, and ciclosporin concentrations and effects (e.g. on renal function) should be carefully monitored during treatment, with further dose adjustment as needed. The ciclosporin dose should be increased again when voriconazole is withdrawn.

Other azoles

The evidence suggests that all the azoles can increase ciclosporin concentrations to a greater or lesser degree. A case report suggests that intravenous miconazole interacts similarly and, in theory, miconazole oral gel might also interact (in high doses it may be sufficiently absorbed to interact systemically). However, many patients might not be affected. Rhabdomyolysis has been reported with the combination of ciclosporin and itraconazole, but four of these cases were complicated by the presence of statins.

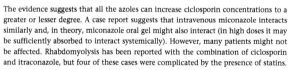

Ciclosporin plasma concentrations and/or effects (e.g. on renal function) should be monitored as a matter of routine, but the frequency of monitoring should be increased and the dose of ciclosporin adjusted accordingly if these azoles are stopped, started, or if the doses are altered. Dose reductions of 50% or more have been reported to be needed with fluconazole and itraconazole.

Azoles + **Cilostazol**

Ketoconazole increases the exposure to cilostazol and its active metabolite, resulting in an overall increase in its pharmacological activity: increased cilostazol adverse effects (such as headache and diarrhoea) might occur. Itraconazole and voriconazole are predicted to interact similarly. Fluconazole, miconazole, and posaconazole might also interact, but probably to a lesser extent.

> The MHRA in the UK advises that the dose of cilostazol should be reduced to 50 mg twice daily when given with ketoconazole or itraconazole. Similar reductions would be advisable for voriconazole, and, the UK and US manufacturers of cilostazol state that the same dose reduction should be extended to fluconazole and miconazole.

Azoles + **Cinacalcet**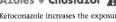

Ketoconazole raises cinacalcet levels 2-fold and increased the incidence of cinacalcet adverse effects. Itraconazole and voriconazole are predicted to interact similarly.

> It may be prudent to monitor parathyroid hormone and serum calcium more frequently if any of these azoles is started or stopped.

Azoles + **Clopidogrel**

Fluconazole or Voriconazole

On the basis of the interaction with the proton pump inhibitors, some predict that fluconazole and voriconazole may theoretically inhibit the conversion of clopidogrel to its active metabolite by CYP2C19.

> The MHRA in the UK, the FDA in the US and the manufacturers advise against the concurrent use of clopidogrel with fluconazole or voriconazole.

Itraconazole or Ketoconazole

In one study, ketoconazole modestly reduced the formation of the active metabolite of clopidogrel, and reduced its antiplatelet effect. Itraconazole has also been reported to reduce the antiplatelet effect of clopidogrel, but only in subjects of one genotype.

> Evidence for an interaction between clopidogrel and these azoles is limited; however, until further data is available some caution is warranted. Bear the possibility of an interaction in mind.

Azoles + **Colchicine**

Ketoconazole increases colchicine exposure and is predicted to increase the risk of colchicine toxicity. Fluconazole, itraconazole, posaconazole, and voriconazole are predicted to interact similarly.

> If any patient is given colchicine with an azole, be alert for colchicine adverse effects (such as nausea, vomiting, and diarrhoea), especially in patients with pre-existing renal impairment. Anticipate the need to reduce the colchicine dose. The US manufacturer makes specific recommendations for colchicine dose reductions in patients taking potent CYP3A4 inhibitors (they name ketoconazole and itraconazole), and moderate CYP3A4 inhibitors (they name fluconazole), or if

they have stopped taking any of these azoles within 2 weeks of starting colchicine. See Colchicine + Macrolides, page 285, for further information. Note that voriconazole is a potent CYP3A4 inhibitor and posaconazole is a moderate CYP3A4 inhibitor, and as such the relevant dosing information might be equally applied to these azoles. Note that the UK and US manufacturers of colchicine contraindicate the concurrent use of colchicine with itraconazole, ketoconazole, or voriconazole in patients with renal or hepatic impairment.

Azoles + Contraceptives ❓

There are isolated reports of breakthrough bleeding and failure of oral combined hormonal contraceptives with fluconazole, itraconazole and ketoconazole. However, fluconazole, itraconazole, ketoconazole and voriconazole have been shown to modestly *increase* the levels of contraceptive steroids. In the case of voriconazole, the increase was considered roughly equivalent to increasing the ethinylestradiol dose from 35 micrograms to 50 micrograms. Intravaginal miconazole slightly increases the levels of ethinylestradiol and etonogestrel during the use of an intravaginal contraceptive ring. Oral combined hormonal contraceptives modestly increase the AUC of voriconazole. Itraconazole appears to increase the exposure to the active metabolite of desogestrel, which might increase the incidence of desogestrel adverse effects. A similar interaction may occur with etonogestrel (when given as the combined hormonal contraceptive vaginal ring or progestogen-only implant).

Although anecdotal reports suggest that these antifungals can rarely make hormonal contraception less reliable, the pharmacokinetic data suggest that, if anything, an *enhanced* effect of the combined hormonal contraceptives is likely. Note that, of all the other drugs proven to decrease the efficacy of combined hormonal contraceptives, all have also been shown to decrease contraceptive steroid levels. Furthermore, the manufacturers do not advise any additional precautions when taking oral contraceptives and azoles. However, some consider that the data warrant consideration being given to the use of additional contraceptive measures. The theoretical teratogenic risk from these azoles may have a bearing on this. The clinical relevance of the increase in voriconazole levels is unclear; however, bear the possibility of increased voriconazole adverse effects in mind on concurrent use. It is unclear if the increase in ethinylestradiol or progestogen exposure will increase the risk of adverse effects; however, until more is known, bear the possibility of an interaction in mind should an increase in contraceptive steroid adverse effects (e.g. nausea and breast tenderness) occur.

Azoles + Corticosteroids ⚠

There is some evidence that itraconazole can increase the exposure to, and/or effects of, oral deflazacort, dexamethasone, methylprednisolone, and to a lesser extent, prednisolone and prednisone, as well as inhaled budesonide and fluticasone. Cases of Cushing's syndrome have been reported. One manufacturer predicts that inhaled beclometasone and ciclesonide might be similarly affected. Similarly, ketoconazole reduces the metabolism and clearance of methylprednisolone, might increase the exposure the active metabolite of ciclesonide, increases the systemic effects of inhaled budesonide and possibly inhaled fluticasone, and markedly increases the exposure to oral budesonide. One manufacturer predicts that inhaled beclometasone might be similarly affected.

Bear a possible interaction in mind if itraconazole or ketoconazole are given to patients receiving any systemic or inhaled corticosteroid as most are metabolised, at least in part, by CYP3A4—see azoles, page 143. Patients should be warned to be alert for any evidence of increased corticosteroid effects (such as moon face, weight gain, hyperglycaemia) and to seek medical advice if these occur. Be alert for the need to reduce the steroid dose; dose reductions of up to 50% have been recommended if ketoconazole is given with methylprednisolone. Note that increased corticosteroid immunosuppression might be undesirable in those with a fungal infection. Some UK manufacturers of inhaled and oral budesonide advise against the concurrent use with itraconazole or ketoconazole. However, if the concurrent use of inhaled or oral budesonide and itraconazole or ketoconazole cannot be avoided, the time interval between giving the two drugs should be as long as possible (for example 12 hours in the case of ketoconazole), and that reducing the budesonide dose should be considered. Adrenal function should also be monitored in patients receiving inhaled budesonide or fluticasone who are also given itraconazole because of the reports of Cushing's syndrome. Similar advice is given for intranasal budesonide, and the UK manufacturer of budesonide rectal foam also advises avoiding the concurrent use of itraconazole or ketoconazole. The manufacturers of ciclesonide suggest that the concurrent use of ketoconazole or itraconazole should be avoided unless the benefits outweigh the risks. Similarly, the manufacturer of fluticasone recommends caution, and, if possible, the avoidance of long-term treatment with itraconazole or ketoconazole. Voriconazole appears to have less of an effect on prednisolone than itraconazole and might therefore be a suitable alternative.

Azoles + Cyclophosphamide

Fluconazole and itraconazole inhibit the metabolism of cyclophosphamide. There is some evidence that, compared with fluconazole, itraconazole might increase cyclophosphamide toxicity.

Until more is known caution is advised when azoles are used in patients taking cyclophosphamide (other than therapies established in randomised clinical studies) being alert for unexpected toxicity or reduced efficacy.

Azoles + Dabigatran

Ketoconazole increases dabigatran exposure. Itraconazole and posaconazole are predicted to interact similarly.

The UK manufacturer of dabigatran contraindicates concurrent use with ketoconazole, whereas the US manufacturer recommends that the dabigatran dose is reduced to 75 mg twice daily in patients being treated for stroke prophylaxis in atrial fibrillation who have moderate renal impairment. Monitor for signs of bleeding or anaemia, and discontinue dabigatran if severe bleeding occurs. The UK manufacturer of dabigatran advises against the concurrent use of posaconazole.

Azoles + Dapoxetine

Fluconazole ▲

Fluconazole is predicted to increase the exposure to dapoxetine. As dapoxetine is also metabolised by CYP2D6, CYP2D6 metaboliser status is predicted to also affect this interaction.

The Swedish manufacturer of dapoxetine recommends a maximum dose of dapoxetine 30 mg on concurrent use with fluconazole.. In patients known to be CYP2D6 extensive metabolisers (which is generally unlikely), the manufacturer advises a maximum dapoxetine dose of 60 mg.

Itraconazole or Ketoconazole

Ketoconazole, a potent CYP3A4 inhibitor, doubles the exposure to dapoxetine. Itraconazole is expected to interact similarly.

The clinical relevance of the increase in dapoxetine exposure is unclear. However, an important adverse reaction of dapoxetine is syncope or orthostatic hypotension, and this is dose-related. Therefore, the manufacturer contraindicates the concurrent use of dapoxetine with ketoconazole or itraconazole. Note that dapoxetine is also metabolised by CYP2D6 and if the patient is known to be a CYP2D6 extensive metaboliser (which is generally unlikely), a 30-mg dose may be used.

Azoles + Darifenacin

Fluconazole and Posaconazole

Fluconazole causes a moderate increase in darifenacin exposure. Posaconazole would be expected to behave similarly.

The UK manufacturers recommend an initial darifenacin dose of 7.5 mg daily in those taking moderate CYP3A4 inhibitors (such as fluconazole or posaconazole), increasing to 15 mg daily if the initial dose is well tolerated. The US manufacturers suggest that no dose adjustment is needed. Bear in mind the possibility of an interaction if antimuscarinic adverse effects (dry mouth, constipation, drowsiness) are increased.

Itraconazole, Ketoconazole and Voriconazole

Ketoconazole markedly increases the exposure to darifenacin by up to 10-fold. Itraconazole and possibly voriconazole would be expected to interact similarly.

The UK manufacturers contraindicate concurrent use whereas the US manufacturers recommend that the daily dose of darifenacin is limited to 7.5 mg daily. It may be prudent to assess adverse effects (such as dry mouth, constipation, and drowsiness) in these patients, and withdraw the drug if it is not tolerated.

Azoles + Digoxin

Itraconazole can cause a marked increase in digoxin levels (usually doubled, but a 6-fold increase was seen in one case). Toxicity may occur unless the digoxin dose is suitably reduced. Ketoconazole and posaconazole are predicted to interact similarly. Itraconazole may have significant negative inotropic effects, and this may oppose the pharmacological effects of digoxin.

Monitor concurrent use for digoxin toxicity (e.g. bradycardia or nausea), taking digoxin levels as necessary. Adjust the dose accordingly. Note that, based on the interaction with itraconazole, the manufacturer of posaconazole advises monitoring digoxin levels.

Azoles + Disopyramide

Itraconazole and ketoconazole are predicted to increase disopyramide levels, which increases the risk of arrhythmias. Other azoles, page 143 are likely to interact similarly, although probably to a greater or lesser extent.

The UK manufacturers of ketoconazole and itraconazole contraindicate concurrent use, whereas the US manufacturer of itraconazole advises caution. If the concurrent use of disopyramide and any azole is essential, monitor the patient for an increase in disopyramide adverse effects (such as dry mouth, blurred vision, urinary retention and nausea).

Azoles + Diuretics

Eplerenone with Fluconazole

Fluconazole increases the AUC of eplerenone 2.2-fold.

The dose of eplerenone should not exceed 25 mg daily. Monitor for an increase in dose-related adverse effects such as hyperkalaemia.

Eplerenone with Itraconazole or Ketoconazole

Ketoconazole increases the AUC of eplerenone 5.4-fold. Itraconazole is predicted to interact similarly.

Concurrent use of either itraconazole or ketoconazole is contraindicated.

Hydrochlorothiazide with Fluconazole

A very brief report describes a slight increase in fluconazole serum exposure in a small group of healthy subjects also given hydrochlorothiazide.

It has been suggested that the fluconazole dose need not be altered, but bear this interaction in mind in case of an unexpected response to treatment.

Azoles + Domperidone

Ketoconazole increases the exposure to domperidone about 3-fold by inhibiting CYP3A4, and further increases the QT-interval prolongation seen with domperidone alone.

Evidence for an interaction between domperidone and the azoles is limited to that with ketoconazole. The increase in the QT interval due to increased domperidone exposure caused by CYP3A4 inhibition alone would probably not be clinically relevant, however when added to the increase in QT interval seen with ketoconazole alone, the overall increase might reach a level at which some concern is warranted. Due to a higher risk of serious cardiac drug reactions, including QTc prolongation, the MHRA in the UK and the European Medicines Agency contraindicate the concurrent use of domperidone with potent CYP3A4 inhibitors (which would include, itraconazole, ketoconazole, posaconazole, and voriconazole).

Azoles + Donepezil

Ketoconazole raises the maximum levels and AUC of donepezil by about 25%, which was not considered to be clinically relevant.

Despite this finding the manufacturer recommends that donepezil should be used with ketoconazole or itraconazole with care.

Azoles + Dopamine agonists

Two patients taking cabergoline had improvements in their Parkinson's disease symptoms while taking itraconazole. In one case a 300% increase in cabergoline levels occurred, and the other patient reduced the dose of her medications without adversely affecting disease control. Bromocriptine is predicted to interact in the same way as cabergoline.

It would be prudent to monitor toxicity and efficacy in any patient taking cabergoline with itraconazole, or similar potent inhibitors of CYP3A4 such as ketoconazole. Similar caution would seem prudent with bromocriptine.

Azoles + Dronedarone ⊗

Ketoconazole very markedly increases dronedarone exposure. Itraconazole and voriconazole are predicted to have a similar effect, while posaconazole might also interact, but to a lesser extent.

Concurrent use of ketoconazole, itraconazole, posaconazole, or voriconazole is contraindicated by the UK manufacturers of dronedarone.

Azoles + Dutasteride ⚠

Potent CYP3A4 inhibitors (itraconazole, ketoconazole) may cause a clinically significant rise in dutasteride levels.

The manufacturers suggest reducing the dosing frequency if increased dutasteride adverse effects occur.

Azoles + Elvitegravir ⚠

Elvitegravir boosted with cobicistat is predicted to increase the plasma concentrations of ketoconazole, itraconazole, and voriconazole.

Monitor for azole adverse effects (e.g. nausea, vomiting, abdominal pain). The US manufacturer of elvitegravir with cobicistat (in a fixed-dose combination also including emtricitabine and tenofovir) recommends a maximum dose of ketoconazole or itraconazole of 200 mg daily; with voriconazole only given if the benefits of use outweigh the risks.

Azoles + Endothelin receptor antagonists

Fluconazole or Voriconazole

Fluconazole is predicted to greatly increase bosentan exposure, increasing bosentan adverse effects, such as hepatotoxicity.

The UK manufacturer of bosentan do not recommend the concurrent use of fluconazole because of the risk of liver toxicity. If both drugs are given, it would seem prudent to monitor the outcome, particularly for any effect on liver function tests.

Itraconazole or Ketoconazole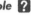

Ketoconazole moderately increases bosentan exposure. Itraconazole is expected to interact similarly.

The manufacturer suggests that no adjustment of the bosentan dose is likely to be required when it is used with ketoconazole (and therefore probably itraconazole). However, because the long-term effects of raised bosentan concentrations are unknown, it would be prudent to monitor the outcome of concurrent use of long courses.

Azoles + Ergot derivatives

Ketoconazole, itraconazole, miconazole, posaconazole, and voriconazole are predicted to increase the concentrations of the ergot derivatives (such as ergotamine, dihydroergotamine, and methysergide), which could result in ergotism. Other azoles, such as fluconazole, might interact similarly, although to a lesser extent.

Concurrent use of ergot derivatives with ketoconazole, itraconazole, miconazole, posaconazole, or voriconazole is generally contraindicated. If concurrent use of ergot derivatives with fluconazole and clotrimazole is unavoidable, advise patients to report any signs of ergotism, such as coldness, numbness or tingling of the hands and feet.

Azoles + Everolimus

Ketoconazole very markedly increases the exposure to everolimus. A report describes reduced everolimus clearance in a patient also given itraconazole, and another patient required a greatly reduced everolimus dose while receiving voriconazole. Posaconazole also increased everolimus concentrations in one patient, but to a lesser extent than voriconazole.

If concurrent use is unavoidable, monitor everolimus concentrations and adverse effects (stomatitis, blood dyscrasias, renal impairment) and consider reducing the everolimus dose, depending on the indication. A large everolimus dose reduction is likely to be needed if given with ketoconazole.

A

Azoles + **Fesoterodine**

Fluconazole or Posaconazole

Fluconazole slightly increases exposure to the active metabolite of fesoterodine (by 27%), with an increase in some minor adverse effects, such as nausea and dizziness. Posaconazole would be expect to interact similarly.

> No fesoterodine dose adjustment is necessary on concurrent use. Bear in mind the possibility of an interaction should an increase in adverse effects occur (e.g. dry mouth, dizziness, insomnia). Concurrent use should be avoided in patients with severe renal impairment, and a maximum fesoterodine dose of 4 mg daily given to those with mild to moderate renal impairment. Concurrent use should also be avoided in patients with moderate or severe hepatic impairment, and a maximum dose of fesoterodine 4 mg daily given to those with mild hepatic impairment.

Itraconazole, Ketoconazole, or Voriconazole

Ketoconazole increases the exposure to fesoterodine about 2.5-fold. Itraconazole and probably voriconazole would be expected to interact similarly.

> The manufacturers state that the dose of fesoterodine should be restricted to 4 mg daily in patients taking these azoles. Concurrent use should be avoided in patients with mild renal or hepatic impairment, and is contraindicated in those with moderate to severe hepatic or renal impairment.

Azoles + **Food**

Some foods increase the absorption of itraconazole capsules or tablets, but appear to decrease the bioavailability of itraconazole solution. Studies with ketoconazole have shown little effect of food on absorption although one found a decrease. Food increases the bioavailability of posaconazole suspension. The bioavailability of voriconazole is slightly reduced by food.

> Itraconazole capsules are best taken with or after food, whereas the acidic solution should be taken at least one hour before food. Similarly, posaconazole should be taken with food. A confusing and conflicting picture is presented by the studies with ketoconazole; however, the UK manufacturer of ketoconazole states that it should always be taken with meals. The manufacturers of voriconazole recommend that it should be taken at least one hour before or at least one to two hours after a meal. Food does not appear to affect fluconazole capsules. Carbonated drinks can increase itraconazole, ketoconazole, and posaconazole bioavailability, see H$_2$-receptor antagonists, page 155, and proton pump inhibitors, page 166.

Azoles + **Galantamine**

Ketoconazole increases the bioavailability of galantamine by 30%, which is predicted to increase galantamine adverse effects (e.g. nausea and vomiting).

> A clinically significant interaction is not expected, however a decrease in the galantamine maintenance dose should be considered in patients who develop galantamine adverse effects. Note that, all azoles, to a greater or lesser extent, inhibit this isoenzyme, and therefore, until more is known, similar caution would seem prudent.

Azoles + H₂-receptor antagonists

H₂-receptor antagonists reduce the absorption of itraconazole, ketoconazole, and posaconazole which seems likely to lead to a reduction in their efficacy.

The manufacturers recommend that if H₂-receptor antagonists are used, itraconazole and ketoconazole should be given with an acidic drink (such as cola), which increase their bioavailability. Itraconazole *solution* would not be expected to be affected, although the US manufacturer advises caution. Posaconazole can also be given with an acidic drink to improve its bioavailability with H₂-receptor antagonists. However, the UK manufacturer currently recommends avoiding concurrent use, unless the benefits outweigh the risk. Fluconazole and voriconazole do not appear to interact and might therefore be suitable alternatives in some cases.

Azoles + Herbal medicines or Dietary supplements

Two weeks of treatment with St John's wort (*Hypericum perforatum*) halved the exposure to a single dose of voriconazole. The UK manufacturer of itraconazole predicts that St John's wort will reduce itraconazole concentrations, increasing the risk of treatment failure.

Patients requiring itraconazole or voriconazole should be asked about current or recent use of St John's wort, because they could be at risk of treatment failure. The manufacturers of voriconazole contraindicate concurrent use and the UK manufacturer of itraconazole advises avoiding St John's wort both during, and for 2 weeks after stopping, St John's wort.

Azoles + HIV-protease inhibitors

Tipranavir with Fluconazole

Fluconazole 100 mg daily slightly increases the exposure to tipranavir boosted with ritonavir.

The UK and US manufacturers of tipranavir state that fluconazole, in doses of greater than 200 mg daily, is not recommended. No dose adjustments are recommended for lower doses of fluconazole.

HIV-protease inhibitors with Itraconazole

Itraconazole increases the concentrations of indinavir, lopinavir boosted with ritonavir, and saquinavir, and might theoretically increase the concentrations of other HIV-protease inhibitors. Some HIV-protease inhibitors might increase itraconazole concentrations leading to adverse effects and case reports support this suggestion.

The UK and US manufacturers of indinavir advise reducing the indinavir dose to 600 mg every 8 hours if it is to be given with itraconazole. The UK manufacturer of saquinavir recommends monitoring for saquinavir toxicity if itraconazole is used but states that no data are available for saquinavir boosted with ritonavir. Most HIV-protease inhibitor manufacturers state that doses of itraconazole greater than 200 mg daily are not recommended with HIV-protease inhibitors boosted with ritonavir. Close monitoring is generally advised: be alert for itraconazole adverse effects (e.g. abdominal pain, dyspepsia). For *unboosted* fosamprenavir, the US manufacturer states that itraconazole doses greater than 400 mg daily might need to be reduced.

Indinavir with Ketoconazole

Ketoconazole raises the AUC of indinavir by 62%.

The UK and US manufacturers of indinavir recommend that the dose of indinavir be reduced to 600 mg every 8 hours when used with ketoconazole.

Other HIV-protease inhibitors with Ketoconazole

Most HIV-protease inhibitors increase the exposure to ketoconazole which might increase its adverse effects. Ketoconazole might slightly increase the exposure to HIV-protease inhibitors, but this is usually not clinically significant. The exception might be indinavir, see above.

Most HIV-protease inhibitor manufacturers state that doses of ketoconazole greater than 200 mg daily are not recommended with HIV-protease inhibitors boosted with ritonavir. Close monitoring is generally advised: be alert for ketoconazole adverse effects (e.g. abdominal pain, dyspepsia). For *unboosted* fosamprenavir, the US manufacturer states that ketoconazole doses greater than 400 mg daily might need to be reduced.

Saquinavir + Miconazole

The UK manufacturer of miconazole oral gel predicts that miconazole might affect saquinavir metabolism.

Although a large proportion of miconazole oral gel (both prescription and non-prescription doses) can be swallowed and therefore achieve systemic absorption sufficient to produce an interaction, saquinavir is usually used boosted with ritonavir, and ritonavir is such a potent CYP3A4 inhibitor it seems unlikely that miconazole would cause an additional effect on saquinavir concentrations.

HIV-protease inhibitors with Posaconazole

Posaconazole appears to increase the exposure to both atazanavir and atazanavir boosted with ritonavir. Posaconazole reduces the exposure to amprenavir (from unboosted fosamprenavir) and unboosted fosamprenavir reduces the exposure to posaconazole.

Patients should be monitored for atazanavir adverse effects and toxicity during concurrent use. Other HIV-protease inhibitors are predicted to interact similarly, and the same precautions are advisable. However, the reduction in amprenavir exposure (from unboosted fosamprenavir) caused by posaconazole seems likely to result in antiviral failure and the UK manufacturer recommends monitoring for a loss of antifungal effects. Until more is known about other HIV-protease inhibitors with posaconazole it might be prudent to monitor both for efficacy and toxicity on their concurrent use.

Ritonavir with Voriconazole

Ritonavir appears to cause a dose-related decrease in voriconazole exposure in most patients, although in some individuals there might be an increase in voriconazole exposure.

Ritonavir, in doses of 400 mg twice daily or more, is contraindicated with voriconazole. Low doses of ritonavir (pharmacokinetic booster doses) should only be given if the benefits outweigh the risks. Consider also, Other HIV-protease inhibitors, below.

Other HIV-protease inhibitors with Voriconazole

The concurrent use of HIV-protease inhibitors with voriconazole might be expected to inhibit the metabolism of both drugs, although no interaction appears to occur with indinavir. Most HIV-protease inhibitors are combined with ritonavir as a pharmacological booster, see also ritonavir with voriconazole, above.

> Until more is known, it would be prudent to monitor both for the possibility of voriconazole adverse effects and for loss of voriconazole efficacy with any other unboosted HIV-protease inhibitors. Be aware that some increase in the concentration of the HIV-protease inhibitor is also theoretically possible if voriconazole is given and it might be prudent to monitor for adverse effects.

Azoles + Ivabradine

Fluconazole

Diltiazem, a moderate inhibitor of CYP3A4, increases the AUC of ivabradine 2- to 3-fold, and reduces the heart rate by an additional 5 bpm. Fluconazole is predicted to interact similarly.

> The manufacturers advise that ivabradine should only be given with fluconazole if the patient's resting heart rate is above 60 bpm, and that the initial ivabradine dose should be reduced to 2.5 mg twice daily, with close monitoring of the heart rate.

Itraconazole or Ketoconazole

Ketoconazole increases ivabradine levels up to 8-fold. Itraconazole is predicted to interact similarly.

> The manufacturer contraindicates the concurrent use of ketoconazole or itraconazole with ivabradine.

Azoles + Lumefantrine

Ketoconazole doubled the exposure to lumefantrine in one study. However, this is within the range of inter-individual variability and no changes in ECG parameters or increases in adverse events were reported.

> This increase is not expected to be clinically relevant, and the UK manufacturer advises that no dose adjustment is necessary when artemether with lumefantrine is used with ketoconazole.

Azoles + Macrolides ❓

Although some moderate pharmacokinetic interactions occur between the azoles and macrolides, most do not appear to be of clinical significance. However, clarithromycin appears to almost double itraconazole levels, whereas erythromycin modestly increases itraconazole levels by about 44%. The manufacturer predicts that posaconazole levels will be increased by clarithromycin and erythromycin. Ketoconazole and itraconazole may increase telithromycin levels by about 52% and 22%, respectively, but no increase in adverse effects occurred.

Monitor the effects of concurrent use of these azoles with clarithromycin or telithromycin. Consider either reducing the dose of the affected drug if adverse effects occur or using a different combination. No dose adjustment is considered necessary when itraconazole is taken with erythromycin.

Azoles + Maraviroc

Ketoconazole markedly increases the exposure to maraviroc. Itraconazole and voriconazole are expected to interact similarly.

The UK and US manufacturers of maraviroc recommend reducing the maraviroc dose to 150 mg twice daily if ketoconazole or itraconazole is also given to patients with normal renal function. In those with renal impairment (creatinine clearance less than 80 mL/minute) in the presence of ketoconazole or itraconazole, the advice in the UK is to increase the maraviroc dose interval to once daily, whereas in the US, maraviroc 150 mg twice daily is recommended for mild and moderate renal impairment, and maraviroc is contraindicated with ketoconazole in those with a creatinine clearance less than 30 mL/minute. A similar interaction might also be expected for voriconazole, and the US HIV guidelines state that consideration should be given to reducing the maraviroc dose to 150 mg twice daily.

Azoles + Mefloquine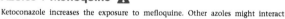

Ketoconazole increases the exposure to mefloquine. Other azoles might interact similarly.

The clinical relevance of this is uncertain, but it might be prudent to exercise caution on the concurrent use of mefloquine and an azole in case of an increase in adverse events. As mefloquine has a long half-life, the manufacturers also advise caution with the use of ketoconazole for up to 15 weeks after a course of mefloquine, particularly with respect to the potential for QT prolongation.

Azoles + Mirtazapine

Ketoconazole is reported to increase the levels and AUC of mirtazapine, although the clinical relevance of this increase is unclear.

The manufacturer of mirtazapine advises caution on concurrent use with potent CYP3A4 inhibitors, such as the azoles, and that a decrease in the dose of mirtazapine may be needed. However, note that the azoles differ in their effects on CYP3A4, see under Azoles, page 143 for further information. Monitor concurrent use for mirtazapine adverse effects (e.g. sedation, fatigue, headache) and adjust the dose as necessary.

A

Azoles + NNRTIs

Delavirdine with Ketoconazole

Ketoconazole appears to increase the minimum plasma concentration of delavirdine by 50%. Delavirdine is predicted to increase ketoconazole exposure.

Monitor for an increase in the adverse effects of delavirdine and ketoconazole if concurrent use is necessary.

Delavirdine with Voriconazole

Voriconazole is predicted to increase the plasma concentration of delavirdine, and delavirdine is predicted to increase the plasma concentrations of voriconazole.

The manufacturers suggest that patients be carefully monitored for evidence of drug toxicity and/or loss of efficacy during concurrent use.

Efavirenz with Itraconazole

Efavirenz appears to slightly decrease itraconazole exposure; however, cases of antifungal treatment failure and subtherapeutic itraconazole concentrations have been reported. The pharmacokinetics of efavirenz are not affected by itraconazole.

The UK and US manufacturers of efavirenz state that alternatives to itraconazole should be considered. If there are no appropriate alternatives, it might be prudent to increase the dose of itraconazole, with increased monitoring for efficacy and toxicity of the combination.

Efavirenz with Ketoconazole

Efavirenz moderately reduces ketoconazole exposure.

The risk of antifungal treatment failure should be considered with concurrent use. Monitor the outcome of concurrent use and increase the ketoconazole dose if necessary.

Efavirenz with Posaconazole

Efavirenz appears to moderately reduce posaconazole exposure. Posaconazole is predicted to increase efavirenz concentrations but no effect was seen in one study.

The UK and US manufacturers of posaconazole advise avoiding concurrent use of efavirenz unless the benefits outweigh the risks. If concurrent use is necessary, monitor for signs of posaconazole treatment failure and/or efavirenz toxicity, and adjust the dose accordingly.

Efavirenz with Voriconazole

Efavirenz moderately decreases voriconazole exposure, and voriconazole slightly increases efavirenz exposure.

The dose of voriconazole should be doubled to 400 mg twice daily, and the efavirenz dose should be halved to 300 mg once daily.

A

Etravirine with Fluconazole

Fluconazole slightly increases etravirine exposure. Etravirine does not affect the pharmacokinetics of fluconazole.

> This interaction seems unlikely to be clinically relevant; nevertheless, the US manufacturer advises caution because of the limited safety data for etravirine at this increased exposure.

Etravirine with Itraconazole

The manufacturers of etravirine predict that itraconazole will increase etravirine concentrations, whereas etravirine is expected to reduce itraconazole concentrations.

> The US manufacturer advises that dose adjustments of itraconazole might be required. However, the UK manufacturer advises that no dose adjustment of either itraconazole or etravirine is required on their concurrent use.

Etravirine with Ketoconazole

The manufacturers of etravirine predict that ketoconazole will increase etravirine concentrations, whereas etravirine is expected to reduce ketoconazole concentrations.

> The US manufacturer advises that dose adjustments of ketoconazole might be required. However, the UK manufacturer states that no dose adjustment of either ketoconazole or etravirine is required on their concurrent use.

Etravirine with Posaconazole

Etravirine concentrations are predicted to be increased by posaconazole.

> The UK manufacturer of etravirine states that no dose adjustment is needed on concurrent use with posaconazole. The US manufacturer predicts that posaconazole concentrations will not be altered by etravirine; however, they still advise that dose adjustments of posaconazole may be needed depending on other concurrent drugs.

Etravirine with Voriconazole

The UK manufacturer of etravirine predicts that the plasma concentrations of both etravirine and voriconazole are likely to be increased on concurrent use, but the effects on the exposure to both drugs are likely to be modest.

> The UK and US manufacturers advise that no dose adjustment of either voriconazole or etravirine is required with concurrent use. However, the US manufacturer advises caution as data on the safety of increased etravirine concentrations is limited. Be alert for any evidence of increased etravirine adverse effects.

Nevirapine with Fluconazole

Fluconazole slightly to moderately increases nevirapine exposure. However, studies have found no increase in adverse effects such as hepatitis, skin rashes, or raised LFTs.

> The UK and US manufacturers advise monitoring for nevirapine adverse effects, although an increase in adverse effects appears to be rare.

Nevirapine with Itraconazole

Nevirapine moderately decreases itraconazole exposure. Itraconazole does not appear to affect the pharmacokinetics of nevirapine.

Monitor itraconazole efficacy carefully and anticipate the need to increase the dose. Note that the US manufacturer of nevirapine advises against concurrent use of itraconazole.

Nevirapine with Ketoconazole

Ketoconazole slightly increases nevirapine exposure, and nevirapine moderately reduces ketoconazole exposure.

The UK and US manufacturers of nevirapine state that ketoconazole should be avoided because of the risk of antifungal treatment failure. If both drugs are necessary monitor antifungal efficacy and increase the ketoconazole dose if necessary.

Nevirapine with Voriconazole

Voriconazole is predicted to increase the plasma concentration of nevirapine, whereas nevirapine is predicted to decrease the plasma concentration of voriconazole.

The UK and US manufacturers suggest that patients be carefully monitored for evidence of drug toxicity and/or loss of efficacy during concurrent use.

Rilpivirine with Itraconazole

Ketoconazole increases the exposure to rilpivirine, and high-dose rilpivirine reduces the minimum concentration and exposure to *ketoconazole*. Itraconazole is predicted to interact similarly.

No dose adjustment of either drug is expected to be necessary on concurrent use; however, given the potential reduction in itraconazole exposure with high-dose rilpivirine the US manufacturer advises that patients should be monitored to ensure the azole remains effective.

Rilpivirine with Ketoconazole

Ketoconazole increases the exposure to rilpivirine, and high-dose rilpivirine reduces the minimum concentration and exposure to ketoconazole.

No dose adjustment of either drug is expected to be necessary on concurrent use; however, given the reduction in ketoconazole exposure with high-dose rilpivirine, the US manufacturer advises that patients should be monitored to ensure the azole remains effective.

Rilpivirine with Posaconazole

Ketoconazole increases the exposure to rilpivirine, and high-dose rilpivirine reduces the minimum concentration and exposure to *ketoconazole*. Posaconazole is predicted to interact similarly.

No dose adjustment of either drug is expected to be necessary on concurrent use; however, given the potential reduction in posaconazole exposure with high-dose rilpivirine the US manufacturer advises that patients should be monitored to ensure the azole remains effective.

Rilpivirine with Voriconazole

Ketoconazole increases the exposure to rilpivirine, and high-dose rilpivirine reduces the minimum concentration and exposure to *ketoconazole*. Voriconazole is predicted to interact similarly.

No dose adjustment of either drug is expected to be necessary on concurrent use; however, given the potential reduction in voriconazole exposure with high-dose rilpivirine the US manufacturer advises that patients should be monitored to ensure the azole remains effective.

Azoles + NRTIs

Didanosine

Itraconazole concentrations might become undetectable if buffered didanosine is taken at the same time. In one case this resulted in treatment failure. A similar interaction would be expected with ketoconazole.

Itraconazole and ketoconazole should be taken at least 2 hours before buffered didanosine. Consider changing to enteric-coated didanosine as it does not appear to affect the absorption of these azoles. Itraconazole *solution* is not expected to be affected by buffered didanosine.

Zidovudine

In one study fluconazole slightly increased the exposure to zidovudine but other studies have found that fluconazole causes only negligible changes in zidovudine pharmacokinetics. Increased zidovudine concentrations, thought to be caused by itraconazole, have been seen in two cases.

Be aware that concurrent use might rarely result in increased zidovudine adverse effects.

Azoles + NSAIDs

Fluconazole increases the AUC of celecoxib by 130% and increases the AUC of the active metabolite of parecoxib (valdecoxib) by 62%. Fluconazole almost doubles flurbiprofen and ibuprofen exposure. Voriconazole increases the levels of and/or exposure to diclofenac and ibuprofen 2-fold.

The manufacturers recommend that half the dose of celecoxib should be used in patients taking fluconazole whereas the US manufacturer suggests starting with the lowest recommended dose. A dose reduction of parecoxib is recommended in patients taking fluconazole. The clinical relevance of the interaction between voriconazole and diclofenac or ibuprofen and fluconazole with ibuprofen or flurbiprofen is unknown but lower doses of these NSAIDs may be adequate to accommodate it.

Azoles + Opioids

Alfentanil or Fentanyl

Some patients experience prolonged and increased alfentanil effects if they are also given fluconazole or voriconazole. Other azoles are expected to interact similarly. Fluconazole and voriconazole inhibit the metabolism of fentanyl. Posaconazole is predicted to interact similarly. There is a case report of a fatality possibly due to the interaction with fluconazole and transdermal fentanyl. Opioid toxicity has been reported when itraconazole was given to a patient with a fentanyl patch, however no interaction was seen in healthy subjects. Note that, at high doses, miconazole oral gel may be absorbed in sufficient quantities to have systemic effects.

A small, single dose of alfentanil is not expected to need adjustment, however, multiple doses or continuous infusions of alfentanil should be given with care. Be alert for evidence of prolonged effects, particularly respiratory depression. It would seem prudent to use similar precautions to those advised for alfentanil if *intravenous* fentanyl is given with any of the azoles, particularly in multiple doses. Several manufacturers of *transdermal* fentanyl do not recommend concurrent use with azoles, unless the patient is closely monitored. Caution should similarly be used if azoles are given concurrently with fentanyl by other routes, such as the *oral transmucosal* route, and a fentanyl dose adjustment should be considered. Close monitoring is recommended.

Buprenorphine

Ketoconazole increases buprenorphine exposure. Itraconazole and voriconazole would also be expected to interact similarly. However, ketoconazole does not appear to affect the pharmacokinetics of *transdermal* buprenorphine.

Monitor for an increase in buprenorphine adverse effects (such as drowsiness, nausea and vomiting) with sublingual or intravenous buprenorphine, and consider a buprenorphine dose reduction as necessary. One manufacturer advises that the dose of sublingual buprenorphine for opioid addiction should be halved when starting ketoconazole, although some manufacturers of sublingual and intravenous buprenorphine recommend avoiding concurrent use. One manufacturer states that no precaution is necessary with ketoconazole in patients using *transdermal* buprenorphine.

Methadone

The metabolism of methadone is reduced by fluconazole, voriconazole, and possibly itraconazole. Other azoles would be expected to interact similarly. A case of torsade de pointes has been reported on concurrent use of itraconazole and methadone.

Patients given an azole with methadone should be monitored for signs of opioid toxicity and a methadone dose alteration should be considered. However, note that the interaction with fluconazole is considered unlikely to be of general clinical significance.

Oxycodone ❓

Itraconazole, ketoconazole, and voriconazole moderately increase the exposure to oxycodone, and miconazole slightly increases the exposure to oxycodone.

The concurrent use of azoles and oxycodone need not be avoided and no oxycodone dose adjustment would generally seem necessary, but be alert for increased adverse effects (such as sedation, constipation, respiratory depression).

Azoles + **Oxybutynin**

Fluconazole and Posaconazole

Moderate CYP3A4 inhibitors, such as fluconazole and posaconazole, are predicted to increase the exposure to oxybutynin.

Bear in mind the possibility of an interaction should any oxybutynin adverse effects occur such as dry mouth, constipation, drowsiness.

Itraconazole, Ketoconazole, and Voriconazole

Single-dose itraconazole causes a small and clinically unimportant increase in the total exposure to oxybutynin and its active metabolite. It is unclear if multiple-dose itraconazole will have similar or greater effect. Ketoconazole can modestly increase the concentration of oxybutynin , although some consider this interaction to be of only minor clinical relevance. Voriconazole would be expected to interact similarly.

The limited evidence available suggests that a clinically relevant interaction is unlikely; however, until more is known, consider this interaction as a cause if oxybutynin adverse effects (dry mouth, constipation, drowsiness) are increased.

Azoles + **Perampanel**

Ketoconazole very slightly increases perampanel exposure. Itraconazole and voriconazole are predicted to interact similarly.

Until more is known, monitor for perampanel adverse effects (dizziness, blurred vision, gait disturbances) and reduce the dose of perampanel according to clinical need.

Azoles + **Phenobarbital**

Itraconazole, Posaconazole, or Voriconazole

Limited evidence suggests phenobarbital causes a large decrease in itraconazole concentrations. Phenobarbital is also predicted to decrease posaconazole and voriconazole concentrations. Note that primidone is metabolised to phenobarbital and therefore might interact similarly with these azoles.

Concurrent use should be avoided unless the benefits are expected to outweigh the risks, although note that the UK and US manufacturers contraindicate the use of voriconazole. If concurrent use is necessary it seems likely that the antifungal dose will need to be increased. It would seem prudent to use other alternatives wherever possible or monitor concurrent use very closely.

Ketoconazole

Phenobarbital (with phenytoin) has been reported to reduce ketoconazole concentrations and its antifungal effects. Note that primidone is metabolised to phenobarbital and therefore might interact similarly.

> Be alert for any signs of a reduced antifungal response. Consider adjusting the dose of ketoconazole.

Azoles + **Phenytoin**

Fluconazole or Miconazole

Phenytoin concentrations are increased by fluconazole, and possibly miconazole, and toxicity has been reported. Fluconazole concentrations are not usually affected by phenytoin, although there is one report of reduced efficacy. Fosphenytoin, a prodrug of phenytoin, might interact similarly.

> Toxicity can develop within 2 to 7 days unless the phenytoin dose is reduced. Monitor phenytoin concentrations closely and reduce the dose appropriately. Also be alert for any evidence of reduced antifungal effects and consider increasing the dose. Note that, at high doses, miconazole oral gel has the potential to interact.

Itraconazole or Ketoconazole

Phenytoin reduces itraconazole, and possibly ketoconazole, concentrations, and treatment failures have occurred. Fosphenytoin, a prodrug of phenytoin, might interact similarly with these azoles.

> Concurrent use of phenytoin and itraconazole (and probably ketoconazole) should be avoided unless the benefits are expected to outweigh the risks. It seems highly likely that these azoles will be ineffective.

Posaconazole or Voriconazole

Phenytoin decreases voriconazole and posaconazole concentrations. Voriconazole increases phenytoin concentrations, while posaconazole appears to have little effect on phenytoin concentrations. . Fosphenytoin, a prodrug of phenytoin, might interact similarly.

> Concurrent use of voriconazole or posaconazole and phenytoin should be avoided unless the benefits outweigh the risks. If both drugs are used, monitor phenytoin concentrations and adverse effects (blurred vision, nystagmus, ataxia or drowsiness) and, if necessary, adjust the dose. The dose of oral voriconazole should be increased from 200 mg to 400 mg twice daily, or from 100 mg to 200 mg twice daily in patients who weigh less than 40 kg, and intravenous voriconazole should be increased from 4 mg/kg to 5 mg/kg twice daily..

Azoles + **Phosphodiesterase type-5 inhibitors**

Ketoconazole increases tadalafil exposure and very markedly increases avanafil and vardenafil exposure, and probably also increases sildenafil exposure. Itraconazole and voriconazole are predicted to interact similarly. Fluconazole, miconazole, and posaconazole might also increase the exposure to phosphodiesterase type-5 inhibitors.

> The UK and US manufacturers of sildenafil recommend that a low starting dose (25 mg) of sildenafil should be used for erectile dysfunction if ketoconazole or itraconazole are used concurrently. The manufacturers state that for pulmonary

hypertension the use of sildenafil with ketoconazole or itraconazole is contra-indicated (UK) or not recommended (US). For tadalafil, when used for erectile dysfunction, the UK manufacturer advises caution and the US manufacturer advises that the 'as needed' dose of tadalafil should not exceed 10 mg in a 72-hour period, or 2.5 mg daily for patients taking ketoconazole (and therefore probably itraconazole). For benign prostatic hyperplasia, the US manufacturer advises that the tadalafil dose should not exceed 2.5 mg daily. For pulmonary hypertension, the UK and US manufacturers state that the concurrent use of tadalafil with ketoconazole or itraconazole should be avoided. The UK manufacturer of vardenafil advises avoiding the concurrent use of ketoconazole or itraconazole in all patients, but specifically contraindicates concurrent use in those over 75-years of age. In contrast, the US manufacturer recommends that the dose of vardenafil should not exceed 5 mg in 24 hours when used with itraconazole or ketoconazole 200 mg daily, or 2.5 mg in 24 hours with itraconazole or ketoconazole 400 mg daily. Similar advice should be used in patients taking these phosphodiesterase type-5 inhibitors with fluconazole, posaconazole, or voriconazole. Note that at the maximum doses, miconazole oral gel is sufficiently absorbed to potentially have systemic effects and it might also interact in the same way. The UK and US manufacturers of avanafil contraindicate concurrent use with potent CYP3A4 inhibitors (e.g. ketoconazole, itraconazole, and voriconazole). The US manufacturer advises that a maximum avanafil dose of 50 mg every 24 hours should not be exceeded with moderate CYP3A4 inhibitors (e.g. fluconazole, and posaconazole) The UK manufacturer however, advises a maximum dose of 100 mg once every 48 hours with moderate CYP3A4 inhibitors.

Azoles + Praziquantel

Ketoconazole almost doubles the exposure to praziquantel, which appears to increase the incidence of mild adverse effects (headache and gastrointestinal adverse effects, including nausea and vomiting).

> Information is limited, but all azoles have the potential to interact, to a greater or lesser extent (see azoles, page 143). It would be prudent to be alert for an increase in the adverse effects of praziquantel, although an increase in efficacy is also possible.

Azoles + Proton pump inhibitors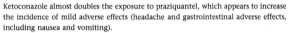

The bioavailability of ketoconazole, itraconazole capsules (but not oral solution), and posaconazole is reduced by omeprazole. Other proton pump inhibitors are expected to behave similarly and a limited number of studies support this suggestion. Voriconazole exposure might be increased by omeprazole. The exposure to esomeprazole and omeprazole is increased or likely to be increased by most azoles, although the extent of the interaction varies.

> An increase in the dose of the azole has been suggested to overcome the reduction in the bioavailability of the affected azoles by the proton pump inhibitors, as has giving ketoconazole or itraconazole capsules with an acidic drink (such as cola), which increases its bioavailability. The manufacturers of posaconazole and one manufacturer of lansoprazole advise avoiding concurrent use. Monitor for antifungal efficacy. Fluconazole, voriconazole and oral itraconazole solution appear to be minimally affected, and they might therefore be alternatives; however, be aware that the levels of some proton pump inhibitors might be

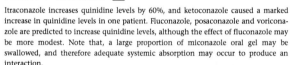
affected by some azoles, see below. The manufacturers of voriconazole recommend halving the dose of omeprazole patients taking omeprazole 40 mg or more, whereas the manufacturers of omeprazole only advise considering a dose adjustment in patients with hepatic impairment or on long-term use. The dose of esomeprazole will only need adjusting in those taking voriconazole if the esomeprazole dose is very high (more than 240 mg). With multiple-dose fluconazole it might be prudent to monitor for proton pump inhibitor adverse effects and consider a dose decrease if these become troublesome. Single-dose fluconazole is unlikely to present a problem.

Azoles + Quinidine

Itraconazole increases quinidine levels by 60%, and ketoconazole caused a marked increase in quinidine levels in one patient. Fluconazole, posaconazole and voriconazole are predicted to increase quinidine levels, although the effect of fluconazole may be more modest. Note that, a large proportion of miconazole oral gel may be swallowed, and therefore adequate systemic absorption may occur to produce an interaction.

The manufacturers of ketoconazole, itraconazole, miconazole, posaconazole and voriconazole contraindicate the concurrent use of quinidine. Therefore, it may be prudent to avoid using fluconazole with quinidine. However if concurrent use is essential, the patient should be very closely monitored and the dose of quinidine reduced accordingly.

Azoles + Ranolazine

Ketoconazole increases the AUC, peak and trough levels, and half-life of ranolazine 2.5- to 4.5-fold. The dose-related adverse effects of ranolazine such as nausea and dizziness were increased by ketoconazole. Further, increases in plasma levels of ranolazine may cause significant QT prolongation and increase the risk of arrhythmias.

The manufacturers of ranolazine contraindicate its use with ketoconazole and other potent CYP3A4 inhibitors. They specifically name itraconazole, posaconazole, and voriconazole.

Azoles + Reboxetine

Ketoconazole decreases the clearance of single-dose reboxetine, without apparently altering its adverse effect profile. Other azoles are predicted to interact similarly.

It has been suggested that caution should be used, and a reduction in reboxetine dose considered, if it is given with ketoconazole. The manufacturers recommend that azoles should not be given with reboxetine as it has a narrow therapeutic index, but this seems overly cautious.

Azoles + Retinoids

The metabolism of tretinoin can be inhibited by single-dose fluconazole and ketoconazole, and the metabolism of alitretinoin can also be inhibited by

A

ketoconazole. Case reports describe tretinoin toxicity with fluconazole and voriconazole.

> The concurrent use of tretinoin with ketoconazole, fluconazole, and voriconazole should be avoided if possible. If one of these azoles is necessary, monitor for tretinoin toxicity (headache, blurred vision), and reduce the tretinoin dose, if appropriate. The UK manufacturer suggests a dose reduction of alitretinoin might be necessary on the concurrent use of ketoconazole. If both drugs are given it may be prudent to monitor for alitretinoin adverse effects (flushing, eye irritation, arthralgia), reducing the dose according to response. There seems to be no evidence regarding an effect of ketoconazole on topical alitretinoin or tretinoin, but as systemic absorption from these formulations is low, no interaction would be expected.

Azoles + Rifabutin

Fluconazole or Miconazole

Fluconazole increases rifabutin concentrations which increases the risk of uveitis. Miconazole oral gel might be absorbed in sufficient quantities to have systemic effects, and it is therefore predicted to interact similarly.

> The concurrent use of rifabutin with fluconazole can be advantageous but because of the increased risk of uveitis, the CSM in the UK states that the dose of rifabutin should be reduced to 300 mg daily. The UK manufacturer of miconazole oral gel advises caution and suggests that rifabutin dose reductions might be necessary on concurrent use.

Itraconazole or Ketoconazole

Rifabutin reduces itraconazole concentrations and reduces its efficacy leading to treatment failure. Itraconazole has been reported to increase rifabutin concentrations: a case of uveitis was attributed to concurrent use. Ketoconazole is predicted to interact similarly.

> Information is sparse, but based on what is known monitor for reduced antifungal activity, raising the azole dose as necessary, and watch for increased rifabutin concentrations and toxicity (in particular uveitis). The manufacturers of itraconazole and ketoconazole do not recommend concurrent use.

Posaconazole

Rifabutin reduces posaconazole concentrations and posaconazole increases the rifabutin concentrations. Adverse effects (headache, back pain, leucopenia, uveitis) have been attributed to the concurrent use of these drugs.

> Concurrent use should be avoided unless the benefits are expected to outweigh the risks. If used together, the efficacy of posaconazole and rifabutin adverse effects should both be closely monitored, particularly full blood counts and uveitis.

Voriconazole

Rifabutin decreases voriconazole concentrations, while voriconazole increases rifabutin concentrations.

> Concurrent use should be avoided unless the benefits are expected to outweigh the

risks. The UK manufacturers recommend that the dose of oral voriconazole should be increased from 200 mg twice daily to 350 mg twice daily (and from 100 to 200 mg twice daily in patients under 40 kg). The intravenous dose should also be increased from 4 to 5 mg/kg twice daily. Patients should be closely monitored for rifabutin adverse effects (e.g. check full blood counts, monitor for uveitis). In the US concurrent use is contraindicated.

Azoles + Rifampicin (Rifampin)

Fluconazole

Rifampicin causes only a negligible decrease in oral fluconazole exposure; however, cases of reduced fluconazole efficacy have been reported and larger effects have been seen with intravenous fluconazole.

Monitor concurrent use and increase the fluconazole dose if necessary (30% has been suggested for some serious infections). This might be especially important during prophylaxis of cryptococcal meningitis with lower doses of fluconazole, such as 200 mg daily.

Other azoles

Rifampicin markedly or very markedly reduces the exposure to itraconazole, ketoconazole and voriconazole and had similar effects on posaconazole in one case. The plasma concentration of rifampicin is reduced by ketoconazole, but is possibly unaffected if the drugs are given 12 hours apart.

The manufacturers do not recommend the concurrent use of itraconazole or ketoconazole with rifampicin and contraindicate voriconazole with rifampicin. The UK manufacturer of posaconazole advises against concurrent use unless the benefit to the patient outweighs the risk. If concurrent use is necessary, monitor closely, being alert for the need to increase the dose of these azoles. With ketoconazole, a rifampicin dose increase might also be needed.

Azoles + Riociguat

Ketoconazole moderately increases riociguat exposure through CYP3A4 inhibition.

The manufacturers of riociguat do not recommend its concurrent use with potent CYP3A4 inhibitors (which would include itraconazole, ketoconazole, and voriconazole). The US manufacturer suggests considering a riociguat starting dose of 0.5 mg three times a day, while the UK manufacturer advises avoiding concurrent use. If azoles and riociguat are used together monitor for any riociguat adverse effects such as hypotension, peripheral oedema, and headache.

Azoles + Rivaroxaban

Ketoconazole increases rivaroxaban exposure. Itraconazole, posaconazole, and voriconazole are predicted to interact similarly.

Concurrent use is not recommended because of the increased bleeding risk. If both drugs are given, monitor closely for signs of bleeding.

Azoles + Roflumilast

Ketoconazole inhibits the metabolism of roflumilast to its active *N*-oxide metabolite but does not affect the overall phosphodiesterase type-4 inhibitory activity to a clinically relevant extent.

> No roflumilast dose adjustments are expected to be necessary if it is given with ketoconazole.

Azoles + Salbutamol (Albuterol) and related bronchodilators

Ketoconazole markedly increases the systemic exposure to inhaled salmeterol, which might result in increased adverse effects of salmeterol. QT-interval prolongation has been reported on concurrent use, even at low doses of salmeterol. Itraconazole and voriconazole are expected to interact similarly.

> Concurrent use of these azoles and salmeterol should be avoided.

Azoles + Sirolimus

Clotrimazole, Fluconazole and Miconazole

Two cases suggest fluconazole causes large increases in sirolimus concentrations. Systemic clotrimazole and miconazole oral gel are predicted to interact similarly.

> Close monitoring of sirolimus plasma concentrations is recommended, with a dose reduction of sirolimus as required. Note that miconazole oral gel may be swallowed in large enough quantities to have a systemic interaction with sirolimus.

Itraconazole, Ketoconazole or Posaconazole

Itraconazole, ketoconazole and posaconazole markedly increase sirolimus plasma concentrations and sirolimus dose reductions of up to 90% have been required in some patients in order to manage this interaction.

> Concurrent use is not recommended by some manufacturers. However, if these azoles are required in a patient taking sirolimus, a pre-emptive sirolimus dose reduction would appear to be prudent, and sirolimus minimum concentrations should be very closely monitored both during use and after the azoles are stopped.

Voriconazole

Voriconazole markedly increases sirolimus exposure.

> These increases are probably too large to be easily accommodated by reducing the dose of the sirolimus. Concurrent use is contraindicated by the UK and manufacturers of voriconazole.

Azoles + Solifenacin

Ketoconazole, a potent CYP3A4 inhibitor, increases solifenacin exposure 2- to 3-fold.

Other potent CYP3A4 inhibitors (e.g. itraconazole and voriconazole) would be expected to have the same effect. Fluconazole and posaconazole, moderate CYP3A4 inhibitors, are also predicted to increase exposure to solifenacin.

It is recommended that the daily dose of solifenacin is limited to 5 mg in patients taking itraconazole, voriconazole, or ketoconazole. In patients taking solifenacin and fluconazole or posaconazole, bear in mind the possibility of an interaction should any solifenacin adverse effects occur, such as dry mouth, constipation, or drowsiness. The concurrent use of solifenacin and potent CYP3A4 inhibitors is contraindicated in patients with severe renal impairment or moderate hepatic impairment.

Azoles + Statins

Atorvastatin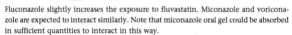

Itraconazole moderately increases atorvastatin exposure. Ketoconazole, posaconazole, and voriconazole would be expected to interact similarly. In theory, fluconazole, particularly in doses above 200 mg daily, could increase atorvastatin exposure, and a case of rhabdomyolysis has been reported with concurrent use. Miconazole would be expected to interact similarly. Note that miconazole oral gel could be absorbed in sufficient quantities to interact in this way.

Avoid the concurrent use of itraconazole, ketoconazole, posaconazole, and voriconazole, if possible. If concurrent use is necessary, close monitoring is recommended, and is specifically advised when atorvastatin doses greater than 20 mg daily (US advice) or 40 mg daily (UK advice) are given. Note that the UK manufacturer of posaconazole contraindicates concurrent use. Because increases in atorvastatin exposure are possible with any azole consider using lower atorvastatin doses in their presence . and advise any patient given atorvastatin with an azole to report any unexplained muscle pain, tenderness, or weakness.

Fluvastatin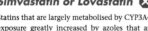

Fluconazole slightly increases the exposure to fluvastatin. Miconazole and voriconazole are expected to interact similarly. Note that miconazole oral gel could be absorbed in sufficient quantities to interact in this way.

The clinical relevance of the slight changes in fluvastatin exposure with fluconazole is unclear. However, because of the potentially serious reactions that can result, any patient given fluvastatin with fluconazole should be told to report any unexplained muscle pain, tenderness or weakness. Similar precautions are warranted for miconazole and voriconazole. Note that the US manufacturer limits the dose of fluvastatin to 20 mg daily if fluconazole is also given.

Simvastatin or Lovastatin ⊗

Statins that are largely metabolised by CYP3A4 (lovastatin and simvastatin) have their exposure greatly increased by azoles that are potent inhibitors of this isoenzyme (itraconazole, ketoconazole, posaconazole, and voriconazole). The drug pairs that have been studied (itraconazole with lovastatin and simvastatin, and posaconazole with simvastatin) have found that the effect is marked to very marked. This interaction has resulted in severe muscle toxicity, including rhabdomyolysis, in a number of cases. Fluconazole (particularly in high dose i.e. greater than 200 mg daily), and miconazole (including the oral gel, which can be absorbed sufficiently to have enzyme-inhibitory effects) are also predicted to interact in the same way, but probably to a lesser extent.

> The concurrent use of itraconazole, ketoconazole, posaconazole, and miconazole oral gel with simvastatin or lovastatin is generally contraindicated. If a short course of these azoles is essential, the statin should be temporarily withdrawn. The UK and US manufacturers of voriconazole recommend considering a dose reduction of lovastatin or simvastatin during concurrent use. Patients taking any azole with these statins should be warned to report promptly any unexplained muscle aches, tenderness, cramps, stiffness, or weakness.

Azoles + Sucralfate

Sucralfate slightly reduces the exposure to ketoconazole, but no appreciable changes appear to occur if ketoconazole is given 2 hours after sucralfate.

> The interaction between sucralfate and ketoconazole is slight and therefore probably of limited clinical importance. Any interaction can be minimised by giving sucralfate 2 to 3 hours before or after ketoconazole.

Azoles + Tacrolimus

When tacrolimus is given orally, its serum concentrations are considerably increased (within 3 days) by oral fluconazole. Oral clotrimazole, itraconazole, ketoconazole, posaconazole, voriconazole, and possibly miconazole oral gel, also increase tacrolimus concentrations. There is some evidence that the concentrations of *intravenous* tacrolimus are less affected by the azoles.

> Monitor tacrolimus concentrations closely if any azole is given and adjust the tacrolimus dose as required. One study specifically examining dose adjustments suggests that fluconazole can be safely used if 60% of the original tacrolimus dose is given. Nearly all patients are expected to need tacrolimus dose reductions if azoles are given: the UK and US manufacturers of posaconazole and voriconazole suggest a reduction of two-thirds. No interaction would be expected if clotrimazole or miconazole are applied to the skin or used intravaginally.

Azoles + Theophylline

In general, no clinically relevant interaction appears to occur between theophylline and the azoles, although a decrease in theophylline concentration has been seen in rare cases with ketoconazole and a small decrease in theophylline clearance and/or an increase in theophylline concentrations have been seen in rare cases with fluconazole.

> A clinically relevant interaction seems unlikely; however, consider an interaction if any unexplained reduction in theophylline efficacy or theophylline adverse effects (such as headache, nausea, tremor) occur, and monitor theophylline concentrations accordingly.

Azoles + Ticagrelor

Ketoconazole markedly increases the exposure to ticagrelor. Itraconazole and voriconazole are predicted to also markedly increase ticagrelor exposure.

> Because the marked increase in exposure can increase the risk of bleeding,

concurrent use of these azoles is contraindicated. The UK and US manufacturers of ticagrelor state that no dose adjustment is necessary on concurrent use with moderate CYP3A4 inhibitors, such as fluconazole or posaconazole.

Azoles + Tolterodine

Tolterodine exposure is increased by ketoconazole, a potent inhibitor of CYP3A4. Itraconazole and voriconazole would be expected to interact similarly. The US manufacturer predicts that miconazole will interact similarly. Fluconazole and posaconazole, moderate inhibitors of CYP3A4, are also predicted to increase the exposure to tolterodine.

> The UK manufacturer advises avoiding concurrent use with potent inhibitors of CYP3A4. The US manufacturer suggests reducing the tolterodine dose to 1 mg twice daily, which seems practical. If potent inhibitors of CYP3A4 are given, monitor carefully for tolterodine adverse effects (dry mouth, constipation, drowsiness), and further reduce the dose or withdraw the drug if it is not tolerated. If fluconazole or posaconazole are given with tolterodine, be alert for an increase in tolterodine adverse effects.

Azoles + Toremifene

The manufacturers of toremifene predict that inhibitors of CYP3A4, such as ketoconazole, might decrease toremifene metabolism, which could lead to toxicity. Itraconazole and voriconazole would be expected to interact similarly.

> Although the clinical relevance of these interactions has not been established, note that CYP3A4 *inducers*, such as *rifampicin (rifampin)*, page 574 have been found to interact, so a pharmacokinetic interaction with CYP3A inhibitors would be expected. It would seem prudent to monitor for toremifene adverse effects (e.g. hot flushes, uterine bleeding, fatigue, nausea, dizziness).

Azoles + Trazodone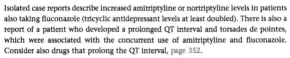

Ketoconazole or itraconazole may inhibit the metabolism of trazodone.

> A lower dose of trazodone should be considered if it is given with these azoles, although in the UK it has been suggested that the combination should be avoided where possible. Monitor for increased trazodone adverse effects such as sedation, if concurrent use is required.

Azoles + Tricyclics ❓

Isolated case reports describe increased amitriptyline or nortriptyline levels in patients also taking fluconazole (tricyclic antidepressant levels at least doubled). There is also a report of a patient who developed a prolonged QT interval and torsades de pointes, which were associated with the concurrent use of amitriptyline and fluconazole. Consider also drugs that prolong the QT interval, page 352.

> The general importance of this interaction is unclear, but bear it in mind in case of an unexpected response to treatment or if tricyclic adverse effects become troublesome. The evidence suggests that other factors (such as renal impairment

and other potentially interacting medications) may be necessary before an interaction occurs.

Azoles + Triptans

Almotriptan

Ketoconazole slightly increases the exposure to almotriptan by about 60%. Itraconazole and probably voriconazole are expected to interact similarly.

The US manufacturers recommend using a starting dose of almotriptan 6.25 mg in patients taking potent CYP3A4 inhibitors, and this would be expected to include ketoconazole, as well as itraconazole and voriconazole.

Eletriptan

Fluconazole moderately increases the exposure to eletriptan by about 2-fold. Ketoconazole markedly increases the exposure to eletriptan by nearly 6-fold. Itraconazole and probably voriconazole are expected to interact similarly to ketoconazole.

Be aware that the effects of eletriptan might be increased in those taking fluconazole. The manufacturers state that the concurrent use of ketoconazole with eletriptan should be avoided. The US manufacturer further recommends that eletriptan should not be given within 72 hours of ketoconazole. Similar precautions should be taken with itraconazole and voriconazole. Other triptans would be expected to have little or no interaction with the azoles and might be suitable alternatives.

Azoles + Ulipristal

Ketoconazole appears to markedly increase the exposure to ulipristal.

The UK manufacturer of low-dose ulipristal for the symptomatic management of fibroids does not recommend its concurrent use with moderate and potent CYP3A4 inhibitors (which would include fluconazole, itraconazole, ketoconazole, posaconazole, and voriconazole). If low-dose ulipristal is given with one of these azoles, monitor for an increase in the adverse effects of ulipristal (such as nausea, abdominal pain, and breast tenderness) or any unexpected outcome occurring during concurrent use. The UK manufacturer of ulipristal for emergency contraception states that CYP3A4 inhibitors are unlikely to have any clinically relevant effects.

Azoles + Warfarin and related oral anticoagulants

Fluconazole causes a dose-related inhibition of the metabolism of warfarin, and increases its anticoagulant effect. Voriconazole interacts similarly. Case reports describe raised INRs and bleeding when fluconazole, ketoconazole, or itraconazole were given with warfarin, acenocoumarol or phenprocoumon. The anticoagulant effects of acenocoumarol, phenindione, phenprocoumon, and warfarin can be greatly increased if miconazole is given orally as a buccal gel, and bleeding can occur. The interaction can also rarely occur with intravaginal miconazole, and possibly with miconazole cream applied to the skin.

Monitor the INR if an azole is given with an indanedione or coumarin and adjust the dose accordingly. Oral miconazole, fluconazole, and voriconazole interfere with the main metabolic pathway of warfarin (and acenocoumarol) and are therefore likely to interact more frequently than the other azoles. Concurrent use of prescription doses of miconazole oral gel should be avoided. The warfarin dose might need to be reduced by about 20% when using fluconazole 50 mg daily, ranging to a reduction of about 70% when using fluconazole 600 mg daily. These larger reductions should be gradual over 5 days or more, although individual variations between patients can be considerable. In general, an interaction with topical azoles seems rare, but it would be prudent to consider monitoring any patient receiving a coumarin if they need to use large amounts of a topical azole, particularly on broken or damaged skin.

Aztreonam

Aztreonam + Warfarin and related oral anticoagulants ❓

Aztreonam occasionally causes a prolongation in prothrombin times, which in theory might possibly be additive with the effects of conventional anticoagulants.

The clinical importance of this interaction is unknown, but bear it in mind in case of an increased response to anticoagulant treatment.

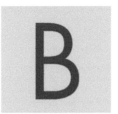

B

Baclofen

Baclofen + Levodopa

Unpleasant adverse effects (hallucinations, confusion, headache, nausea) and worsening of the symptoms of parkinsonism have occurred in patients taking levodopa who were also given baclofen.

Information is limited, but what is known suggests that baclofen should be used cautiously in patients taking levodopa.

Baclofen + Lithium

Two patients with Huntington's chorea showed an aggravation of their hyperkinetic symptoms within a few days of starting lithium and baclofen. One patient took lithium first, the other baclofen.

The clinical significance of this interaction is unclear. Bear it in mind in case of an unexpected response to treatment and consider stopping one of the drugs if hyperkinesis develops.

Baclofen + NSAIDs

An isolated report describes baclofen toxicity (confusion, disorientation, bradycardia, blurred vision, hypotension and hypothermia) in a patient who took ibuprofen. It appeared that the toxicity was caused by ibuprofen-induced acute renal impairment leading to baclofen accumulation.

The general importance of this interaction is likely to be very small. There appears to be no information about baclofen and other NSAIDs, and little reason for avoiding concurrent use.

Baclofen + Tricyclics ❓

An isolated report describes a patient with multiple sclerosis taking baclofen, who was unable to stand within a few days of starting to take nortriptyline, and later imipramine.

The UK manufacturer of baclofen warns that the effect of baclofen may be potentiated by tricyclic antidepressants, resulting in pronounced muscular hypotonia; however, this case report appears to be the only documentation to suggest that a clinically relevant interaction occurs.

B

Balsalazide

Balsalazide + Digoxin

Because digoxin levels can be reduced by up to 50% by *sulfasalazine* the manufacturers cautiously suggest that an interaction may occur with balsalazide. However, no interactions appear to have been reported.

The manufacturer of balsalazide recommends that plasma levels of digoxin should be monitored in patients starting balsalazide.

Benzodiazepines

Benzodiazepines + Beta blockers

Only small and clinically unimportant pharmacokinetic interactions occur between most benzodiazepines and beta blockers, but there is limited evidence that some psychomotor tests might possibly be impaired in patients taking some benzodiazepines with beta blockers, in particular diazepam with metoprolol.

The current evidence does not seem to justify any particular caution, but bear this interaction in mind in case of an unexpected response to treatment.

Benzodiazepines + Bicalutamide

Bicalutamide slightly increases the exposure to midazolam, but this does not appear to increase its sedative effects.

The manufacturers advise caution on concurrent use; however, the likelihood of a clinically relevant interaction seems small.

Benzodiazepines + Calcium-channel blockers

Diltiazem and verapamil moderately increase midazolam exposure. The effects are likely to be greater with oral than intravenous midazolam. This also occurs with triazolam and diltiazem, and is predicted to occur with triazolam and verapamil. Alprazolam is expected to interact similarly, although to a lesser extent than midazolam.

Monitor the outcome of concurrent use. Benzodiazepine effects such as sedation may persist for several hours. Consider using a lower initial dose of midazolam or triazolam. It has been suggested that the usual dose of midazolam should be reduced at least 50%. Other benzodiazepines seem generally unlikely to be affected

B

to a clinically relevant extent (although not all combinations have been studied) and might therefore provide suitable alternatives.

Benzodiazepines + **Carbamazepine**

Alprazolam, Midazolam, or Triazolam

Carbamazepine markedly reduces midazolam exposure, almost abolishing its effects. Carbamazepine also moderately increases alprazolam clearance. A patient had a reduction of more than 50% in plasma alprazolam concentrations when given carbamazepine, and this led to a deterioration in his clinical condition. Triazolam is expected to interact similarly to midazolam.

> Expect to need to use a much larger dose of midazolam in the presence of carbamazepine. An alternative hypno-sedative might be needed. The dose of alprazolam and possibly triazolam might also need to be adjusted.

Other benzodiazepines ❓

The use of benzodiazepines with carbamazepine is common, although some evidence suggests that the effects of the benzodiazepines are sometimes reduced (clobazam, clonazepam, diazepam, etizolam, zolpidem, and zopiclone). Nitrazepam is predicted to be similarly affected.

> No action is generally needed, but be aware that sometimes the effects of the benzodiazepines might be reduced.

Benzodiazepines + **Cobicistat**

Midazolam or Triazolam ❌

Cobicistat very markedly increases the exposure to *oral* midazolam, and triazolam is expected to be similarly affected. *Parenteral* midazolam is expected to interact similarly, although possibly to a lesser extent.

> The US manufacturer of elvitegravir boosted with cobicistat (in a fixed-dose combination also including emtricitabine and tenofovir disoproxil fumarate) contraindicates concurrent use with triazolam and *oral* midazolam. *Parenteral* midazolam should only be used with close monitoring for respiratory depression and/or prolonged sedation, and facilities for immediate resuscitation. Consider reducing the dose of parenteral midazolam, especially if more than a single dose of midazolam is administered.

Other benzodiazepines ⚠

The US manufacturer of elvitegravir boosted with cobicistat (in a fixed-dose combination also including emtricitabine and tenofovir disoproxil fumarate) predicts that it might increase the exposure to benzodiazepines.

> Monitor for benzodiazepine adverse effects (such as sedation, respiratory depression) and adjust the dose as needed.

Benzodiazepines + Digoxin

Digoxin toxicity occurred in two elderly patients, and rises in serum digoxin levels have been seen in others, when they were given alprazolam. This interaction seems to occur particularly in patients over 65 years of age.

Given the range of benzodiazepines available it would seem sensible to avoid alprazolam in patients on digoxin. If concurrent use is necessary, monitor heart rate and digoxin levels, and reduce the digoxin dose as necessary. There is no evidence to suggest a clinically significant interaction with other benzodiazepines.

Benzodiazepines + Disulfiram

An isolated and unconfirmed report describes temazepam toxicity, possibly due to disulfiram. The serum concentrations of chlordiazepoxide and diazepam are increased by disulfiram, and some patients might experience increased drowsiness.

If sedation occurs, reduce the dose of the benzodiazepine if necessary. Other benzodiazepines that are metabolised similarly might interact in the same way but this needs confirmation. Alprazolam, lorazepam, and oxazepam appear to be non-interacting alternatives, but they might still have additive effects with disulfiram on drowsiness.

Benzodiazepines + Felbamate

Felbamate appears to increase the metabolism of clobazam (in the presence of enzyme-inducing antiepileptics).

The clinical significance of this interaction is unknown. Both drugs have CNS effects and therefore it would seem prudent to be aware that additive sedative or other adverse effects might occur.

Benzodiazepines + H$_2$-receptor antagonists ✓

The plasma concentrations of many of the benzodiazepines and related drugs appear to be increased by cimetidine, but normally this appears to be of little or no clinical importance and only the occasional patient might experience an increase in adverse effects (sedation).

In general no clinically significant interaction occurs, but note that individual patients might rarely experience increased adverse effects such as sedation. If a patient develops increased benzodiazepine effects, reduce the benzodiazepine dose: a dose reduction of one-third or increased dosing intervals (twice daily instead of three times daily) have been suggested for alprazolam. Consider changing to a non-interacting benzodiazepine (such as lorazepam, lormetazepam, oxazepam, or temazepam), or to a non-interacting H$_2$-receptor antagonist (such as ranitidine, famotidine, nizatidine, or roxatidine).

Benzodiazepines + **Herbal medicines or Dietary supplements**

Kava

A man taking alprazolam became semicomatose a few days after starting to take kava.

> The clinical importance of this isolated case report is uncertain, but bear it in mind in case of an unexpected response to treatment.

St John's wort (Hypericum perforatum)

Long-term use of St John's wort decreases alprazolam and oral midazolam exposure. Triazolam and zopiclone are expected to interact similarly. St John's wort preparations taken as a single dose, or containing low-hyperforin levels, appear to have less of an effect. Single doses of intravenous midazolam do not appear to be affected to a clinically relevant extent.

> Until more is known about the interacting constituents of St John's wort and the amount necessary to provoke an interaction, monitor patients receiving alprazolam and oral midazolam concurrently for any signs of reduced efficacy and increase the dose if needed. Similar caution would seem prudent in patients taking zopiclone or triazolam with St John's wort: the manufacturer states that the zopiclone dose might need to be increased on concurrent use.

Benzodiazepines + **HIV-protease inhibitors**

Midazolam and Triazolam

The HIV-protease inhibitors appear to dramatically increase the exposure to, and effects of, midazolam and triazolam. Increased and prolonged sedation is expected to occur.

> The concurrent use of *oral* midazolam and HIV-protease inhibitors is contra-indicated. The UK manufacturers of the HIV-protease inhibitors state that *intravenous* midazolam can be used with close monitoring within an intensive care unit or similar setting so that the appropriate management of respiratory depression is available. They also suggest that dose reductions should be considered. The authors of one study suggest that continuous intravenous midazolam doses should be reduced by 50%, but they do not consider dose adjustments to single intravenous doses necessary. The US manufacturers similarly contraindicate the concurrent use of midazolam with HIV-protease inhibitors; however, some do not always differentiate between oral or intravenous midazolam. Triazolam would be expected to interact in the same way as midazolam, and therefore the UK and US manufacturers generally contraindicate its use.

Other benzodiazepines

Interactions between other HIV-protease inhibitors and benzodiazepines are variable, although the concentrations of alprazolam, clorazepate, diazepam, estazolam, flurazepam, zolpidem, and zopiclone are most commonly predicted to be increased.

> Clorazepate, diazepam, estazolam, and flurazepam are contraindicated by the UK manufacturer of ritonavir and indinavir, but cautioned by the US manufacturer of ritonavir. The US manufacturer of fosamprenavir and the UK and US manufac-

turers of saquinavir also suggest the possibility of an interaction with clorazepate, diazepam, and flurazepam, and suggest that careful monitoring is needed, with dose adjustments as required. Alprazolam is contraindicated by the UK and US manufacturers of indinavir, whereas the manufacturers of saquinavir and the US manufacturer of fosamprenavir advise caution. Note that the manufacturer of ritonavir also cautions alprazolam during initial use, before induction of alprazolam metabolism develops. The manufacturer of ritonavir notes that zolpidem can be given concurrently with careful monitoring for excessive sedative effects and consideration of reducing the dose of zolpidem. Zopiclone might be similarly affected.

Benzodiazepines + Isoniazid

Isoniazid reduces the clearance of both diazepam and triazolam. Some increase in their effects would be expected.

The decreases in clearance are slight and unlikely to result in increased effects; however, bear the possibility in mind if problems occur when starting isoniazid in patients taking diazepam or triazolam. Clotiazepam and oxazepam appear to be non-interacting alternatives.

Benzodiazepines + Lamotrigine

Lamotrigine appears to lower clonazepam plasma concentrations by about 40% in some patients.

The general significance of this interaction is unclear. Both drugs have CNS effects and therefore it would seem prudent to be aware that additive sedative or other adverse effects might occur.

Benzodiazepines + Levodopa

On rare occasions it seems that the therapeutic effects of levodopa can be reduced by chlordiazepoxide, diazepam or nitrazepam, but this is not an established interaction.

There is no need to avoid concurrent use, but bear these reports in mind in case of an unexpected response to treatment.

Benzodiazepines + Lithium

Neurotoxicity and increased serum lithium levels were reported in 5 patients when they took clonazepam with lithium. Increased serum-lithium levels have been described in one patient taking bromazepam and lithium and an isolated case of hypothermia has been reported during the concurrent use of lithium and diazepam.

It has been recommended that lithium levels should be measured more frequently if clonazepam is added, and the effects of concurrent use should be well monitored. This general significance of the isolated cases is unclear and concurrent use need not be avoided, but bear these cases in mind should any unexpected adverse effects occur.

B

Benzodiazepines + Macrolides

Alprazolam, Brotizolam, Midazolam, Triazolam or Zopiclone ⚠

The exposure to midazolam and triazolam, and their resulting effects, are markedly increased by clarithromycin, telithromycin, and moderately increased and prolonged by erythromycin. The same interaction has been seen to a limited extent with josamycin and roxithromycin, but not with azithromycin. Not all macrolides will interact, see macrolides, page 474. The exposure to other benzodiazepines, such as alprazolam, brotizolam, and zopiclone is moderately increased by erythromycin, and so would be expected to be similarly affected by these other macrolides.

> Monitor for increased sedation, and warn patients about the increase in effects such as sedation and counsel them against driving or undertaking other skilled tasks. The dose of midazolam should be reduced 50 to 75% when these antibacterials are used if excessive adverse effects (marked drowsiness, memory loss) are to be avoided. High doses of intravenous midazolam given long-term will need to be carefully titrated: one Australian manufacturer suggests an initial 50% reduction in dose in the presence of the interacting macrolides. Similar precautions are warranted for triazolam, but smaller dose reductions or monitoring should be adequate with the other interacting hypnotics. Single bolus doses of intravenous midazolam probably do not need adjusting.

Other benzodiazepines ✓

Erythromycin has only a negligible to slight effect on the metabolism of diazepam, flunitrazepam, nitrazepam, and zaleplon.

> The manufacturer of zaleplon states that patients should be advised that increased sedation is possible with erythromycin, although a dose adjustment is usually not required. A clinically significant interaction is unlikely with these other benzodiazepines.

Benzodiazepines + MAOIs ❓

Isolated case reports describe adverse reactions (chorea, severe headache, facial flushing, massive oedema, and prolonged coma), which have been attributed to interactions between phenelzine and chlordiazepoxide, clonazepam or nitrazepam, and between isocarboxazid and chlordiazepoxide.

> The case reports of adverse interactions appear to be isolated, and it is by no means certain that all the responses were in fact due to drug interactions. They seem unlikely to be of general significance.

Benzodiazepines + Melatonin ❓

The CNS effects of benzodiazepines and related hypnotics might be additive with those of melatonin.

> It would be wise to be aware that increased drowsiness is a possibility if melatonin is given with a benzodiazepine, especially those that are longer-acting. Warn all patients of the potential effects, and counsel against driving or undertaking other skilled tasks.

Benzodiazepines + Mirtazapine

The sedative effects of mirtazapine are increased by the benzodiazepines.

> Patients should be warned that the sedative effects of benzodiazepines in general may be potentiated by concurrent use with mirtazapine. Note that the US manufacturer actually recommends that patients taking mirtazapine avoid the use of diazepam and similar drugs, but this is probably overly cautious.

Benzodiazepines + Modafinil

Modafinil reduces the exposure to triazolam: midazolam, and possibly alprazolam, may be similarly affected. Armodafinil, the *R*-isomer of modafinil, reduces midazolam exposure, and might also affect the metabolism of other similarly metabolised benzodiazepines, such as triazolam and possibly alprazolam. In contrast, diazepam exposure is predicted to be increased by modafinil and armodafinil.

> Monitor to ensure that the benzodiazepine effects are adequate, and, in the case of diazepam, not excessive. Dose adjustments of the benzodiazepines might be necessary on concurrent use.

Benzodiazepines + Moxonidine

Moxonidine increases the cognitive impairment caused by lorazepam. Sedation and dizziness may occur with moxonidine alone, which the manufacturers suggest may be additive with the effects of benzodiazepines.

> The degree of impairment will depend on the individual patient. However, warn all patients of the potential effects, and counsel against driving or undertaking other skilled tasks.

Benzodiazepines + NNRTIs

Delavirdine

Delavirdine is predicted to increase the exposure to alprazolam, midazolam, and triazolam by inhibiting CYP3A4.

> The concurrent use of delavirdine with alprazolam, midazolam, or triazolam is contraindicated.

Efavirenz

Efavirenz appears to increase the metabolism of midazolam. Triazolam and, to a lesser extent, alprazolam would be expected to interact similarly. In contrast, the manufacturers of efavirenz suggest that competition with midazolam for metabolism by CYP3A4 could inhibit midazolam metabolism resulting in prolonged sedation and respiratory depression.

> The study suggests that patients should be monitored for midazolam and probably triazolam efficacy: increase the dose as necessary. However, based on their prediction, the manufacturers of efavirenz contraindicate concurrent use, but note that competition for metabolism rarely results in clinically relevant increases in the concentrations of either of the two drugs involved.

B

Etravirine

Etravirine is predicted to increase diazepam exposure by inhibiting CYP2C19.

> The UK manufacturer of etravirine suggests that alternatives to diazepam should be considered, whereas the US manufacturer suggests reducing the diazepam dose as necessary.

Nevirapine

Nevirapine is predicted to decrease the exposure to midazolam by inducing CYP3A4; triazolam and, to a lesser extent, alprazolam are predicted to be similarly affected.

> Monitor for benzodiazepine efficacy and increase the dose as necessary.

Benzodiazepines + Opioids

As would be expected, increased sedative and respiratory depressant effects may occur in patients given opioids with benzodiazepines; rarely, hypotension has occurred in patients given intravenous opioids and benzodiazepines. Minor pharmacokinetic interactions may occur, but there is insufficient evidence to suggest that any of these are of general significance.

> Concurrent use is common and is usually beneficial. However, additive adverse effects can occur and the degree of impairment will depend on the individual patient. However, warn all patients of the potential effects, and counsel against driving or undertaking other skilled tasks. Be aware that hypotension may occur if intravenous opioids are given with benzodiazepines.

Benzodiazepines + Phenobarbital

Clobazam and clonazepam appear to reduce the clearance of primidone, and toxicity has been seen, however some studies found no interaction. Phenobarbital and primidone reduce the plasma concentrations of some benzodiazepines, including clobazam and clonazepam. However, caution might be necessary with benzodiazepines, such as midazolam, triazolam, and alprazolam, which are primarily metabolised by CYP3A4. Similarly, the manufacturer of zopiclone notes that the concurrent use of phenobarbital might decrease the plasma concentrations of zopiclone. Additive adverse effects such as sedation might occur during the initial use of a benzodiazepine and phenobarbital. More serious effects (hallucinations, violent behaviour) have been reported, but appear rare.

> These interactions do not appear to be of general clinical significance, but bear it in mind in the event of an unexpected response to treatment. Adverse effects such as sedation might be more evident when benzodiazepines are given with barbiturates, particularly in the initial stages of treatment, and careful dose adjustment might be required. It might be prudent to be alert for primidone adverse effects in patients also given clobazam or clonazepam. Indicators of phenobarbital and primidone toxicity include drowsiness, ataxia, and dysarthria.

Benzodiazepines + Phenytoin

Midazolam

Phenytoin reduces the exposure to midazolam by about 95%. The effects of midazolam were also reduced. Fosphenytoin, a prodrug of phenytoin, would be expected to interact similarly.

Expect to need to use a much larger dose of midazolam in the presence of phenytoin. An alternative hypnotic may be needed.

B

Other benzodiazepines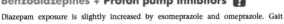

Reports are inconsistent: benzodiazepines can cause serum phenytoin concentrations to increase (chlordiazepoxide, clobazam, clonazepam, diazepam), occasionally resulting in toxicity; or decrease (clonazepam, diazepam); or remain unaltered (alprazolam, clonazepam). In addition, phenytoin might reduce the serum concentrations of clobazam, clonazepam, diazepam, and oxazepam. Zopiclone is predicted to be similarly affected. Fosphenytoin, a prodrug of phenytoin, seems likely to have similar effects on benzodiazepine metabolism.

Monitor the outcome of concurrent use and consider monitoring phenytoin concentrations so that undesirable changes can be detected. Warn the patient to be alert for indicators of phenytoin toxicity (blurred vision, nystagmus, ataxia or drowsiness). Be aware that the benzodiazepine might be less effective than expected and consider a dose increase if required.

Benzodiazepines + **Pregabalin**

The manufacturer notes that there was no clinically relevant pharmacokinetic interaction between pregabalin and lorazepam, and that concurrent use caused no clinically important effect on respiration. However, they note that pregabalin may potentiate the effects of lorazepam (presumably sedation). All benzodiazepines seem likely to increase sedation when given with pregabalin.

The degree of impairment will depend on the individual patient. However, warn all patients of the potential effects, and counsel against driving or undertaking other skilled tasks.

Benzodiazepines + **Probenecid**

Probenecid reduces the clearance of lorazepam and nitrazepam. Increased therapeutic and adverse effects (sedation) might be expected. There seems to be no direct information of an interaction with other benzodiazepines, but those that are metabolised like lorazepam and nitrazepam might also interact.

Monitor the outcome of concurrent use for increased sedation and decrease the benzodiazepine dose if this becomes troublesome. Limited evidence suggests that temazepam does not interact.

Benzodiazepines + **Proton pump inhibitors**

Diazepam exposure is slightly increased by esomeprazole and omeprazole. Gait disturbances (attributed to benzodiazepine toxicity) occurred in 2 patients given omeprazole with triazolam and lorazepam, or with flurazepam. Another patient taking diazepam and omeprazole became wobbly and sedated.

The increase in diazepam exposure is probably unlikely to be clinically relevant in most patients. Nevertheless the case reports suggest that some patients given omeprazole or esomeprazole with diazepam might experience increased benzo-

diazepine effects (sedation, unstable gait). Dexlansoprazole, lansoprazole, pantoprazole, or rabeprazole appear not to interact with diazepam to a clinically
relevant extent and could be suitable alternatives. Information regarding other
benzodiazepines appears to be limited to case reports and no general conclusions
can be drawn.

Benzodiazepines + Rifampicin (Rifampin)

Rifampicin causes a very marked decrease in oral midazolam and triazolam exposure; a
marked decrease in nitrazepam, zaleplon, and zopiclone exposure; and a moderate
decrease in diazepam, lorazepam, intravenous midazolam, and zolpidem exposure.
Benzodiazepines that are metabolised similarly (e.g. alprazolam, chlordiazepoxide,
flurazepam) are expected to interact in the same way.

The effects of these benzodiazepines might be almost completely abolished if
rifampicin is given. Consider increasing the benzodiazepine dose, although the
increase with some is so large that an alternative benzodiazepine should be used
instead: temazepam appears to be a non-interacting alternative.

Benzodiazepines + Rufinamide

Rufinamide reduces the exposure to triazolam by 36%. Alprazolam and midazolam
would be expected to interact similarly.

Be alert for a reduction in the effects of triazolam, alprazolam and midazolam, and
adjust the dose if necessary. The manufacturers recommend monitoring for
2 weeks after starting, stopping, or changing the dose of rufinamide.

Benzodiazepines + Sodium oxybate

The UK and US manufacturers state that sodium oxybate should not be given in
combination with sedative hypnotics, and the UK manufacturer specifically advises
against the concurrent use of benzodiazepines because of the possibility of an
increased risk of respiratory depression.

Be aware that concurrent use might increase CNS depression, including respiratory
depression. Warn all patients of the potential effects, and counsel against driving
or undertaking other skilled tasks.

Benzodiazepines + SSRIs

Fluvoxamine

Fluvoxamine moderately increases the exposure to alprazolam, bromazepam, and
diazepam.

The doses of alprazolam, bromazepam, and diazepam should be reduced, probably
by half, in the presence of fluvoxamine to avoid adverse effects (drowsiness,
reduced psychomotor performance and memory). Furthermore, some US manufacturers recommend avoiding the use of fluvoxamine with diazepam as substantial diazepam accumulation could occur. Warn all patients of the potential effects,
and counsel caution with driving or undertaking other skilled tasks.

Other SSRIs ❓

On the whole, no clinically significant interaction appears to occur between the SSRIs and the benzodiazepines or related drugs, such as zaleplon or zolpidem. There is some limited evidence to support the suggestion that sedation is likely to be increased by the concurrent use of SSRIs and benzodiazepines and related drugs, such as cloral hydrate. Rare cases of hallucinations have been seen with zolpidem and some SSRIs.

> No particular precaution is necessary on concurrent use but remember that the degree of sedation will depend on the individual patient and drug combination. Warn all patients of the potential effects, and counsel caution with driving or undertaking other skilled tasks.

B

Benzodiazepines + Teduglutide ❓

Teduglutide might increase the absorption of other drugs given concurrently, although evidence for this appears limited to an association with altered mental status in patients also taking benzodiazepines. The manufacturers state that the possibility of this effect should be considered, particularly for those drugs a narrow therapeutic range or where the dose is titrated against effect (they specifically name the benzodiazepines), as dose adjustments might be required.

> Until more is known it would seem prudent to consider the possibility of an interaction if the adverse effects of these drugs increase in patients given teduglutide.

Benzodiazepines + Theophylline ❓

Aminophylline and theophylline appear to antagonise the effects of benzodiazepines (mainly sedative effects, but possibly also anxiolytic effects). The extent of the interaction will depend on the benzodiazepine used, the dose used, and the individual patient.

> The extent to which these xanthines actually reduce the anxiolytic effects of the benzodiazepines remains uncertain but be alert for reduced benzodiazepine effects.

Benzodiazepines + Tricyclics ⚠️

The concurrent use of tricyclic antidepressants and benzodiazepines is not uncommon, and normally appears to be uneventful. However, there have been reports of increased drowsiness and incoordination following the use of the combination.

> No particular action is necessary but remember that the degree of sedation will depend on the individual patient and drug combination. Warn all patients of the potential effects, and counsel caution with driving or undertaking other skilled tasks.

Benzodiazepines + Valproate ❓

Valproate increases lorazepam exposure, and possibly also increases diazepam concentrations, while clobazam appears to increase valproate concentrations. Clonazepam clearance might increase and valproate clearance might decrease during concurrent use; increased adverse effects have been seen. The concurrent use of a benzodiazepine and valproate might enhance sedation.

> The general significance of these interactions is not established and concurrent use can be beneficial. However, the UK manufacturer recommends reducing the dose of lorazepam. It would seem prudent to monitor the concurrent use of valproate and a benzodiazepine for adverse effects, particularly sedation, and adjust treatment according to clinical need.

Beta blockers

Beta blockers + Bupropion ⚠

Bupropion is predicted to decrease the metabolism of metoprolol; a case report describes patient taking metoprolol developed bradycardia and hypotension when bupropion was also given.

> The manufacturers of bupropion recommend that if metoprolol is added to existing treatment with bupropion, doses at the lower end of the range should be used. If bupropion is added to existing treatment with metoprolol, decreased doses of metoprolol should be considered. These precautions seem prudent, especially in patients with heart failure, where raised beta blocker levels seem most likely to cause an adverse effect.

Beta blockers + Calcium-channel blockers

Diltiazem ⚠

The cardiac depressant effects of diltiazem and beta blockers are additive, although concurrent use can be beneficial. A number of patients, usually those with pre-existing ventricular failure or conduction abnormalities, have developed serious and potentially life-threatening bradycardia. Note that additive hypotensive effects are likely, see antihypertensives, page 97, but in most cases this is likely to be desirable.

> Monitor the outcome of concurrent use for additive haemodynamic effects (e.g. bradycardia, hypotension or heart failure). Note that an interaction has been reported to occur from within a few hours of starting treatment to after 2 years of concurrent use.

Nifedipine or Nisoldipine ❓

Isolated cases of severe hypotension and heart failure have been seen in patients taking beta blockers with nifedipine or nisoldipine. Patients with impaired left ventricular function (which is a caution for the use of nifedipine) and/or those taking high-dose beta blockers are most at risk. Note that all cases of an interaction involved short-acting nifedipine (which is now considered unsuitable in angina or hypertension) or when extended-release nifedipine was crushed. Note that additive hypotensive effects are likely, see antihypertensives, page 97, but in most cases this is likely to be desirable.

> Be aware that concurrent use may result in additive haemodynamic effects (e.g.

hypotension or heart failure). However, the combination of a dihydropyridine-type calcium-channel blocker and a beta blocker is generally beneficial.

Verapamil

The cardiac depressant effects of verapamil and beta blockers are additive, and although concurrent use can be beneficial, serious cardiodepression (bradycardia, asystole, sinus arrest) sometimes occurs. An adverse interaction can occur even with beta blockers given as eye drops. Note that additive hypotensive effects are likely, see antihypertensives, page 97.

Concurrent use should only be undertaken if the patient can initially be closely monitored. The doses should be carefully titrated to effect. It has been suggested that verapamil injections should not be given to patients recently given beta blockers because of the risk of hypotension and asystole. The UK manufacturer of verapamil contraindicates its intravenous use in those receiving intravenous beta blockers.

Other calcium-channel blockers

The use of beta blockers with felodipine, isradipine, lacidipine, nicardipine, and nimodipine normally appears to be useful and safe. Changes in the pharmacokinetics of the beta blockers and calcium-channel blockers may also occur, but these changes do not appear to be clinically important. Note that additive hypotensive effects are likely, see antihypertensives, page 97, but in most cases this is likely to be desirable.

Be aware that concurrent use may result in additive haemodynamic effects (e.g. hypotension or heart failure). However, the combination of a dihydropyridine-type calcium-channel blocker and a beta blocker is generally beneficial.

Beta blockers + Ciclosporin (Cyclosporine)

Carvedilol might modestly increase ciclosporin concentrations in some patients. In general, atenolol, and metoprolol do not appear to interact with ciclosporin.

The available data suggests that ciclosporin dose reductions of 10 to 20% might be necessary to maintain ciclosporin concentrations at the target level. It would therefore be prudent to monitor ciclosporin concentrations if carvedilol is started or stopped, but also to be aware changes appear to be gradual and that it could take some months for the full extent of the effect to become clear. It appears that no ciclosporin dose adjustment would be expected to be needed in patients taking metoprolol and atenolol.

Beta blockers + Clonidine ⚠

The use of clonidine with beta blockers can be therapeutically valuable, but a sharp and serious rise in blood pressure (rebound hypertension) can follow the sudden withdrawal of clonidine, which may be worsened by the presence of a beta blocker. Note that additive hypotensive effects are likely, see antihypertensives, page 97.

Control this adverse effect by stopping the beta blocker several days before starting a gradual withdrawal of clonidine. A successful alternative is to replace the clonidine and the beta blocker with labetalol, which is both an alpha blocker and a beta blocker: the patient may experience tremor, nausea, apprehension and

B

palpitations, but no serious blood pressure rise or headaches occur. If a hypertensive episode develops, re-introduction of oral or intravenous clonidine may be one way to stabilise the situation. It is clearly important to emphasise to patients taking clonidine and beta blockers that they must keep taking both drugs.

Beta blockers + Contraceptives ❓

The plasma concentrations of metoprolol are increased in women taking combined hormonal contraceptives, but the clinical importance of this is probably very small. Acebutolol, oxprenolol, and propranolol pharmacokinetics are minimally affected by contraceptives. Oral combined hormonal contraceptives are associated with increased blood pressure and might antagonise the efficacy of antihypertensive drugs, see Antihypertensives + Contraceptives, page 98.

No action needed.

Beta blockers + Digoxin ❓

The concurrent use of digoxin and a beta blocker may result in additive bradycardia; one case has been reported in a 91-year-old patient taking digoxin and timolol eye drops. In general there appears to be no pharmacokinetic interaction between digoxin and beta blockers. However, carvedilol appears to increase the bioavailability of digoxin (14% increase in AUC seen in adults, cases suggest a doubling of levels in children).

Normally uneventful, no immediate action needed. If bradycardia does occur dose adjustment may be necessary, and this seems more likely in children. It has been suggested that the dose of digoxin should be reduced by at least 25% in children given carvedilol, with further adjustments as required.

Beta blockers + Disopyramide ⚠️

Severe bradycardia has been described after the use of disopyramide with beta blockers including practolol, pindolol and metoprolol. A patient given disopyramide and intravenous sotalol developed asystole (see also drugs that prolong the QT interval, page 352).

Although an interaction appears rare, fatalities have been reported. The US manufacturers of disopyramide suggest that the combination of disopyramide and beta blockers should generally be avoided, except in the case of life-threatening arrhythmias unresponsive to a single drug.

Beta blockers + Donepezil ❓

The concurrent use of donepezil and a beta blocker may increase the risk of bradycardia.

Although it appears that the increased risk of bradycardia is probably low, it would be prudent to be alert for bradycardia if a beta blocker is given with donepezil.

Beta blockers + **Dronedarone**

Sotalol

Additive bradycardia may occur if dronedarone is taken with any beta blocker, see below. Additive QT-prolonging effects are likely on the concurrent use of sotalol and dronedarone (see drugs that prolong the QT interval, page 352).

The concurrent use of dronedarone and sotalol is generally contraindicated.

Other Beta blockers

Additive bradycardia may occur if dronedarone is taken with any beta blocker, although in one study the additional increase in the negative inotropic effects seen as a consequence was modest. In addition, dronedarone increases the AUC of metoprolol and propranolol, and is also likely to interact with other beta blockers that are similarly metabolised: this may further contribute to bradycardia.

The manufacturers recommend an initial low dose of the beta blocker. Increase the beta blocker dose only when an ECG confirms no excessive bradycardia or heart block. In patients already taking a beta blocker when starting dronedarone, an ECG should be performed and the dose adjusted if necessary.

Beta blockers + **Ergot derivatives**

The use of ergot derivatives (e.g. ergotamine) with beta blockers is normally safe and beneficial, but there are a handful of reports of adverse interactions (severe peripheral vasoconstriction and hypertension).

Interactions seem rare. Nevertheless, some manufacturers of ergotamine advise that concurrent use with beta blockers should be avoided. At the very least it would be prudent to be alert for any signs of an adverse response, particularly those suggestive of reduced peripheral circulation (such as coldness, numbness or tingling of the hands and feet).

Beta blockers + **Flecainide**

The concurrent use of flecainide and beta blockers may have additive cardiac depressant effects. An isolated case of bradycardia and fatal AV block has been reported during the use of flecainide with sotalol, and bradycardia has been reported in a patient taking flecainide and timolol eye drops.

Careful monitoring has been recommended if beta blockers are given with flecainide: monitor for bradycardia.

Beta blockers + **Galantamine** ❓

The concurrent use of galantamine and a beta blocker may increase the risk of bradycardia.

Although it appears that the increased risk of bradycardia is probably low, it would be prudent to be alert for bradycardia if a beta blocker is given with galantamine.

B

Beta blockers + H₂-receptor antagonists

No clinically significant interaction appears to occur between the beta blockers and cimetidine, although the blood levels of some extensively metabolised beta blockers (labetalol, metoprolol, nebivolol, pindolol and propranolol) can be doubled by cimetidine. Isolated case reports describe bradycardia with atenolol, an irregular heart beat with metoprolol, and hypotension with labetalol, in patients also taking cimetidine.

> Normally the beta blockers are considered to have a wide therapeutic range, and so raises in levels are generally well tolerated, even in patients with heart failure. Those with impaired liver function may be more at risk of an interaction with cimetidine. In this type of patient be alert for effects such as hypotension. Note that other H₂-receptor antagonists (e.g. famotidine, nizatidine and ranitidine) do not appear to interact and so may be suitable alternatives.

Beta blockers + HIV-protease inhibitors

Ritonavir

Ritonavir (including ritonavir used in low dose as a pharmacokinetic enhancer) is predicted to increase plasma levels of metoprolol, propranolol and timolol, and other similarly metabolised beta blockers (by inhibiting CYP2D6). In addition, the situation with propranolol may be more complicated as ritonavir may theoretically *reduce* propranolol levels by inducing glucuronidation and CYP1A2, by which propranolol is also partially metabolised.

> This interaction is likely to be of limited clinical relevance for most patients; however until more is known, it may be prudent to monitor for an increase in beta blocker adverse effects such as shortness of breath, hypotension and bradycardia, and reduce the dose of the beta blocker, or withdraw it, as appropriate. The interaction is most likely to be of significance in patients with heart failure. The pharmacokinetic outcome of the concurrent use of propranolol and ritonavir is unclear; however, bear the possibility of both reduced and increased effects in mind. Note that saquinavir boosted with ritonavir have been associated with QT prolongation, see Drugs that prolong the QT interval, page 352 for further information.

Tipranavir

Tipranavir (with ritonavir) is predicted to increase metoprolol levels. Serious adverse effects such as bradycardia and arrhythmias may occur.

> It may be prudent to monitor for symptoms such as shortness of breath, hypotension and bradycardia, and reduce the dose of metoprolol or withdraw the beta blocker as appropriate. Note that the UK manufacturer of tipranavir contraindicates concurrent use when metoprolol is used for heart failure.

Beta blockers + Hydralazine

Plasma levels of propranolol and other extensively metabolised beta blockers (metoprolol, oxprenolol) are increased by hydralazine, but an increase in adverse effects does not seem to have been reported.

> Concurrent use is usually valuable in the treatment of hypertension. Note that

additive hypotensive effects are likely, see antihypertensives, page 97. No particular precautions seem to be necessary unless an undesirably large decrease in blood pressure occurs.

Beta blockers + Inotropes and Vasopressors

The hypertensive effects of adrenaline (epinephrine) can be markedly increased in patients taking non-selective beta blockers such as propranolol. A severe and potentially life-threatening hypertensive reaction and/or marked bradycardia can develop. Cardioselective beta blockers such as atenolol and metoprolol interact minimally. Dobutamine would be expected to interact in the same way as adrenaline, but some studies and case reports suggest that paradoxical effects may occur. The pressor effects of noradrenaline (norepinephrine) appear to be diminished by the beta blockers. Some evidence suggests anaphylactic shock in patients taking beta blockers may be resistant to treatment with adrenaline (epinephrine).

Patients taking non-selective beta blockers such as propranolol should only be given adrenaline (epinephrine) in very reduced doses because of the marked bradycardia and hypertension that can occur. A less marked effect is likely with the cardioselective beta blockers such as atenolol and metoprolol. Local anaesthetics such as those used in dental surgery usually contain very low concentrations of adrenaline (e.g. 5 to 20 micrograms/mL, i.e. 1:200 000 to 1:50 000) and only small volumes are usually given, so that an undesirable interaction is unlikely. There appears to be less evidence about the other inotropes and vasopressors, but it would seem prudent to monitor blood pressure with both dobutamine and noradrenaline (norepinephrine) titrating doses as necessary.

Beta blockers + Lidocaine

The plasma concentrations of lidocaine after intravenous, and possibly oral, use can be increased by the concurrent use of propranolol, which has resulted in toxicity in isolated cases. Nadolol and penbutolol possibly interact similarly, but there is uncertainty about metoprolol. Concurrent use might increase the risk of adverse cardiac effects such as bradycardia.

It would seem prudent to monitor the concurrent use of any beta blocker and lidocaine for cardiac depressant effects. Note that the UK manufacturer of propranolol states that concurrent use should be avoided.

Beta blockers + Lumefantrine

The manufacturer of a preparation containing artemether and lumefantrine notes that *in vitro* lumefantrine significantly inhibits CYP2D6. They therefore contraindicate any drug that is metabolised by CYP2D6, and they name metoprolol.

This seems very restrictive as metoprolol is not contraindicated with proven CYP2D6 inhibitors. Until more is known, it would be prudent to at least monitor the effects of concurrent use. Note that, additive QT-prolonging effects are likely with the artemether component and sotalol, see drugs that prolong the QT interval, page 352.

B

Beta blockers + Moxonidine

Beta blockers can exacerbate the rebound hypertension that follows the withdrawal of clonidine, page 189. Moxonidine is predicted to interact similarly, although there appear to be no reports of an interaction.

Moxonidine is reported to have less affinity for central alpha-receptors than clonidine and therefore would be expected to present less of a risk. However, to be on the safe side the manufacturers advise that any beta blocker should be stopped first, followed by the moxonidine a few days later. Note that additive hypotensive effects are likely, see antihypertensives, page 97.

Beta blockers + NSAIDs

There is evidence to suggest that most NSAIDs can increase blood pressure in patients taking antihypertensives, although some studies have not found the increase to be clinically relevant. However, various small studies have found some evidence of reduced beta blocker effects, either for hypertension or heart failure, particularly with indometacin.

Only some patients are affected. Nevertheless, some have suggested that the use of NSAIDs should be kept to a minimum in patients taking antihypertensives, whereas, others suggest that the interaction is, generally, not clinically relevant. Consider monitoring blood pressure if an NSAID is started or stopped. Note that NSAIDs should generally be avoided in those with heart failure.

Beta blockers + Pasireotide

Bradycardia is a common adverse effect of pasireotide, which might be additive with the effects of other drugs that affect heart rate, such as the beta blockers. Sotalol has a high risk, and pasireotide has some risk, of prolonging the QT interval, which might lead to the potentially fatal torsade de pointes arrhythmia. Dangerous QT prolongation is likely if they are used together see Drugs that prolong the QT interval, page 352 for further information.

It would seem prudent to monitor potassium concentrations closely. If bradycardia develops consider adjusting the dose of the beta blocker, according to clinical need. Avoid concurrent use with sotalol.

Beta blockers + Phenobarbital

The plasma levels and the effects of beta blockers that are mainly metabolised in the liver (e.g. alprenolol, metoprolol, timolol) are reduced by phenobarbital and other barbiturates. The extent of any interaction is likely to vary between different pairs of barbiturates and beta blockers.

A reduced response is possible with the hepatically metabolised beta blockers, although the interaction between phenobarbital and timolol was not clinically significant in one study. Consider an interaction if the response to the beta blocker is less than anticipated. Beta blockers that are mainly excreted unchanged in the urine (e.g. atenolol, nadolol) would not be expected to be affected by the barbiturates and may therefore be suitable alternatives in some cases.

Beta blockers + Pilocarpine

The concurrent use of oral pilocarpine and beta blockers is said to be associated with a risk of conduction disorders (presumably bradycardia). Systemic adverse effects with pilocarpine eye drops are rare, although cardiac adverse effects have been reported with excessive use.

> Although palpitations are said to be common with the use of oral pilocarpine there appear to be no published reports to suggest that the concurrent use of a beta blocker presents an additional risk.

B

Beta blockers + Propafenone

Carvedilol, Metoprolol, Nebivolol, Propranolol and Timolol

Plasma metoprolol and propranolol concentrations can be markedly increased by propafenone. Toxicity has developed in some cases. Propafenone and the beta blockers also have negative inotropic effects, see below.

> Information is limited. Anticipate the need to reduce the dose of metoprolol and propranolol, and monitor closely for adverse effects. It is possible that other beta blockers that undergo liver metabolism will interact similarly. Consider the potential for adverse cardiac effects on the concurrent use of propafenone.

Other Beta blockers

Propafenone and the beta blockers have negative inotropic effects, which could be additive and result in unwanted cardiodepression.

> Consider the potential for adverse cardiac effects (such as bradycardia, hypotension) if propafenone is given with a beta blocker.

Beta blockers + Quinidine ⚠

Isolated reports describe marked bradycardia and orthostatic hypotension in patients given a beta blocker with quinidine. Quinidine can raise plasma metoprolol, propranolol, and timolol levels, but the clinical relevance of this is uncertain. Additive QT-prolonging effects are likely with sotalol, see drugs that prolong the QT interval, page 352.

> Beta blockers are considered to have a wide therapeutic range, and increases in levels are generally well tolerated. However, patients with heart failure may be more at risk of adverse effects (e.g. shortness of breath, bradycardia, hypotension). Care is advised as both quinidine and the beta blockers have negative inotropic effects, which could be additive and result in unwanted cardiodepression. Note that, additive QT-prolonging effects are likely with quinidine and sotalol, see drugs that prolong the QT interval, page 352.

Beta blockers + Ranolazine ⚠

Ranolazine increases the levels of metoprolol by about 80%.

> The effects of any interaction are not expected to be clinically relevant in most

B

patients although some caution would be advised in patients with heart failure. Consider an interaction if an increase in metoprolol adverse effects (such as bradycardia, hypotension) occurs, and decrease the dose accordingly.

Beta blockers + Rifampicin (Rifampin) [?]

Rifampicin increases the clearance of bisoprolol, carvedilol, celiprolol, metoprolol, propranolol and tertatolol, and reduces their plasma levels. Similar but smaller effects have been seen when atenolol is given with rifampicin, but a case report suggests that occasionally the effects may be large enough to be of clinical relevance. The effects of rifampicin on propranolol appear more pronounced.

The clinical significance of this interaction is uncertain but probably small. However, bear it in mind in case of an unexpected response to treatment. Consider increasing the dose of the beta blocker if there is any evidence that the therapeutic response is inadequate.

Beta blockers + Rivastigmine [?]

The concurrent use of rivastigmine and a beta blocker may increase the risk of bradycardia.

Although it appears that the increased risk of bradycardia is probably low, it would be prudent to be alert for bradycardia if a beta blocker is given with rivastigmine.

Beta blockers + SSRIs [?]

Fluoxetine can increase pindolol and carvedilol exposure, and possibly increases metoprolol and propranolol exposure. Paroxetine appears to increase carvedilol exposure and might increase metoprolol exposure, resulting in increased beta-blocking effects. Citalopram and escitalopram might also increase metoprolol concentrations. Fluvoxamine probably markedly increases propranolol concentrations (a case report of bradycardia suggests that this may be relevant in some patients), but does not alter the pharmacokinetics of atenolol, although slight bradycardia and hypotension were reported.

The clinical relevance of these potential interactions is unclear, but be aware that there are a few isolated reports of AV block with metoprolol and paroxetine and severe bradycardia with the use of a beta blocker and fluoxetine, or fluvoxamine. An interaction seems more likely to be important in those given metoprolol for heart failure; in which case the UK manufacturer of paroxetine suggests avoiding concurrent use, and the UK manufacturer of escitalopram advises caution and possible dose adjustments. Pharmacokinetic interactions might occur between other combinations of beta blockers and SSRIs, but any effect is generally modest, and there is no evidence to suggest that clinically relevant adverse effects occur as a result. However, consider an interaction as a cause if bradycardia or undesirable hypotension develop. If problems arise, the interaction can apparently be avoided by giving a beta blocker which is not extensively metabolised (such as atenolol) . Alternatively, sertraline and citalopram seem to be less likely than the other SSRIs to interact with extensively metabolised beta blockers. Remember that fluoxetine and particularly its metabolite have long half-lives so that this interaction might occur for some days after the fluoxetine has been stopped. Note that sotalol and

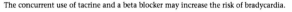

some SSRIs can prolong the QT interval, see Drugs that prolong the QT interval, page 352 for further information.

Beta blockers + Tacrine

The concurrent use of tacrine and a beta blocker may increase the risk of bradycardia.

Although it appears that the increased risk of bradycardia is probably low, it would be prudent to be alert for bradycardia if a beta blocker is given with tacrine.

Beta blockers + Terbinafine

In vitro studies suggest that terbinafine is an inhibitor of CYP2D6. It might therefore be expected to increase the plasma concentrations of other drugs that are substrates of this isoenzyme. The manufacturers suggest that the concentrations of some beta blockers might be raised. Carvedilol, metoprolol, nebivolol, propranolol and timolol are all metabolised, at least in part, by CYP2D6.

Until more is known it would seem wise to be aware of the possibility of an increase in beta blocker adverse effects if any of these drugs is given with terbinafine and consider a dose reduction if necessary. The interaction is most likely to be of clinical significance when drugs such as metoprolol are given for heart failure.

Beta blockers + Triptans

No clinically important interaction occurs between most triptans and beta blockers, but the exposure to rizatriptan is increased by propranolol by about 70%.

If propranolol is also given the manufacturers recommend a rizatriptan dose reduction to 5 mg, with a maximum of two or three doses in 24 hours. In the UK, the manufacturer of rizatriptan also recommends that dosing should be separated by 2 hours, but the basis for this is unclear, as a study found that this does not modify the interaction.

Beta blockers + Zileuton

Zileuton appears to increase the exposure to propranolol (by CYP1A2 inhibition), and this has led to a decrease in heart rate.

The US manufacturer of zileuton recommends monitoring concurrent use, presumably for bradycardia, and decreasing the dose of propranolol if necessary. Until more is known, this seems prudent. The manufacturer also extends caution to the other beta blockers. However, as propranolol is the only beta blocker known to be metabolised by CYP1A2, an interaction between zileuton and the other beta blockers seems unlikely.

B

Bexarotene

Due to the low systemic exposure to bexarotene after topical use, any increases that occur with CYP3A4 inhibitors are unlikely to be sufficient to result in adverse effects with a low to moderate intensity topical bexarotene regimen.

Bexarotene + Contraceptives

The US manufacturer suggests that bexarotene might theoretically increase the metabolism of oral or other systemic hormonal contraceptives, thereby reducing both their serum concentrations and their efficacy.

The UK and US manufacturers of bexarotene advise that additional non-hormonal contraception (such as a barrier method) should be used to avoid the risk of contraceptive failure during treatment with, and for at least one month after stopping, bexarotene. They state that this is particularly important because if contraceptive failure were to occur, the foetus might be exposed to the teratogenic effects of bexarotene.

Bexarotene + Corticosteroids

The manufacturers say that, in theory, dexamethasone may reduce bexarotene levels.

This interaction does not appear to have been studied in patients, so the clinical importance of this prediction is unknown. However note that clinically relevant interactions occurring as a result of dexamethasone inducing CYP3A4 appear rare.

Bexarotene + Fibrates

A population analysis of patients with cutaneous T-cell lymphoma found that gemfibrozil substantially increased the plasma concentration of oral bexarotene, leading to dose-limiting hypertriglyceridaemia.

The UK and US manufacturers of bexarotene state that concurrent use should be avoided.

Bexarotene + Food

Oral administration of bexarotene with a fat-containing meal resulted in an increase of about 50% in its maximum plasma concentration, when compared with administration of bexarotene with a glucose solution.

It is therefore recommended that bexarotene capsules are taken with food.

Bexarotene + Grapefruit juice

The manufacturers say that, in theory, grapefruit juice may raise bexarotene levels.

This interaction does not appear to have been studied in patients, so the clinical importance of this prediction is unknown.

Bexarotene + HIV-protease inhibitors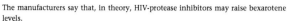

The manufacturers say that, in theory, HIV-protease inhibitors may raise bexarotene levels.

This interaction does not appear to have been studied in patients, so the clinical importance of this prediction is unknown.

Bexarotene + Macrolides

The manufacturers say that, in theory, clarithromycin and erythromycin may raise bexarotene levels.

This interaction does not appear to have been studied in patients, so the clinical importance of this prediction is unknown. If this prediction is clinically relevant other macrolides may also interact, although it seems unlikely that they all will, see macrolides, page 474.

Bexarotene + NNRTIs

The concurrent use of bexarotene and efavirenz is predicted to reduce the concentrations of both drugs: reduced efficacy of both drugs has been seen in one case.

Monitor the efficacy and concentrations of both efavirenz and bexarotene on concurrent use. Topical bexarotene is unlikely to interact.

Bexarotene + Phenobarbital

The manufacturers say that, in theory, phenobarbital (and therefore probably primidone) may reduce bexarotene levels.

This interaction does not appear to have been studied in patients, so the clinical importance of this prediction is unknown.

Bexarotene + Phenytoin

The manufacturers say that, in theory, phenytoin (and therefore probably fosphenytoin) may reduce bexarotene levels.

This interaction does not appear to have been studied in patients, so the clinical importance of this prediction is unknown.

Bexarotene + Rifampicin (Rifampin) ?

The manufacturers say that, in theory, rifampicin may reduce bexarotene levels.

This interaction does not appear to have been studied in patients, so the clinical importance of this prediction is unknown.

Bexarotene + Statins ?

Bexarotene appears to decrease atorvastatin exposure, whereas atorvastatin does not appear to affect bexarotene exposure. Simvastatin and lovastatin might be similarly affected.

Bear the possibility of an interaction in mind should the statin become ineffective: a dose increase might be needed.

B

Bexarotene + Tamoxifen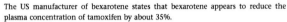

The US manufacturer of bexarotene states that bexarotene appears to reduce the plasma concentration of tamoxifen by about 35%.

The clinical significance of this is unknown; however, bear it in mind should any unexpected decrease in tamoxifen efficacy occur.

Bexarotene + Vitamin A

Bexarotene is related to vitamin A.

In patients taking bexarotene vitamin A supplements should be limited to 15 000 units or less daily to avoid potentially additive toxic effects.

Bicalutamide

Bicalutamide + Calcium-channel blockers

The manufacturers of bicalutamide predict that it might increase the plasma concentrations of the calcium-channel blockers by inhibiting their metabolism by CYP3A4.

The manufacturers of bicalutamide advise caution on concurrent use; although, as bicalutamide only weakly inhibits CYP3A4, this seems overly cautious.

Bicalutamide + Ciclosporin (Cyclosporine)

The manufacturers predict that bicalutamide might increase the plasma concentrations of ciclosporin by inhibiting its metabolism by CYP3A4.

The manufacturers of bicalutamide advise monitoring of ciclosporin plasma concentrations and effects on concurrent use; although, as bicalutamide only weakly inhibits CYP3A4, this seems overly cautious.

Bicalutamide + H₂-receptor antagonists

The manufacturer of bicalutamide predicts that inhibitors of CYP3A4 might increase the plasma concentrations of bicalutamide, which can increase the risk of adverse effects: they specifically name cimetidine.

The manufacturer advises caution as bicalutamide adverse effects might be increased. However, as steady-state concentrations of bicalutamide are highly variable and cimetidine is only a weak inhibitor of CYP3A4, any increase seems unlikely to be clinically relevant.

Bicalutamide + Warfarin and related oral anticoagulants ?

The manufacturers state that bicalutamide might interact with warfarin by displacing it from its protein binding sites, a mechanism that, as a sole cause of interactions, has now largely been discredited. To date, there appear to be no published or confirmed cases of an interaction.

Despite this, the manufacturer of bicalutamide recommends that the prothrombin time be carefully monitored when it is given with coumarins, adjusting the dose when necessary.

Bisphosphonates

Bisphosphonates + Food ⚠

The absorption of the bisphosphonates is reduced by food.

Recommendations on the timing of administration of bisphosphonates in relation to food and other drugs vary. Alendronate should be taken with plain (not mineral) water, after an overnight fast, at least 30 minutes before the first food of the day. Clodronate should be given at least 1 hour before or after food. Ibandronate should be given with plain water on an empty stomach at least 30 minutes to 1 hour before the first food of the day. Risedronate should be given at least 30 minutes before the first food or drink of the day or at least 2 hours from any food or drink during the day, and at least 30 minutes before bedtime. Etidronate and tiludronate should be given on an empty stomach at least 2 hours before or after food.

Bisphosphonates + Iron ⚠

The oral absorption of bisphosphonates is significantly reduced by aluminium/ magnesium hydroxide. Other polyvalent cations, such as iron, are expected to interact similarly.

Bisphosphonates should be prevented from coming into contact with iron. Recommendations on the timing of administration of bisphosphonates in relation to food and other drugs varies. Alendronate should be taken with plain (not mineral) water, after an overnight fast at least 30 minutes before taking the first dose of iron. Clodronate should probably be taken at least 1 hour before or after iron. Ibandronate should be taken with plain water on an empty stomach at least 30 minutes to 1 hour before iron. Risedronate should be taken at least 30 minutes before taking the first dose of iron or at least 2 hours from any iron doses during the rest of the day, and at least 30 minutes before bedtime. Etidronate and tiludronate should be taken on an empty stomach at least 2 hours apart from iron.

Bisphosphonates + NSAIDs ❓

There is conflicting information as to whether the concurrent use of NSAIDs in patients taking alendronate increases the risk of gastrointestinal adverse effects. In clinical studies, no increased risk has been reported with concurrent use of NSAIDs with ibandronate and risedronate. Indometacin increases tiludronate bioavailability about 2-fold. NSAIDs may exacerbate the renal impairment sometimes seen with clodronate; zoledronate is predicted to interact similarly.

Guidance regarding alendronate is conflicting: some consider that it should not be given to patients taking NSAIDs, others urge caution and others say that there is no evidence of increased gastrointestinal toxicity on concurrent use. It would seem sensible to monitor the concurrent use of alendronate and NSAIDs carefully. The manufacturer of ibandronate advises caution if it is given with an NSAID. The manufacturer advises that indometacin and tiludronate should be given 2 hours apart. Some bisphosphonates alone may cause renal impairment. Renal function should be assessed before giving a bisphosphonate and this would seem particularly important in those taking NSAIDs.

Bisphosphonates + Zinc ⚠

The oral absorption of bisphosphonates is significantly reduced by aluminium/magnesium hydroxide. Other polyvalent cations, such as zinc, are expected to interact similarly.

Bisphosphonates should be prevented from coming into contact with zinc. Recommendations on the timing of administration of bisphosphonates in relation to food and other drugs varies. Alendronate should be taken with plain (not mineral) water, after an overnight fast at least 30 minutes before taking the first dose of zinc. Clodronate should probably be taken at least 1 hour before or after zinc. Ibandronate should be taken with plain water on an empty stomach at least 30 minutes to 1 hour before zinc. Risedronate should be taken at least 30 minutes before taking the first dose of zinc or at least 2 hours from any zinc doses during the rest of the day, and at least 30 minutes before bedtime. Etidronate and tiludronate should be taken on an empty stomach at least 2 hours apart from zinc.

Bupropion

Bupropion + Carbamazepine ⚠

Carbamazepine decreases the maximum plasma levels and AUC of bupropion by about 81 to 96%. The AUC of the active metabolite of bupropion, hydroxybupropion, is increased by 50%.

Monitor for any evidence of reduced efficacy (which is likely) and/or increased toxicity (due to the increased exposure to the metabolite). Note that bupropion is contraindicated in patients with seizure disorders.

Bupropion + Clopidogrel

Clopidogrel increases the AUC of bupropion by 60% and decreases the AUC of its active metabolite, hydroxybupropion, by about 50%.

> The clinical relevance of these modest changes is unclear. It would seem prudent to monitor for increased bupropion adverse effects (lightheadedness, gastrointestinal effects) and/or efficacy, adjusting the dose as necessary.

Bupropion + Dextromethorphan

Bupropion may reduce the metabolism of dextromethorphan in some patients.

> Dextromethorphan is generally considered to have a wide therapeutic range and its dose is not individually titrated; therefore, the interaction with bupropion is unlikely to be clinically relevant. Nevertheless, it is possible that some patients might become more sensitive to the adverse effects of dextromethorphan while taking bupropion. Note that dextromethorphan is widely found in non-prescription preparations such as cough suppressants.

Bupropion + Flecainide

The manufacturers warn that bupropion may raise flecainide levels (by inhibiting CYP2D6). This seems a reasonable prediction as other CYP2D6 substrates are affected by bupropion in this way.

> If flecainide is added to treatment with bupropion, doses at the lower end of the range should be used. If bupropion is added to existing treatment, decreased doses should be considered.

Bupropion + Herbal medicines or Dietary supplements ❓

Mania and dystonia have been reported in patients taking St John's wort (*Hypericum perforatum*) and bupropion.

> No general conclusions can be drawn from these isolated reports.

Bupropion + HIV-protease inhibitors ⚠

Ritonavir, both at doses used to boost the concentrations of other HIV-protease inhibitors and at higher doses, *decreases* the exposure to bupropion and its active metabolite: reduced efficacy might be expected. Lopinavir and tipranavir, both boosted with ritonavir, interact similarly. This is the opposite effect to that which was originally predicted. It seems likely that other HIV-protease inhibitors boosted with ritonavir will interact similarly.

> In patients taking ritonavir, or other HIV-protease inhibitors boosted with ritonavir, it would seem prudent to start bupropion at the recommended starting dose and titrate to effect. Nevertheless, because of the original *in vitro* data, the UK and US manufacturers of bupropion state that the recommended doses should not be exceeded. On the basis of the findings with ritonavir, it is not possible to predict

what will occur clinically with nelfinavir-containing regimens. In this case, it would seem prudent to start bupropion at the lowest recommended dose and titrate to effect.

Bupropion + Levodopa

The manufacturer says that the concurrent use of bupropion and levodopa should be undertaken with caution because limited clinical data suggests a higher incidence of undesirable effects (nausea, vomiting, excitement, restlessness, postural tremor).

Good monitoring is advisable and patients should be given small initial bupropion doses, which should be increased gradually.

Bupropion + MAOIs

In theory, bupropion toxicity may be enhanced by the MAOIs and concurrent use could lead to severe hypertension, but there appears to be no evidence to suggest that this occurs in practice.

Some manufacturers state that concurrent use is contraindicated with and for 2 weeks after the use of an MAOI.

Bupropion + Moclobemide

In theory, the concurrent use of bupropion and moclobemide could lead to severe hypertension, but there appears to be no evidence to suggest that this occurs in practice.

Some manufacturers state that concurrent use is contraindicated with and for 24 hours after stopping moclobemide.

Bupropion + NNRTIs

Efavirenz reduces the exposure to bupropion by about 50%. Nevirapine might interact similarly.

Monitor concurrent use to ensure bupropion remains effective, and consider increasing the bupropion dose as necessary. Note that the UK and US manufacturers of bupropion advise against exceeded the maximum licensed dose.

Bupropion + Opioids

The analgesic effects of codeine, and probably also hydrocodone, are predicted to be reduced or abolished by bupropion.

Monitor for analgesic efficacy and consider using an alternative to codeine or hydrocodone in the case of reduced efficacy.

Bupropion + **Phenobarbital**

Carbamazepine decreases the maximum plasma levels and AUC of bupropion by about 81 to 96%. The AUC of the active metabolite of bupropion, hydroxybupropion, is increased by 50%. The manufacturers predict that phenobarbital (and therefore probably primidone) will interact similarly.

> Monitor for any evidence of reduced efficacy (which is likely) and/or increased toxicity (due to the increased exposure to the metabolite). Note that bupropion is contraindicated in patients with seizure disorders.

Bupropion + **Phenytoin**

Carbamazepine decreases the maximum plasma levels and AUC of bupropion by about 81 to 96%. The AUC of the active metabolite of bupropion, hydroxybupropion, is increased by 50%. The manufacturers predict that phenytoin (and therefore possibly fosphenytoin) will interact similarly.

> Monitor for any evidence of reduced efficacy (which is likely) and/or increased toxicity (due to the increased exposure to the metabolite). Note that bupropion is contraindicated in patients with seizure disorders.

Bupropion + **Propafenone**

The manufacturers warn that bupropion may raise propafenone levels (by inhibiting CYP2D6). This seems a reasonable prediction as other CYP2D6 substrates are affected by bupropion in this way.

> If propafenone is added to treatment with bupropion, doses at the lower end of the range should be used. If bupropion is added to existing treatment, decreased doses should be considered.

Bupropion + **Rifampicin (Rifampin)**

Rifampicin markedly reduces the AUC of both bupropion and its active metabolite hydroxybupropion. Reduced efficacy might be anticipated on concurrent use.

> Monitor the efficacy of bupropion in any patient requiring rifampicin, and titrate the bupropion dose as necessary.

Bupropion + **SSRIs**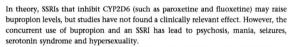

In theory, SSRIs that inhibit CYP2D6 (such as paroxetine and fluoxetine) may raise bupropion levels, but studies have not found a clinically relevant effect. However, the concurrent use of bupropion and an SSRI has lead to psychosis, mania, seizures, serotonin syndrome and hypersexuality.

> Concurrent use should be well monitored. The manufacturers recommend that drugs that are metabolised by CYP2D6 (most SSRIs are, but fluoxetine, paroxetine and sertraline have been specifically named) should be given with bupropion with caution and initiated at the lower end of the dose range. If bupropion is given to a patient already taking a drug metabolised by CYP2D6, the need to decrease the dose of this drug should be considered. Note that because the SSRIs can reduce the

seizure threshold consideration should be given to reducing the dose of bupropion to a maximum of 150 mg daily for smoking cessation.

B

Bupropion + Tamoxifen

Paroxetine reduces the metabolism of tamoxifen to one of its active metabolites (by inhibiting CYP2D6): this might decrease the efficacy of tamoxifen and possibly increase the risk of breast cancer recurrence. The MHRA predicts that other CYP2D6 inhibitors (they name bupropion) could possibly interact similarly.

The European Medicines Agency and the MHRA in the UK state that concurrent of CYP2D6 inhibitors use should be avoided whenever possible in patients taking tamoxifen, and they specifically name bupropion. Consider alternatives to tamoxifen in patients clearly benefiting from bupropion.

Bupropion + Ticlopidine

Ticlopidine increases the AUC of bupropion and decreases the AUC of its active metabolite, hydroxybupropion; both by about 85%.

The clinical relevance of these modest changes is unclear. It would seem prudent to monitor for increased bupropion adverse effects (lightheadedness, gastrointestinal effects) and efficacy, adjusting the dose as necessary.

Bupropion + Tricyclics

Bupropion may increase the levels of the tricyclics, including desipramine, imipramine, and nortriptyline. Adverse effects including confusion, lethargy and unsteadiness have been reported with nortriptyline and bupropion. A seizure occurred in two patients given trimipramine or clomipramine with bupropion.

It would be prudent to be alert for increased tricyclic adverse effects if bupropion is also given, reducing the tricyclic dose as necessary. Note that a maximum bupropion dose of 150 mg daily is recommended if it is given with other drugs that reduce the seizure threshold, such as the tricyclics.

Bupropion + Valproate

A study found that the AUC of the active metabolite of bupropion was almost doubled when bupropion was given with valproate. An increase in valproate levels of almost 30% was seen in one patient and visual and auditory hallucinations have been reported in another patient, which resolved when bupropion was stopped.

Monitor for any evidence of increased toxicity (due to the raised bupropion metabolites or valproate). Note that bupropion is contraindicated in patients with seizure disorders.

Bupropion + Venlafaxine

Bupropion appears to increase the plasma concentration of venlafaxine, sometimes leading to serotonergic adverse effects (tension, agitation, insomnia).

Consider reducing the venlafaxine dose if adverse effects become troublesome.

Buspirone

Buspirone + Calcium-channel blockers

Diltiazem and verapamil moderately to markedly increase the exposure to buspirone which increases the likelihood of adverse effects.

It would seem prudent to reduce the buspirone dose, or start buspirone at a lower dose. The US manufacturer suggests adjusting the buspirone dose according to response.

Buspirone + Carbamazepine

Rifampicin can markedly reduce the exposure to buspirone, reducing its effects. Carbamazepine is predicted to interact similarly.

Monitor concurrent use to ensure buspirone remains effective: the US manufacturer states that if a patient has been titrated to a stable dose of buspirone, a dose adjustment might be necessary to avoid reduced anxiolytic activity.

Buspirone + Cobicistat

Cobicistat is predicted to increase buspirone concentrations.

Monitor for buspirone adverse effects (such as dizziness, muscle pain, tachycardia), and adjust the buspirone dose if necessary.

Buspirone + Corticosteroids

Rifampicin can markedly reduce the exposure to buspirone (by inducing CYP3A4), reducing its effects. The US manufacturer of buspirone predicts that dexamethasone will interact similarly. However, dexamethasone rarely appears to cause clinically significant interactions by this mechanism.

Until more is known, consider the possibility of an interaction if buspirone efficacy appears reduced in patients given dexamethasone: the US manufacturer states that if a patient has been titrated to a stable dose of buspirone, a dose adjustment might be necessary to avoid reduced anxiolytic activity.

B

Buspirone + **Grapefruit juice**

Large amounts of grapefruit juice markedly increase buspirone exposure about 4-fold, but a only minor increase in effects appears to occur.

Be alert for an increase in buspirone adverse effects in patients drinking large amounts of grapefruit juice: the US manufacturer suggests that patients should avoid drinking large quantities of grapefruit juice.

Buspirone + **Herbal medicines or Dietary supplements**

A patient taking buspirone developed marked CNS adverse effects after starting to take herbal medicines including St John's wort (*Hypericum perforatum*), melatonin, and *Ginkgo biloba*. Serotonin syndrome, page 580 has been reported in a patient who took buspirone with St John's wort (*Hypericum perforatum*).

The general significance of these cases is unclear, but they highlight the importance of considering the adverse effects of herbal medicines when they are used with conventional medicines.

Buspirone + **HIV-protease inhibitors**

Ritonavir, and possibly indinavir, are predicted to reduce the metabolism of buspirone. A single case report describes Parkinson-like symptoms attributed to this interaction.

The UK manufacturer of buspirone recommends that a lower dose of buspirone 2.5 mg twice daily should be used with potent inhibitors of CYP3A4, such as ritonavir and other HIV-protease inhibitors.

Buspirone + **Linezolid**

Linezolid has weak, reversible MAO-inhibitory properties and it is therefore possible that it may interact with buspirone in the same way as the non-selective MAOIs (see Buspirone + MAOIs, page 209), although to a much lesser extent.

The manufacturers of linezolid contraindicate its use with buspirone, unless facilities are available for close observation and monitoring of blood pressure. In addition, the US manufacturer advises that patients should only receive linezolid with buspirone if they are observed for signs of serotonin syndrome, page 580.

Buspirone + **Macrolides**

In one study the exposure to buspirone was increased about 6-fold by erythromycin, which resulted in psychomotor impairment and an increase in adverse effects. Clarithromycin and telithromycin might therefore increase buspirone exposure to a greater extent than erythromycin.

Reduce the buspirone dose: for clarithromycin and telithromycin, the manufacturers recommend that the dose should be reduced to 2.5 mg twice daily (UK) or even once daily (US). For erythromycin, the manufacturers suggest a starting dose of buspirone 2.5 mg twice daily. Other macrolides might also interact, although it seems unlikely that all macrolides will, see macrolides, page 474.

Buspirone + MAOIs

Elevated blood pressure has been reported in patients taking buspirone with either phenelzine or tranylcypromine. All non-selective MAOIs could, theoretically, interact similarly.

The manufacturers of buspirone recommend that it should not be used concurrently with any MAOI. One US manufacturer of tranylcypromine contraindicates concurrent use and states that at least 10 days should elapse between stopping the MAOI and starting buspirone.

Buspirone + Phenobarbital

Rifampicin can markedly reduce the exposure to buspirone, reducing its effects. Phenobarbital and primidone would be expected to interact similarly.

Monitor concurrent use to ensure buspirone remains effective: the US manufacturer states that if a patient has been titrated to a stable dose of buspirone, a dose adjustment might be necessary to avoid reduced anxiolytic activity.

Buspirone + Phenytoin

Rifampicin can markedly reduce the exposure to buspirone, reducing its effects. Phenytoin and fosphenytoin would be expected to interact similarly.

Monitor concurrent use to ensure buspirone remains effective: the US manufacturer states that if a patient has been titrated to a stable dose of buspirone, a dose adjustment might be necessary to avoid reduced anxiolytic activity.

Buspirone + Rifampicin (Rifampin)

Rifampicin can markedly reduce the exposure to buspirone , reducing its effects.

If both drugs are used be alert for the need to increase the buspirone dose, although the extent of this interaction is so great that this might not be effective, and therefore it would be prudent to consider alternatives to buspirone, where possible.

Buspirone + SSRIs 🔲

Isolated reports describe the development of serotonin syndrome, page 580 on the concurrent use of buspirone and an SSRI. The combination of buspirone and fluoxetine can be effective, but cases of atypical dystonia, a reduction in buspirone efficacy, seizures and worsening of symptoms have been reported. Fluvoxamine increases the exposure to buspirone about 3-fold; however, no increase in adverse effects was reported.

The general importance of these adverse reactions is not well understood. There would seem to be little reason for avoiding concurrent use; however, bear them in mind when buspirone is given with an SSRI.

Busulfan

Busulfan + Metronidazole ⚠

Metronidazole increases the minimum concentration of high-dose busulfan and increases its toxicity.

High-dose busulfan should not be given at the same time as metronidazole. If metronidazole is given to a patient taking conventional dose busulfan, the UK manufacturer recommends weekly blood counts to detect any increase in toxicity.

Busulfan + Phenytoin ❓

Phenytoin increases the clearance of busulfan and reduces its AUC by about 20%. Subtherapeutic levels of phenytoin may occur in the presence of busulfan.

The changes in busulfan clearance are relatively small, but nevertheless it has been suggested that phenytoin should be avoided in patients taking busulfan. The UK manufacturer of parenteral busulfan found no evidence that phenytoin increased its clearance whereas another suggests using a benzodiazepine instead of phenytoin for prophylaxis. The US manufacturer of parenteral busulfan gives a dose assuming that phenytoin will also be given, and notes that if other antiepileptics are used instead, the busulfan plasma levels may be increased and monitoring is recommended. If both drugs are given monitor closely to ensure that busulfan remains effective, and that phenytoin levels remain therapeutic.

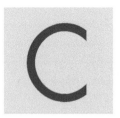

Calcium-channel blockers

Both verapamil and diltiazem are principally metabolised by CYP3A4, and also inhibit this isoenzyme. They are therefore affected by drugs that induce or inhibit CYP3A4, and also themselves affect drugs metabolised by CYP3A4. Many of the dihydropyridine-type calcium-channel blockers are also metabolised by CYP3A4, and are affected by inducers or inhibitors of this isoenzyme. However, they do not generally inhibit CYP3A4 or other isoenzymes to a clinically relevant extent. The exception is perhaps nicardipine, which may cause a clinically relevant inhibition of CYP3A4.

Calcium-channel blockers + Calcium-channel blockers ⚠

Plasma levels of both nifedipine and diltiazem are increased by concurrent use and blood pressure is reduced accordingly. Verapamil is predicted to interact similarly with nifedipine. Amlodipine levels are raised by diltiazem (and therefore possibly verapamil). There are isolated reports of intestinal occlusion attributed to the concurrent use of nifedipine and diltiazem. If nimodipine is used with another calcium-channel blocker, additive reductions in blood pressure are likely.

> Monitor blood pressure on concurrent use and adjust the dose or stop one calcium-channel blocker as appropriate. The clinical use of two calcium-channel blockers is rarely justified and consideration should be given to stopping one or other of the drugs, as appropriate.

Calcium-channel blockers + Carbamazepine

Diltiazem or Verapamil ⚠

Both diltiazem and verapamil can increase carbamazepine concentrations, causing toxicity.

> Monitor carbamazepine concentrations and adjust the dose accordingly to avoid toxicity. A 50% reduction in the dose of carbamazepine has been suggested if diltiazem is to be used. Indicators of carbamazepine toxicity include nausea, vomiting, ataxia, and drowsiness.

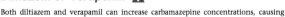

Nimodipine

The plasma concentration of nimodipine is reduced by carbamazepine.

> The UK manufacturer of nimodipine contraindicates its concurrent use with carbamazepine because of the possibility of a large reduction in its bioavailability.

Other calcium-channel blockers

The plasma concentrations of felodipine, nifedipine, and nilvadipine are decreased by carbamazepine, probably as a result of CYP3A4 induction. The majority of calcium-channel blockers are metabolised by CYP3A4, and carbamazepine would therefore be expected to decrease their exposure to some extent.

> Monitor the outcome of concurrent use (e.g. blood pressure), being aware that the dose of the calcium-channel blocker might need to be increased. Oxcarbazepine interacts to a lesser extent and might be suitable alternative in some patients.

Calcium-channel blockers + Ciclosporin (Cyclosporine)

Lercanidipine

Lercanidipine slightly increases ciclosporin concentrations, whereas ciclosporin greatly increases lercanidipine concentrations: taking ciclosporin 3 hours after lercanidipine might minimise this effect. Combined use of calcium-channel blockers and ciclosporin increases the risk of gingival overgrowth.

> The UK manufacturer of lercanidipine contraindicates concurrent use. If it is essential, consider separating the doses by 3 hours and monitor for lercanidipine adverse effects in particular hypotension. Consider an interaction if unexplained increases in ciclosporin concentrations or gingival hypertrophy occur.

Other calcium-channel blockers

Diltiazem, nicardipine, and verapamil greatly increase the plasma concentration of ciclosporin, but also appear to possess kidney protective effects. Amlodipine has modestly increased ciclosporin concentrations in some studies, but not in others, and it might also have kidney protective properties. A single case describes elevated plasma concentrations of ciclosporin caused by nisoldipine. Nifedipine also appears to have kidney protective effects and normally appears not to interact, but increases and decreases in ciclosporin plasma concentrations have been seen in a few patients. Combined use of calcium-channel blockers and ciclosporin increases the risk of gingival overgrowth.

> Ciclosporin plasma concentrations and/or effects (e.g. on renal function) should be well monitored (especially with diltiazem, nicardipine, and verapamil) and dose reductions made as necessary. With diltiazem and verapamil, the ciclosporin dose can apparently be reduced by about 25 to 50%. Take care not to substitute one diltiazem product for another after the patient has been stabilised because there is evidence that differences in their bioequivalence can alter the extent of the interaction. The UK manufacturer of ciclosporin specifically recommends avoiding nifedipine in patients who develop gingival overgrowth whilst taking ciclosporin. It might be prudent to apply this to all calcium-channel blockers, when possible.

Calcium-channel blockers + **Cilostazol**

Diltiazem or Verapamil

Diltiazem slightly increases the exposure to cilostazol. Verapamil would be expected to interact similarly.

> Monitor concurrent use for cilostazol adverse effects (such as headache and diarrhoea). Diltiazem and verapamil are both moderate CYP3A4 inhibitors, and the UK and US manufacturers of cilostazol suggest reducing the its dose to 50 mg twice daily when given with any CYP3A4 inhibitor.

Other calcium-channel blockers

The UK manufacturer notes that the concurrent use of cilostazol with dihydropyridine calcium-channel blockers increases the incidence of palpitations and peripheral oedema.

> Monitor the outcome of concurrent use for an increase in these adverse effects.

Calcium-channel blockers + **Cobicistat**

Cobicistat is predicted to increase the plasma concentrations of calcium-channel blockers.

> Monitor for calcium-channel blocker adverse effects (such as oedema, hypotension, headache, flushing), and adjust the calcium-channel blocker dose if needed.

Calcium-channel blockers + **Colchicine**

Diltiazem and verapamil increase the exposure to colchicine. Colchicine toxicity has been seen in one patient after colchicine was given to a patient taking verapamil.

> Until more information is available, if any patient is given colchicine with diltiazem or verapamil, monitor for signs of colchicine toxicity (such as nausea, vomiting, diarrhoea, myopathy, and pancytopenia), particularly in patients with pre-existing hepatic or renal impairment. Additionally, anticipate the need to reduce the colchicine dose. The US manufacturer of colchicine also advises specific dose reductions in patients taking moderate CYP3A4 inhibitors, such as diltiazem or verapamil, or if they have stopped taking such drugs within 2 weeks of starting colchicine (see Colchicine + Macrolides, page 285 for further information).

Calcium-channel blockers + **Corticosteroids**

Diltiazem increases the exposure to intravenous and oral methylprednisolone. The metabolism of oral prednisone is also reduced by diltiazem. Cases of adrenal insufficiency have been described on the concurrent use of diltiazem with inhaled budesonide, and verapamil with inhaled fluticasone.

> Monitor the concurrent use of diltiazem or verapamil and methylprednisolone for an increase in corticosteroid adverse effects (e.g. fluid retention, hypertension and hyperglycaemia). Monitor the effects of the concurrent use of diltiazem or verapamil with inhaled fluticasone or budesonide on adrenal function for any

C

signs of excessive corticosteroid effects. Similar precautions would seem sensible in patients taking oral budesonide with these calcium-channel blockers.

Calcium-channel blockers + Dapoxetine

Diltiazem and verapamil are predicted to increase the exposure to dapoxetine. As dapoxetine is also metabolised by CYP2D6, CYP2D6 metaboliser status is predicted to also affect this interaction.

The Swedish manufacturer of dapoxetine recommends a maximum dose of dapoxetine 30 mg on the concurrent use of diltiazem or verapamil). In CYP2D6 extensive metabolisers (which is generally unlikely to be known), the manufacturer advises a maximum dapoxetine dose of 60 mg.

Calcium-channel blockers + Darifenacin

Erythromycin causes a moderate increase in darifenacin exposure. Other moderate inhibitors of CYP3A4 such as diltiazem and verapamil are expected to interact similarly. In addition, verapamil is predicted to increase darifenacin exposure by inhibiting P-glycoprotein, and so might have a greater effect than diltiazem.

The UK manufacturer recommends an initial dose of darifenacin 7.5 mg daily in those taking moderate CYP3A4 inhibitors, increasing the dose to 15 mg daily if the dose is well tolerated. However the US manufacturers suggest that no dose adjustments are necessary with these calcium-channel blockers. Bear in mind the possibility of an interaction if antimuscarinic effects (dry mouth, constipation, drowsiness) are increased. Note that verapamil also inhibits P-glycoprotein, and the UK manufacturer of darifenacin advises that the concurrent use of P-glycoprotein inhibitors, such as verapamil, should be avoided.

Calcium-channel blockers + Digoxin

Diltiazem

Serum digoxin levels were found to be unchanged by diltiazem in a number of studies but other studies describe increases ranging from 20 to 85%. Additive bradycardia and heart block may also occur with concurrent use.

All patients taking digoxin with diltiazem should be well monitored for signs of over-digitalisation or additive adverse effects (e.g. bradycardia), and digoxin dose reductions should be made if necessary.

Verapamil

Serum digoxin levels are increased by about 40% by verapamil 160 mg daily, and by about 70% by verapamil 240 mg daily. Digoxin toxicity may develop if the dose is not reduced. Deaths have occurred as a result of this interaction. There is a risk of additive bradycardia and conduction disturbances when cardiac glycosides are given with verapamil.

An initial 30 to 50% digoxin dose reduction has been recommended. The interaction develops within 2 to 7 days, approaching or reaching a maximum within 14 days or so. Monitor digoxin levels and for signs of digoxin toxicity (such

as nausea, vomiting, visual disturbances, confusion) as well as cardiac conduction disorders during this period.

Other calcium-channel blockers

Felodipine, isradipine, lacidipine, lercanidipine, and nicardipine do not alter digoxin exposure, although small increases in maximum digoxin concentrations have been seen with some of these calcium-channel blockers. Nisoldipine might cause a minor rise in minimum digoxin concentrations. The situation with nitrendipine is uncertain but it possibly causes only a small rise in digoxin exposure. Serum digoxin concentrations are normally unchanged or increased only to a small extent by the concurrent use of nifedipine; however, a few studies describe increases ranging from 45 to 66%.

Bear this interaction in mind if patients are given digoxin with one of these calcium-channel blockers. The possibility of a serious interaction seems small, but if undesirable bradycardia or other symptoms of over-digitalisation occur, consider measuring digoxin concentrations, and reduce the digoxin dose as necessary.

Calcium-channel blockers + Disopyramide

Profound hypotension and collapse has occurred in a small number of patients taking verapamil with disopyramide.

The UK manufacturer warns about giving disopyramide with verapamil (because of additive negative inotropic effects), although in some specific circumstances the combination may be beneficial. However, the US manufacturer advises that until more data is available, disopyramide should not be given within 48 hours before or 24 hours after verapamil. If concurrent used is necessary, monitor closely.

Calcium-channel blockers + Diuretics

Mild to moderate inhibitors of CYP3A4 (such as diltiazem and verapamil) cause up to a 3-fold increase in eplerenone levels, which increases the risks of hyperkalaemia.

It is generally recommended that the dose of eplerenone should not exceed 25 mg daily in patients taking diltiazem or verapamil. Note that additive hypotensive effects are likely when calcium-channel blockers are given with any diuretic, see antihypertensives, page 97.

Calcium-channel blockers + Donepezil

The risk of adverse effects, including bradycardia, might be increased if a centrally-acting anticholinesterase is given with a calcium-channel blocker. Although not specifically stated, only the calcium-channel blockers that have effects on heart rate (that is, diltiazem and verapamil) would be expected to be implicated.

Be alert for bradycardia on the concurrent use of donepezil and diltiazem or verapamil and adjust treatment if necessary.

Calcium-channel blockers + **Dronedarone**

The manufacturers state that diltiazem and verapamil slightly increase dronedarone exposure. Dronedarone also slightly increases diltiazem and verapamil exposure, although in one study, no increase in hypotension, bradycardia or heart failure occurred. Additive cardiac depression of the sinus and AV nodes might occur on concurrent use.

The UK and US manufacturers of dronedarone advise that diltiazem and verapamil should be started at a low dose in patients taking dronedarone, and the dose should only be increased after an ECG has been checked. If dronedarone is started in a patient already taking these calcium-channel blockers, they advise that a baseline ECG should be done and the dose of the calcium-channel blocker should be adjusted if needed.

Calcium-channel blockers + **Dutasteride**

In one study diltiazem and verapamil were found to decrease the clearance of dutasteride by 44% and 37%, respectively. However, this was not thought to be clinically significant due to the wide therapeutic range of dutasteride.

No action needed, although bear this interaction in mind if dutasteride adverse effects are troublesome. If this occurs, consider decreasing the dosing frequency of dutasteride.

Calcium-channel blockers + **Everolimus**

Increased concentrations of both everolimus and verapamil can occur on concurrent use. Diltiazem might be expected to increase everolimus concentrations. One Australian manufacturer predicts that nicardipine will increase everolimus concentrations.

Monitor everolimus concentrations and adverse effects (stomatitis, blood dyscrasias, renal impairment). Adjust the everolimus dose as needed, depending on the indication. Monitor for verapamil adverse effects (hypotension, flushing, oedema), and adjust the dose if required.

Calcium-channel blockers + **Fesoterodine**

Fluconazole slightly increased the exposure to the active metabolite of fesoterodine, and an increase in some minor adverse effects, such as nausea and dizziness, occurred. Diltiazem and verapamil would be expected to interact similarly.

No fesoterodine dose adjustment is necessary on concurrent use. Bear in mind the possibility of an interaction should any adverse effects occur (e.g. dry mouth, dizziness, insomnia). Concurrent use should be avoided in patients with severe renal impairment, and a maximum fesoterodine dose of 4 mg daily given to those with mild to moderate renal impairment. Concurrent use should also be avoided in those with moderate to severe hepatic impairment, and a maximum fesoterodine dose of 4 mg daily given to those with mild hepatic impairment.

Calcium-channel blockers + **Flecainide**

Although flecainide and verapamil have been used together successfully, serious and potentially life-threatening cardiogenic shock and asystole have been seen in a few patients. This is probably because the cardiac depressant effects of the two drugs can be additive.

> This interaction might not be of clinical importance in most patients, however those with poor cardiac reserve could be more susceptible. If both drugs are used, monitor the outcome carefully.

Calcium-channel blockers + **Food**

Some modified-release preparations of felodipine, nifedipine, and nisoldipine show markedly increased levels when given with food, particularly high-fat food. The bioavailability of lercanidipine is markedly increased and the absorption of manidipine is improved by food. Food modestly decreases the rate and extent of absorption of nimodipine capsules and food also modestly decreases the peak level of nicardipine.

> The manufacturers of *Vascalpha* (felodipine), *Adalat CC* (nifedipine) and *Sular* (nisoldipine) recommend that they are taken on an empty stomach or with a light meal, avoiding high-fat meals. Because of the potential increase in peak plasma concentrations, the manufacturers of lercanidipine advise giving it before meals (at least 15 minutes before has been recommended). The US manufacturer of nimodipine capsules recommends taking them not less than one hour before or 2 hours after meals. It has been recommended that manidipine and *Cardene SR* (nicardipine) should be taken with food. Consider also Grapefruit juice, page 217.

Calcium-channel blockers + **Galantamine**

The risk of adverse effects, including bradycardia, might be increased if a centrally-acting anticholinesterase is given with a calcium-channel blocker. Although not specifically stated, only the calcium-channel blockers that have effects on heart rate (that is, diltiazem and verapamil) would be expected to be implicated.

> Be alert for bradycardia on the concurrent use of galantamine and diltiazem or verapamil and adjust treatment if necessary.

Calcium-channel blockers + **Grapefruit juice**

Grapefruit juice moderately increases the exposure to felodipine, manidipine, and nisoldipine, and alters their haemodynamic effects. The bioavailability of nicardipine, nifedipine, nimodipine, nitrendipine, and verapamil is increased without significantly altering haemodynamic effects (some ECG changes were seen with verapamil), whereas the bioavailability of amlodipine and diltiazem is only minimally affected.

> Several UK manufacturers of felodipine state that it should not be taken with grapefruit juice. It has been suggested that whole grapefruit or products made from grapefruit peel, such as marmalade, should also be avoided in patients taking felodipine. The UK manufacturer of lercanidipine and one manufacturer of verapamil also contraindicate grapefruit juice, although another manufacturer of verapamil suggests that this interaction appears to be of little clinical relevance in the majority of patients. Generally speaking, studies suggest that the concurrent use of grapefruit juice and most calcium-channel blockers other than felodipine,

C

and possibly manidipine, nifedipine or nisoldipine, need not be avoided. However it would be worth checking the diet of any patient who complains of increased or excessive adverse effects with any calcium-channel blocker (e.g. hypotension, headache, flushing, oedema). Any problems can be solved either by avoiding grapefruit juice, or, where possible, by swapping the calcium-channel blocker for one less likely to interact (although note that cases have been reported with amlodipine, which is generally considered as unlikely to interact). Note that some studies suggest that the effects of grapefruit juice can persist for several days, and this should be taken into account when adjusting treatment.

Calcium-channel blockers + H₂-receptor antagonists ⚠

The plasma levels of diltiazem, felodipine, isradipine, lacidipine, nifedipine, nimodipine, nisoldipine, nitrendipine and possibly verapamil and lercanidipine, are increased by cimetidine.

If cimetidine is given with a calcium-channel blocker monitor for an increase in the calcium-channel blocker effects (such as hypotension, flushing, headache, peripheral oedema). If necessary, a dose reduction should be considered and the following dose adjustments have been suggested, in general, 30 to 50% decreases have been suggested, but any decrease should be based on patient response. In theory, all calcium-channel blockers may interact similarly, although some evidence suggests that amlodipine does not interact.

Calcium-channel blockers + Herbal medicines or Dietary supplements ⚠

St John's wort (*Hypericum perforatum*) reduces the bioavailability of verapamil by 80% and nifedipine by 45%. Other calcium-channel blockers would be expected to interact similarly.

Patients taking St John's wort with nifedipine or verapamil should have their blood pressure and heart rate monitored to ensure the calcium-channel blocker is still effective, and the dose should be adjusted if needed. There appears to be no information about other calcium-channel blockers, but as they are all metabolised by CYP3A4, to a greater or lesser extent, it would seem prudent to monitor concurrent use carefully. If an interaction occurs it may be prudent to use an alternative class of drugs (ACE inhibitors, angiotensin II receptor antagonists and beta blockers are not known to be affected by CYP3A4), or advise against the use of St John's wort.

Calcium-channel blockers + HIV-protease inhibitors ⚠

The HIV-protease inhibitors, particularly ritonavir, are predicted to increase the exposure to the calcium-channel blockers, to varying degrees: case reports describe adverse effects (hypotension, oedema, acute renal failure) on the concurrent use of a number of different HIV-protease inhibitor and calcium-channel blocker pairs.

If a HIV-protease inhibitor and a calcium-channel blocker are given, monitor for toxicity, such as hypotension, dizziness, flushing, oedema and palpitations,

reducing the dose of the calcium-channel blocker if necessary. Note that the UK manufacturer of lercanidipine contraindicates the concurrent use of strong inhibitors of CYP3A4; this would include most, if not all HIV-protease inhibitors. The initial dose of diltiazem should be reduced by 50% with subsequent dose titration and ECG monitoring when given with atazanavir. Consider alternative antihypertensives, such as ACE inhibitors and diuretics, which are primarily eliminated renally.

Calcium-channel blockers + Ivabradine

Diltiazem, a moderate inhibitor of CYP3A4, increases the AUC of ivabradine 2-to 3-fold, and additive bradycardia occurs on concurrent use. Verapamil is predicted to interact similarly.

The manufacturer advise avoiding the concurrent use of diltiazem or verapamil with ivabradine.

Calcium-channel blockers + Lithium

The concurrent use of lithium and verapamil can be uneventful, but neurotoxicity (ataxia, movement disorders, tremors) with unchanged lithium levels has been reported in a few patients. Reduced and increased lithium levels have also occurred with verapamil. An acute parkinsonian syndrome and marked psychosis has been seen in at least one patient taking lithium and diltiazem. Reduced lithium clearance, and one possible case of increased lithium levels have been reported with nifedipine.

The clinical significance of this interaction is unclear, as there is good evidence of uncomplicated treatment. Given the unpredictable changes in levels it may be prudent to consider monitoring lithium in patients also given verapamil, and considering an interaction as a possible cause if unexpected adverse effects develop with diltiazem or nifedipine.

Calcium-channel blockers + **Macrolides**

Lercanidipine ✕

Because ketoconazole increases the exposure to lercanidipine 15-fold, the UK manufacturer predicts that other CYP3A4 inhibitors, such as erythromycin, will interact similarly.

The UK manufacturer of lercanidipine contraindicates concurrent use with erythromycin.

Other calcium-channel blockers ⚠

Erythromycin moderately increases the exposure to felodipine. Cases reports and retrospective analyses suggest that the use of clarithromycin, erythromycin, or telithromycin with calcium-channel blockers, including diltiazem, felodipine, nifedipine, and verapamil, increases the risk of toxicity and adverse effects, such as hypotension and QT prolongation. Note that the calcium-channel blockers are all metabolised by CYP3A4, so all have the potential to interact. Reports also suggest that the cardiac toxicity of erythromycin might be increased by verapamil, and diltiazem, and it has been suggested that erythromycin should not be used with diltiazem and verapamil. However a serious interaction seems rare.

> Monitor concurrent use. Anticipate the need to reduce the calcium-channel blocker dose if erythromycin or clarithromycin, or possibly also telithromycin, is added and adverse effects become troublesome (such as hypotension, dizziness, flushing and palpitations).

Calcium-channel blockers + Magnesium

Pregnant women have developed bilateral hand contractures or muscular weakness and then paralysis, after receiving intravenous magnesium sulfate, either alone, or with nifedipine or amlodipine. Profound hypotension occurred in two women when nifedipine was added to magnesium sulfate and methyldopa. However a larger retrospective study did not find an increase in risk of neuromuscular effects or of hypotension on concurrent use of nifedipine. Other calcium-channel blockers would be expected to interact similarly, but this has not been studied. One UK manufacturer of magnesium sulfate injection states that concurrent use of nimodipine might very rarely lead to a calcium ion imbalance which could result in abnormal muscle function.

> One UK manufacturer of nifedipine advises particular caution when it is used in combination with intravenous magnesium sulfate in pregnant women, and recommends careful monitoring of blood pressure. Plasma calcium and magnesium should also be carefully monitored when using intravenous magnesium sulfate in pregnancy. The interaction would not be expected with oral magnesium compounds because these have a low risk of causing hypermagnesaemia.

Calcium-channel blockers + NNRTIs

Efavirenz decreases the bioavailability of diltiazem by increasing its metabolism by CYP3A4; other calcium-channel blockers are expected to interact similarly. Delavirdine is predicted to inhibit the metabolism of the calcium-channel blockers.

> Monitor the outcome of concurrent use (e.g. blood pressure) and adjust the calcium-channel blocker dose as necessary. If dose titration of the calcium-channel blocker proves difficult it may be prudent, where possible, to try an alternative class of drugs. ACE inhibitors, angiotensin II receptor antagonists, and beta blockers are not known to be affected by CYP3A4 and therefore may be suitable alternatives in some cases.

Calcium-channel blockers + NSAIDs

There is evidence that most NSAIDs can increase blood pressure in patients taking antihypertensives, although some studies have not found the increase to be clinically relevant. Individual patients may experience more significant effects. Some small pharmacokinetic interactions may occur, but they do not appear to be clinically relevant.

> Only some patients are affected. Nevertheless, some have suggested that the use of NSAIDs should be kept to a minimum in patients taking antihypertensives, whereas others suggest that the interaction is, generally, not clinically relevant. Consider monitoring blood pressure if an NSAID is started or stopped.

Calcium-channel blockers + Oxybutynin

Ketoconazole, a potent CYP3A4 inhibitor, moderately increased oxybutynin concentrations, however the pharmacokinetics of its active metabolite were unchanged. Moderate CYP3A4 inhibitors, such as verapamil and diltiazem, are predicted to increase the exposure to oxybutynin. Further evidence suggests interactions between oxybutynin and CYP3A4 inhibitors are not clinically relevant, however manufacturers advise an increase in oxybutynin concentration cannot be ruled out.

> Bear in mind the possibility of an interaction if an increase in antimuscarinic adverse effects (dry mouth, constipation, drowsiness) occurs.

Calcium-channel blockers + Pasireotide

Bradycardia is a common adverse effect of pasireotide, which might be additive with the effects of other drugs that affect heart rate, such as diltiazem or verapamil. *In vitro*, pasireotide has been shown to be a substrate of P-glycoprotein and therefore the manufacturers predict that potent P-glycoprotein inhibitors, such as verapamil, will increase pasireotide concentrations.

> If bradycardia develops, consider adjusting the dose of the calcium-channel blocker, according to clinical need. Monitor for pasireotide adverse effects (such as abdominal pain, diarrhoea, and myalgia) and reduce the pasireotide dose if these become troublesome.

Calcium-channel blockers + Phenobarbital

Nimodipine or Isradipine

The plasma concentration of nimodipine is greatly decreased by phenobarbital through induction of CYP3A4. Isradipine is expected to be similarly affected by phenobarbital. Note that primidone is metabolised to phenobarbital and is expected to interact similarly.

> The UK manufacturer of nimodipine contraindicates concurrent use with phenobarbital, and the UK manufacturer of isradipine advises against concurrent use. If concurrent use is necessary, monitor the outcome, being aware that the dose of the calcium-channel blocker might need to be increased.

Other calcium-channel blockers ⚠

Phenobarbital greatly decreases the plasma concentration and/or increases the clearance of felodipine, nifedipine, and verapamil, probably by inducing CYP3A4. Other calcium-channel blockers are expected to interact similarly with phenobarbital. Note that primidone is metabolised to phenobarbital and is expected to interact similarly.

> Monitor the outcome of concurrent use (e.g. blood pressure), being aware that the dose of calcium-channel blocker might need to be increased. Given the size of the reductions seen it might be prudent to consider alternatives (ACE inhibitors, angiotensin II receptor antagonists, and beta blockers are not known to be affected by CYP3A4).

Calcium-channel blockers + **Phenytoin**

A case report describes neurological toxicity when a patient taking phenytoin (with carbamazepine) was given isradipine. Case reports also describe phenytoin toxicity in patients given diltiazem or nifedipine. Nisoldipine and felodipine plasma concentrations are greatly reduced by phenytoin. Case reports suggest that nimodipine and verapamil concentrations can also be reduced by phenytoin: other calcium-channel blockers are expected to be similarly affected. Fosphenytoin, a prodrug of phenytoin, might interact similarly.

> A considerable increase in the dose of the calcium-channel blocker will probably be needed when given with phenytoin and it would be prudent to consider alternatives. The UK manufacturer of nimodipine contraindicates the concurrent use with phenytoin, while the UK manufacturer of isradipine and the US manufacturer of nisoldipine advise against concurrent use. If it is essential, monitor to ensure the calcium-channel blocker remains effective. Monitor for signs of phenytoin toxicity (blurred vision, nystagmus, ataxia, drowsiness) when diltiazem is given with phenytoin: the dose of phenytoin might need to be reduced to avoid toxicity.

Calcium-channel blockers + **Phosphodiesterase type-5 inhibitors**

Diltiazem and verapamil are predicted to increase the exposure to the phosphodiesterase type-5 inhibitors.

> Be alert for an increase in phosphodiesterase type-5 inhibitor adverse effects (such as headache, flushing, and visual disturbances). Consider giving a smaller starting dose of sildenafil, tadalafil, or vardenafil on concurrent use with diltiazem or verapamil. The US manufacturer advises that a maximum avanafil dose of 50 mg every 24 hours should not be exceeded with moderate CYP3A4 inhibitors, such as diltiazem and verapamil. The UK manufacturer however, advises a maximum dose of 100 mg once every 48 hours with moderate CYP3A4 inhibitors.

Calcium-channel blockers + **Quinidine**

Verapamil

Verapamil reduces the clearance of quinidine and in one patient the serum quinidine levels doubled and quinidine toxicity developed. Concurrent use has resulted in dizziness, blurred vision, atrioventricular block and a significant lowering of blood pressure.

> A reduction in the dosage of quinidine (of up to 50%) may be needed to avoid toxicity. Monitor for an increase in quinidine adverse effects (e.g. nausea, diarrhoea, tinnitus).

Other calcium-channel blockers

The quinidine levels of a number of patients have increased when nifedipine was stopped, but no interaction has occurred in others. One study even suggests that quinidine serum levels may be slightly raised by nifedipine. Nifedipine levels may be modestly raised by quinidine. One study with diltiazem found that it did not interact with quinidine, whereas another found that diltiazem increased the quinidine AUC by

51%, with resulting significant increases in QTc and PR intervals, and a significant decrease in heart rate and diastolic blood pressure.

Monitor for quinidine adverse effects (e.g. nausea, diarrhoea, tinnitus) and, with nifedipine, for nifedipine adverse effects (e.g. hypotension, flushing, oedema). Adjust the doses of both drugs as necessary.

Calcium-channel blockers + Ranolazine

Verapamil and diltiazem increase ranolazine levels 2.2-fold and 2.4-fold, respectively, which increases the risk of QT prolongation and potentially life-threatening arrhythmias. However, concurrent use may be beneficial.

The UK manufacturer states that lower ranolazine doses and careful dose titration may be needed. The US manufacturer recommends that the dose of ranolazine should be limited to 500 mg twice daily. Monitor for adverse effects (nausea, dizziness) and reduce the dose of ranolazine if needed.

Calcium-channel blockers + Rifampicin (Rifampin)

The plasma concentrations of diltiazem, nifedipine, nilvadipine, verapamil and possibly those of barnidipine, isradipine, lercanidipine, manidipine, nicardipine, nimodipine, and nisoldipine are greatly reduced by rifampicin. They might become therapeutically ineffective unless their doses are increased. All calcium-channel blockers would be expected to be affected by rifampicin.

Increase the frequency of blood pressure monitoring and adjust the antihypertensive dose, or use an alternative drug, as necessary. Note that some UK manufacturers of nifedipine and nimodipine contraindicate their use with rifampicin, and some manufacturers of diltiazem and isradipine advise avoiding concurrent use.

Calcium-channel blockers + Rivastigmine

The risk of adverse effects, including bradycardia, might be increased if a centrally-acting anticholinesterase is given with a calcium-channel blocker. Although not specifically stated, only the calcium-channel blockers that have effects on heart rate (that is, diltiazem and verapamil) would be expected to be implicated.

Be alert for bradycardia on the concurrent use of rivastigmine and diltiazem or verapamil and adjust treatment if necessary.

Calcium-channel blockers + Sirolimus

Diltiazem and verapamil increase sirolimus concentrations. Nicardipine is predicted to interact similarly. Sirolimus caused a small increase in verapamil concentrations in one study.

The UK and US manufacturers of sirolimus recommend whole blood monitoring and possible sirolimus dose adjustments if these calcium-channel blockers are used concurrently. The clinical relevance of the modest increase in verapamil concentrations is uncertain, but bear it in mind if an increase in verapamil adverse effects occurs (e.g. hypotension, flushing and oedema).

Calcium-channel blockers + **Solifenacin**

Diltiazem and verapamil are predicted to increase the exposure to solifenacin.

> Bear in mind the possibility of an interaction should any solifenacin adverse effects occur, such as dry mouth, constipation, drowsiness.

Calcium-channel blockers + **Statins**

Amlodipine

Steady-state amlodipine slightly increases simvastatin exposure.

> It seems unlikely that the increase in exposure to simvastatin will be clinically relevant, and problems with combinations of statins and dihydropyridine-type calcium-channel blockers are rare. Nevertheless, a maximum simvastatin dose of 20 mg daily in patients taking amlodipine is recommended. Advise patient to report any unexplained muscle pain, tenderness, or weakness.

Diltiazem or Verapamil

Diltiazem moderately increases lovastatin and simvastatin exposure, and verapamil moderately increases simvastatin exposure. Isolated cases of rhabdomyolysis have occurred as a result of these interactions. Diltiazem slightly to moderately increases atorvastatin exposure and there are isolated cases of rhabdomyolysis with the combination.

> In patients taking verapamil, a maximum simvastatin dose of 20 mg daily (UK advice) or 10 mg daily (US advice), and a maximum dose of 40 mg daily of lovastatin is recommended. For diltiazem, the dose of simvastatin should not exceed 20 mg daily (UK advice) or 10 mg daily (US advice). The UK manufacturer advises that a lower dose of atorvastatin should be considered if diltiazem or verapamil are also given, with close monitoring at the start of treatment or if the dose of diltiazem or verapamil is changed. Patients should be told to be alert for any signs of possible rhabdomyolysis (i.e. otherwise unexplained muscle tenderness, pain, or weakness or dark coloured urine).

Calcium-channel blockers + **Tacrine**

The risk of adverse effects, including bradycardia, might be increased if a centrally-acting anticholinesterase is given with a calcium-channel blocker. Although not specifically stated, only the calcium-channel blockers that have effects on heart rate (that is, diltiazem and verapamil) would be expected to be implicated.

> Be alert for bradycardia on the concurrent use of tacrine and diltiazem or verapamil and adjust treatment if necessary.

Calcium-channel blockers + **Tacrolimus**

Nifedipine causes a small increase in tacrolimus concentrations and also appears to be kidney protective. Large increases in tacrolimus concentrations have been reported in a few cases with diltiazem, although a study found no interaction. Cases of increased tacrolimus concentrations have been reported on the concurrent use of amlodipine, felodipine, and nicardipine. Verapamil, and possibly nilvadipine, are predicted to interact similarly.

> Tacrolimus concentrations and/or effects (e.g. on renal function) should be monitored as a matter of routine, but consider increasing monitoring if one of these calcium-channel blockers is started or stopped.

Calcium-channel blockers + Theophylline

Giving calcium-channel blockers to patients taking theophylline normally has no adverse effect on the control of asthma, despite the small or modest alterations that occur in theophylline concentrations with diltiazem, felodipine, nifedipine and verapamil. However, there are isolated case reports of unexplained theophylline toxicity in 2 patients given nifedipine and 2 patients given verapamil. Aminophylline might interact similarly.

> A clinically relevant interaction is generally unlikely; however, consider the possibility of an interaction in the case of any unexplained theophylline adverse effects (such as headache, nausea, tremor). If this occurs, monitor theophylline concentrations and adjust the dose of theophylline or aminophylline if indicated.

Calcium-channel blockers + Ticagrelor

Diltiazem moderately increases the exposure to ticagrelor, whereas ticagrelor does not affect the plasma concentrations of diltiazem. Verapamil might increase ticagrelor exposure. Concurrent use of ticagrelor with these calcium-channel blockers might cause additive bradycardia.

> Monitor for increased ticagrelor effects (e.g. bleeding) and be aware of a possible increased risk of bradycardia.

Calcium-channel blockers + Tizanidine

Diltiazem and verapamil are predicted to increase the exposure to tizanidine, increasing its hypotensive and sedative effects.

> The UK and US manufacturers suggest that concurrent use should be avoided. Until more is known be alert for adverse effects such as bradycardia, hypotension, and drowsiness.

Calcium-channel blockers + Tolterodine

Moderate CYP3A4 inhibitors, such as verapamil and diltiazem, are predicted to increase the exposure to tolterodine.

> Bear in mind the possibility of an interaction if an increase in antimuscarinic adverse effects (dry mouth, constipation, drowsiness) occurs.

Calcium-channel blockers + Tricyclics

Diltiazem and verapamil can increase imipramine levels, possibly accompanied by undesirable ECG changes. Two isolated reports describe increased nortriptyline and trimipramine levels in 2 patients given diltiazem. It has been suggested that the postural hypotension that may occur in patients taking tricyclics could be exacerbated by the use of antihypertensives.

The general importance of this interaction is unclear, but bear it in mind in case of an unexpected response to treatment. Warn patients about the possibility of postural hypotension.

Calcium-channel blockers + Ulipristal

Moderate inhibitors of CYP3A4, such as diltiazem and verapamil, are predicted to moderately increase the exposure to ulipristal.

The UK manufacturer of low-dose ulipristal for the symptomatic management of uterine fibroids does not recommend its concurrent use with moderate CYP3A4 inhibitors. If low-dose ulipristal is given with diltiazem or verapamil, monitor for an increase in the adverse effects of ulipristal (for example nausea, abdominal pain, and breast tenderness) or any unexpected outcome occurring during concurrent use. The UK manufacturer of ulipristal for emergency contraception states that CYP3A4 inhibitors are unlikely to have any clinically relevant effects.

Calcium-channel blockers + Valproate

In a group of patients taking sodium valproate, the AUC of nimodipine was found to be about 50% higher than in a control group not taking sodium valproate.

Monitor concurrent use carefully, bearing in mind it may be necessary to adjust the dose of nimodipine.

Capecitabine

Capecitabine + Folates

A patient died after treatment with capecitabine possibly because the concurrent use of folic acid enhanced capecitabine toxicity. The maximum tolerated dose of capecitabine is decreased by folinic acid.

The UK manufacturers say that the maximum tolerated capecitabine dose when used alone in the intermittent regimen is $3\,g/m^2$, but it is reduced to $2\,g/m^2$ if folinic acid 30 mg twice daily is also given. Consider the use of folate supplements as a contributory factor in the case of troublesome capecitabine adverse effects.

Capecitabine + Phenytoin

Phenytoin toxicity occurred in a patient given capecitabine. Fosphenytoin, a prodrug of phenytoin, may interact similarly.

As the interaction of capecitabine with phenytoin is in line with the way fluorouracil interacts, it would seem prudent to warn the patient to monitor for signs of phenytoin toxicity (blurred vision, nystagmus, ataxia or drowsiness). Take phenytoin levels and adjust the dose as necessary.

Capecitabine + **Warfarin and related oral anticoagulants**

Capecitabine has been reported to markedly increase the anticoagulant effects of phenprocoumon and warfarin: in one study the INR in response to warfarin was almost doubled by capecitabine. The interaction may occur within several days or even after months of concurrent use.

> The INR should be more frequently monitored in patients taking capecitabine with these and other coumarins. Note that, from a disease perspective, when treating venous thromboembolic disease in patients with cancer, warfarin is generally inferior (higher risk of major bleeds and recurrent thrombosis) to low-molecular-weight heparins.

Carbamazepine

Carbamazepine is extensively metabolised by CYP3A4 to the active 10,11-epoxide metabolite, which is then further metabolised. Concurrent use of CYP3A4 inhibitors or inducers can therefore lead to toxicity or reduced efficacy. However, importantly, carbamazepine also induces CYP3A4 and so induces its own metabolism (auto-induction). Because of this, it is important that drug interaction studies are multiple-dose and carried out at steady state. Auto-induction also means that moderate inducers of CYP3A4 might have less effect on steady-state carbamazepine concentrations than expected. Carbamazepine can also act as an inhibitor of CYP2C19.

Carbamazepine + **Caspofungin** ▲

Population pharmacokinetic data suggests that carbamazepine might reduce caspofungin concentrations.

> The UK manufacturer recommends that consideration should be given to increasing the dose of caspofungin from 50 mg daily to 70 mg daily in adults and to 70 mg/m² daily (maximum 70 mg daily) in children, whereas the US manufacturer specifically states that the higher dose should be used.

Carbamazepine + **Ciclosporin (Cyclosporine)** ▲

Carbamazepine greatly reduces ciclosporin concentrations.

> Ciclosporin concentrations and/or effects (e.g. on renal function) should be monitored as a matter of routine, but it would be prudent to increase monitoring and adjust the ciclosporin dose as needed if carbamazepine is stopped, started, or the dose altered.

Carbamazepine + **Cilostazol** ⚠

The UK manufacturer of cilostazol predicts that inducers of CYP2C19 and CYP3A4 (they name carbamazepine) might alter the antiplatelet efficacy of cilostazol.

> The UK manufacturer advises monitoring the concurrent use of carbamazepine for an alteration in the antiplatelet effects of cilostazol.

Carbamazepine + **Clopidogrel** ⊗

On the basis of the interaction with the proton pump inhibitors, page 274, some predict that carbamazepine may theoretically inhibit the conversion of clopidogrel to its active metabolite by CYP2C19.

> The MHRA in the UK and the manufacturers advise that concurrent use should be avoided.

Carbamazepine + **Cobicistat** ⊗

Carbamazepine is predicted to decrease cobicistat plasma concentrations, which might reduce its efficacy. Cobicistat is predicted to increase carbamazepine concentrations.

> The US manufacturer of elvitegravir with cobicistat (in a fixed-dose combination also including emtricitabine and tenofovir) contraindicates concurrent use. Consider an alternative to carbamazepine.

Carbamazepine + **Contraceptives**

Combined hormonal contraceptives, oral progestogen-only contraceptives, and probably emergency hormonal contraceptives and progestogen-only implants, are less reliable during treatment with carbamazepine. Breakthrough bleeding and spotting can take place and unintended pregnancies have occurred. Controlled studies have shown that carbamazepine can reduce contraceptive steroid concentrations (both oestrogens and progestogens).

> Because of the consequences of an unwanted pregnancy, especially with drugs that can cause foetal abnormalities, adjustments should be made. For general advice on the use of enzyme inducers, such as carbamazepine, and hormonal contraceptives, see contraceptives, page 288.

Carbamazepine + **Corticosteroids**

The clearance of methylprednisolone and prednisolone is increased in patients taking carbamazepine. Dexamethasone clearance is also increased, and therefore the results of the dexamethasone adrenal suppression test may be invalid in those taking carbamazepine. More study is needed but it is likely that other corticosteroids such as hydrocortisone and prednisone may also be affected.

> Patients taking carbamazepine are likely to need increased doses of dexamethasone, methylprednisolone or prednisolone. Prednisolone is less affected than methylprednisolone and may therefore be preferred in some situations.

Carbamazepine + **Dabigatran**

Carbamazepine, a P-glycoprotein inducer, is predicted to decrease the exposure to dabigatran, which would be expected to affect its anticoagulant effects.

> The UK and US manufacturers advise avoiding concurrent use. If this is unavoidable, monitor for efficacy.

C

Carbamazepine + **Danazol**

Serum carbamazepine levels can be doubled by danazol and carbamazepine toxicity may occur.

> Consider monitoring carbamazepine levels and adjust the dose if necessary. Carbamazepine toxicity may present as nausea, vomiting, ataxia or drowsiness.

Carbamazepine + **Darifenacin**

The manufacturers predict that CYP3A4 inducers, such as carbamazepine, may decrease darifenacin levels.

> Monitor the outcome of concurrent use to ensure that darifenacin is effective and adjust the dose if necessary.

Carbamazepine + **Desmopressin**

Drugs that can cause water retention or hyponatraemia (e.g. carbamazepine) may have an additive effect with desmopressin: water overload and/or hyponatraemia may occur.

> The increased risk may be small, with severe complications being rare; however, it would be prudent to exercise caution on concurrent use, with more frequent monitoring of serum sodium.

Carbamazepine + **Diuretics**

Because St John's wort (*Hypericum perforatum*) decreases the AUC of eplerenone by 30% the manufacturers say that more potent enzyme inducers (such as carbamazepine) may have a greater effect on eplerenone.

> Concurrent use is not recommended by the manufacturers.

Carbamazepine + **Dronedarone**

Carbamazepine is predicted to reduce dronedarone exposure.

> The UK and US manufacturers of dronedarone advise that the concurrent use of carbamazepine should be avoided.

Carbamazepine + Elvitegravir

Carbamazepine is predicted to decrease elvitegravir plasma concentrations, which might reduce its efficacy.

The US manufacturer of elvitegravir with cobicistat (in a fixed-dose combination also including emtricitabine and tenofovir) contraindicates concurrent use. Consider an alternative to carbamazepine.

C

Carbamazepine + Eslicarbazepine

Carbamazepine slightly reduces the exposure to eslicarbazepine. It has also been noted that the frequency of adverse effects (such as double vision, abnormal coordination, and dizziness) were higher in patients taking both eslicarbazepine and carbamazepine, compared with those not taking carbamazepine.

Until further data is available, it would be prudent to monitor concurrent use for an increase in adverse effects and/or a reduced response to eslicarbazepine. Adjust the eslicarbazepine dose as indicated.

Carbamazepine + Ethosuximide

Some, but not all studies suggest that carbamazepine reduces ethosuximide levels by about 20% and reduces its half-life by about 50%.

The concurrent use of antiepileptics is common and often advantageous and a clinically relevant interaction seems unlikely in most patients. Nevertheless, consider monitoring concurrent use for potential ethosuximide toxicity and to ensure adequate seizure control.

Carbamazepine + Everolimus

Carbamazepine is predicted to reduce the bioavailability and increases the clearance of everolimus.

If concurrent use is unavoidable, increase the everolimus dose according to the indication for use, and monitor everolimus concentrations closely.

Carbamazepine + Exemestane

Rifampicin (rifampin) reduces the exposure to exemestane. Carbamazepine is predicted to interact similarly.

Monitor concurrent use for exemestane efficacy. The US manufacturer suggests doubling the exemestane dose to 50 mg daily in patients taking *phenytoin* or *rifampicin*: similar dose adjustments might be necessary with carbamazepine.

Carbamazepine + Fesoterodine

Rifampicin reduces the levels of the active metabolite of fesoterodine by about 75%. Carbamazepine is predicted to interact similarly.

Concurrent use is not recommended by the UK manufacturer, whereas the US manufacturer states that no fesoterodine dose adjustments are recommended. If both drugs are given it would be prudent to monitor for fesoterodine efficacy.

Carbamazepine + Gestrinone

The manufacturers warn that carbamazepine may increase the metabolism of gestrinone and thereby reduce its effects.

The clinical significance of this warning is unclear and there appear to be no reports of an interaction in practice; however, be aware that gestrinone might be less effective if carbamazepine is given concurrently.

Carbamazepine + Grapefruit juice ⚠

Grapefruit juice increases carbamazepine levels by about 40%. A case of possible carbamazepine toxicity has been seen in a man taking carbamazepine after he started to eat grapefruit.

The manufacturers advise monitoring levels and adjusting the dose of carbama-zepine as necessary. If monitoring is not practical, or regular intake of grapefruit is not desired, it would seem prudent to avoid grapefruit or grapefruit juice.

Carbamazepine + H₂-receptor antagonists

The serum levels of those taking long-term carbamazepine may transiently increase, possibly accompanied by an increase in adverse effects, for the first few days after starting to take cimetidine, but these adverse effects rapidly disappear.

An increase in carbamazepine adverse effects (nausea, headache, dizziness, fatigue, drowsiness, ataxia, an inability to concentrate, a bitter taste) may be seen, and patients should be warned. However, because the serum levels are only transiently increased the adverse effects normally disappear by the end of a week. Ranitidine appears to be a non-interacting alternative to cimetidine, and oxcarbazepine appears to be a non-interacting alternative to carbamazepine.

Carbamazepine + Herbal medicines or Dietary supplements ⊘

St John's wort (*Hypericum perforatum*) modestly increased the clearance of single-dose carbamazepine in one study, but had no effect on multiple-dose carbamazepine in another study.

Before the publication of these studies the CSM in the UK had advised that patients taking carbamazepine should not take St John's wort. This advice was based on predicted pharmacokinetic interactions. In the light of the above studies, this advice may no longer apply, although concurrent use should probably still be monitored to ensure adequate carbamazepine levels and efficacy.

Carbamazepine + HIV-protease inhibitors

Case reports suggest that ritonavir markedly increases carbamazepine concentrations and toxicity. Cases have also been reported with lopinavir boosted with ritonavir, saquinavir with ritonavir, and nelfinavir. Darunavir boosted with ritonavir also appears to increase carbamazepine exposure. Carbamazepine reduces indinavir concentrations and efficacy, reduces tipranavir concentrations (when given boosted with ritonavir), and would also be expected to decrease the concentrations of other HIV-protease inhibitors. However, darunavir concentrations (when given boosted with ritonavir) are not affected by carbamazepine even though the concentrations of the ritonavir are reduced.

Avoid concurrent use where possible (mainly because of the risk of antiviral treatment failure): some manufacturers contraindicate concurrent use. If carbamazepine and an HIV-protease inhibitor must be used then extremely close monitoring of both HIV-protease inhibitor concentrations and/or efficacy and carbamazepine concentrations and/or adverse effects is warranted. Indicators of carbamazepine toxicity include nausea, vomiting, ataxia, and drowsiness. The authors of one report suggest that amitriptyline or gabapentin would be possible alternatives for carbamazepine when used for pain, or valproic acid or lamotrigine for carbamazepine when used for seizures. However, note that ritonavir might increase the concentrations of some tricyclics, page 439.

Carbamazepine + HRT

The hormones in HRT are similar to those used in hormonal contraceptives, page 228, and so may be affected by enzyme-inducing drugs, such as carbamazepine, in the same way.

The clinical significance of any interaction is unclear; however, consider the possibility of reduced HRT efficacy on concurrent use. This effect is most noticeable where HRT is prescribed for menopausal vasomotor symptoms, but might be difficult to detect where the indication is osteoporosis. The interaction is not relevant to HRT applied locally for menopausal vaginitis.

Carbamazepine + 5-HT$_3$-receptor antagonists

A preliminary report of a controlled study reported a marked reduction in ondansetron exposure in patients taking long-term carbamazepine, when compared with control subjects. The Australian manufacturer of tropisetron states that drugs known to induce hepatic enzymes might lower tropisetron concentrations: carbamazepine would be expected to interact in this way.

The US manufacturer of ondansetron states that no ondansetron dose adjustment is necessary on concurrent use with carbamazepine; however, it may be prudent to monitor the outcome of concurrent use to assess ondansetron efficacy, increasing the ondansetron dose if necessary. Until more is known, it would seem prudent to use similar caution with the concurrent use of tropisetron and carbamazepine.

Carbamazepine + Isoniazid

Carbamazepine levels are markedly and rapidly increased by isoniazid, and toxicity can occur. *Rifampicin (rifampin)* has been reported both to augment and negate this interaction. Limited evidence suggests that carbamazepine may potentiate isoniazid hepatotoxicity.

> Carbamazepine toxicity can develop quickly (within 1 to 5 days) and also seems to disappear quickly if isoniazid is withdrawn. Monitor concurrent use and reduce the carbamazepine dose as necessary. Carbamazepine toxicity may present as nausea, vomiting, ataxia or drowsiness.

Carbamazepine + Lacosamide ❓

Although population pharmacokinetic data has suggested that carbamazepine modestly reduces lacosamide exposure, several pharmacokinetic studies have found that no clinically relevant interaction occurs.

> A clinically relevant pharmacokinetic interaction is not expected. However, the manufacturers advise caution if lacosamide is given with drugs known to be associated with PR prolongation, and they name carbamazepine, although note that the UK manufacturer also reports that one study did not find an increase in PR prolongation on concurrent use.

Carbamazepine + Lamotrigine ❓

Most studies have found that lamotrigine has no effect on the pharmacokinetics of carbamazepine or its active epoxide metabolite. However, some studies have found that lamotrigine increases the serum concentrations of carbamazepine-epoxide. Carbamazepine decreases lamotrigine concentrations. Toxicity has been seen irrespective of changes in levels.

> Patients should be well monitored if lamotrigine is added, and the carbamazepine dose reduced if CNS adverse effects occur. Carbamazepine induces the metabolism of lamotrigine, and the recommended starting dose and long-term maintenance dose of lamotrigine in patients already taking carbamazepine is twice that of patients receiving lamotrigine monotherapy. However, if they are also taking valproate in addition to carbamazepine, the lamotrigine dose should be reduced.

Carbamazepine + Levothyroxine ❓

Clinical hypothyroidism can occur in patients taking levothyroxine when they start carbamazepine.

> Be alert for any evidence of changes in thyroid status if carbamazepine is added or withdrawn from patients taking levothyroxine. Monitor thyroid function if an interaction is suspected, and adjust the levothyroxine dose accordingly.

Carbamazepine + Lithium ⚠️

Although the combined use of lithium and carbamazepine is beneficial in many patients, mild to severe neurotoxicity is reported to have developed in some, and possibly sinus node dysfunction in others.

> Monitor the outcome of concurrent use carefully, but note that signs of toxicity have developed even with lithium levels within the normal range. If severe

neurotoxicity develops the lithium treatment should be discontinued promptly, whatever the lithium level. Risk factors appear to be a history of neurotoxicity with lithium therapies and compromised medical or neurological functioning.

Carbamazepine + Macrolides

Erythromycin or Telithromycin

Erythromycin raises carbamazepine levels by as much as 5-fold, which has resulted in toxicity in several cases. Telithromycin is predicted to interact similarly.

Avoid the concurrent use of carbamazepine and erythromycin unless carbamazepine levels can be closely monitored and suitable dose reductions made. Symptoms commonly begin within 24 to 72 hours of starting erythromycin. In most cases toxicity resolves within 5 days of stopping the erythromycin. Carbamazepine toxicity may present as nausea, vomiting, ataxia or drowsiness. The manufacturers of telithromycin recommend avoiding concurrent use during and for up to 2 weeks after carbamazepine treatment. If concurrent use is essential monitor carbamazepine levels and adjust the dose as necessary.

Other macrolides

Clarithromycin raises carbamazepine levels by 20 to 50%, despite dose reductions of up to 40%. Several cases of toxicity have been seen.

Monitor carbamazepine levels and adjust the dose accordingly. It has been recommended that carbamazepine doses are reduced by 30 to 50% and patients monitored within 3 to 5 days of starting clarithromycin. Carbamazepine toxicity may present as nausea, vomiting, ataxia or drowsiness.

Carbamazepine + MAOIs

MAOIs and carbamazepine have been used together, uneventfully and successfully, and there appear to be no reports of an interaction. However, because carbamazepine is structurally related to the tricyclics, page 491, which should be avoided with MAOIs, the manufacturers of carbamazepine suggest avoiding concurrent use.

Avoid concurrent use. MAOIs should be discontinued at least 2 weeks before carbamazepine is started, although this may be over-cautious. Note that, rarely, the MAOIs have been seen to cause convulsions and they should therefore be used cautiously in patients with epilepsy.

Carbamazepine + Maraviroc

Carbamazepine is predicted to reduce the exposure to maraviroc.

The US HIV guidelines do not recommend concurrent use. If concurrent use is necessary, The UK and US manufacturers, and the US HIV guidelines, recommend increasing the maraviroc dose to 600 mg twice daily if carbamazepine also given.

Carbamazepine + Mebendazole

Carbamazepine appears to lower the plasma concentration of mebendazole.

When treating systemic worm infections it might be necessary to increase the mebendazole dose in patients taking carbamazepine. Monitor the outcome of concurrent use. This interaction is of no importance when mebendazole is used for intestinal worm infections where its action is a local effect on the worms in the gut.

C

Carbamazepine + Melatonin

One manufacturer predicts that carbamazepine may increase the metabolism of melatonin (by inducing CYP1A2), thereby decreasing its levels. However, note that carbamazepine is not a particularly potent inducer of this isoenzyme.

No action needed.

Carbamazepine + Methylphenidate

Limited evidence suggests that carbamazepine may decrease methylphenidate levels.

It would seem wise to monitor the response to methylphenidate treatment carefully in patients taking carbamazepine. Note that the manufacturer states that methylphenidate should be used with caution in patients with epilepsy, as it can, rarely, cause an increase in seizure frequency. If seizure frequency increases, methylphenidate should be discontinued.

Carbamazepine + Mirtazapine

Carbamazepine decreases the AUC and maximum plasma levels of mirtazapine, by 63% and 44%, respectively. Mirtazapine does not appear to affect the pharmacokinetics of carbamazepine.

Monitor concurrent use to assess mirtazapine efficacy, and adjust the dose accordingly. Note that, mirtazapine can lower the seizure threshold, and therefore its use should be carefully considered in patients with epilepsy.

Carbamazepine + NNRTIs

Carbamazepine reduces the concentrations of delavirdine, efavirenz, and nevirapine, and is predicted to reduce the concentrations of etravirine and rilpivirine. This would be expected to lead to treatment failure. Efavirenz reduces carbamazepine concentrations, and nevirapine is predicted to interact similarly.

The use of an NNRTI with carbamazepine is not recommended, or should be undertaken with caution. Use an alternative to carbamazepine if possible or monitor NNRTI plasma concentrations (where possible) to establish antiviral efficacy. Note that efavirenz can itself cause seizures and caution is recommended in patients with a history of convulsions.

Carbamazepine + **Opioids**

Dextropropoxyphene (Propoxyphene)

Dextropropoxyphene increases carbamazepine concentrations. Several cases of toxicity have been seen.

Monitor carbamazepine concentrations and adjust the dose if necessary. Consider using a non-interacting analgesic as an alternative. Carbamazepine toxicity can present as nausea, vomiting, ataxia, or drowsiness.

Other opioids

Carbamazepine appears to increase fentanyl requirements, reduce the serum concentrations of tramadol and methadone (opiate withdrawal seen), and reduce buprenorphine efficacy.

Be alert for the need to increase opioid doses. It might be necessary to give methadone twice daily to prevent withdrawal symptoms towards the end of the day. One UK manufacturer of buprenorphine and one US manufacturer of tramadol advises avoiding the concurrent use of carbamazepine. Note that tramadol should be avoided in patients with a history of epilepsy.

Carbamazepine + **Orlistat**

The MHRA in the UK suggests that the absorption of antiepileptics might be decreased by orlistat, leading to a loss of seizure control.

Although an interaction has not been established, the MHRA advises that patients should be monitored for changes in the severity or frequency of convulsions, and consideration given to separating the administration of orlistat and the antiepileptic.

Carbamazepine + **Perampanel** ⚠

Carbamazepine decreases perampanel concentrations.

Monitor for perampanel efficacy and increase the perampanel dose if necessary.

Carbamazepine + **Phenobarbital** ⚠

Carbamazepine serum concentrations are reduced to some extent by phenobarbital, but the concentrations of its active metabolite are increased; seizure control remains unaffected. In children, phenobarbital clearance is decreased by carbamazepine. Primidone seems to interact similarly.

This interaction seems to be of little clinical importance as seizure control is not affected. However, it would be prudent to monitor phenobarbital concentrations in children also given carbamazepine as changes in clearance might affect dose requirements.

Carbamazepine + **Phenytoin**

Some reports describe increases in serum phenytoin concentrations, with toxicity, whereas others describe decreases in phenytoin concentrations, when given with carbamazepine. Genetic differences in the metabolism of these drugs might be an explanation for the differences. Decreases in carbamazepine concentrations, sometimes with increases in carbamazepine-10,11–epoxide concentrations, have also been described. Fosphenytoin is a prodrug of phenytoin, and might interact similarly.

> Monitor antiepileptic concentrations during concurrent use (where possible including carbamazepine-10,11–epoxide, the active metabolite of carbamazepine) so that steps can be taken to avoid the development of toxicity or lack of efficacy. Not all patients appear to have an adverse interaction, and, at present, it does not seem possible to identify those potentially at risk.

Carbamazepine + **Phosphodiesterase type-5 inhibitors**

Carbamazepine is predicted to reduce the exposure to the phosphodiesterase type-5 inhibitors by inducing CYP3A4.

> It might be prudent to follow the same advice for rifampicin: if standard doses of these phosphodiesterase type-5 inhibitors are not effective for erectile dysfunction in patients taking carbamazepine, it would seem sensible to try a higher dose with close monitoring. For pulmonary hypertension, the UK manufacturer of sildenafil states that sildenafil efficacy should be closely monitored, with the sildenafil dose increased as necessary, whereas the manufacturers of tadalafil for pulmonary hypertension do not recommend the concurrent use of carbamazepine. The UK and US manufacturers of avanafil contraindicate concurrent use with all CYP3A4 inducers.

Carbamazepine + **Praziquantel**

Carbamazepine markedly reduces the exposure to praziquantel, but whether this results in neurocysticercosis treatment failures is unclear; one study found that concurrent use was still effective.

> When treating systemic worm infections such as neurocysticercosis some authors have advised increasing the praziquantel dose from 25 to 50 mg/kg if carbamazepine is being taken, but in one study this dose was not effective. Note that the recommended dose of praziquantel for neurocysticercosis is 50 mg/kg daily in 3 divided doses. The interaction with carbamazepine is of no importance when praziquantel is used for intestinal worm infections (where its action is a local effect on the worms in the gut).

Carbamazepine + **Ranolazine**

Rifampicin (rifampin) reduces ranolazine levels by 95%, and loss of efficacy is expected. Carbamazepine is predicted to interact in the same way as rifampicin.

> The manufacturers recommend avoiding concurrent use. In the absence of any information on the magnitude of the effect of carbamazepine on ranolazine levels, this seems prudent.

Carbamazepine + **Retigabine (Ezogabine)**

Retigabine clearance is increased by carbamazepine but retigabine does not affect carbamazepine pharmacokinetics.

> The clinical importance of this interaction is unknown, but bear it in mind in the case of an unexpected response to treatment.

C

Carbamazepine + **Rivaroxaban**

Carbamazepine is predicted to decrease the exposure to rivaroxaban, and therefore decrease its anticoagulant effects.

> Given the likely clinical risk of reduced rivaroxaban efficacy, it would seem prudent to consider using an alternative drug; however, if this is not possible, consider closely monitoring the prothrombin time to ensure the anticoagulant effect of rivaroxaban is maintained. The US manufacturer of rivaroxaban advises avoiding concurrent use.

Carbamazepine + **Roflumilast**

Rifampicin (rifampin) increases the metabolism of roflumilast to its active metabolite, roflumilast *N*-oxide, but decreases the overall bioavailability of roflumilast *N*-oxide, resulting in a decrease in its phosphodiesterase inhibitory effects. Carbamazepine might interact similarly.

> Monitor concurrent use to ensure that roflumilast is effective, and consider increasing the dose of roflumilast, according to clinical need.

Carbamazepine + **Sirolimus**

Carbamazepine is predicted to reduce sirolimus concentrations.

> The UK and US manufacturers of sirolimus recommend avoiding concurrent use. It would seem prudent to increase the frequency of monitoring of sirolimus concentrations during concurrent use and adjust the sirolimus dose as necessary.

Carbamazepine + **Solifenacin**

The manufacturers predict that CYP3A4 inducers, such as carbamazepine, will reduce solifenacin levels.

> Monitor the outcome of concurrent use to ensure that solifenacin is effective and adjust the dose if necessary.

Carbamazepine + **SSRIs**

Fluvoxamine or Fluoxetine

Case reports indicate that carbamazepine concentrations can be increased by fluoxetine (by up to 60%) and fluvoxamine (concentration doubled). Toxicity might develop. The use of carbamazepine with an SSRI has, rarely, led to effects such as hyponatraemia, serotonin syndrome, and parkinsonism.

> It would be prudent to monitor carbamazepine concentrations and be alert for the need to reduce the carbamazepine dose if used concurrently with fluoxetine or fluvoxamine. Carbamazepine toxicity might present as nausea, vomiting, ataxia, or drowsiness. The UK manufacturer of fluoxetine suggests that carbamazepine should be started at, or adjusted towards, the lower end of the dose range in those taking fluoxetine, and caution is needed if fluoxetine has been taken during the previous 5 weeks. Note that SSRIs can reduce the seizure threshold and so should be used with caution in patients with epilepsy.

Other SSRIs

Citalopram, paroxetine, and sertraline concentrations might be reduced by carbamazepine. The use of carbamazepine with an SSRI has, rarely, led to effects such as hyponatraemia, serotonin syndrome, and parkinsonism.

> Be aware that some SSRIs might be less effective in the presence of carbamazepine and consider a dose increase if necessary. Note that SSRIs can reduce the seizure threshold and so should be used with caution in patients with epilepsy.

Carbamazepine + Statins

Carbamazepine moderately reduces simvastatin exposure. Other statins metabolised in the same way as simvastatin (lovastatin, and to a lesser extent, atorvastatin) might be similarly affected.

> A simvastatin dose increase seems likely to be necessary. Monitor concurrent use to check that simvastatin is effective. Until more is known it would seem prudent to follow the same advice for lovastatin and probably atorvastatin.

Carbamazepine + Tacrolimus

Carbamazepine appears to decrease tacrolimus concentrations.

> Monitor the concentrations and effects of tacrolimus (e.g. on renal function) more frequently in a patient given carbamazepine, and adjust the dose as necessary.

Carbamazepine + Tetracyclines

Doxycycline levels are reduced and may fall below the accepted therapeutic minimum in patients taking carbamazepine long-term.

> It has been suggested that the doxycycline dose could be doubled to counteract this interaction. Other tetracyclines appear not to interact and may therefore be suitable alternatives.

Carbamazepine + Theophylline

Case reports suggest that carbamazepine might moderately increase theophylline clearance. Another single case report and a pharmacokinetic study suggest that carbamazepine exposure might be slightly reduced by theophylline. Aminophylline would be expected to interact similarly.

It would be prudent to be alert for any reduction in the effects of theophylline and/or carbamazepine on concurrent use. If an interaction is suspected, monitor theophylline concentrations and increase the aminophylline or theophylline dose as necessary.

Carbamazepine + Tiagabine ⚠

The plasma concentrations of tiagabine may be reduced 1.5- to 3-fold by carbamazepine.

The manufacturers recommend that tiagabine 30 to 45 mg (in divided doses) should be given to patients taking enzyme-inducing antiepileptics such as carbamazepine. A lower maintenance dose of 15 to 30 mg should be given to patients who are not taking enzyme-inducing drugs.

Carbamazepine + Ticagrelor ⚠

Carbamazepine is predicted to decrease ticagrelor exposure.

If concurrent use is unavoidable, be alert for reduced ticagrelor efficacy.

Carbamazepine + Topiramate ⚠

Topiramate concentrations might be reduced by carbamazepine. Carbamazepine pharmacokinetics are not affected by topiramate. However, one report suggests that the toxicity seen when topiramate was added to the maximum tolerated doses of carbamazepine might respond to a reduction in the carbamazepine dose.

Topiramate dose adjustments are unlikely to be needed. Reduce the carbamazepine dose should any carbamazepine adverse effects occur. Indicators of carbamazepine toxicity include nausea, vomiting, ataxia, and drowsiness.

Carbamazepine + Toremifene ⚠

Carbamazepine can reduce the exposure of toremifene.

Monitor concurrent use to ensure toremifene remains effective. The UK manufacturer of toremifene suggests that the toremifene dose might need to be doubled in the presence of carbamazepine.

Carbamazepine + Trazodone

A single case report describes a moderate rise in carbamazepine levels in a patient given trazodone. Carbamazepine may moderately decrease trazodone levels.

Monitor trazodone efficacy and increase the dose as needed. The clinical significance of the rise in carbamazepine levels is likely to be small. However, if indicators of carbamazepine toxicity (nausea, vomiting, ataxia, drowsiness) develop, consider an interaction as a possible cause.

Carbamazepine + Tricyclics ⚠

The levels of amitriptyline, desipramine, doxepin, imipramine and nortriptyline, but possibly not clomipramine, can be reduced (halved or more) by the concurrent use of carbamazepine but there is evidence to suggest that this is not necessarily clinically important. The tetracyclic, mianserin, may be similarly affected. In contrast, raised clomipramine levels have been seen in patients taking carbamazepine and an isolated report describes carbamazepine toxicity in a patient shortly after starting desipramine.

Bear this interaction in mind in case of a reduced response to a tricyclic. Note that the tricyclics can lower the convulsive threshold and should therefore be used with caution in patients with epilepsy.

Carbamazepine + Ulipristal ⚠

The UK and US manufacturers of ulipristal predict that CYP3A4 inducers, such as carbamazepine, might reduce the plasma concentration of ulipristal and reduce its efficacy.

The US manufacturer of ulipristal gives no specific advice about how to manage this potential interaction, whereas the UK manufacturer advises that ulipristal should not be used for emergency contraception in women taking CYP3A4 inducers (such as carbamazepine), or who have stopped taking an enzyme inducer within the last 2 to 3 weeks. Until more is known, this advice seems prudent.

Carbamazepine + Vaccines ❓

Carbamazepine levels rose modestly 14 days after influenza vaccination in one study. A case report describes carbamazepine toxicity and markedly increased carbamazepine levels in a teenager 13 days after influenza vaccination.

The moderate increase in carbamazepine levels seen in the study is unlikely to have much clinical relevance. However, the case report of markedly increased carbamazepine levels introduces a note of caution. Carbamazepine toxicity may present as nausea, vomiting, ataxia or drowsiness.

Carbamazepine + Valproate ❓

Carbamazepine concentrations are usually only minimally affected by sodium valproate, valproic acid, or valpromide, although a larger increase in the concentrations of its active epoxide metabolite might occur. Carbamazepine might reduce the concentrations of sodium valproate, and. concurrent use might increase the incidence of sodium valproate-induced hepatotoxicity.

Monitor valproate concentrations, and adjust the dose if necessary. Consider an interaction if hepatotoxicity occurs. Also monitor for carbamazepine toxicity (due to increased carbamazepine-epoxide concentrations), which might present as nausea, vomiting, ataxia, or drowsiness.

Carbamazepine + Vitamin D

The long-term use of *phenytoin* can disturb vitamin D and calcium metabolism, which may result in osteomalacia. There are a few reports of patients taking vitamin D supplements who responded poorly to vitamin replacement while taking *phenytoin*. Limited evidence suggests that carbamazepine may interact similarly.

Monitor the outcome of concurrent use. Larger doses of vitamin D may be needed.

Carbamazepine + Warfarin and related oral anticoagulants ⚠

The anticoagulant effects of warfarin can be markedly reduced (by around 50% in many reports) by carbamazepine. Cases of this interaction have been seen with phenprocoumon and acenocoumarol.

Monitor the INR if carbamazepine is added to warfarin therapy. Continue monitoring until the carbamazepine dose is stabilised. Also monitor the INR if carbamazepine is withdrawn as the effects of warfarin may become excessive within a week. Similar precautions would be prudent with the other coumarins.

Carbamazepine + Zonisamide ❓

Carbamazepine can cause a small to moderate reduction in the levels of zonisamide, and zonisamide has been reported to cause increases, decreases or no changes to carbamazepine serum levels.

The clinical importance of this interaction is unknown, but be aware of the possibility of changes in the levels of both drugs if they are given together.

Carbimazole

Carbimazole + Digoxin ⚠

Carbimazole slightly lowers digoxin levels in euthyroid subjects. However, the drug-disease interaction that also occurs is probably of more importance. Hyperthyroid subjects are relatively resistant to the effects of digoxin and so need higher doses. As treatment with carbimazole progresses and they become euthyroid, the dose of digoxin will need to be decreased.

Monitor digoxin levels and for digoxin adverse effects (such as bradycardia, nausea, vomiting), adjusting the digoxin dose as necessary, until the patient is euthyroid.

Carbimazole + Theophylline ⚠

Thyroid function affects theophylline metabolism: in hyperthyroidism it is increased. Correction of thyroid function (e.g. with carbimazole) decreases theophylline metabolism, and so smaller doses are needed. Two case reports describe theophylline toxicity in patients being treated for hyperthyroidism. Aminophylline would be expected to interact similarly.

Monitor the outcome of adjusting thyroid status on the theophylline concentration (this may take weeks or months to stabilise) and adjust the dose of theophylline or aminophylline as necessary.

Carbimazole + **Warfarin and related oral anticoagulants**

Hyperthyroidism increases the metabolism of the clotting factors. Correction of hyperthyroidism therefore alters anticoagulant requirements. Increased coumarin requirements have been seen in patients given carbimazole.

Close monitoring of the INR is advisable for any patient taking an oral anticoagulant until their thyroid hormone levels are stabilised.

Caspofungin

Caspofungin + **Ciclosporin (Cyclosporine)**

Ciclosporin slightly increases the AUC of caspofungin and this might result in increased liver enzymes (AST and ALT of up to 3-fold in one study).

The manufacturer advises that ciclosporin and caspofungin should only be used if the benefits outweigh the risks of treatment, and if they are used, close monitoring of liver enzymes is recommended.

Caspofungin + **NNRTIs**

Population pharmacokinetic data suggests that efavirenz and nevirapine might reduce caspofungin concentrations.

The UK manufacturer recommends that consideration should be given to increasing the dose of caspofungin from 50 mg daily to 70 mg daily in adults and to 70 mg/m² daily (maximum 70 mg daily) in children, whereas the US manufacturer specifically states that the higher dose should be used.

Caspofungin + **Phenytoin**

Population data suggests that phenytoin might reduce caspofungin concentrations. Although the mechanism for this effect is not fully understood it would seem prudent to expect fosphenytoin, a prodrug of phenytoin, to interact similarly.

The UK manufacturer recommends that consideration should be given to increasing the dose of caspofungin from 50 mg daily to 70 mg daily in adults and to 70 mg/m² daily (maximum 70 mg daily) in children, whereas the US manufacturer specifically states that the higher dose should be used.

Caspofungin + **Rifampicin (Rifampin)**

Rifampicin initially increases the minimum concentration of caspofungin, but after 2 weeks the minimum concentration of caspofungin decreases, and is about 30% lower than in patients not receiving rifampicin. Antifungal treatment failure has been seen in a patient taking rifampicin with caspofungin (70 mg on the first day then 50 mg daily).

> The UK manufacturer recommends that consideration should be given to increasing the dose of caspofungin from 50 mg daily to 70 mg daily in adults and to 70 mg/m² daily (maximum 70 mg daily) in children, whereas the US manufacturer specifically states that the higher dose should be used. However, close monitoring is still required because of the isolated report of treatment failure even at the higher dose.

Caspofungin + **Tacrolimus**

Caspofungin slightly decreases trough tacrolimus levels by 26%. Tacrolimus does not affect the pharmacokinetics of caspofungin.

> Tacrolimus levels and/or effects (e.g. on renal function) should be monitored as a matter of routine, but it is advisable to increase monitoring if caspofungin is started or stopped, and adjust the dose of tacrolimus if required.

Cephalosporins

Cephalosporins + **Ciclosporin (Cyclosporine)**

Isolated reports suggest that ceftazidime, ceftriaxone, and latamoxef might increase ciclosporin concentrations, whereas one report suggests that ceftazidime, ceftriaxone, and cefuroxime do not, although ceftazidime caused a deterioration in some measures of renal function.

> Information about these cephalosporins is very limited. The general relevance of these reports is uncertain, but bear them in mind in the event of declining renal function.

Cephalosporins + **Contraceptives**

A few anecdotal cases of combined hormonal contraceptive failure have been reported with the cephalosporins. The interaction (if such it is) appears to be very rare indeed.

> It is possible that the anecdotal cases of contraceptive failure with antibacterials are indistinguishable from the normal accepted failure rate and no special precautions are required. Historically UK guidelines cautiously advised that additional contraceptive precautions were necessary; however, it is now advised that no additional precautions are needed, which is in line with the advice given by a number of other authorities. For further information on the use of antibacterials with contraceptives, see contraceptives, page 288.

Cephalosporins + H₂-receptor antagonists

Ranitidine and famotidine modestly reduce the bioavailability of cefpodoxime proxetil. Ranitidine (with sodium bicarbonate) reduces the bioavailability of cefuroxime axetil, but not if it is taken with food. As it is thought that a change in gastric pH is responsible for this interaction it would seem likely that all H₂-receptor antagonists will interact similarly.

> The clinical importance of the interaction with cefpodoxime has not been studied, but the manufacturer recommends that it should be given at least 2 hours before H₂-receptor antagonists. As long as cefuroxime is taken with food (as is recommended), any interaction is minimal.

Cephalosporins + Heparin

Although a number of cephalosporins have been associated with an increased risk of bleeding, in one study cefamandole did not appear to increase the anticoagulant effects of prophylactic doses of heparin.

> Any interaction most usually occurs after about 3 days. Routine monitoring should be adequate to detect any adverse reaction.

Cephalosporins + Mycophenolate

A selective bowel decontamination regimen of cefuroxime (with nystatin and tobramycin) appears to modestly reduce mycophenolate bioavailability, although the clinical relevance of these reductions has not been assessed.

> Until further information is available, it would seem prudent to monitor the outcome of concurrent use, and for a short period after stopping the antibacterial, to ensure that mycophenolate remains effective.

Cephalosporins + Probenecid

Overall, probenecid reduces the clearance, raises the serum levels and sometimes prolongs the half-lives of some, but not all, cephalosporins.

> No special precautions are normally needed. However, be aware that elevated serum levels of some cephalosporins (such as cefaloridine and cefalotin) might possibly increase the risk of nephrotoxicity.

Cephalosporins + Proton pump inhibitors

Ranitidine and *famotidine* modestly reduce the bioavailability of cefpodoxime proxetil. *Ranitidine* (with sodium bicarbonate) reduces the bioavailability of cefuroxime axetil, although not if taken with food. As it is thought that a change in gastric pH is responsible for this interaction it would seem likely that the proton pump inhibitors will interact similarly.

> The clinical relevance of these effects are unclear. However, as long as cefuroxime is taken with food (as is recommended), any interaction is minimal.

Cephalosporins + **Warfarin and related oral anticoagulants**

Cephalosporins and related beta lactams with an N-methylthiotetrazole or similar side-chain can occasionally cause bleeding when they are used alone. These effects could therefore be additive with those of the coumarins. The cephalosporins implicated include cefalotin, cefamandole, cefazolin, cefoperazone, cefotetan, cefotiam, and ceftriaxone. Isolated case reports describe over-anticoagulation in patients taking a coumarin or indanedione and a cephalosporin that does not possess an N-methylthiotetrazole side chain (such as cefaclor, cefixime, cefradine, and cefuroxime.)

> It would seem prudent to monitor the INR on concurrent use, particularly in the early stages of treatment, and adjust the anticoagulant dose accordingly. If dose alterations are needed further INR monitoring will be required when the cephalosporin is stopped.

Chloramphenicol

Chloramphenicol + **Ciclosporin (Cyclosporine)**

Case reports describe increased ciclosporin concentrations in patients also given chloramphenicol. A small study supports these findings.

> Ciclosporin concentrations and/or effects (e.g. on renal function) should be monitored as a matter of routine, but it would be prudent to increase monitoring if chloramphenicol is started or stopped. Adjust the dose of ciclosporin as necessary. It seems doubtful that there will be enough chloramphenicol absorbed from eye drops to interact with ciclosporin, but this needs confirmation.

Chloramphenicol + **Clopidogrel**

On the basis of the interaction with the proton pump inhibitors, some predict that chloramphenicol may theoretically inhibit the conversion of clopidogrel to its active metabolite by CYP2C19.

> The MHRA in the UK and the manufacturers advise that concurrent use should be avoided.

Chloramphenicol + **Contraceptives**

One or two cases of combined hormonal contraceptive failure have been reported with chloramphenicol. These isolated cases are anecdotal and unconfirmed, and the interaction (if such it is) appears to be very rare indeed.

> It is possible that the anecdotal cases of contraceptive failure with antibacterials are indistinguishable from the normal accepted failure rate and no special precautions are required. Historically UK guidelines cautiously advised that additional contraceptive precautions were necessary; however, it is now advised that no additional precautions are needed, which is in line with the advice given

by a number of other authorities. For further information on the use of antibacterials with contraceptives, see contraceptives, page 288.

Chloramphenicol + Iron

In addition to the serious and potentially fatal bone marrow depression that can occur with chloramphenicol, it may also cause a milder, reversible bone marrow depression, which can oppose the treatment of anaemia with iron.

It has been suggested that chloramphenicol doses of 25 to 30 mg/kg are usually adequate for treating infections without running the risk of elevating serum levels to 25 micrograms/mL or more, which is when this type of marrow depression can occur. Monitor the effects of using iron concurrently. Where possible it would be preferable to use a different antibacterial.

Chloramphenicol + Paracetamol (Acetaminophen)

Although there is limited evidence to suggest that paracetamol may affect chloramphenicol pharmacokinetics its validity has been criticised. Evidence of a clinically relevant interaction appears lacking.

No action needed. It would seem prudent to be aware of the potential for interaction, especially in malnourished patients, but routine monitoring would appear unnecessary without further evidence.

Chloramphenicol + Phenobarbital

Studies in children show that phenobarbital can markedly reduce chloramphenicol levels. An isolated case describes markedly increased phenobarbital levels in an adult caused by the use of chloramphenicol. Note that primidone is metabolised to phenobarbital and therefore may interact similarly.

Concurrent use should be well monitored to ensure that chloramphenicol levels are adequate. Make appropriate dose adjustments as necessary. The case of raised phenobarbital levels is of uncertain importance.

Chloramphenicol + Phenytoin

Phenytoin levels can be raised two- to fourfold by the concurrent use of systemic chloramphenicol, and phenytoin toxicity may occur. Evidence from children suggests that phenytoin may reduce or raise chloramphenicol levels. Fosphenytoin, a prodrug of phenytoin, may interact similarly.

Monitor concurrent use for phenytoin toxicity (blurred vision, nystagmus, ataxia or drowsiness), monitoring levels and reducing the dose of phenytoin as necessary. The use of a single prophylactic dose of phenytoin or fosphenytoin may be an exception to this. Also monitor for chloramphenicol efficacy and toxicity. It is doubtful if enough chloramphenicol is absorbed from eye drops or ointments for an interaction to occur.

Chloramphenicol + **Rifampicin (Rifampin)**

Case reports describe markedly reduced chloramphenicol levels in children also given rifampicin. There is a risk that chloramphenicol levels will become subtherapeutic.

It is unclear if a dose increase of chloramphenicol is appropriate as some consider that increasing the chloramphenicol dose may possibly expose the patient to a greater risk of bone marrow aplasia. It has been suggested that rifampicin prophylaxis should be delayed in patients with invasive *Haemophilus influenzae* infections until the end of chloramphenicol treatment.

Chloramphenicol + **Tacrolimus**

A marked rise in tacrolimus levels has been reported in several patients also given systemic chloramphenicol.

Tacrolimus levels and/or effects (e.g. on renal function) should be monitored as a matter of routine, but it may be prudent to increase monitoring if systemic chloramphenicol is started or stopped. It seems doubtful if a clinically relevant interaction will occur with topical chloramphenicol because the dose and the systemic absorption is small, but this needs confirmation.

Chloramphenicol + **Vitamin B$_{12}$**

In addition to the serious and potentially fatal bone marrow depression that can occur with systemic chloramphenicol, it may also cause a milder, reversible bone marrow depression, which can oppose the treatment of anaemia with iron or vitamin B$_{12}$.

It has been suggested that chloramphenicol doses of 25 to 30 mg/kg are usually adequate for treating infections without running the risk of elevating serum levels to 25 micrograms/mL or more, which is when this type of marrow depression can occur. Monitor the effects of using iron or vitamin B$_{12}$ concurrently. Where possible it would be preferable to use a different antibacterial.

Chloramphenicol + **Warfarin and related oral anticoagulants**

Some limited, and poor quality evidence suggests that the anticoagulant effects of acenocoumarol can be increased by oral chloramphenicol. An isolated report attributes a marked INR rise in a patient taking warfarin to the use of chloramphenicol eye drops.

This interaction is not established but it would be prudent to be aware that increases in INR are possible and consider increasing the frequency of INR monitoring. The interaction with chloramphenicol eye drops seems unlikely to be generally relevant.

Chloroquine

Chloroquine + Ciclosporin (Cyclosporine)

Three transplant patients had rapid increases in ciclosporin concentrations, with evidence of nephrotoxicity in two of them, when they were given chloroquine. Note that hydroxychloroquine might interact similarly. When low-dose ciclosporin is given for rheumatoid arthritis, neither chloroquine nor hydroxychloroquine appear to contribute to the known adverse effects of ciclosporin on creatinine and renal function.

> Ciclosporin concentrations and/or effects (e.g. on renal function) should be monitored as a matter of routine, but it might be prudent to increase monitoring if chloroquine, or hydroxychloroquine, is started or stopped. Adjust the dose of ciclosporin as necessary.

Chloroquine + Digoxin

The levels of digoxin were found to be markedly increased by 70% in two elderly patients when they took hydroxychloroquine. A similar increase has been seen with chloroquine in *dogs*.

> The clinical significance of this interaction is uncertain, but it would seem sensible to be aware of this potential interaction if both drugs are used.

Chloroquine + H$_2$-receptor antagonists

Cimetidine reduces the metabolism and halves the clearance of chloroquine. Hydroxychloroquine is expected to be similarly affected.

> The clinical importance of this interaction is uncertain, but it would seem prudent to be alert for any signs of chloroquine or hydroxychloroquine toxicity on concurrent use. Ranitidine might be a suitable alternative as it does not appear to interact with chloroquine.

Chloroquine + Kaolin

Kaolin reduces the absorption of chloroquine by about 30%. Hydroxychloroquine is predicted to interact similarly.

> The clinical significance of this reduction is unclear, but one way to minimise any possible effect on chloroquine absorption is to separate the doses of chloroquine and kaolin as much as possible (at least 2 to 3 hours) to minimise the interaction.

Chloroquine + Lanthanum

The manufacturers of lanthanum predict that the absorption of drugs that are affected by gastric pH will be altered by lanthanum. They name chloroquine and hydroxy-chloroquine, but note that these drugs appear to interact due to altered absorption rather than changes in gastric pH.

> The manufacturers recommend separating dosing by at least 2 hours.

Chloroquine + **Leflunomide**

The manufacturers say that the concurrent use of leflunomide and chloroquine or hydroxychloroquine has not yet been studied, but it would be expected to increase the risk of serious adverse reactions (haematological toxicity or hepatotoxicity).

The manufacturers advise avoiding concurrent use. As the active metabolite of leflunomide has a long half-life of 1 to 4 weeks a washout with colestyramine or activated charcoal is recommended by the manufacturers if patients are to be switched to other DMARDs.

Chloroquine + **Mefloquine**

In theory there is an increased risk of convulsions if mefloquine is given with chloroquine, but no cases appear to have been reported. The manufacturers suggest that concurrent use increases the risks of ECG abnormalities. Note that hydroxy-chloroquine might interact similarly.

Caution is advised on concurrent use.

Chloroquine + **Penicillamine**

The concurrent use of chloroquine and penicillamine may result in increased toxicity, possibly as a result of increased penicillamine levels.

If problems occur consider this drug interaction as a possible cause. Note that chloroquine, hydroxychloroquine and penicillamine are associated with serious haematological adverse effects, and therefore the US manufacturer suggests that the use of penicillamine with either of these drugs should be avoided.

Chloroquine + **Praziquantel**

Chloroquine reduces praziquantel exposure, which would be expected to reduce its efficacy in systemic worm infections such as schistosomiasis. Note that hydroxy-chloroquine might interact similarly.

It has been suggested that an increased dose of praziquantel should be considered in the presence of chloroquine, particularly in anyone who does not respond to initial treatment. This interaction is not of importance when praziquantel is used for intestinal worm infections (where its action is a local effect on the worms in the gut).

Ciclosporin (Cyclosporine)

Ciclosporin (Cyclosporine) + **Cobicistat**

The US manufacturer of elvitegravir boosted with cobicistat (in a fixed-dose combination also including emtricitabine and tenofovir) predicts that it will increase the plasma concentrations of ciclosporin.

Monitor the concentrations and effects (e.g. on renal function) of ciclosporin more frequently when starting or stopping elvitegravir with cobicistat, and adjust the ciclosporin dose as necessary.

Ciclosporin (Cyclosporine) + **Colchicine**

Ciclosporin increases colchicine exposure. A number of cases of serious muscle disorders (myopathy, rhabdomyolysis), some with multiple organ failure, have been seen when colchicine and ciclosporin were given concurrently. Ciclosporin toxicity has also been seen rarely.

If both drugs are necessary, monitor closely for signs of colchicine toxicity (such as nausea, vomiting, myopathy and pancytopenia) and reduce the colchicine dose or interrupt treatment at the earliest signs of myopathy. The US manufacturer gives the following specific advice for colchicine dose reductions in patients taking P-glycoprotein inhibitors, such as ciclosporin, or if they have stopped taking any of these drugs within 2 weeks of starting colchicine:

- For the treatment of gout, the dose of colchicine should be reduced to a single dose of 600 micrograms. The dose should not be repeated within 3 days.
- For gout prophylaxis, the dose of colchicine should be reduced to 300 micrograms daily (if the initial dose was 600 micrograms twice daily) or 300 micrograms on alternate days (if the initial dose was 600 micrograms daily).
- For familial Mediterranean fever, a maximum total daily dose of colchicine 600 micrograms (which can be given as 300 micrograms twice daily) is recommended.

Patients should be reminded to report any unexplained muscle pain, tenderness, or weakness, or dark urine. Note that both the US and UK manufacturers of colchicine contraindicate the concurrent use of ciclosporin in patients with renal or hepatic impairment.

Ciclosporin (Cyclosporine) + **Contraceptives**

Isolated reports describe hepatotoxicity and increased ciclosporin concentrations in two patients taking ciclosporin when given oral combined hormonal contraceptives. A couple of reports also describe some increase in ciclosporin concentrations with norethisterone.

The interactions between ciclosporin and hormonal contraceptives or norethisterone are unconfirmed and of uncertain clinical relevance. There is insufficient evidence to recommend increased monitoring, but be aware of the potential for an interaction in case of an unexpected response to treatment.

Ciclosporin (Cyclosporine) + **Corticosteroids**

Some evidence suggests that ciclosporin levels may be raised by corticosteroids (2-fold by methylprednisolone) or reduced (10 to 20% reduction with prednisone). Ciclosporin can moderately increase corticosteroid levels, which may lead to symptoms of overdose (cushingoid symptoms such as steroid-induced diabetes, osteonecrosis of the hip joints). Convulsions have also been described during concurrent use.

Concurrent use is common and advantageous but be alert for any evidence of increased ciclosporin and corticosteroid effects.

Ciclosporin (Cyclosporine) + Co-trimoxazole

A large-scale study has found that co-trimoxazole was effective and well tolerated in patients taking ciclosporin, although a 15% increase in serum creatinine concentrations was noted. Interstitial nephritis, granulocytopenia and thrombocytopenia have been reported in a few patients.

> Serious interactions between ciclosporin and co-trimoxazole seem rare and so no additional monitoring would seem to be necessary, at least for low-dose prophylactic co-trimoxazole. However, the manufacturer recommends close monitoring of renal function with concurrent use; this would seem a prudent precaution.

Ciclosporin (Cyclosporine) + Dabigatran

Ciclosporin is predicted to increase the exposure to dabigatran.

> The UK manufacturer of dabigatran contraindicates concurrent use. If it is unavoidable, monitor for signs of bleeding or anaemia, and discontinue dabigatran if severe bleeding occurs.

Ciclosporin (Cyclosporine) + Danazol

Large increases in ciclosporin concentrations (3-fold in one case) have been seen in patients taking danazol.

> Ciclosporin concentrations and/or effects (e.g. on renal function) should be monitored as a matter of routine, but it might be prudent to increase monitoring on concurrent use with danazol, and dose adjustments made as necessary.

Ciclosporin (Cyclosporine) + Digoxin

Ciclosporin causes 3- to 4-fold rises in digoxin levels in some patients.

> The effects of concurrent use should be monitored very closely for digoxin adverse effects (such as bradycardia, nausea, visual disturbances), and the digoxin dose should be adjusted according to levels.

Ciclosporin (Cyclosporine) + Diuretics

Potassium-sparing diuretics

The concurrent use of ciclosporin with potassium-sparing diuretics, such as amiloride, spironolactone, and eplerenone, might increase potassium concentrations. The use of both ciclosporin and diuretics might increase the risk of hyperuricaemia and gout.

> Monitor potassium concentrations and renal function if a potassium-sparing diuretic is given. The US manufacturers of eplerenone advise avoiding concurrent use, whereas the UK manufacturers advise caution. The continued use of diuretics after the initial stages of transplantation should be carefully evaluated in patients at high risk of gout.

Thiazide diuretics

Isolated cases of nephrotoxicity have been described in patients taking ciclosporin with either amiloride/hydrochlorothiazide or metolazone. The concurrent use of ciclosporin with thiazides might increase serum magnesium concentrations. The use of both ciclosporin and diuretics might increase the risk of hyperuricaemia and gout.

The general importance of these adverse interactions is not clear. It seems likely that routine monitoring of electrolytes (including magnesium concentrations) will detect any adverse effects. The continued use of diuretics after the initial stages of transplantation should be carefully evaluated in patients at high risk of gout.

Ciclosporin (Cyclosporine) + Dronedarone

Ketoconazole, a potent inhibitor of CYP3A4, markedly increases dronedarone exposure. The US manufacturer of dronedarone predicts that ciclosporin will have a similar effect; however, note that ciclosporin is not usually considered to be a potent CYP3A4 inhibitor.

The US manufacturer of dronedarone contraindicates the concurrent use of ciclosporin.

Ciclosporin (Cyclosporine) + Endothelin receptor antagonists

Ambrisentan

Ciclosporin moderately increases ambrisentan exposure. Ambrisentan has no clinically significant effect on the pharmacokinetics of ciclosporin.

The UK and US manufacturers of ambrisentan recommend a maximum dose of 5 mg daily on the concurrent use of ciclosporin. Monitor for an increase in ambrisentan adverse effects such as constipation, flushing, and fluid retention.

Bosentan ⊗

Bosentan decreases ciclosporin concentrations, and ciclosporin greatly increases bosentan concentrations: increased liver toxicity might occur.

Concurrent use is contraindicated.

Ciclosporin (Cyclosporine) + Etoposide

High-dose ciclosporin markedly raises etoposide levels and increases the suppression of white blood cell production. Severe toxicity has been reported in one patient.

Some have suggested reducing the dose of etoposide by 40 or 50%. The use of high-dose ciclosporin for multidrug resistant tumour modulation remains experimental and should only be used in clinical studies. Concurrent use should be very well monitored.

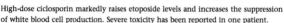

Ciclosporin (Cyclosporine) + Everolimus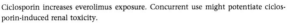

Ciclosporin increases everolimus exposure. Concurrent use might potentiate ciclosporin-induced renal toxicity.

Monitor renal function and everolimus concentrations and adjust the immunosuppressant doses as necessary. In kidney transplant patients, everolimus is licensed for use with reduced-dose ciclosporin. In renal cell carcinoma patients, consider reducing the everolimus dose to 5 mg daily or on alternate days.

Ciclosporin (Cyclosporine) + Ezetimibe

Exposure to ezetimibe is moderately increased by ciclosporin, although one patient with renal impairment had a much larger increase in ezetimibe exposure. Ezetimibe very slightly increases ciclosporin exposure.

The small increase in ciclosporin exposure is not usually considered to be clinically relevant in most patients; however, the UK and US manufacturers advise monitoring ciclosporin concentrations. It has been suggested that ezetimibe should be started at 5 mg daily in patients receiving ciclosporin with careful monitoring of lipid concentrations if the dose is increased.

Ciclosporin (Cyclosporine) + Fibrates

The use of bezafibrate with ciclosporin has resulted in significantly increased serum creatinine concentrations. Reductions, no change, or increased ciclosporin concentrations have also been seen. The use of fenofibrate has also been associated with reduced renal function and possibly reduced ciclosporin concentrations. Three studies found no pharmacokinetic interaction between ciclosporin and gemfibrozil while a fourth found gemfibrozil caused a reduction in ciclosporin concentrations and an increase in serum creatinine in some patients.

Ciclosporin concentrations and effects (e.g. on renal function) should be monitored as a matter of routine, but it may be prudent to increase monitoring if a fibrate (particularly bezafibrate or fenofibrate) is started or stopped. Adjust the dose of ciclosporin as necessary and consider dose reduction, or withdrawal of the fibrate, should significant renal impairment occur.

Ciclosporin (Cyclosporine) + Grapefruit and other fruit juices ✕

Grapefruit juice, and possibly pomelo juice, but not cranberry or orange juices, can increase the bioavailability of oral ciclosporin. Purple grape juice reduced the bioavailability of ciclosporin in one study.

The interaction between grapefruit juice and ciclosporin is established and clinically important. In general, grapefruit juice should be avoided, and the US manufacturers also suggest avoiding whole grapefruit. There is insufficient evidence to recommend avoiding pomelo juice or pomelo fruit when taking ciclosporin but bear this potential interaction in mind. Similarly, the importance of the reduction in bioavailability of ciclosporin seen with purple grape juice is also unclear. Until more is known, it would be prudent to bear this potential interaction in mind.

Ciclosporin (Cyclosporine) + Griseofulvin

An isolated report describes decreased ciclosporin concentrations in a patient given griseofulvin, whereas another report found no interaction.

> This interaction is unconfirmed and of uncertain general significance. There is insufficient evidence to recommend increased monitoring, but be aware of the potential for an interaction in the case of an unexpected response to treatment.

C

Ciclosporin (Cyclosporine) + H₂-receptor antagonists

Although some reports suggest that cimetidine can rarely increase ciclosporin concentrations, the majority of the information suggests no interaction occurs. Ranitidine, and probably famotidine, do not appear to affect ciclosporin concentrations. Note that an increase in serum creatinine concentration has been seen with the concurrent use of ciclosporin and cimetidine or ranitidine, but this does not appear to be related to renal toxicity or reduced renal function. Isolated cases of thrombocytopenia and hepatotoxicity have been reported with ranitidine and ciclosporin.

> There is little to suggest that concurrent use should be avoided, but good initial monitoring is possibly advisable with cimetidine.

Ciclosporin (Cyclosporine) + Herbal medicines or Dietary supplements

Alfalfa and/or Black cohosh ⊗

An isolated report describes acute rejection and vasculitis after a renal transplant patient taking ciclosporin started supplements containing black cohosh and alfalfa.

> The evidence of for this interaction is limited, but as the effects in this case were so severe, it would seem prudent to avoid concurrent use, particularly in patients taking ciclosporin for serious indications such as organ transplantation. For indications such as eczema, psoriasis or rheumatoid arthritis, although avoidance would be prudent, short-term concurrent use is likely to be less hazardous and patients should be counselled about the possible risks (i.e. loss of disease control) should they wish to take alfalfa or black cohosh with ciclosporin.

Geum chiloense

A single case report describes a large, rapid increase in the ciclosporin concentrations of a man after he drank an infusion of *Geum chiloense*.

> There is insufficient evidence to make any strong recommendations, but be aware of the potential for an interaction.

Red yeast rice (Monascus purpureus)

Red yeast rice has been reported to cause rhabdomyolysis in a kidney transplant patient taking ciclosporin.

> Ciclosporin is well known to interact with the statins, and this interaction appeared to be mediated by a statin-like component in the red yeast rice. Patients

should report any unexplained muscle pain, tenderness or weakness if they take red yeast rice with ciclosporin.

St John's wort (Hypericum perforatum)

Large reductions in ciclosporin blood concentrations (resulting in transplant rejection in some cases) can occur within a few weeks of starting St John's wort.

The advice of the CSM in the UK is that patients receiving ciclosporin should avoid or stop taking St John's wort. In the latter situation, the ciclosporin blood concentrations should be well monitored and the dose adjusted as necessary. Some evidence suggests that increased monitoring will be needed for at least 2 weeks after the St John's wort is stopped. It is possible to accommodate this interaction by increasing the ciclosporin dose, but this raises the costs of an already expensive drug and might be difficult to adequately manage.

Ciclosporin (Cyclosporine) + HIV-protease inhibitors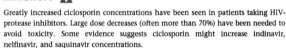

Greatly increased ciclosporin concentrations have been seen in patients taking HIV-protease inhibitors. Large dose decreases (often more than 70%) have been needed to avoid toxicity. Some evidence suggests ciclosporin might increase indinavir, nelfinavir, and saquinavir concentrations.

Ciclosporin concentrations should be carefully monitored and the dose adjusted accordingly if HIV-protease inhibitors are also given. The clinical importance of the effects of ciclosporin on some HIV-protease inhibitors is unclear, although in one study the effect was not sustained.

Ciclosporin (Cyclosporine) + Lanreotide

Octreotide causes a reduction in ciclosporin concentrations and inadequate immuno-suppression might result. Lanreotide is predicted to interact similarly.

Ciclosporin concentrations and effects (e.g. on renal function) should be monitored as a matter of routine, but it might be prudent to increase monitoring if lanreotide is started or stopped.

Ciclosporin (Cyclosporine) + Macrolides

Ciclosporin concentrations can be greatly increased by clarithromycin , erythromycin (intravenous erythromycin seems to have less effect than oral), josamycin , and possibly midecamycin. Telithromycin is predicted to interact similarly. Although major studies have found no interaction with azithromycin, there have been two isolated case reports of increased ciclosporin plasma concentrations in patients given azithromycin.

Ciclosporin plasma concentrations and effects (e.g. on renal function) should be monitored as a matter of routine, but it might be prudent to increase monitoring if macrolides are started or stopped. A ciclosporin dose reduction of about 35% has been suggested when using erythromycin or clarithromycin concurrently. With erythromycin, also consider increased monitoring if the route of administration is changed. Other macrolides might also interact, although it seems unlikely that they all will, see macrolides, page 474.

Ciclosporin (Cyclosporine) + Methotrexate

Previous or concurrent treatment with methotrexate might increase the risk of liver and other toxicity, but effective and valuable concurrent use has also been reported. Ciclosporin causes a modest increase in methotrexate concentrations but methotrexate does not appear to affect the pharmacokinetics of ciclosporin.

Patients receiving ciclosporin should routinely be monitored for renal adverse effects, and those receiving methotrexate routinely monitored for hepatotoxicity. If both drugs are given concurrently, it could be worth increasing the frequency of this monitoring to aid rapid detection of any adverse effects. The dose of either drug might need to be reduced.

Ciclosporin (Cyclosporine) + Metoclopramide

Metoclopramide very slightly increases the exposure to ciclosporin and increases its blood concentrations.

The clinical importance of this interaction is uncertain. Concurrent use should be well monitored to ensure that any increase in ciclosporin maximum concentrations does not increase adverse effects.

Ciclosporin (Cyclosporine) + Modafinil

Ciclosporin concentrations were reported to be reduced by modafinil in one patient. Armodafinil, the *R*-isomer of modafinil, would be expected to interact in a similar way to modafinil.

This seems to be the only reported case of an interaction between ciclosporin and modafinil, however, a clinically relevant interaction seems possible, as ciclosporin has a narrow therapeutic range. It would seem prudent to anticipate a reduction in ciclosporin concentrations if modafinil or armodafinil is used, although as the effects would generally be expected to be slight, ciclosporin dose adjustments might not always be necessary.

Ciclosporin (Cyclosporine) + NRTIs

Ciclosporin-induced renal impairment might increase entecavir exposure.

Until more is known, it would be prudent to monitor renal function closely on concurrent use.

Ciclosporin (Cyclosporine) + NNRTIs

Efavirenz, and to a lesser extent nevirapine, appear to decrease the levels of ciclosporin. The ciclosporin levels of one patient dramatically decreased following the addition of efavirenz. Etravirine is also predicted to interact in this way. In contrast, delavirdine is predicted to inhibit the metabolism of ciclosporin and increase its levels.

> Although there is limited information, it is in line with the way these drugs are known to interact. It would seem prudent to closely monitor ciclosporin levels in any patient given an NNRTI, adjusting the ciclosporin dose as necessary.

Ciclosporin (Cyclosporine) + NSAIDs

NSAIDs sometimes reduce renal function in individual patients, which is reflected in increases in serum creatinine concentrations and possibly in changes in ciclosporin concentrations, but concurrent use can also be uneventful. Diclofenac concentrations can be doubled by ciclosporin.

> Concurrent use in rheumatoid arthritis need not be avoided but renal function should be closely monitored. The UK manufacturer of ciclosporin also recommends close monitoring of liver function, because hepatotoxicity is a potential adverse effect of both drugs. It is difficult to generalise about what will or will not happen if any particular NSAID is given. It has been recommended that doses at the lower end of the range for diclofenac should be used initially, and it has been suggested that lower than usual doses should be considered for other NSAIDs.

Ciclosporin (Cyclosporine) + Octreotide

Octreotide causes a reduction in ciclosporin concentrations and inadequate immunosuppression might result.

> Ciclosporin concentrations and effects (e.g. on renal function) should be monitored as a matter of routine, but it might be prudent to increase monitoring if octreotide is started or stopped. An increase in the ciclosporin dose of around 50% has been suggested and the serum concentrations monitored daily.

Ciclosporin (Cyclosporine) + Orlistat

The absorption of ciclosporin is reduced by orlistat (by more than 50% in some cases) and cases of low concentrations have been reported with both formulations (*Neoral* and *Sandimmun*). A non-significant episode of acute graft rejection has been reported with *Neoral*.

> It has been suggested that the effects of the interaction can be reduced by using the microemulsion formulation of ciclosporin (*Neoral*); however, close monitoring is still required because there is still a risk of subtherapeutic concentrations. Some recommend avoiding concurrent use. The US manufacturer recommends taking ciclosporin at least 3 hours after orlistat to reduce the chance of an interaction. However, there is evidence that separation of doses does not avoid the interaction.

Ciclosporin (Cyclosporine) + Oxcarbazepine

Oxcarbazepine appears to decrease ciclosporin concentrations.

> Monitor the concentrations and effects (e.g. on renal function) of ciclosporin more

frequently if oxcarbazepine is started or stopped, adjusting the ciclosporin dose as necessary.

Ciclosporin (Cyclosporine) + Pasireotide

Pasireotide might decrease ciclosporin exposure. *In vitro*, pasireotide has been shown to be a substrate of P-glycoprotein and therefore the manufacturers predict that potent P-glycoprotein inhibitors such as ciclosporin will increase pasireotide concentrations.

It would seem prudent to monitor ciclosporin concentrations, adjusting the dose of ciclosporin as necessary. Also monitor for pasireotide adverse effects (such as abdominal pain, diarrhoea, and myalgia) and reduce the pasireotide dose if these become troublesome.

Ciclosporin (Cyclosporine) + Phenobarbital

Ciclosporin concentrations are greatly reduced by phenobarbital. As primidone is metabolised to phenobarbital it seems likely that it will interact similarly.

Ciclosporin concentrations and effects (e.g. on renal function) should be monitored as a matter of routine, but it would be prudent to increase monitoring if phenobarbital or primidone are stopped, started, or the dose altered, adjusting the ciclosporin dose as necessary.

Ciclosporin (Cyclosporine) + Phenytoin

Ciclosporin concentrations are greatly reduced by phenytoin. Fosphenytoin, a prodrug of phenytoin, would be expected to interact similarly.

Ciclosporin concentrations and effects (e.g. on renal function) should be monitored as a matter of routine, but it would be prudent to increase monitoring if phenytoin is stopped, started, or the dose altered, adjusting the ciclosporin dose as necessary.

Ciclosporin (Cyclosporine) + Propafenone

In an isolated report, propafenone caused a notable increase in the ciclosporin concentrations of a patient.

The general importance of this isolated report is unknown. Nevertheless, the UK manufacturer of propafenone advises caution on concurrent use, and that the dose of ciclosporin should be reduced if ciclosporin toxicity occurs.

Ciclosporin (Cyclosporine) + Proton pump inhibitors ❓

Omeprazole does not usually appear to affect ciclosporin concentrations, but isolated reports describe both increases and decreases in ciclosporin concentrations upon concurrent use.

The concurrent use of ciclosporin and omeprazole need not be avoided, but it would be prudent to consider the possibility of an interaction if patients taking higher doses of omeprazole have otherwise unexplained changes in ciclosporin concentrations.

Ciclosporin (Cyclosporine) + Quinolones

Ciclosporin concentrations are normally unchanged by the use of ciprofloxacin, but increased concentrations and nephrotoxicity might occur in a small number of patients. Some evidence suggests increased ciclosporin concentrations might develop in patients given norfloxacin and levofloxacin, but other studies found no change. There is also some evidence that the immunosuppressant effects of ciclosporin are reduced by ciprofloxacin.

No pharmacokinetic interaction usually occurs between ciclosporin and these quinolones, but as very occasionally and unpredictably an increase in serum ciclosporin concentrations and/or nephrotoxicity has occurred, it would be prudent to bear these interactions in mind on concurrent use.

Ciclosporin (Cyclosporine) + Ranolazine

The concurrent use of ciclosporin and ranolazine may lead to increased levels of both ranolazine and ciclosporin.

Information is limited, but it would seem prudent to monitor the levels of both drugs on concurrent use. The manufacturers advise careful dose titration when starting ranolazine. Patients already taking ranolazine and started on ciclosporin should be monitored for adverse effects (nausea, dizziness) and the dose of ranolazine reduced if needed.

Ciclosporin (Cyclosporine) + Rifabutin

A case report suggests that rifabutin increases the clearance of ciclosporin by about 20%.

Evidence for an interaction is limited, however the UK manufacturer of rifabutin and the CSM in the UK warn about the possibility of an interaction: consider increasing the monitoring of ciclosporin concentrations and effects (e.g. on renal function) if rifabutin is started or stopped, adjusting the ciclosporin dose as necessary.

Ciclosporin (Cyclosporine) + Rifampicin (Rifampin)

Ciclosporin concentrations are greatly reduced (in one case within a single day) by the concurrent use of rifampicin. Transplant rejection can rapidly develop if the ciclosporin dose is not increased.

Ciclosporin concentrations and effects (e.g. on renal function) should be monitored as a matter of routine, but it is essential to increase monitoring if rifampicin is started or stopped. If the concurrent use of rifampicin is essential, increase the ciclosporin dose appropriately: 3- to 5-fold dose increases (sometimes increasing the dose frequency from two to three times daily) have proven to be effective, with daily monitoring.

Ciclosporin (Cyclosporine) + Sevelamer

Sevelamer did not appear to alter ciclosporin levels in one study; however, a case report describes a large reduction in ciclosporin concentrations within 6 days of starting sevelamer.

The manufacturers of sevelamer advise that ciclosporin should be taken at least 1 hour before, or 3 hours after, sevelamer. Consider close monitoring of ciclosporin concentrations, particularly when sevelamer is started or stopped.

Ciclosporin (Cyclosporine) + Statins

Simvastatin, Pitavastatin, or Rosuvastatin

Ciclosporin moderately increases the exposure to pitavastatin and markedly to very markedly increases the exposure to rosuvastatin and simvastatin. Ciclosporin concentrations are unaffected by pitavastatin and rosuvastatin and increased to a small extent by simvastatin.

The concurrent use of ciclosporin and these statins is generally contraindicated, although note that the US manufacturer recommends limiting the dose of rosuvastatin to 5 mg daily. If the concurrent use of ciclosporin and either of these statins is considered unavoidable, patients should be closely monitored and they should be told to report any unexplained muscle pain, tenderness, or weakness or dark coloured urine.

Other statins

Ciclosporin moderately to very markedly increases the exposure to atorvastatin, fluvastatin, lovastatin, and pravastatin, and for some of the statins this had led to the development of serious myopathy (rhabdomyolysis) accompanied by renal failure. The plasma concentrations of ciclosporin appear not to be affected by fluvastatin, lovastatin or pravastatin, but some slight changes have been seen with atorvastatin.

The concurrent use of ciclosporin and these statins should be avoided, where possible. If concurrent use is necessary, monitor the outcome closely, a precautionary recommendation being to start (or reduce) the statin at the lowest daily dose, appropriate to the patient's condition. The manufacturers recommend the following statin doses in patients also taking ciclosporin: atorvastatin 10 mg daily (UK); fluvastatin 20 mg daily (US); lovastatin 20 mg daily; and pravastatin 20 mg daily (UK, titrated to 40 mg daily) or 10 mg daily (US, titrated to 20 mg daily). Patients should be told to report any unexplained muscle pain, tenderness, or weakness or dark coloured urine. If myopathy does occur, withdrawing the statin has been shown to resolve the symptoms. It might also be prudent to monitor ciclosporin concentrations more closely in the presence of atorvastatin.

Ciclosporin (Cyclosporine) + Sulfinpyrazone

Sulfinpyrazone can reduce ciclosporin concentrations, and this has led to transplant rejection in some cases, which developed over a period of several months.

If sulfinpyrazone is added to established treatment with ciclosporin, it would be prudent to increase monitoring of ciclosporin concentrations and be alert for the need to increase the ciclosporin dose. Be aware that the two cases of transplant rejection occurred after 4 months and 7 months of taking ciclosporin with sulfinpyrazone, therefore long-term monitoring would be a prudent precaution.

Ciclosporin (Ciclosporine) + Sulfonamides

In isolated cases, sulfadiazine given orally, or sulfadimidine given intravenously with trimethoprim, have caused a decrease in ciclosporin concentrations. Sulfametoxydiazine possibly caused a minor reductions in ciclosporin concentrations in one case.

These interactions are not firmly established. Until more information is available it would be prudent to check ciclosporin concentrations if any sulphonamide is added to established treatment with ciclosporin.

Ciclosporin (Ciclosporine) + Terbinafine

Terbinafine causes a small, usually clinically unimportant reduction in ciclosporin concentrations (maximum blood concentration reduced by 14%).

No action is generally needed; however, bear the possibility of an interaction in mind, particularly in patients whose ciclosporin concentrations are at the lower end of the therapeutic range.

Ciclosporin (Ciclosporine) + Ticagrelor

Ciclosporin might increase ticagrelor exposure.

The UK manufacturer of ticagrelor recommends that concurrent use is avoided, but if both drugs are given, monitor for increased ticagrelor effects (e.g. bleeding).

Ciclosporin (Ciclosporine) + Ticlopidine

Three case reports describe decreases in ciclosporin concentrations, and one study noted that minimum ciclosporin concentrations were halved by ticlopidine. However, the interaction was not confirmed in a later randomised, controlled study.

Information appears to be limited however, the controlled study used a low dose of ticlopidine and just 2 weeks of concurrent use, whereas in the other study and reports the interaction was noted after a few months of concurrent use. For this reason, it would be prudent to closely monitor ciclosporin concentrations, both when ticlopidine is first added, and for the first few months of concurrent use.

Ciclosporin (Ciclosporine) + Ursodeoxycholic acid (Ursodiol)

Ursodeoxycholic acid unpredictably increases the absorption and concentrations of ciclosporin in some, but not all, patients.

Ciclosporin concentrations and effects (e.g. on renal function) should be monitored as a matter of routine, but it would be prudent to increase monitoring if ursodeoxycholic acid is started or stopped. Adjust the dose of ciclosporin as necessary.

Ciclosporin (Cyclosporine) + Vaccines

The body's immune response is suppressed by ciclosporin. The antibody response to vaccines may be reduced, and the use of live attenuated vaccines may result in generalised infection.

For many inactivated vaccines even the reduced response seen is considered clinically useful and, in the case of renal transplant patients, influenza vaccination is actively recommended. If a vaccine is given, it may be prudent to monitor the response, so that alternative prophylactic measures can be considered where the response is inadequate. Note that even where effective antibody titres are produced, these may not persist as long as in healthy subjects, and more frequent booster doses may be required. The use of live vaccines is generally considered to be contraindicated. Ideally vaccines should take place before immunosuppressive treatment is started, and live vaccines should not be given for up to 6 months after treatment has stopped.

Ciclosporin (Cyclosporine) + Vancomycin

Vancomycin appears to increase the risk of nephrotoxicity when it is given with ciclosporin.

Renal function should be routinely monitored when either drug is given; however, it may be prudent to increase the frequency of monitoring if both drugs are given.

Ciclosporin (Cyclosporine) + Vitamins

Ciclosporin concentrations were increased by vitamin E (water-soluble formulation) in two studies, while another study found that ciclosporin exposure was modestly decreased. Other studies have also found modestly reduced ciclosporin concentrations with vitamin E combined with vitamin C, with or without betacarotene.

Ciclosporin concentrations and/or effects (e.g. on renal function) should be monitored as a matter of routine, but until more is known consider increasing monitoring if vitamin E is started or stopped, adjusting the dose of ciclosporin as necessary. In addition, it might be prudent to question patients about their intake of vitamin supplements before starting or when taking ciclosporin, particularly if a sudden or unexplained reduction in stable ciclosporin concentrations occurs.

Ciclosporin (Cyclosporine) + Warfarin and related oral anticoagulants

A case report describes reduced ciclosporin concentrations and reduced warfarin efficacy in patients given both drugs concurrently. A further report describes an increase in serum ciclosporin concentrations when an unnamed anticoagulant was given. Other reports describe increased or decreased acenocoumarol effects and decreased ciclosporin concentrations in two patients given both drugs.

Information is limited to a few reports, and both drugs should be monitored as a matter of routine. However, consider these cases in the event of an unexpected response to treatment.

Cilostazol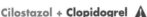

Cilostazol + **Clopidogrel**

Clopidogrel has no clinically relevant effect on the pharmacokinetics of cilostazol, and concurrent use does not alter the platelet count, aPTT, or prothrombin time. The addition of cilostazol to clopidogrel does not appear to further increase the bleeding time relative to clopidogrel alone.

> Although cilostazol does not appear to increase the risk of bleeding seen with clopidogrel alone, the UK manufacturer of cilostazol advises caution on concurrent use. Combinations of antiplatelet drugs are commonly used and can be clinically beneficial; however, be aware of the increased risk of bleeding. Note, the European Medicines Agency contraindicates the use of cilostazol with two or more antiplatelet drugs or anticoagulants.

Cilostazol + **Dipyridamole**

The concurrent use of cilostazol and dipyridamole might theoretically increase the risk of bleeding.

> Although combinations of antiplatelet drugs are commonly used and can be clinically beneficial in some indications, be aware of the increased risk of bleeding.

Cilostazol + **Dabigatran**

The concurrent use of antiplatelet drugs with dabigatran can theoretically increase the risk of bleeding.

> The manufacturers do not recommend concurrent use. If both drugs are essential, patients should be closely monitored for signs and symptoms of bleeding.

Cilostazol + **Ergot derivatives** 🛆

The UK manufacturer predicts that cilostazol will increase the levels of drugs that are metabolised by CYP3A4 and they name the ergot derivatives. This might increase the risk of ergotism.

> It would be prudent to be alert for any signs of an adverse response, particularly those suggestive of reduced peripheral circulation (coldness, numbness or tingling of the hands and feet).

Cilostazol + **Food** 🛆

Food slightly increases the bioavailability of cilostazol and almost doubles its maximum plasma levels, which may increase adverse effects.

> The manufacturer recommends that cilostazol should be taken 30 minutes before or 2 hours after food.

Cilostazol + Herbal medicines or Dietary supplements

Ginkgo biloba

A study found no significant increase in the antiplatelet effects of single doses of cilostazol when a single dose of *Ginkgo biloba* was added. However, the bleeding time was significantly increased, although none of the subjects developed any significant adverse effects.

> The evidence is too slim to advise patients taking cilostazol to avoid *Ginkgo biloba*. However, as with any two drugs that a affect platelet function some caution (e.g. reporting any evidence of bleeding) would be prudent if *Ginkgo biloba* is used with cilostazol.

St John's wort (Hypericum perforatum)

The UK manufacturer of cilostazol predicts that inducers of CYP3A4 (they name St John's wort) might alter the antiplatelet efficacy of cilostazol.

> The UK manufacturer advises monitoring the concurrent use of St John's wort for an alteration in the antiplatelet effects of cilostazol.

Cilostazol + HIV-protease inhibitors

The HIV-protease inhibitors are predicted to increase the exposure of cilostazol and its active metabolite, and to increase its overall pharmacological effect.

> Increased cilostazol adverse effects (such as headache and diarrhoea) might occur. The UK and US manufacturers suggest considering reducing the dose of cilostazol to 50 mg twice daily.

Cilostazol + Macrolides

Erythromycin increases the exposure of cilostazol but appears to have no clinically relevant effect on the exposure of its active metabolite. Other macrolides might also interact, although it seems unlikely that they all will, see macrolides, page 474.

> Increased cilostazol adverse effects (such as headache and diarrhoea) might occur. The UK and US manufacturers suggest considering reducing the dose of cilostazol to 50 mg twice daily.

Cilostazol + Phenobarbital

The UK manufacturer of cilostazol predicts that inducers of CYP2C19 and CYP3A4 might alter the antiplatelet efficacy of cilostazol. It seems likely that this will include phenobarbital. Primidone is metabolised to phenobarbital and would be expected to interact similarly.

> The UK manufacturer advises monitoring the concurrent use of enzyme inducers (such as phenobarbital and primidone) for an alteration in the antiplatelet effects of cilostazol.

Cilostazol + **Phenytoin**

The UK manufacturer of cilostazol predicts that inducers of CYP2C19 and CYP3A4 (they name phenytoin) might alter the antiplatelet efficacy of cilostazol. Fosphenytoin is a prodrug of phenytoin and would be expected to interact similarly.

> The UK manufacturer advises monitoring the concurrent use of phenytoin (and therefore fosphenytoin) for an alteration in the antiplatelet effects of cilostazol.

C

Cilostazol + **Prasugrel**

The concurrent use of cilostazol and prasugrel might theoretically increase the risk of bleeding.

> Although combinations of antiplatelet drugs are commonly used and can be clinically beneficial, be aware of the increased risk of bleeding.

Cilostazol + **Proton pump inhibitors**

Omeprazole increases the bioavailability of cilostazol (and its main active metabolite) and increases its pharmacological activity. Esomeprazole might interact similarly.

> The UK manufacturer of cilostazol predicts that an increase in cilostazol adverse effects (such as headache and diarrhoea) might occur on concurrent use, and along with the MHRA in the UK and the US manufacturer, they advise that a cilostazol dose reduction to 50 mg twice daily should be considered, depending on efficacy and tolerability.

Cilostazol + **Rifampicin (Rifampin)**

The UK manufacturer of cilostazol predicts that inducers of CYP2C19 and CYP3A4 (they name rifampicin) might alter the antiplatelet efficacy of cilostazol.

> The UK manufacturer advises monitoring the concurrent use of rifampicin for an alteration in the antiplatelet effects of cilostazol.

Cilostazol + **Rivaroxaban**

The concurrent use of rivaroxaban and cilostazol might increase the risk of bleeding.

> Advise patients to be aware of increased bruising or prolonged bleeding, and to seek medical advice if this occurs.

Cilostazol + **SSRIs**

The US manufacturer of cilostazol predicts that fluoxetine, fluvoxamine and sertraline will increase the exposure to cilostazol, by inhibiting CYP3A4. However these SSRIs only weakly inhibit CYP3A4 (at most). The bleeding risk associated with antiplatelet drugs (such as cilostazol) might be further increased by the concurrent use of an SSRI, although the data appears to be conflicting.

> In general, the manufacturers of the SSRIs advise caution on the concurrent use of

drugs that affect platelet function. Consider giving gastroprotective drugs in those at high risk of gastrointestinal bleeding (e.g. the elderly, those with a history of gastrointestinal bleeding, patients taking multiple antiplatelet drugs). Advise patients to report any signs of excessive bleeding. A clinically relevant *pharmacokinetic* interaction seems unlikely. Nevertheless, the US manufacturer advises caution and suggests considering reducing the dose of cilostazol to 50 mg twice daily.

Cilostazol + Statins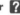

Cilostazol moderately increases the exposure to lovastatin; simvastatin would be expected to be similarly affected.

It has been suggested that statin dose reductions may be needed on concurrent use, but this seems over-cautious. Patients given a statin should be counselled regarding myopathy (e.g. report any unexplained muscle pain, tenderness, or weakness) and it would seem prudent to reinforce this if cilostazol is also given.

Cilostazol + Ticagrelor

The concurrent use of cilostazol and ticagrelor might theoretically increase the risk of bleeding.

Although combinations of antiplatelet drugs are commonly used and can be clinically beneficial in some indications, be aware of the increased risk of bleeding.

Cilostazol + Ticlopidine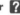

The concurrent use of cilostazol and ticlopidine might theoretically increase the risk of bleeding.

Although combinations of antiplatelet drugs are commonly used and can be clinically beneficial in some indications, be aware of the increased risk of bleeding.

Cilostazol + Warfarin and related oral anticoagulants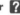

Cilostazol does not appear to have a clinically relevant effect on the pharmacokinetics or pharmacodynamics of warfarin. Nevertheless, as with other antiplatelet drugs, concurrent use might increase the bleeding risk.

The UK manufacturer advises that the concurrent use of cilostazol and oral anticoagulants should be used with caution and that monitoring should be carried out more frequently to reduce the possibility of bleeding. Further, note that use of cilostazol in patients receiving two or more additional antiplatelet drugs or anticoagulants is contraindicated.

Cinacalcet

Cinacalcet + **Dextromethorphan**

Cinacalcet very markedly increases dextromethorphan levels.

This is not expected to be of clinical significance as dextromethorphan has a wide
therapeutic range and its dose is not individually titrated, but bear this interaction
in mind in the case of an unexpected response to treatment. Remember that many
non-proprietary cough preparations contain dextromethorphan.

Cinacalcet + **Food**

Cinacalcet absorption is increased by food (AUC increased by 68%).

Cinacalcet should be taken with food or shortly after a meal to maximise
absorption.

Cinacalcet + **HIV-protease inhibitors**

Ketoconazole raises cinacalcet levels 2-fold and increased the incidence of cinacalcet
adverse effects, probably by inhibiting the metabolism of cinacalcet by CYP3A4. Other
potent CYP3A4 inhibitors, such as the HIV-protease inhibitors, are predicted to
interact similarly.

It may be prudent to monitor parathyroid hormone and serum calcium more
frequently in any patient receiving a HIV-protease inhibitor.

Cinacalcet + **Macrolides**

Ketoconazole raises cinacalcet levels 2-fold and increased the incidence of cinacalcet
adverse effects, probably by inhibiting the metabolism of cinacalcet by CYP3A4. Other
potent CYP3A4 inhibitors, such as some macrolides, are predicted to interact similarly,
although they differ in their ability to inhibit CYP3A4, see macrolides, page 474.

It may be prudent to monitor parathyroid hormone and serum calcium more
frequently if a macrolide that potently inhibits CYP3A4 is started or stopped. The
manufacturers specifically mention erythromycin and telithromycin.

Cinacalcet + **Opioids**

The analgesic effects of codeine, and probably also hydrocodone, are predicted to be
reduced or abolished by cinacalcet.

Monitor for analgesic efficacy and consider using an alternative to codeine or
hydrocodone in the case of reduced efficacy.

Cinacalcet + Quinolones

Ciprofloxacin may decrease the clearance (and therefore increase the levels) of cinacalcet, by inhibiting its metabolism by CYP1A2.

It may be prudent to monitor parathyroid hormone and serum calcium more frequently if ciprofloxacin is started or stopped, adjusting the cinacalcet dose as needed. Note that other quinolones may also interact similarly, although they differ in their ability to inhibit CYP1A2, see quinolones, page 564.

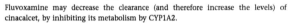

Cinacalcet + Rifampicin (Rifampin)

Rifampicin is predicted to decrease cinacalcet levels by inducing its metabolism by CYP3A4. This seems a reasonable prediction as potent CYP3A4 inhibitors raise cinacalcet levels.

It may be prudent to monitor parathyroid hormone and serum calcium more frequently if rifampicin is started or stopped, increasing the cinacalcet dose as needed.

Cinacalcet + SSRIs

Fluvoxamine may decrease the clearance (and therefore increase the levels) of cinacalcet, by inhibiting its metabolism by CYP1A2.

It may be prudent to monitor parathyroid hormone and serum calcium more frequently if fluvoxamine is started or stopped, adjusting the cinacalcet dose as needed.

Cinacalcet + Tamoxifen ✕

Paroxetine reduces the metabolism of tamoxifen to one of its active metabolites (by inhibiting CYP2D6): this might decrease the efficacy of tamoxifen and possibly increase the risk of breast cancer recurrence. The MHRA predicts that other CYP2D6 inhibitors could possibly interact similarly.

The European Medicines Agency and the MHRA in the UK state that concurrent of CYP2D6 inhibitors use should be avoided whenever possible in patients taking tamoxifen, and they specifically name cinacalcet. Consider alternatives to tamoxifen in patients clearly benefiting from cinacalcet.

Cinacalcet + Tricyclics

Cinacalcet increases the AUC of desipramine 3.6-fold. Other tricyclics are likely to be similarly affected.

Dose reductions of the tricyclic are likely to be needed if cinacalcet is also given. If starting a tricyclic in a patient taking cinacalcet it would seem prudent to start at the lowest dose and titrate upwards carefully. Monitor closely for adverse effects such as dry mouth, urinary retention and constipation.

Clindamycin

Clindamycin + **Contraceptives**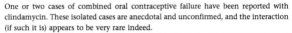

One or two cases of combined oral contraceptive failure have been reported with clindamycin. These isolated cases are anecdotal and unconfirmed, and the interaction (if such it is) appears to be very rare indeed.

It is possible that the anecdotal cases of contraceptive failure with antibacterials are indistinguishable from the normal accepted failure rate and no special precautions are required. Historically UK guidelines cautiously advised that additional contraceptive precautions were necessary; however, it is now advised that no additional precautions are needed, which is in line with the advice given by a number of other authorities. For further information on the use of antibacterials with contraceptives, see contraceptives, page 288.

Clomethiazole

Clomethiazole + **H₂-receptor antagonists**

Increased sedation appears to occur when clomethiazole is given with cimetidine. Ranitidine does not appear to affect the pharmacokinetics of clomethiazole.

The clinical relevance of these relatively modest effects with the concurrent use of cimetidine is probably small. Ranitidine might therefore provide a useful alternative to cimetidine if an interaction were to occur.

Clonidine

Clonidine + **Inotropes and Vasopressors**

Studies suggest that pretreatment with clonidine decreases the blood pressure response to small doses of dopamine and can increase the blood pressure responses to dobutamine, ephedrine and phenylephrine.

The exact outcome of the concurrent use of clonidine and these drugs is not clear. It has been suggested that the effects may be different at different doses of dopamine. Some suggest that the increase in pressor response is unlikely to be clinically significant. If dobutamine, ephedrine, or phenylephrine are given with clonidine, be aware that they may have a greater than expected effect.

Clonidine + **Levodopa**

Limited evidence suggests that the control of Parkinson's disease with levodopa may be impaired by clonidine.

Be alert for a reduction in the control of the Parkinson's disease during concurrent use. The effects of this interaction appear to be reduced if antimuscarinic drugs are also being used. Be aware that, as with all antihypertensives, additive hypotensive effects may occur with levodopa, see antihypertensives, page 97.

Clonidine + Methylphenidate

Much publicised fears about the serious consequences of using methylphenidate with clonidine appear to be unfounded. There is some evidence to suggest that concurrent use can be both safe and effective.

No action needed.

Clonidine + Tricyclics

The tricyclic antidepressants reduce or abolish the antihypertensive effects of clonidine and a case report describes a hypertensive crisis as a result of this interaction.

This interaction is not seen in all patients. Avoid concurrent use unless the effects on blood pressure can be monitored. Increasing the dose of clonidine seems to be an effective way of managing this interaction.

Clopidogrel

Clopidogrel + Dabigatran

The concurrent use of antiplatelet drugs with dabigatran might theoretically increase the risk of bleeding.

The UK manufacturer of dabigatran does not recommend concurrent use. If both drugs are essential, patients should be closely monitored for signs and symptoms of bleeding.

Clopidogrel + Dipyridamole

The concurrent use of clopidogrel with dipyridamole might theoretically increase the risk of bleeding.

Although combinations of antiplatelet drugs are commonly used and can be clinically beneficial in some indications, be aware of the increased risk of bleeding.

Clopidogrel + Duloxetine

The bleeding risk associated with antiplatelet drugs such as clopidogrel might be further increased by the concurrent use of an SSRI, although the data appears to be conflicting. SNRIs (e.g. duloxetine) are expected to interact similarly.

The UK manufacturers of duloxetine advise caution on concurrent use in patients taking antiplatelet drugs (such as clopidogrel). Consider giving gastroprotective drugs in those at high risk of gastrointestinal bleeding (e.g. the elderly, those with a history of gastrointestinal bleeding, patients taking multiple antiplatelet drugs). Advise patients to report any signs of excessive bleeding.

Clopidogrel + H₂-receptor antagonists ⊗

Cimetidine may theoretically inhibit the conversion of clopidogrel to its active metabolite by CYP2C19. Limited retrospective evidence suggests that cimetidine might possibly reduce the cardiovascular benefit of clopidogrel (increase the risk of cardiovascular adverse events), although one retrospective study found no increased cardiovascular risk on concurrent use.

Until more is known, it may be prudent to use an alternative H₂-receptor antagonist, such as ranitidine, which does not affect CYP2C19.

Clopidogrel + Heparin ⚠

The antiplatelet effects of clopidogrel are not altered by heparin. Nevertheless, the concurrent use of heparin with antiplatelet drugs such as clopidogrel may increase the risk of bleeding. Furthermore, concurrent use may contribute to the development of epidural or spinal haematoma after epidural anaesthesia.

The concurrent use of clopidogrel and heparin may be beneficial in specific indications (such as acute coronary syndromes), but it would still be prudent to be aware of the increased risk of bleeding and be alert for any signs of this. If they are used together, the manufacturers recommend caution or careful clinical and laboratory monitoring. Unless specifically indicated, concurrent use should probably be avoided. Extreme caution is needed if concurrent use is considered appropriate in patients undergoing epidural anaesthesia.

Clopidogrel + Herbal medicines or Dietary supplements ⚠

Ginkgo biloba alone has been associated with bleeding, platelet and clotting disorders, and there are isolated reports of serious adverse reactions after its concurrent use with clopidogrel. However, a single-dose study found no increase in adverse effects when *Ginkgo biloba* was given with clopidogrel.

The evidence is too slim to advise patients taking clopidogrel to avoid *Ginkgo biloba*. However, as with any two drugs that affect platelet function some caution (e.g. reporting any evidence of bleeding) would be prudent if *Ginkgo biloba* is used with clopidogrel.

Clopidogrel + Laropiprant ❓

Laropiprant appears to cause a transitory increase in the prolongation of bleeding time and inhibition of platelet aggregation caused by clopidogrel. Laropiprant had no clinically relevant effect on the prolongation of bleeding time and inhibition of platelet aggregation caused by aspirin, but it might increase the bleeding time if it is given with both aspirin and clopidogrel.

Clopidogrel is often used in combination with antiplatelet doses of aspirin. It would seem prudent to be alert for signs of bleeding whenever clopidogrel is used with laropiprant.

Clopidogrel + Low-molecular-weight heparins

Although in various large clinical studies in patients with acute coronary syndrome or myocardial infarction, most patients received LMWHs and clopidogrel without an obvious difference in the rate of bleeding, concurrent use may increase the risks of bleeding and case reports describe occasional serious bleeding events, including the development of spinal haematoma and retroperitoneal bleeding.

The concurrent use of clopidogrel and a LMWH may be beneficial in specific indications (such as acute coronary syndromes), but it would still be prudent to be aware of the increased risk of bleeding and be alert for any signs of this. If they are used together, the manufacturers recommend caution or careful clinical and laboratory monitoring. Unless specifically indicated, concurrent use of a LMWH with clopidogrel should probably be avoided because of the possible risk of increased bleeding. Extreme caution is needed if concurrent use is considered appropriate in patients undergoing epidural anaesthesia.

Clopidogrel + Macrolides

Limited data suggests that erythromycin slightly reduces the antiplatelet effects of clopidogrel. Clarithromycin and telithromycin may possibly interact similarly.

An interaction is not established and the clinical outcome of the slight reduction in antiplatelet effects is unclear. However, until further data are available, it would seem prudent to consider the possibility of a reduced antiplatelet effect in response to clopidogrel in patients taking macrolides that are potent inhibitors of CYP3A4 (such as erythromycin, clarithromycin and telithromycin).

Clopidogrel + Moclobemide

On the basis of the interaction with the proton pump inhibitors, page 274, some predict that moclobemide may theoretically inhibit the conversion of clopidogrel to its active metabolite by CYP2C19.

The MHRA in the UK and the manufacturers advise that concurrent use should be avoided.

Clopidogrel + NNRTIs

On the basis of the interaction with the proton pump inhibitors, page 274, some predict that etravirine may theoretically inhibit the conversion of clopidogrel to its active metabolite by CYP2C19. However, note that etravirine is only a weak inhibitor of CYP2C19.

The manufacturers of etravirine advise that concurrent use should be avoided.

Clopidogrel + NSAIDs ❓

Clopidogrel increases the risk of bleeding (including gastrointestinal bleeding) and there is evidence that this may be further increased with NSAIDs.

> If concurrent use is necessary, patients should be monitored for signs of excessive bleeding and advised to report signs of excessive bleeding. Consider giving additional gastrointestinal prophylaxis such as an H_2-receptor antagonist or a proton pump inhibitor (but see also Clopidogrel + Proton pump inhibitors, page 274) in patients at risk of gastrointestinal ulceration and bleeding. Note that the need for any NSAID should be very carefully considered as NSAIDs (particularly coxibs and diclofenac, but also other non-selective NSAIDs) are associated with an increased thrombotic/cardiovascular risk, particularly when used at high doses and for long-term treatment. Therefore coxibs and diclofenac are contraindicated, and other NSAIDs should generally be avoided, in those with ischaemic heart disease, cerebrovascular disease, or peripheral artery disease. Diclofenac is also contraindicated in those with congestive heart failure.

Clopidogrel + Oxcarbazepine ✕

On the basis of the interaction with the proton pump inhibitors, some predict that oxcarbazepine may theoretically inhibit the conversion of clopidogrel to its active metabolite by CYP2C19.

> The MHRA in the UK and the manufacturers advise that concurrent use should be avoided.

Clopidogrel + Proton pump inhibitors

Esomeprazole or Omeprazole

High-dose omeprazole almost halves the exposure to the active metabolite of clopidogrel and reduces the antiplatelet action of clopidogrel. Findings from the numerous retrospective studies looking at the clinical relevance of the interaction of omeprazole and esomeprazole with clopidogrel are conflicting: some studies suggest that concurrent use might reduce the efficacy of clopidogrel and increase the risk of adverse cardiovascular effects, while others have found no such interaction. Further prospective studies are needed to confirm an interaction. The mechanism for the interaction between the proton pump inhibitors and clopidogrel is not yet established. At present, the most plausible mechanism is that omeprazole (and therefore probably its isomer, esomeprazole) inhibit the conversion of clopidogrel to its active metabolite by CYP2C19.

> The concurrent use of clopidogrel with omeprazole or esomeprazole should be avoided: this is advised by the MHRA in the UK, the FDA in the US, and the European Medicines Agency. If a proton pump inhibitor is essential in a patient taking clopidogrel, a proton pump inhibitor other than omeprazole or esomeprazole should be considered. Gastroprotective drugs other than the proton pump inhibitors, such as antacids or H_2-receptor antagonists (except cimetidine, page 272), might also be suitable alternatives to omeprazole or esomeprazole, where clinically appropriate. Consider also the patient's possible risk factors for gastrointestinal bleeding versus the possibility of clopidogrel treatment failure.

Other proton pump inhibitors

Evidence for an interaction between clopidogrel and lansoprazole, pantoprazole, and rabeprazole is mostly based on retrospective data, some of which is contradictory, and does not appear to fit with the known lack of a clinically relevant CYP2C19 inhibitory effect of these proton pump inhibitors.

A clinically relevant interaction would not be expected, although ideally prospective studies are needed to confirm this.

Clopidogrel + **Quinolones**

On the basis of the interaction with the proton pump inhibitors, some predict that ciprofloxacin may theoretically inhibit the conversion of clopidogrel to its active metabolite by CYP2C19. However, there do not appear to be any clinically relevant interactions with ciprofloxacin as a result of this mechanism.

The MHRA in the UK and the manufacturers advise that concurrent use should be avoided.

Clopidogrel + **Rifampicin (Rifampin)**

Rifampicin moderately induces the metabolism of clopidogrel to its active metabolite, and slightly increases its antiplatelet effects; however, it is unclear if this results in an increase in beneficial cardiovascular effects and/or an increase in the bleeding risk with clopidogrel.

Until further data are available on the clinical outcomes of this interaction, bear this interaction in mind should any otherwise unexplained bleeding occur in a patient taking both drugs.

Clopidogrel + **Rivaroxaban**

The concurrent use of rivaroxaban and clopidogrel led to an increase in bleeding time in some patients. The pharmacokinetics of both drugs were not affected.

Advise patients to be aware of increased bruising or prolonged bleeding, and to seek medical advice if this occurs.

Clopidogrel + **SSRIs**

Fluoxetine and Fluvoxamine ⚠

On the basis of the interaction of clopidogrel with the proton pump inhibitors, page 274, some predict that fluoxetine and fluvoxamine might theoretically inhibit the conversion of clopidogrel to its active metabolite by CYP2C19. However, note that fluoxetine only weakly inhibits CYP2C19. The SSRIs can increase the risk of upper gastrointestinal bleeding and the risk might be further increased by the concurrent use of clopidogrel.

Although an interaction by CYP2C19 seems unlikely, the MHRA in the UK advises against the concurrent use of clopidogrel with fluoxetine or fluvoxamine. If concurrent use is essential, consideration should be given to the prescribing of gastroprotective drugs such as an H_2-receptor antagonist or a proton pump inhibitor (but see also Clopidogrel + Proton pump inhibitors, page 274) in those at high risk of gastrointestinal bleeding, such as elderly patients, patients taking multiple antiplatelets or those with a history of gastrointestinal bleeding. Advise patients to report any signs of bleeding.

Other SSRIs ❓

The bleeding risk associated with antiplatelet drugs such as clopidogrel might be further increased by the concurrent use of an SSRI, although the data appears to be conflicting.

> In general, the manufacturers of the SSRIs advise caution on concurrent use in patients taking antiplatelet drugs (such as clopidogrel). Consideration should be given to the prescribing of gastroprotective drugs such as an H_2-receptor antagonist or a proton pump inhibitor (but see also Clopidogrel + Proton pump inhibitors, page 274) in those at high risk of gastrointestinal bleeding, such as elderly patients or those with a history of gastrointestinal bleeding. Advise patients to report any signs of bleeding.

Clopidogrel + Statins ✅

Atorvastatin had no clinically relevant effect on the pharmacokinetics or antiplatelet effect of clopidogrel in controlled studies. Similarly, pravastatin, rosuvastatin, and possibly lovastatin, do not to alter the antiplatelet effect of clopidogrel. Simvastatin and fluvastatin also appear not to interact with clopidogrel, although one study showed some reduction in its antiplatelet effect. Nevertheless, clinical outcome data from numerous retrospective analyses of large studies, and from two randomised studies, does not support an interaction with any of these other statins.

> Although an interaction between clopidogrel and some statins has been seen in some studies, the majority of the evidence supports the conclusion that no interaction would be expected to occur in clinical use.

Clopidogrel + Ticagrelor ❓

The concurrent use of clopidogrel and ticagrelor might theoretically increase the risk of bleeding.

> Although combinations of antiplatelet drugs are commonly used and can be clinically beneficial in some indications, be aware of the increased risk of bleeding.

Clopidogrel + Ticlopidine ❌

On the basis of the interaction with the proton pump inhibitors, page 274, some predict that ticlopidine may theoretically inhibit the conversion of clopidogrel to its active metabolite by CYP2C19.

> The MHRA in the UK and the manufacturers advise that concurrent use should be avoided. However, note that, ticlopidine, like clopidogrel, is a thienopyridine antiplatelet drug, and it is not usually used with clopidogrel because it has the same mechanism of action.

Clopidogrel + Venlafaxine ❓

The bleeding risk associated with antiplatelet drugs such as clopidogrel might be further increased by the concurrent use of an SSRI, although the data appears to be conflicting. SNRIs (e.g. venlafaxine) are expected to interact similarly.

> The UK manufacturer of venlafaxine advises caution on concurrent use in patients taking antiplatelet drugs (such as clopidogrel). Consider giving gastroprotective drugs in those at high risk of gastrointestinal bleeding (e.g. the elderly, those with a history of gastrointestinal bleeding, patients taking multiple antiplatelet drugs). Advise patients to report any signs of excessive bleeding.

Clopidogrel + Warfarin and related oral anticoagulants ❓

Clopidogrel does not appear to have a clinically relevant effect on the pharmacokinetics or pharmacodynamics of warfarin. Nevertheless, the concurrent use of clopidogrel, either with warfarin or when given with warfarin and aspirin, increases the bleeding risk.

> The concurrent use of warfarin and clopidogrel increases the risk of bleeding and so both drugs should only be given when there is a clear indication for concurrent use. The lowest effective INR should be targeted and the combination used for the shortest duration possible. Monitor for signs of bleeding and check bleeding times as necessary. Consideration should be given to the prescribing of gastroprotective drugs such as an H_2-receptor antagonist or a proton pump inhibitor, but see also Clopidogrel + Proton pump inhibitors, page 274. Note that, in the UK, the manufacturers actually state that concurrent use is not recommended, whereas the US manufacturers just recommend caution.

Cobicistat

Cobicistat + Colchicine ⚠

The US manufacturer of elvitegravir boosted with cobicistat (in a fixed-dose combination also including emtricitabine and tenofovir) predicts that it will increase the plasma concentrations of colchicine.

> If any patient is given colchicine and cobicistat, be alert for colchicine adverse effects such as nausea, vomiting, and diarrhoea, especially in patients with pre-existing renal impairment. In the US, it is generally recommended that the dose of colchicine be reduced as follows:
>
> - For the treatment of gout, the dose of colchicine should be reduced to a single dose of 600 micrograms, with a further 300-microgram dose one hour later. The dose should not be repeated within 3 days.
> - For gout prophylaxis, the dose of colchicine should be reduced to 300 micrograms daily (if the initial dose was 600 micrograms twice daily) or on alternate days (if the initial dose was 600 micrograms daily).
> - For familial Mediterranean fever, a maximum total daily dose of colchicine 600 micrograms is recommended.

Cobicistat + **Corticosteroids**

Dexamethasone

The US manufacturer of elvitegravir boosted with cobicistat (in a fixed-dose combination also including emtricitabine and tenofovir) predicts that dexamethasone might decrease cobicistat plasma concentrations by inducing CYP3A4; however, dexamethasone rarely appears to cause clinically significant interactions by this mechanism.

If both drugs are given, monitor outcome for reduced efficacy.

Fluticasone

Cobicistat (given to boost elvitegravir) is predicted to increase the systemic concentrations of inhaled or intranasal fluticasone.

Monitor for fluticasone adverse effects. Alternative corticosteroids should be used, particularly in the longer term.

Cobicistat + **Dapoxetine**

Cobicistat is predicted to increase dapoxetine exposure.

Concurrent use is contraindicated if CYP2D6 status is unknown (likely). In patients known to be CYP2D6 extensive metabolisers, the manufacturer advises a maximum dapoxetine dose of 30 mg. Monitor for dapoxetine adverse effects, especially dose-related syncope or orthostatic hypotension.

Cobicistat + **Disopyramide**

The US manufacturer of elvitegravir boosted with cobicistat (in a fixed-dose combination also including emtricitabine and tenofovir) predicts that cobicistat will increase disopyramide concentrations.

Monitor for disopyramide adverse effects (dry mouth, blurred vision, urinary retention, ECG changes) and adjust the disopyramide dose if necessary.

Cobicistat + **Domperidone**

Potent CYP3A4 inhibitors, such as cobicistat, are predicted to increase the exposure to domperidone, which might increase the risk of QT-interval prolongation, possibly leading to the potentially fatal torsade de pointes arrhythmia.

The MHRA in the UK and the European Medicines Agency contraindicate the concurrent use of domperidone with potent CYP3A4 inhibitors.

Cobicistat + **Dronedarone**

Cobicistat is predicted to increase dronedarone exposure.

Avoid concurrent use.

Cobicistat + **Endothelin receptor antagonists**

Cobicistat is predicted to increase bosentan concentrations.

Stop bosentan for 36 hours, start elvitegravir with cobicistat for 10 days, and then restart bosentan 62.5 mg daily or on alternate days, as tolerated. Starting bosentan in a patient taking elvitegravir with cobicistat: give bosentan 62.5 mg daily or on alternate days, as tolerated.

Cobicistat + **Ergot derivatives**

The US & UK manufacturers of elvitegravir with cobicistat (in a fixed-dose combination also including emtricitabine and tenofovir disoproxil fumarate) predicts it will increase ergot derivative concentrations.

Concurrent use is contraindicated.

Cobicistat + **Ethosuximide**

The US manufacturer of elvitegravir with cobicistat (in a fixed-dose combination also including emtricitabine and tenofovir) predicts that it will increase the plasma concentration of ethosuximide.

Monitor concurrent use for ethosuximide adverse effects (such as nausea, vomiting, ataxia, dizziness).

Cobicistat + **Flecainide**

The US manufacturer of elvitegravir boosted with cobicistat (in a fixed-dose combination also including emtricitabine and tenofovir) predicts that cobicistat will increase flecainide concentrations.

Monitor for flecainide adverse effects (dizziness, nausea, and tremor) and adjust the flecainide dose if necessary.

Cobicistat + **Herbal medicines or Dietary supplements**

St John's wort (*Hypericum perforatum*) is predicted to decrease cobicistat plasma concentrations, which might reduce its efficacy.

The US manufacturer of elvitegravir boosted with cobicistat (in a fixed-dose combination also including emtricitabine and tenofovir) contraindicates concurrent use.

Cobicistat + **Lidocaine** ⚠

The US manufacturer of elvitegravir boosted with cobicistat (in a fixed-dose combination also including emtricitabine and tenofovir) predicts that cobicistat will increase lidocaine concentrations.

Monitor for lidocaine adverse effects (bradycardia, hypotension, pins and needles) and adjust the lidocaine dose if necessary.

Cobicistat + **Macrolides**

Clarithromycin ❓

The US manufacturer of elvitegravir with cobicistat (in a fixed-dose combination also including emtricitabine and tenofovir) predicts that both cobicistat and clarithromycin concentrations will be increased on concurrent use.

> No dose adjustment is necessary in patients with normal renal function. However, in patients with a creatinine clearance of 50 to 60 mL/minute, the clarithromycin dose should be halved when given with cobicistat. Further dose reductions are not given as cobicistat should be discontinued if creatinine clearance decreases below 50 mL/minute.

Telithromycin ⚠️

The US manufacturer of elvitegravir with cobicistat (in a fixed-dose combination also including emtricitabine and tenofovir) predicts that both cobicistat and telithromycin concentrations will be increased on concurrent use.

> Monitor concurrent use for telithromycin adverse effects (such as diarrhoea, dizziness and headache).

Cobicistat + **Maraviroc** ⚠️

Cobicistat is predicted to increase the exposure to maraviroc.

> Monitor for maraviroc adverse effects (such as diarrhoea, nausea, asthenia, anaemia). Consider reducing the maraviroc dose to 150 mg daily on concurrent use.

Cobicistat + **Mexiletine** ⚠️

The US manufacturer of elvitegravir boosted with cobicistat (in a fixed-dose combination also including emtricitabine and tenofovir) predicts that cobicistat will increase mexiletine concentrations.

> Monitor for mexiletine adverse effects (nausea, tremor, hypotension) and adjust the mexiletine dose if necessary.

Cobicistat + **Oxcarbazepine** ❌

Oxcarbazepine is predicted to decrease cobicistat plasma concentrations, which might reduce its efficacy.

> The US manufacturer of elvitegravir with cobicistat (in a fixed-dose combination also including emtricitabine and tenofovir) contraindicates concurrent use. Consider an alternative to oxcarbazepine.

Cobicistat + **Phenobarbital** ❌

Phenobarbital is predicted to decrease cobicistat plasma concentrations, which might reduce its efficacy. Primidone is metabolised to phenobarbital and might therefore interact similarly.

The US manufacturer of elvitegravir with cobicistat (in a fixed-dose combination also including emtricitabine and tenofovir) contraindicates concurrent use. Consider an alternative to phenobarbital.

Cobicistat + Phenytoin

Phenytoin is predicted to decrease cobicistat plasma concentrations, which might reduce its efficacy. Fosphenytoin, a prodrug of phenytoin, might interact similarly.

The US manufacturer of elvitegravir with cobicistat (in a fixed-dose combination also including emtricitabine and tenofovir) contraindicates concurrent use. Consider an alternative to phenytoin.

Cobicistat + Phosphodiesterase type-5 inhibitors

Cobicistat is predicted to increase the plasma concentrations of the phosphodiesterase type-5 inhibitors, resulting in an increase in their adverse events, including hypotension, syncope, visual disturbances, and priapism.

Monitor for phosphodiesterase type-5 inhibitors-related adverse events. The US manufacturers of elvitegravir with cobicistat (in a fixed-dose combination also including emtricitabine and tenofovir disoproxil fumarate) make the following recommendations: When phosphodiesterase type-5 inhibitors are being used for pulmonary arterial hypertension:

● The use of **sildenafil** is contraindicated;
● In patients already taking elvitegravir with cobicistat (for at least one week), start **tadalafil** at 20 mg daily, and increase the dose to 40 mg daily based on tolerability;
● In patients already taking **tadalafil**, stop tadalafil at least 24 hours before starting elvitegravir with cobicistat. After at least one week, restart tadalafil at 20 mg daily, increasing to 40 mg daily based on individual tolerability.

When phosphodiesterase type-5 inhibitors are being used for erectile dysfunction the recommended doses for use with elvitegravir boosted with cobicistat are:

● **Sildenafil** at a single dose not exceeding 25 mg in 48 hours;
● **Tadalafil** at a single dose not exceeding 10 mg in 72 hours;
● **Vardenafil** at a single dose not exceeding 2.5 mg in 72 hours.

The UK and US manufacturers of avanafil contraindicate concurrent use with potent CYP3A4 inhibitors, such as cobicistat.

Cobicistat + Propafenone

The US manufacturer of elvitegravir boosted with cobicistat (in a fixed-dose combination also including emtricitabine and tenofovir) predicts that cobicistat will increase propafenone concentrations.

Monitor for propafenone adverse effects (hypotension, bradycardia, dizziness, dry mouth) and adjust the propafenone dose if necessary.

Cobicistat + Quinidine

The US manufacturer of elvitegravir boosted with cobicistat (in a fixed-dose combination also including emtricitabine and tenofovir) predicts that cobicistat will increase quinidine concentrations.

Monitor for quinidine adverse effects (nausea, diarrhoea, tinnitus) and adjust the quinidine dose if necessary.

Cobicistat + Salbutamol (Albuterol) and related bronchodilators ⊗

Cobicistat (given to boost elvitegravir) is predicted to increase the systemic concentrations of inhaled salmeterol, increasing the risk of cardiovascular adverse events (such as QT prolongation, palpitations, and sinus tachycardia).

Avoid concurrent use.

Cobicistat + Sirolimus ⚠

The US manufacturer of elvitegravir boosted with cobicistat (in a fixed-dose combination also including emtricitabine and tenofovir) predicts that it will increase the plasma concentrations of sirolimus.

Monitor the concentrations and effects (e.g. on renal function) of sirolimus more frequently when starting or stopping elvitegravir with cobicistat, and adjust the sirolimus dose as necessary.

Cobicistat + SSRIs ⚠

The US manufacturer of elvitegravir boosted with cobicistat (in a fixed-dose combination also including emtricitabine and tenofovir) states that the plasma concentrations of SSRIs might be increased on concurrent use.

Monitor concurrent use for SSRI adverse effects (such as nausea, diarrhoea, dry mouth) and titrate the SSRI dose as tolerated.

Cobicistat + Statins

Lovastatin and Simvastatin ⊗

Cobicistat (given to boost elvitegravir) is predicted to increase lovastatin and simvastatin concentrations.

Avoid concurrent use.

Atorvastatin ⚠

Cobicistat (given to boost elvitegravir) is predicted to increase atorvastatin concentrations.

Give the lowest atorvastatin starting dose and titrate carefully, monitoring for any unexplained muscle pains or weakness.

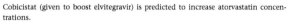

Cobicistat + Tacrolimus

The US manufacturer of elvitegravir boosted with cobicistat (in a fixed-dose combination also including emtricitabine and tenofovir) predicts that it will increase the plasma concentrations of tacrolimus.

Monitor the concentrations and effects (e.g. on renal function) of tacrolimus more frequently when starting or stopping elvitegravir with cobicistat, and adjust the tacrolimus dose as necessary.

C

Cobicistat + Ticagrelor

Cobicistat is predicted to markedly increase ticagrelor exposure.

Because the marked increase in exposure increases the risk of bleeding, concurrent use is contraindicated.

Cobicistat + Trazodone

Cobicistat (given to boost elvitegravir) is predicted to increase trazodone concentrations.

Avoid concurrent use if possible. If it is necessary, titrate the trazodone dose carefully and monitor for trazodone adverse effects.

Cobicistat + Ulipristal

Potent inhibitors of CYP3A4, such as cobicistat, are predicted to markedly increase the exposure to ulipristal.

The UK manufacturer of low-dose ulipristal for the symptomatic management of uterine fibroids does not recommend its concurrent use with potent CYP3A4 inhibitors. If low-dose ulipristal is given with cobicistat, monitor for an increase in the adverse effects of ulipristal (for example nausea, abdominal pain, and breast tenderness) or any unexpected outcome occurring during concurrent use. The UK manufacturer of ulipristal for emergency contraception states that CYP3A4 inhibitors are unlikely to have any clinically relevant effects.

Colchicine

Colchicine + Digoxin

Isolated cases of myopathy and rhabdomyolysis have been attributed to the concurrent use of colchicine and digoxin.

The US manufacturer of colchicine suggests careful monitoring of patients on concurrent use, especially during the initiation of treatment, being alert for signs of muscle pain, tenderness, or weakness. However, this advice seems overly cautious, and standard monitoring of colchicine treatment would seem sufficient. Very limited evidence suggests that colchicine does not affect digoxin concentrations.

Colchicine + Fibrates

Case reports suggest that the current use of fibrates and colchicine can result in rhabdomyolysis or neuromyopathy.

Information is limited, although rhabdomyolysis is associated with both colchicine and the fibrates. Suspect this interaction in any patient taking these drugs who presents with muscle pain or a raised creatinine kinase concentration.

Colchicine + Grapefruit juice ⚠

Grapefruit juice is predicted to increase colchicine exposure and a case report describes toxicity; however one study found no interaction.

Evidence for an interaction is limited, but some individuals might be affected. The US manufacturer recommends that the dose of colchicine be reduced in patients taking moderate CYP3A4 inhibitors, such as colchicine: see Colchicine + Macrolides, page 285 for detailed recommendations on colchicine dose adjustment in these patients. However, note that as the effect of grapefruit juice is likely to vary with different batches of the juice, it might be prudent to avoid grapefruit juice altogether.

Colchicine + HIV-protease inhibitors ⚠

Ritonavir increases the exposure to colchicine. Other HIV-protease inhibitors are predicted to interact similarly.

If any patient is given colchicine and a HIV-protease inhibitor, be alert for colchicine adverse effects (such as nausea, vomiting, and diarrhoea), and anticipate the need to reduce the colchicine dose. The UK and US manufacturers of colchicine contraindicate its concurrent use with HIV-protease inhibitors in patients with hepatic or renal impairment. The US manufacturer makes the following specific recommendations for colchicine dose reductions in patients taking potent CYP3A4 inhibitors (they name the HIV-protease inhibitors, with the exception of unboosted amprenavir and fosamprenavir), or if they have stopped taking these drugs within 2 weeks of starting colchicine:

- For the treatment of gout, the dose of colchicine should be reduced to a single dose of 600 micrograms, with a further 300-microgram dose one hour later. The dose should not be repeated within 3 days.
- For gout prophylaxis, the dose of colchicine should be reduced to 300 micrograms daily (if the initial dose was 600 micrograms twice daily) or on alternate days (if the initial dose was 600 micrograms daily).
- For familial Mediterranean fever, a maximum total daily dose of colchicine 600 micrograms is recommended.

The US manufacturer makes the following specific recommendations for colchicine dose reductions in patients taking moderate CYP3A4 inhibitors (they name unboosted amprenavir and fosamprenavir), or if they have stopped taking these drugs within 2 weeks of starting colchicine:

- The dose of colchicine should be reduced in the treatment of gout to 1.2 mg as a single dose. The dose should not be repeated within 3 days.
- For gout prophylaxis, the dose of colchicine should be halved, from 600 micrograms twice daily to 300 micrograms twice daily, or from 600 micrograms daily to 300 micrograms daily.

- For familial Mediterranean fever, a maximum total daily dose of colchicine 1.2 mg is recommended.

Colchicine + Macrolides

Clarithromycin and azithromycin increase the exposure to colchicine, to varying extents. Several case reports describe acute life-threatening colchicine toxicity, some of which were fatal, caused by the concurrent use of erythromycin or clarithromycin.

Information on this interaction is limited, but it appears that azithromycin, erythromycin, and clarithromycin can provoke acute colchicine toxicity, at the very least in pre-disposed individuals. Telithromycin is predicted to interact similarly. If any patient is given colchicine and a macrolide, monitor for colchicine toxicity (such as nausea, vomiting, diarrhoea, myopathy, and pancytopenia), and anticipate the need to reduce the colchicine dose, especially in patients with pre-existing renal impairment. Note that the UK and US manufacturers of colchicine contraindicate the concurrent use of colchicine with clarithromycin or telithromycin in patients with renal or hepatic impairment. The US manufacturer makes specific recommendations for reducing the colchicine dose in patients taking potent CYP3A4 inhibitors (such as clarithromycin or telithromycin), or if they have stopped taking these drugs within 2 weeks of starting colchicine:

- For the treatment of gout, the dose of colchicine should be reduced to a single dose of 600 micrograms, with a further 300-microgram dose one hour later. The dose should not be repeated within 3 days;
- For gout prophylaxis, the dose of colchicine should be reduced to 300 micrograms daily (if the initial dose was 600 micrograms twice daily) or on alternate days (if the initial dose was 600 micrograms daily);
- For familial Mediterranean fever, a maximum total daily dose of colchicine 600 micrograms (which can be given as 300 micrograms twice daily) is recommended.

The US manufacturer of colchicine also advises the following dose reductions in patients taking moderate CYP3A4 inhibitors, (such as erythromycin) or if they have stopped taking it within 2 weeks of starting colchicine:

- For the treatment of gout, the dose of colchicine should be reduced to a single dose of 1.2 mg. The dose should not be repeated within 3 days;
- For gout prophylaxis, the dose of colchicine should be reduced to 300 micrograms twice daily or 600 micrograms daily (if the initial dose was 600 micrograms twice daily) or 300 micrograms daily (if the initial dose was 600 micrograms daily);
- For familial Mediterranean fever, a maximum total daily dose of colchicine 1.2 mg (which can be given as 600 micrograms twice daily) is recommended.

Colchicine + Quinidine

Quinidine is predicted to increase colchicine exposure and toxicity.

Consider an interaction in the case of otherwise unexplained colchicine toxicity (e.g. diarrhoea, vomiting). Concurrent use is contraindicated in renal or hepatic impairment. The US manufacturer makes specific recommendations for colchicine dose reductions in patients taking P-glycoprotein inhibitors, such as quinidine. See Ciclosporin (Cyclosporine) + Colchicine, page 251 for further information.

Colchicine + **Ranolazine** ⚠

Ranolazine is predicted to increase colchicine exposure and toxicity.

Consider an interaction in the case of otherwise unexplained colchicine toxicity (e.g. diarrhoea, vomiting). Concurrent use is contraindicated in renal or hepatic impairment. The US manufacturer makes specific recommendations for colchicine dose reductions in patients taking P-glycoprotein inhibitors, such as ranolazine. See Ciclosporin (Cyclosporine) + Colchicine, page 251 for more details.

Colchicine + **Statins** ❓

Case reports describe myopathy or rhabdomyolysis in patients given colchicine and atorvastatin, fluvastatin, lovastatin, pravastatin, or simvastatin. It seems possible that this reaction could occur with colchicine and any statin.

Although this interaction is rare, and not established (many patients were taking higher than recommended doses of colchicine), it is serious. All patients taking statins should be warned about the symptoms of myopathy and told to report muscle pain or weakness. It would be prudent to reinforce this advice if they are given colchicine.

Colestyramine and related drugs

Note that it is generally recommended that other drugs are given one hour before or 4 hours after colestipol, one hour before or 4 to 6 hours after colestyramine, and at least 4 hours before colesevelam. Interactions have therefore only been included where information suggests that different actions may be appropriate.

Colestyramine and related drugs + **Diuretics**

Loop diuretics ⚠

The 4-hour diuretic response to furosemide can be reduced by 58% and 77% by colestipol and colestyramine, respectively.

Furosemide should be given 2 to 3 hours before taking colestyramine or colestipol to minimise this interaction.

Thiazides ⚠

The absorption of hydrochlorothiazide and chlorothiazide can be reduced by more than one-third if colestipol is given concurrently. Colestyramine also reduces the absorption of hydrochlorothiazide by more than two-thirds.

Separating the doses of hydrochlorothiazide and colestyramine by 4 hours can reduce, but not totally overcome the effects of this interaction. Even with a dosing separation, the possibility of this interaction should be considered in patients who have a reduced response to this diuretic.

Colestyramine and related drugs + **Leflunomide**

Studies have shown that colestyramine reduces the levels of the active metabolite of leflunomide by up to 65% after 48 hours.

Patients taking leflunomide should not be given colestyramine unless it is needed to remove the leflunomide from the body more quickly, such as in overdose or when switching to another DMARD.

Colestyramine and related drugs + **Mycophenolate**

Colestyramine modestly reduces the AUC of mycophenolic acid after administration of mycophenolate.

The clinical importance of this reduction has not been assessed but it would seem prudent to confirm that the immunosuppressant effects remain adequate in the presence of colestyramine. Separating the administration is not likely to eliminate this interaction, as colestyramine affects the enterohepatic recirculation of mycophenolate. Note that the US manufacturers of mycophenolate advise avoiding the concurrent use of colestyramine and other drugs that bind to bile acids (e.g. colestipol).

Colestyramine and related drugs + **NSAIDs**

Giving colestyramine even three or more hours after oral sulindac, piroxicam, or tenoxicam markedly reduced their plasma levels. Colestyramine, given after the NSAID, markedly reduces the levels of *intravenous* meloxicam or tenoxicam.

It is usually recommended that other drugs are given one hour before or 4 to 6 hours after colestyramine. However, meloxicam, piroxicam, sulindac, and tenoxicam undergo enterohepatic recirculation and so the interaction cannot be entirely avoided by separating the doses. Therefore it may be best to avoid using these NSAIDs with colestyramine.

Colestyramine and related drugs + **Raloxifene**

The manufacturers report that the concurrent use of colestyramine reduced the absorption of raloxifene by about 60%, due to an interruption in enterohepatic cycling.

Separating administration is unlikely to be effective as the interaction is via enterohepatic circulation. It is recommended that these two drugs should not be used concurrently. Other drugs, such as colestipol, are expected to interact similarly.

Colestyramine and related drugs + **Valproate**

Colestyramine causes a small 20% reduction in the absorption of valproate.

The fall in absorption is small and probably of very limited clinical importance, but the interaction can apparently be totally avoided by separating administration by 3 hours. Note that it is usually recommended that other drugs are given one hour before or 4 to 6 hours after colestyramine. Colesevelam does not appear to interact, and may therefore be a suitable alternative in some patients.

Colestyramine and related drugs + Vitamin D

The UK and US manufacturers of calcitriol, and the UK manufacturer of colecalciferol, state that colestyramine might reduce their absorption.

> Separate the dosing administration: it is normally recommended to avoid taking the affected drug at least one hour before or 4 to 6 hours after colestyramine.

Colestyramine and related drugs + Warfarin and related oral anticoagulants ⚠

The anticoagulant effects of phenprocoumon and warfarin can be reduced by colestyramine. An isolated and unexplained report describes a paradoxical increase in the effects of warfarin. Other coumarins are expected to interact similarly. The manufacturers warn that long-term colestyramine or colestipol can reduce vitamin K absorption and can cause hypoprothrombinaemia, and this may affect the anticoagulant effects of both coumarins and indanediones.

> If the concurrent use of colestyramine and a coumarin is thought necessary, prothrombin times should be monitored and the dose of the anticoagulant increased appropriately. Giving the colestyramine 4 to 6 hours after the anticoagulant has been shown to minimise the effects of this interaction; however, case reports suggest that, despite a dose separation, an interaction is still possible. Bear in mind that long-term colestyramine and colestipol can reduce vitamin K absorption and can cause hypoprothrombinaemia. This might result in an increased effect of warfarin, but there is little evidence to suggest that this is clinically relevant.

Contraceptives

As HRT contains many of the same hormones as the contraceptives, studies with contraceptives may be applicable to HRT and *vice versa*, although the relative doses should be borne in mind. Similar careful extrapolations may be made between studies with contraceptives and HRT, systemic oestrogens or progestogens.

General advice for use with antibacterials

The interactions between combined hormonal contraceptives and non-enzyme inducing antibacterials is not established and controversial. Almost all of the evidence suggesting that antibacterials might cause combined hormonal contraceptive failure is anecdotal with no controls, and the very limited evidence with controls shows no increase in risk. Moreover, data from over 20 studies have not shown any clinically important pharmacokinetic interaction or reduction in the suppression of ovulation by the contraceptive. The total number of failures is extremely small when viewed against the number of women worldwide using oral combined hormonal contraceptives, and it seems likely that the anecdotal cases of contraceptive failure with broad-spectrum antibacterials are indistinguishable from the accepted contraceptive failure rate. The contraceptive efficacy of the various progestogen-only contraceptive methods (tablets, implants, injections, IUDs) is also not affected by antibacterials that do not induce liver enzymes. Despite the limited evidence, a cautious approach has historically been adopted in, for example, the UK, where it was advised that additional contraceptive precautions were necessary. However, after a review of all the evidence, in 2011 the UK Faculty of Sexual and Reproductive Healthcare (FSRH, formerly the FFPRHC) updated their guidance on hormonal contraceptives and drug interactions, to advise that additional contraceptive precautions are not required during or after short courses of antibacterials (non-enzyme inducing). They note that, should the antibacterials and/or the illness cause vomiting or diarrhoea, then the usual additional precautions relating to these conditions should be observed. This approach is the one most readily justified from the available evidence.

General advice for use with enzyme-inducing drugs

In the UK in 2011, the Faculty of Sexual and Reproductive Healthcare (FSRH) issued guidance on the use of drugs that induce liver enzymes with combined hormonal contraceptives (tablets, patch and vaginal ring) and progestogen-only hormonal contraceptives, including emergency hormonal contraceptives. They recommend that women taking these drugs should preferably change to a contraceptive method unaffected by enzyme-inducing drugs (that is, copper IUDs, the levonorgestrel-releasing intrauterine system, or depot progestogen-only injections). Alternatively, for women who wish to use a **combined hormonal contraceptive**, they provide advice for both the short-term and the long-term concurrent use of enzyme-inducing drugs:

- *Short-term use (less than 2 months).* Women using the contraceptive patch, vaginal ring, and standard-strength tablet containing at least 30 micrograms of ethinylestradiol should use additional contraceptive precautions, such as condoms, while taking an enzyme-inducing drug and for 28 days after it has been stopped. In addition, to minimise the risk of contraceptive failure, an extended or tricycling regimen with a shortened hormone-free interval of 3 to 4 days is recommended. For those who do not wish to use additional contraceptive precautions, the same ethinylestradiol dose adjustments as recommended for the long-term use of enzyme-inducing drugs is advised, see below.

- *Long-term use (greater than 2 months).* Women using the contraceptive patch, vaginal ring, and standard-strength tablet containing at least 30 micrograms of ethinylestradiol should use an ethinylestradiol dose of at least 50 micrograms daily, during the concurrent use of an enzyme-inducing drug, and for 28 days after it has been stopped. This preparation should be used in an extended or tricycling regimen, with a shortened pill-free interval of 4 days. If breakthrough bleeding occurs, then the dose of ethinylestradiol may be increased in 10-microgram increments up to a maximum of 70 micrograms daily. Alternatively, additional non-hormonal methods of contraception, such as condoms, can be used, or the contraceptive can be switched to one unaffected by enzyme-inducing drugs. Note that, for those using the patch or vaginal ring, the use of more than one patch or vaginal ring is not recommended. The WHO also advise using a combined hormonal contraceptive containing a minimum of 30 micrograms of ethinylestradiol; however, this is lower than the FSRH guidelines of 50 micrograms. Although a 30-microgram dose of ethinylestradiol would seem adequate for weak enzyme inducers, such as topiramate, it is probably not sufficient for potent inducers, such as phenytoin or carbamazepine and related drugs.

- The **progestogen-only implant** may be continued with *short* courses of enzyme inducers. For *short-term use (less than 2 months)*, additional methods of contraception (such as condoms) should also be used by patients using the progestogen-only

C

implant, both when taking the liver enzyme inducers and for at least 28 days after stopping the enzyme-inducing drug. Alternatively, the FSRH state that women could be offered a one-off injection of medroxyprogesterone acetate to cover the period of risk. Alternatives to the progestogen-only implant should be considered with long-term (greater than 2 months) use of liver enzyme inducers, such as progestogen-only injections, the copper IUD or the levonorgestrel intra-uterine system. However, note that the WHO acknowledge that enzyme-inducing antiepileptics may decrease the efficacy of progestogen implants, and that the use of other contraceptives should be encouraged, in their 2009 guidance they advised that progestogen-only implants containing levonorgestrel or etonogestrel may generally be used in women taking enzyme inducers.

- **Oral progestogen-only contraceptives** are not recommended for use with enzyme inducers, and alternative methods of contraception (such as progestogen-only contraceptive depot injections or the levonorgestrel intrauterine system) are advised.

- For women requiring **progestogen-only** *emergency* hormonal contraception while taking enzyme-inducing drugs or within 28 days of stopping them, a copper IUD is the most effective method. In women who decline or who are not eligible for a copper IUD, a single 3-mg dose of levonorgestrel should be given (double the usual dose).

- Copper or levonorgestrel-releasing intrauterine devices (**IUDs**) and **depot progestogen-only injections** (medroxyprogesterone and norethisterone) are preferred alternative contraceptive methods, particularly for women requiring hormonal contraception who are likely to be taking the enzyme inducer in the long-term, as these are unaffected by liver enzyme inducers.

Contraceptives + Co-trimoxazole

In controlled studies, ovulation suppression/contraceptive steroid concentrations were not adversely affected when non-enzyme inducing antibacterials were given with combined hormonal contraceptives. However, rarely, contraceptive failure has been attributed to the concurrent use of various sulfonamides, and trimethoprim.

The pharmacokinetic and pharmacodynamic evidence indicates that co-trimoxazole is not likely to reduce the effectiveness of combined hormonal contraceptives. It is possible that these case reports of contraceptive failure are coincidental, and fit within the normal failure rate of combined hormonal contraceptives. Historically UK guidelines cautiously advised that additional contraceptive precautions were necessary; however, it is now advised that no additional precautions are needed, which is in line with the advice given by a number of other authorities. For more information on the use of antibacterials with contraceptives, see contraceptives, page 288.

Contraceptives + Danazol

There is a theoretical risk that the effects of both danazol and hormonal contraceptives might be altered or reduced on concurrent use.

As danazol can cause virilisation of a female foetus, the manufacturer advises that reliable non-hormonal contraceptive methods should be used while taking danazol, and, by inference, the avoidance of hormonal contraceptives.

Contraceptives + Diuretics

Drospirenone, which is given as the progestogen component of oral combined hormonal contraceptives, might increase the risk of hyperkalaemia when given with other drugs that can cause hyperkalaemia such as potassium-sparing diuretics and aldosterone antagonists.

The risk of hyperkalaemia appears to be low, especially if renal function is normal. However, the UK manufacturer recommends that potassium levels should be monitored during the first cycle in women who regularly take a potassium-sparing diuretic or an aldosterone antagonist. This is particularly important where risk factors for hyperkalaemia exist (e.g. renal impairment). The US manufacturer also advises considering monitoring potassium levels on the concurrent use of drospirenone-containing contraceptives with these drugs. For women with severe renal impairment, the UK manufacturer contraindicates the use of drospirenone-containing contraceptives, whereas, in the US, its use in renal impairment [to any degree] is contraindicated. Note that hormonal contraceptives are generally cautioned or contraindicated in some of the patient groups who may be treated with a diuretic, and oestrogens (usually in larger doses than those present in combined hormonal contraceptives) can raise blood pressure, which may antagonise the effects of diuretics. However, the effects on blood pressure are far greater with the high-dose contraceptives that were used historically, and the risks appear to be smaller with the newer low-dose contraceptives. The risks with progestogen-only contraceptives seem to be low.

Contraceptives + Endothelin receptor antagonists

Bosentan reduces the levels of ethinylestradiol and norethisterone given as a combined hormonal contraceptive, which may result in contraceptive failure. The contraceptive efficacy of oral progestogen-only contraceptives, the progestogen-only implant and emergency hormonal contraceptives (both progestogen-only and combined hormonal preparations) are also expected to be reduced.

The clinical relevance of the reduction in contraceptive steroid exposure is uncertain; however, as the risk of contraceptive failure might be increased in some patients, and in addition, as bosentan is potentially teratogenic, effective contraception is required. In the UK, the Faculty of Sexual and Reproductive Healthcare (FSRH) include bosentan in their 2011 guidance on the use of enzyme inducers with combined hormonal contraceptives: see contraceptives, page 288, for details of this guidance.

Contraceptives + Eslicarbazepine

Combined hormonal contraceptives and possibly oral progestogen-only contraceptives are less reliable during treatment with eslicarbazepine. Breakthrough bleeding and spotting can take place. Controlled studies have shown that eslicarbazepine can reduce contraceptive steroid concentrations; this could lead to a reduction in contraceptive efficacy. The contraceptive efficacy of the progestogen-only implant and emergency hormonal contraceptives (both progestogen-only and combined hormonal preparations) are also expected to be reduced.

The increase in failure rate appears small, but because of the consequences of an unwanted pregnancy, especially with drugs that might cause foetal abnormalities, adjustments should be made. For additional advice on the use of enzyme inducers, such as eslicarbazepine, and hormonal contraceptives, see contraceptives, page 288.

Contraceptives + Felbamate 🅰

Felbamate increased the clearance of gestodene from an oral combined hormonal contraceptive in one study, but ovulation remained suppressed. Felbamate does not appear to have a clinically relevant effect on the pharmacokinetics of ethinylestradiol (from an oral combined hormonal contraceptive).

> A reduction in the contraceptive efficacy of gestodene-containing oral combined hormonal contraceptives cannot be ruled out. If both drugs are used tell patients to report any changes in bleeding.

Contraceptives + Fusidate ✅

One or two cases of oral combined hormonal contraceptive failure have been reported with fusidate. These isolated cases are anecdotal and unconfirmed, and the interaction (if such it is) appears to be very rare.

> It is possible that the anecdotal cases of contraceptive failure with antibacterials are indistinguishable from the normal accepted failure rate and no special precautions are required. Historically UK guidelines cautiously advised that additional contraceptive precautions were necessary; however, it is now advised that no additional precautions are needed, which is in line with the advice given by a number of other authorities. For guidance on the use of antibacterials with contraceptives. For further information on the use of antibacterials with contraceptives, see contraceptives, page 288.

Contraceptives + Gestrinone ⚠

There is a theoretical risk that the effects of both gestrinone and hormonal contraceptives might be altered or reduced on concurrent use. Note that high doses of gestrinone have been shown to be embryotoxic in some *animal* species.

> Avoid concurrent use. The manufacturers strongly emphasise the importance of using barrier methods of contraception while taking gestrinone.

Contraceptives + Griseofulvin ⚠

The effects of oral combined hormonal contraceptives may possibly be disturbed (either inter-menstrual bleeding or amenorrhoea) if griseofulvin is taken concurrently. There are a few isolated reports of women taking oral contraceptives who became pregnant while taking griseofulvin. The situation with progestogen-only oral contraceptives is not clear, but it has been suggested that they are not the contraceptive of choice in those taking griseofulvin because of increased menstrual irregularities. The manufacturers of the levonorgestrel intra-uterine system predicts that CYP3A4 inducers (they name griseofulvin) might reduce its contraceptive reliability; however, the available evidence does not seem to support this prediction. Furthermore, griseofulvin is not an established enzyme inducer.

> The risk of contraceptive failure is uncertain but probably very small. However, as

griseofulvin is potentially teratogenic it has been recommended that, for maximal contraceptive protection, additional contraceptives measures (such as a barrier method) should be used with oral combined hormonal contraceptives or oral progestogen-only contraceptives during and for one month after taking griseoful- vin.

Contraceptives + Heparin

Drospirenone, which is given as the progestogen component of oral combined hormonal contraceptives, might increase the risk of hyperkalaemia when given with other drugs that can cause hyperkalaemia such as heparin.

The risk of hyperkalaemia appears to be low, especially if renal function is normal. In the US, it is recommended that consideration be given to monitoring potassium levels during the first cycle in women [with normal renal function] who regularly take heparin, whereas the UK manufacturer recommends that the potassium level is measured during the first cycle or month of treatment in women with mild or moderate renal impairment only. For women with severe renal impairment, the UK manufacturer contraindicates the use of drospirenone-containing contracep- tives, whereas, in the US, its use in renal impairment [to any degree] is contraindicated. In patients at higher risk of developing hyperkalaemia (e.g. in renal impairment) it is generally recommended that potassium levels are measured during the first cycle of treatment with drospirenone.

Contraceptives + Herbal medicines or Dietary supplements

St John's wort (*Hypericum perforatum*) might cause small decreases in the concentra- tions of desogestrel, ethinylestradiol, and norethisterone from oral combined hormo- nal contraceptives, although there is some evidence that an extract with low hyperforin content might not interact. Both breakthrough bleeding and oral hormonal contraceptive failure have been seen in women taking St John's wort. In two cases, the failure of *emergency* hormonal contraception has been attributed to the use of St John's wort, and in one case the contraceptive efficacy of an oral progestogen- only contraceptive was reduced. Progestogen-only implants have also reportedly been affected.

The effect of St John's wort on contraceptive steroid concentrations appears to be very small, and would probably not be relevant in many women. However, as it is not known who is particularly likely to be at risk, women using hormonal contraceptives should generally avoid St John's wort. The MHRA in the UK specifically advises that all patients taking hormonal contraceptives for the prevention of pregnancy (except IUDs, but probably including emergency hormonal contraceptives) should not take herbal products that contain St John's wort. In the UK, the Faculty of Sexual and Reproductive Healthcare (FSRH) include St John's wort in their 2011 guidance on the use of enzyme inducers with combined hormonal contraceptives. If concurrent use is considered essential, see contraceptives, page 288 for general advice on the use of enzyme inducers, such as St John's wort, and contraceptives.

Contraceptives + HIV-protease inhibitors ⚠

Ritonavir and nelfinavir, given alone, markedly reduce the exposure of ethinylestradiol. Similarly, HIV-protease inhibitors boosted with ritonavir markedly (darunavir, fosamprenavir, lopinavir and tipranavir) or modestly (atazanavir) reduce ethinylestradiol exposure. Conversely, *unboosted* atazanavir, amprenavir, and indinavir *increase* the exposure to ethinylestradiol. Progestogens are also affected, with a number of HIV-protease inhibitors (darunavir, fosamprenavir, lopinavir) boosted with ritonavir slightly reducing norethisterone exposure. It is therefore possible that some HIV-protease inhibitors could reduce the contraceptive efficacy of progestogen-only oral contraceptives containing norethisterone. The efficacy of emergency hormonal contraceptives and the progestogen-only implant might also be decreased. In contrast, tipranavir boosted with ritonavir slightly *increases* norethisterone exposure and atazanavir boosted with ritonavir increases the AUC of the active metabolite of norgestimate by 85%.

In the UK, the Faculty of Sexual and Reproductive Healthcare (FSRH) Clinical Effectiveness Unit include ritonavir and HIV-protease inhibitors boosted with ritonavir in their 2011 guidance on the use of enzyme inducers with hormonal contraceptives. For the use of enzyme-inducers (which could include the use of HIV-protease inhibitors for post-exposure prophylaxis) in those who choose a combined hormonal contraceptive, the advice is to use a standard-strength preparation (30 or 35 micrograms of ethinylestradiol), with additional contraceptive precautions such as condoms, see contraceptives, page 288, for further details on this guidance. In the absence of barrier methods, standard-strength preparations may not be sufficiently effective given the reductions in ethinylestradiol exposure that occur, and at least 50 micrograms (as advised by the FSRH) is likely to be necessary. Note that the manufacturers of fosamprenavir actually advise alternative non-hormonal methods of contraception because of the risk of raised liver enzymes, as well as the decrease in hormone exposure. The UK manufacturer of atazanavir boosted with ritonavir states that as there is no information on the concurrent use of other progestogens, preparations with progestogens other than norgestimate should be avoided.

Contraceptives + Isoniazid

Two cases of oral combined hormonal contraceptive failure have been reported with isoniazid. However, there is evidence that isoniazid does not cause contraceptive failure when used in combination with other antimycobacterials (without rifampicin (rifampin)). These isolated cases are anecdotal and unconfirmed, and the interaction (if such it is) appears to be very rare.

No additional contraceptive precautions would be expected to be required in women taking combined hormonal contraceptives and requiring isoniazid. Historically UK guidelines cautiously advised that additional contraceptive precautions were necessary; however, 2011 guidelines advise that no additional precautions are needed, which is in line with the advice given by a number of other authorities, see contraceptives, page 288, for further discussion.

Contraceptives + Lamotrigine ⚠

In one study, lamotrigine for 2 weeks did not alter the levels of ethinylestradiol and levonorgestrel or the suppression of ovulation in women taking an oral combined hormonal contraceptive. However, another study of 6 weeks' use found a slight reduction in levonorgestrel exposure, and some loss in suppression of FSH and LH, but no evidence of ovulation. Combined hormonal contraceptives reduce the levels of lamotrigine, which can lead to a decrease in seizure control, and, conversely, an increase in lamotrigine exposure with a risk of toxicity during the hormone free week.

The manufacturers suggest that reduced contraceptive efficacy cannot be ruled out. If an oral combined hormonal contraceptive (and probably the combined hormonal contraceptive patch and vaginal ring) is used as the only form of contraception, they advise that women should be alert for signs of breakthrough bleeding. However, on the basis of the available evidence, the UK Faculty of Sexual and Reproductive Healthcare (FSRH) 2011 guideline the on drug interactions with hormonal contraceptives does not advise the use of additional contraception when combined hormonal contraceptives [any form] are used with lamotrigine. In addition, because of the cyclical effect of the contraceptive on lamotrigine exposure, the FSRH 2011 guideline does not usually recommend the use of combined hormonal contraceptives with lamotrigine monotherapy. However, if concurrent use is necessary and a combined hormonal contraceptive (oral, patch or vaginal ring) is started in women already taking lamotrigine, as monotherapy or with other drugs that are *not* strong inducers or inhibitors of lamotrigine glucuronidation, the maintenance dose of lamotrigine may need to be increased by as much as twofold, according to clinical response. It has been suggested that the cyclical nature of the interaction could be overcome by using a combined hormonal contraceptive as an extended regimen or continuously without a hormone-free (e.g. a pill-free) interval. For women already taking lamotrigine with strong inducers of lamotrigine glucuronidation, such as carbamazepine or phenytoin, no lamotrigine dose adjustment is necessary when hormonal contraceptives are started. Changes in lamotrigine doses also appear unlikely to be needed in those given hormonal contraceptives and already taking lamotrigine with valproate, which is a strong inhibitor of lamotrigine glucuronidation.

Contraceptives + Levothyroxine

Oral HRT (conjugated oestrogens) appears to increase the requirement for levothyroxine in some patients. A similar effect might therefore be expected with oral combined hormonal contraceptives, which include oestrogens.

It would be prudent to monitor thyroid function several months after starting or stopping oral oestrogens to check levothyroxine requirements.

Contraceptives + Macrolides

Controlled studies have not shown the macrolides clarithromycin, dirithromycin, roxithromycin and telithromycin to have any effect on contraceptive steroid concentrations and/or suppression of ovulation in women given combined hormonal contraceptives. Moreover, *increases* in contraceptive steroid concentrations have been seen with erythromycin and clarithromycin. Nevertheless, isolated cases of contraceptive failure have been attributed to erythromycin or spiramycin. Conversely, in two studies of contraceptive failures in dermatology patients, no pregnancies were identified in a total of 74 women taking erythromycin with an oral contraceptive.

Historically UK guidelines cautiously advised that additional contraceptive precautions were necessary; however, it is now advised that no additional precautions are needed, which is in line with the advice given by a number of

other authorities. For further information on the use of antibacterials with
contraceptives, see contraceptives, page 288.

Contraceptives + MAO-B inhibitors

In a small study, the bioavailability of selegiline was markedly higher (mean of about
20-fold) in women taking oral combined hormonal contraceptives than in those not
taking contraceptives.

The manufacturers of selegiline advise avoiding concurrent use. If concurrent use
is necessary, monitor for increased selegiline adverse effects (such as nausea,
constipation, hypotension and diarrhoea).

Contraceptives + Metronidazole

Isolated cases of oral combined hormonal contraceptive failure have been reported
with metronidazole. The interaction (if such it is) appears to be very rare. In controlled
studies, metronidazole did not affect contraceptive steroid concentrations and/or
ovulation suppression.

It is possible that the anecdotal cases of contraceptive failure with antibacterials
are indistinguishable from the normal accepted failure rate and no special
precautions are required. Historically UK guidelines cautiously advised that
additional contraceptive precautions were necessary; however, it is now advised
that no additional precautions are needed, which is in line with the advice given
by a number of other authorities. For further information on the use of
antibacterials with contraceptives, see contraceptives, page 288.

Contraceptives + Modafinil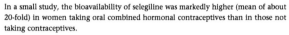

Modafinil slightly reduced the exposure to ethinylestradiol, from an oral combined
hormonal contraceptive; this may reduce contraceptive efficacy. The contraceptive
efficacy of oral progestogen-only contraceptives, the progestogen-only implant and
emergency hormonal contraceptives (both progestogen-only and combined hormonal
preparations) are also expected to be reduced. Armodafinil, the *R*-isomer of modafinil,
would be expected to interact similarly.

These small changes may be sufficient to cause the failure of combined hormonal
contraceptives in rare cases, and should be borne in mind due to the potential
teratogenicity of modafinil. For additional advice on the use of enzyme inducers,
such as modafinil, and hormonal contraceptives, see contraceptives, page 288. The
manufacturers recommend that additional or alternative methods should be used
during and for one (US) or 2 months (UK) after stopping modafinil and for
one month after stopping armodafinil (US), which seems overly cautious.

Contraceptives + Nitrofurantoin

One or two cases of combined oral contraceptive failure have been reported with
nitrofurantoin. These isolated cases are anecdotal and unconfirmed, and the
interaction (if such it is) appears to be very rare.

It is possible that the anecdotal cases of contraceptive failure with antibacterials are indistinguishable from the normal accepted failure rate and no special precautions are required. Historically UK guidelines cautiously advised that additional contraceptive precautions were necessary; however, it is now advised that no additional precautions are needed, which is in line with the advice given by a number of other authorities. For further information on the use of antibacterials with contraceptives, see contraceptives, page 288.

Contraceptives + NNRTIs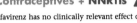

Efavirenz has no clinically relevant effect on ethinylestradiol exposure, but decreases the exposure to the active metabolites of norgestimate, from an oral combined hormonal contraceptive. Nevirapine modestly reduces ethinylestradiol and norethisterone exposure from an oral combined hormonal contraceptive, which could reduce the efficacy of contraception. The efficacy of emergency hormonal contraceptives and progestogen-only implants or injections may also be reduced by efavirenz and nevirapine.

In the UK, the Faculty of Sexual and Reproductive Healthcare (FSRH) include both efavirenz and nevirapine in their 2011 guidance on the use of enzyme inducers with hormonal contraceptives; see contraceptives, page 288, for details of this guidance. Note that whatever other methods of contraception are being used, barrier methods are always advisable to reduce the risk of HIV transmission.

Contraceptives + NSAIDs

A study in women taking ethinylestradiol and norethisterone-containing oral contraceptives found that the addition of etoricoxib increased the exposure to ethinylestradiol by 50 to 60%, but the rise in norethisterone exposure was not clinically relevant. Drospirenone may increase the risk of hyperkalaemia if it is given to patients with other drugs which increase potassium levels such as NSAIDs (although this is rare). A few early reports suggest that the very occasional failure of copper IUDs to prevent pregnancy may have been due to an interaction with NSAIDs.

There would appear to be no reason for avoiding concurrent use but the manufacturers of etoricoxib suggest that this increase in ethinylestradiol levels should be considered when choosing a hormonal contraceptive. It may be appropriate to use a contraceptive with a low 20 microgram dose of ethinylestradiol or the vaginal ring. Note also that coxibs alone are associated with an increased risk of thrombotic events. It is generally recommended that potassium levels are measured during the first cycle of treatment with drospirenone. The evidence is insufficient to justify general precautions if NSAIDs are given to women using copper IUDs.

Contraceptives + Orlistat

Studies suggest that orlistat does not alter the suppression of ovulation in women taking oral combined hormonal contraceptives. However, an isolated pregnancy has occurred in a woman taking an oral combined hormonal contraceptive with orlistat, and the UK manufacturer says that severe orlistat-induced diarrhoea might be a risk for this.

The manufacturers recommend additional contraceptive measures (presumably barrier methods) if severe diarrhoea occurs. Oral contraceptives, both combined or progestogen-only, might be expected to be affected, whereas the contraceptive effect of the combined hormonal contraceptive given as a *patch* is said not to be affected by diarrhoea.

Contraceptives + **Oxcarbazepine**

Combined hormonal contraceptives and possibly oral progestogen-only contraceptives are less reliable during treatment with oxcarbazepine. Breakthrough bleeding and spotting can take place. Controlled studies have shown that oxcarbazepine can reduce contraceptive steroid levels; this may lead to a reduction in contraceptive efficacy. The contraceptive efficacy of the progestogen-only implant and emergency hormonal contraceptives (both progestogen-only and combined hormonal preparations) are also expected to be reduced.

The increase in failure rate appears small, but because of the consequences of an unwanted pregnancy, especially with drugs that may cause foetal abnormalities, adjustments should be made. For additional advice on the use of enzyme inducers, such as oxcarbazepine, and hormonal contraceptives, see contraceptives, page 288.

Contraceptives + **Penicillins**

Failure of oral combined hormonal contraceptives has been attributed to the concurrent use of penicillins, but the interaction (if such it is) appears to be very rare. Controlled studies have not shown any effect of ampicillin or amoxicillin on contraceptive steroid concentrations and the suppression of ovulation in women given these contraceptives.

It is possible that the anecdotal cases of contraceptive failure with antibacterials are indistinguishable from the normal accepted failure rate and no special precautions are required. Historically UK guidelines cautiously advised that additional contraceptive precautions were necessary; however, it is now advised that no additional precautions are needed, which is in line with the advice given by a number of other authorities. For further information on the use of antibacterials with contraceptives, see contraceptives, page 288.

Contraceptives + **Perampanel**

Perampanel 12 mg daily decreases levonorgestrel exposure (from an oral combined hormonal contraceptive) which might decrease contraceptive efficacy. Lower doses of perampanel do not appear to affect levonorgestrel exposure.

In 2013, the UK Faculty of Sexual and Reproductive Healthcare (FSRH) issued a statement on the use of perampanel (at any dose) with combined hormonal, or progesterone-only, contraceptives, which recommends the same advice as for women taking other enzyme-inducing drugs with these contraceptives; see contraceptives, page 288.

Contraceptives + **Phenobarbital**

Combined hormonal contraceptives, and possibly progestogen-only oral contraceptives, are less reliable during treatment with phenobarbital. Inter-menstrual breakthrough bleeding and spotting can take place, and pregnancies have occurred. Controlled studies have shown that phenobarbital can reduce contraceptive steroid concentrations. Similarly, emergency hormonal contraceptives and progestogen-only implants are considered to be less effective in those taking phenobarbital. Note that primidone is metabolised to phenobarbital and might therefore interact similarly.

The increase in failure rate appears small, but because of the consequences of an unwanted pregnancy, especially with drugs that may cause foetal abnormalities, adjustments should be made. For additional advice on the use of enzyme inducers, such as phenobarbital or primidone and hormonal contraceptives, see contraceptives, page 288.

C

Contraceptives + **Phenytoin**

Combined hormonal contraceptives, and possibly progestogen-only oral contraceptives and progestogen-only implants, are less reliable during treatment with phenytoin. Inter-menstrual breakthrough bleeding and spotting can take place, and pregnancies have occurred. Controlled studies have shown that phenytoin can reduce contraceptive steroid concentrations (both progestogens and oestrogens). Similarly, emergency hormonal contraceptives are considered to be less effective in those taking phenytoin. Fosphenytoin, a prodrug of phenytoin, might interact similarly.

The increase in failure rate appears small, but because of the consequences of an unwanted pregnancy, especially with drugs that may cause foetal abnormalities, adjustments should be made. For general advice on the use of enzyme inducers, such as phenytoin, and hormonal contraceptives, see contraceptives, page 288.

Contraceptives + **Potassium**

Drospirenone, which is given as the progestogen component of oral combined hormonal contraceptives, might increase the risk of hyperkalaemia when given with other drugs that can cause hyperkalaemia such as potassium supplements.

The risk of hyperkalaemia appears to be low, especially if renal function is normal. In the US, it is recommended that consideration be given to monitoring potassium levels during the first cycle in women [with normal renal function] who regularly take a potassium supplement, whereas the UK manufacturer recommends that the potassium level is measured during the first cycle or month of treatment in women with mild or moderate renal impairment only. For women with severe renal impairment, the UK manufacturer contraindicates the use of drospirenone-containing contraceptives, whereas, in the US, its use in renal impairment [to any degree] is contraindicated. In patients at higher risk of developing hyperkalaemia (e.g. in renal impairment) it is generally recommended that potassium levels are measured during the first cycle of treatment with drospirenone.

Contraceptives + **Quinolones**

Ciprofloxacin, moxifloxacin, and ofloxacin have been shown not to affect the pharmacokinetics of oral combined hormonal contraceptives in controlled studies. Contraceptive failure does not appear to have been reported, and ovarian suppression is not affected.

It is possible that the anecdotal cases of contraceptive failure with antibacterials are indistinguishable from the normal accepted failure rate and no special precautions are required. Historically UK guidelines cautiously advised that additional contraceptive precautions were necessary; however, it is now advised that no additional precautions are needed, which is in line with the advice given by a number of other authorities. For further information on the use of antibacterials with contraceptives, see contraceptives, page 288.

Contraceptives + Retinoids ❓

The pharmacokinetics and/or ovulation suppressant effect of oral combined hormonal contraceptives are not affected by acitretin, alitretinoin, etretinate, isotretinoin, or tazarotene, all given orally. The adverse effects of isotretinoin on lipids might be additive with those of oral contraceptives.

Because the retinoids are established human teratogens, it is very important that women taking them systemically do not become pregnant. The oral combined hormonal contraceptive should be started one month before the oral retinoid is given, and continued for one month after stopping alitretinoin, isotretinoin, and tretinoin, for 2 years after stopping etretinate, and for at least 2 years (UK manufacturer) or 3 years (US manufacturer and British Association of Dermatologists) after stopping acitretin. In the US, it is standard practice to mandate that a second form of contraception, such as a barrier method, should also be used, and this is also advised by the British Association of Dermatologists for isotretinoin, and is also preferred by the UK manufacturers of alitretinoin and isotretinoin. Some consider that *parenteral* progestogen-only contraceptives (depot injections, implants, the levonorgestrel-releasing intra-uterine system) might be preferable contraceptives, as these are more effective contraceptives than oral combined hormonal contraceptives. Note that *oral* progestogen-only contraceptives are generally not considered reliable enough for use with teratogenic drugs. The currently available formulations of tazarotene are for *topical* use, and, on the basis of the data for *oral* tazarotene, these would not be expected to interact with combined hormonal contraceptives. The manufacturers advise that women of child bearing age should use adequate contraception while using topical tazarotene, because of the theoretical teratogenic risk.

Contraceptives + Rifabutin ⚠

Combined hormonal contraceptives and progestogen-only oral contraceptives are considered to be less reliable during treatment with rifabutin. Contraceptive steroid exposure and the ovulation suppressant effects of oral combined hormonal contraceptives are reduced by rifabutin. Emergency hormonal contraceptives are considered to be less effective in those taking rifabutin and progestogen-only implants are also expected to be less effective.

For general advice on the use of enzyme inducers, such as rifabutin, and hormonal contraceptives, see contraceptives, page 288.

Contraceptives + **Rifampicin (Rifampin)**

Rifampicin reduces contraceptive steroid exposure and reduces the ovulation suppressant effect of oral combined hormonal contraceptives. Combined hormonal contraceptives are less reliable during treatment with rifampicin: breakthrough bleeding and spotting are common, and pregnancies have occurred. Progestogen-only oral contraceptives, progestogen-only implants and emergency hormonal contraceptives are therefore considered to be less effective in those taking rifampicin.

> The interaction between the combined hormonal contraceptives and rifampicin is well documented, well established and clinically important. For advice on the use of enzyme inducers, such as rifampicin, and contraceptives, see contraceptives, page 288.

Contraceptives + **Rufinamide**

Rufinamide very slightly decreases ethinylestradiol and norethisterone exposure from an oral combined hormonal contraceptive; this may reduce contraceptive efficacy. The contraceptive efficacy of oral progestogen-only contraceptives, the progestogen-only implant and emergency hormonal contraceptives (both progestogen-only and combined hormonal preparations) are also expected to be reduced.

> These small changes may be sufficient to cause the failure of combined hormonal contraceptives in rare cases. In the UK, the Faculty of Sexual and Reproductive Healthcare (FSRH) include rufinamide in their 2011 guidance on the use of enzyme inducers with combined hormonal contraceptives, see contraceptives, page 288, for details of this guidance.

Contraceptives + **Sulfonamides**

In controlled studies, ovulation suppression/contraceptive steroid concentrations were not adversely affected by giving non-enzyme-inducing antibacterials (including a sulfonamide) with combined hormonal contraceptives. However, rarely, contraceptive failure has been attributed to the concurrent use of sulfonamides.

> It is possible that the anecdotal cases of contraceptive failure with antibacterials are indistinguishable from the normal accepted failure rate and no special precautions are required. Historically UK guidelines cautiously advised that additional contraceptive precautions were necessary; however, it is now advised that no additional precautions are needed, which is in line with the advice given by a number of other authorities. For further information on the use of antibacterials with contraceptives, see contraceptives, page 288.

Contraceptives + **Tacrolimus**

The UK manufacturer of tacrolimus states that, during clinical use, ethinylestradiol has been shown to increase the concentration of tacrolimus to a minor extent, and *in vitro* data suggests that gestodene and norethisterone might do the same. Tacrolimus has the potential to interfere with the metabolism of hormonal contraceptives.

> A clinically relevant pharmacokinetic interaction seems unlikely. Nevertheless, the UK manufacturer states that care should be taken when deciding upon contraceptive measures in patients also taking tacrolimus.

Contraceptives + **Tetracyclines**

Contraceptive failure has been attributed to a tetracycline in several reported cases, some of which specified long-term antibacterial use. The interaction (if such it is) appears to be very rare. Controlled studies have not found that tetracyclines affect contraceptive steroid concentrations (from tablets, the patch or the vaginal ring).

> It is possible that the anecdotal cases of contraceptive failure with antibacterials are indistinguishable from the normal accepted failure rate and no special precautions are required. Historically UK guidelines cautiously advised that additional contraceptive precautions were necessary; however, it is now advised that no additional precautions are needed, which is in line with the advice given by a number of other authorities. For further information on the use of antibacterials with contraceptives, see contraceptives, page 288.

Contraceptives + **Tizanidine**

Combined hormonal contraceptives moderately increase tizanidine exposure, and might increase its hypotensive and adverse effects.

> A clinical response or adverse effect with tizanidine might occur at lower doses of tizanidine in patients taking oral combined hormonal contraceptives, therefore during dose titration, individual doses should be reduced. Monitor for tizanidine adverse effects such as bradycardia, hypotension, and drowsiness.

Contraceptives + **Topiramate**

Ethinylestradiol levels may be reduced by high-dose topiramate (400 to 800 mg daily), increasing the risk of breakthrough bleeding in women taking oral combined hormonal contraceptives; contraceptive efficacy may be reduced. Lower therapeutic doses of topiramate (50 to 100 mg daily) appear to only slightly affected the pharmacokinetics of oral combined hormonal contraceptives. The contraceptive efficacy of oral progestogen-only contraceptives, the progestogen-only implant and emergency hormonal contraceptives (both progestogen-only and combined hormonal preparations) are also expected to be reduced.

> Topiramate is a weak enzyme inducer and the very small changes seen with lower therapeutic doses of topiramate would generally not be considered clinically relevant. However, with higher doses, the possibility of contraceptive failure in some women cannot be excluded. Therefore, in the UK, the Faculty of Sexual and Reproductive Healthcare (FSRH) 2011 guidance on the concurrent use of liver enzyme inducers with combined hormonal contraceptives includes topiramate in their list of enzyme-inducing drugs, but only at doses of 200 mg daily or more. For general advice on the concurrent use of topiramate (at doses greater than 200 mg daily) and hormonal contraceptives, see contraceptives, page 288. As topiramate is teratogenic, the manufacturers state that the concurrent use of adequate contraception (not specified) is required in women of child-bearing age.

Contraceptives + **Trimethoprim**

In controlled studies, ovulation suppression/contraceptive steroid concentrations were not adversely affected when non-enzyme inducing antibacterials were given with combined hormonal contraceptives. However, rarely, contraceptive failure has been attributed to the concurrent use of trimethoprim.

It is possible that the anecdotal cases of contraceptive failure with antibacterials are indistinguishable from the normal accepted failure rate and no special precautions are required. Historically UK guidelines cautiously advised that additional contraceptive precautions were necessary; however, it is now advised that no additional precautions are needed, which is in line with the advice given by a number of other authorities. For further information on the use of antibacterials with contraceptives, see contraceptives, page 288.

Contraceptives + Ulipristal

The UK manufacturers note that ulipristal acetate binds to the progesterone receptor with high affinity, and therefore could theoretically interfere with the action of progestogen-containing products. They state that it might reduce the efficacy of combined hormonal contraceptives and progestogen-only contraceptives.

The UK and US manufacturers of ulipristal recommend that, after using ulipristal as emergency contraception, a reliable barrier method of contraception should be used until the next menstrual period starts. In addition, the UK manufacturer specifically states that the concurrent use of ulipristal acetate and emergency hormonal contraception containing levonorgestrel is not recommended. When ulipristal is given for the symptomatic management of fibroids, the UK manufacturer advises that concurrent use of ulipristal with any progestogen-containing products is not recommended, and such products should not be taken within 12 days of stopping ulipristal.

Contraceptives + Ursodeoxycholic acid (Ursodiol)

Ursodeoxycholic acid does not affect the bioavailability of ethinylestradiol. However, oestrogens might decrease the effectiveness of ursodeoxycholic acid by increasing the elimination of cholesterol in bile.

The manufacturers suggest that concurrent use should be avoided.

Contraceptives + Warfarin and related oral anticoagulants

Acenocoumarol dose requirements appear to be about 20% lower during the use of a combined hormonal contraceptive. An isolated report describes a marked increase in the INR of a woman taking warfarin when she was given emergency contraception with levonorgestrel. In contrast, the anticoagulant effects of phenprocoumon were slightly decreased by oral contraceptives.

Direct information is limited. Combined hormonal contraceptives are usually contraindicated in patients with thromboembolic disorders. However, if they are used be aware that the anticoagulant response may be affected.

Corticosteroids

Corticosteroids + Digoxin

Corticosteroids can cause potassium loss, which increases the risk of digoxin toxicity.

Monitor concurrent use for digoxin adverse effects (e.g. bradycardia). Consider monitoring potassium levels. No problems of this kind would usually be expected with corticosteroids used topically or by inhalation, because the amounts absorbed are likely to be relatively small.

Corticosteroids + Diuretics

Both loop or thiazide diuretics and corticosteroids can reduce potassium levels, which can lead to life-threatening cardiac arrhythmias. The extent of this interaction will depend on the drugs used and the patient. One study reported hypokalaemia in 31% of patients given a potassium-depleting diuretic and a corticosteroid. Naturally occurring corticosteroids such as cortisone and hydrocortisone cause the greatest potassium loss. Fludrocortisone can also cause hypokalaemia. The synthetic corticosteroids (glucocorticoids) have a less marked potassium-depleting effect and are therefore less likely to cause problems. These include betamethasone, dexamethasone, prednisolone, prednisone and triamcinolone.

Consider monitoring potassium levels, based on the severity of the patient's condition, the number of potassium-depleting drugs used, and any predisposing disease states.

Corticosteroids + Elvitegravir

The US manufacturer of elvitegravir boosted with cobicistat (in a fixed-dose combination also including emtricitabine and tenofovir) predicts that dexamethasone might decrease cobicistat plasma concentrations by inducing CYP3A4; however, dexamethasone rarely appears to cause clinically significant interactions by this mechanism.

If both drugs are given, monitor outcome for reduced efficacy.

Corticosteroids + Everolimus

Some manufacturers predict that dexamethasone, prednisone, and prednisolone might reduce everolimus bioavailability

The UK and US manufacturers advise avoiding concurrent use. If it is essential, increase the everolimus dose according to the indication for use, and monitor everolimus concentrations closely.

Corticosteroids + Grapefruit juice

Grapefruit juice moderately increases budesonide concentrations.

One UK manufacturer of budesonide states that regular ingestion of grapefruit or grapefruit juice should be avoided in connection with budesonide administration, but if this is not possible, the time interval between ingestion of grapefruit (or its juice) and taking oral budesonide should be as long as possible, and a reduction of the budesonide dose should be considered. Another UK manufacturer of oral and rectal budesonide also recommends avoiding concurrent use.

Corticosteroids + Herbal medicines or Dietary supplements

Constituents of liquorice can delay the clearance of prednisolone and hydrocortisone. Liquorice, if given in large quantities with corticosteroids, may cause additive hypokalaemia.

The clinical significance of this interaction is unclear however it may be prudent to monitor the concurrent use of liquorice and corticosteroids, especially if liquorice ingestion is prolonged or if large amounts are taken as additive effects on water and sodium retention, and potassium depletion may occur.

Corticosteroids + HIV-protease inhibitors ⚠

Numerous cases of Cushing's syndrome have been seen in patients given inhaled or intranasal fluticasone with ritonavir, and several cases have been reported with inhaled, intranasal, and oral budesonide. Ritonavir increases the plasma concentration of intranasal fluticasone, and might reduce the clearance of prednisone, prednisolone, and some other corticosteroids. Ritonavir and nelfinavir might increase the exposure to the active metabolite of ciclesonide and possibly beclometasone. Other HIV-protease inhibitors are expected to interact similarly. Several cases of cushingoid adverse effects and adrenal suppression have been reported in patients taking HIV-protease inhibitors boosted with ritonavir, such as atazanavir, indinavir, and lopinavir, when they were also given epidural, intra-articular, or intramuscular injections of triamcinolone. Dexamethasone is predicted to reduce the plasma concentrations of indinavir, saquinavir, and possibly darunavir.

If concurrent use is necessary, monitor for signs of corticosteroid overdose such as fluid retention, hypertension and hyperglycaemia: the need for a dose reduction of the corticosteroid should be borne in mind. The problem may take months to manifest itself with inhaled corticosteroids. Consider changing to inhaled beclometasone, which is likely to be less affected; however, note that some UK manufacturers predict that inhaled beclomethasone might also interact and they caution concurrent use. The clinical outcome of the reductions in HIV-protease inhibitor concentrations with dexamethasone is unclear, particularly as dexamethasone rarely appears to cause clinically significant interactions by this mechanism. However, it would seem prudent to monitor antiviral efficacy if these combinations are used until further information is available.

Corticosteroids + Macrolides ⚠

Clarithromycin and erythromycin can reduce the clearance of methylprednisolone, thereby increasing both its therapeutic and adverse effects. Other macrolides might also interact, although it seems unlikely that they all will, see macrolides, page 474. An isolated case of Cushing's syndrome has been reported in a patient taking long-term clarithromycin after using inhaled budesonide.

> Appropriate methylprednisolone dose reductions (based on symptoms) might be needed to avoid the development of corticosteroid adverse effects. In general concurrent use need not be avoided, but it would be prudent to monitor for corticosteroid adverse effects (such as moon face, weight gain, hyperglycaemia). In most cases the interaction should be manageable by reducing the corticosteroid dose until the macrolide is withdrawn. Bear the case report in mind should a patient taking inhaled corticosteroids develop otherwise unexpected cushingoid adverse effects. Prednisolone seems to be a non-interacting alternative, except possibly in those also taking enzyme inducers (e.g. phenobarbital, page 307).

Corticosteroids + Methotrexate

Dexamethasone may increase the acute hepatotoxicity of high-dose methotrexate.

> Monitor the outcome of concurrent use: full blood count and liver function tests are likely to already be monitored.

Corticosteroids + Mifepristone

The UK manufacturer of mifepristone states that the efficacy of corticosteroids (including inhaled corticosteroids) is expected to be reduced in the 3 to 4 days following the use of mifepristone.

> Patients taking corticosteroids should be monitored in the 3 to 4 days following the use of mifepristone, and consideration given to increasing the corticosteroid dose. The US manufacturer contraindicates the use of mifepristone in those receiving long-term corticosteroids.

Corticosteroids + Nasal decongestants

Ephedrine increased the clearance of dexamethasone by 40% in one study, but the clinical effect of this is unknown. The manufacturers of betamethasone predict that it will be similarly affected.

> Monitor the outcome of concurrent use to ensure dexamethasone efficacy. Adjust the dose as necessary.

Corticosteroids + NSAIDs

Corticosteroids may increase the incidence and/or severity of ulceration associated with NSAIDs, and increase the possibility of gastrointestinal bleeding.

> Concurrent use need not be avoided, but be aware that the risks are increased. Consider the use of mucosal protectants such as H_2-receptor antagonists or proton pump inhibitors, particularly in at-risk patients (e.g. the elderly).

Corticosteroids + **Phenobarbital**

The therapeutic effects of systemic dexamethasone, hydrocortisone, methylprednisolone, prednisolone and prednisone are decreased by phenobarbital. Primidone and
some other corticosteroids probably interact similarly, although direct evidence is
lacking. The dexamethasone adrenal suppression test may be expected to be unreliable
in those taking phenobarbital.

Prednisone and prednisolone appear to be less affected and therefore may be
preferred. Monitor concurrent use to ensure corticosteroid efficacy and increase
the corticosteroid dose as necessary.

C

Corticosteroids + **Phenytoin**

The therapeutic effects of dexamethasone, fludrocortisone, methylprednisolone,
prednisolone, prednisone (and probably other glucocorticoids) can be greatly reduced
by phenytoin. One study suggested that dexamethasone might modestly increase the
serum concentration of phenytoin, but another study and two case reports suggest
that an important *decrease* can occur. The results of the dexamethasone adrenal
suppression test may prove to be unreliable in those taking phenytoin. Fosphenytoin,
a prodrug of phenytoin, might interact similarly with these corticosteroids.

The significance of the reduction in corticosteroid concentrations will depend on
the disease the corticosteroid is prescribed for. Monitor the outcome of concurrent
use closely, especially in transplant patients. The interaction can be managed by
increasing the steroid dose, changing the steroid to one that is less affected by
phenytoin (possibly prednisone or prednisolone), or changing to a non-interacting antiepileptic (e.g. valproate), as appropriate. Consider monitoring phenytoin
concentrations if dexamethasone is given. An interaction seems unlikely with
corticosteroids given topically, by inhalation, intra-articular injection, or enema.

Corticosteroids + **Rifabutin**

The UK manufacturers and the CSM in the UK predict that rifabutin might decrease
the exposure to, and effects of, the corticosteroids.

. Monitor the outcome of concurrent use to ensure corticosteroid efficacy, and
increase the dose accordingly. Note that systemic corticosteroids are usually
considered as contraindicated, or only to be used with great care, in patients with
active or quiescent tuberculosis. Topical preparations are not likely to be affected.

Corticosteroids + **Rifampicin (Rifampin)**

The effects of cortisone, dexamethasone, fludrocortisone, hydrocortisone, methylprednisolone, prednisolone, and prednisone can be markedly reduced by rifampicin.

The need to increase the doses of these corticosteroids should be expected if
rifampicin is also given. Other corticosteroids are predicted to be similarly
affected. Note that systemic corticosteroids are usually considered as contraindicated, or only to be used with great care, in patients with active or quiescent
tuberculosis. Topical preparations are not likely to be affected.

Corticosteroids + **Salbutamol (Albuterol) and related bronchodilators** ❓

Beta₂ agonists, such as salbutamol and terbutaline, can cause hypokalaemia. This can be increased by other potassium-depleting drugs such as the corticosteroids. In severe cases the risk of serious cardiac arrhythmias could be increased.

> The CSM in the UK advises monitoring potassium in severe asthma, because of the probability of multiple potassium-depleting drugs being used, and because some conditions predispose these patients to hypokalaemia (e.g. hypoxia). Consider monitoring based on the severity of the patient's condition, and the number of potassium-depleting drugs used. Note that the combined use of beta₂-agonists and corticosteroids in asthma is usually beneficial.

Corticosteroids + **Tacrolimus** ❓

The concurrent use of tacrolimus and corticosteroids is very common but some evidence suggests that methylprednisolone and prednisolone or prednisone might alter tacrolimus pharmacokinetics.

> The concurrent use of tacrolimus and corticosteroids is advantageous, but be alert for any evidence of altered tacrolimus concentrations and/or effects. Increased monitoring of tacrolimus concentrations when corticosteroid doses are altered would seem to be a prudent measure.

Corticosteroids + **Theophylline** ❓

Theophylline and corticosteroids have established roles in the management of asthma and their concurrent use is common and beneficial. There are isolated reports of increases in theophylline concentration (sometimes associated with toxicity) when oral or parenteral corticosteroids are given, but other studies have found no changes. The general clinical importance of these findings is uncertain. Both theophylline and corticosteroids can cause hypokalaemia, which may be additive. There do not appear to be any data on the effect of inhaled corticosteroids on the clearance of theophylline.

> From the study data available, it would seem that, in general, a clinically relevant pharmacokinetic interaction is unlikely to occur. The CSM in the UK advises monitoring potassium concentrations in severe asthma, because of the probability of multiple potassium-depleting drugs being used, and because some conditions predispose these patients to hypokalaemia (e.g. hypoxia).

Corticosteroids + **Ticagrelor** ❓

The UK and US manufacturers of ticagrelor predict that dexamethasone might decrease its exposure.

> A clinically relevant interaction seems unlikely. However, consider an interaction if reduced ticagrelor efficacy occurs on concurrent use.

Corticosteroids + Vaccines

Patients who are immunised with live vaccines while receiving immunosuppressive doses of corticosteroids may develop generalised, possibly life-threatening, infections.

It has been recommended that live vaccination should be postponed for at least 3 months after high-dose corticosteroids are stopped. Adult patients taking the equivalent of 40 mg of prednisolone daily for more than one week would generally be considered to be immunosuppressed.

Corticosteroids + Warfarin and related oral anticoagulants

High-dose corticosteroids increase the anticoagulant effects of the coumarins and indanediones: raised INRs and bleeding have been reported. Only small increases or decreases in anticoagulation appear to occur when low to moderate doses of corticosteroids are given with oral anticoagulants.

Monitor the anticoagulant effect if high-dose corticosteroids are started or stopped in patients taking oral anticoagulants. Consider an interaction with lower doses if any unexplained changes in anticoagulant control occur. Note that corticosteroids are associated with a weak increase in peptic ulceration and gastrointestinal bleeding, and the risk of this could theoretically be increased if over-anticoagulation occurs.

Co-trimoxazole

Co-trimoxazole is a combination product containing sulfamethoxazole and trimethoprim.

Co-trimoxazole + Dapsone

The levels of both dapsone and trimethoprim are possibly raised by concurrent use. Both increased efficacy and, rarely, dapsone toxicity have been seen. Note that co-trimoxazole contains trimethoprim.

Be alert for evidence of dapsone toxicity (methaemoglobinaemia). No adverse effects would be expected if topical dapsone is used in a patient taking oral trimethoprim.

Co-trimoxazole + Digoxin ⚠

Digoxin levels can be increased by about 22% by trimethoprim, but some individuals may show a much greater rise.

Monitor for digoxin adverse effects (such as bradycardia, nausea, vomiting) if trimethoprim is given, and consider measuring digoxin levels, particularly in the elderly. Adjust the dose as necessary. Trimethoprim is a constituent of co-trimoxazole but it is not known whether prophylactic doses of co-trimoxazole

(160 mg of trimethoprim a day from a 960-mg dose of co-trimoxazole) will interact to a clinically significant degree. An interaction would seem likely with high-dose co-trimoxazole, and care is needed in the elderly with any co-trimoxazole dose.

Co-trimoxazole + Methotrexate

Several cases of severe bone marrow depression (some of which were fatal) have been reported in patients given low-dose methotrexate and co-trimoxazole. Pancytopenia has also been reported in a few patients given co-trimoxazole shortly after stopping methotrexate.

Low-dose co-trimoxazole is commonly given without problem to patients taking methotrexate as prophylaxis of pneumocystis pneumonia. This type of patient should be having regular blood monitoring as a matter of course. However, the situation with higher doses of either drug is potentially more hazardous. Some have recommended avoiding the combination. If both drugs must be used, the haematological picture should be very closely monitored because the outcome can be life-threatening.

Co-trimoxazole + Phenytoin

Phenytoin concentrations can be increased by co-trimoxazole. Phenytoin toxicity might develop in some cases. Fosphenytoin is a prodrug of phenytoin and therefore has the potential to be similarly affected.

The risk of toxicity appears small and is most likely in those with phenytoin concentrations at the top end of the range. Monitor phenytoin concentrations and adjust the dose accordingly. Indicators of phenytoin toxicity include blurred vision, nystagmus, ataxia, or drowsiness.

Co-trimoxazole + Procainamide

Trimethoprim causes a marked increase in the plasma levels of procainamide and its active metabolite, N-acetylprocainamide. Note that co-trimoxazole contains trimethoprim.

Anticipate the need to reduce the procainamide dose if trimethoprim is given to patients taking procainamide.

Co-trimoxazole + Pyrimethamine

Serious pancytopenia and megaloblastic anaemia have occasionally occurred in patients given pyrimethamine and co-trimoxazole.

Caution should be used in prescribing the combination, especially in the presence of other drugs (e.g. methotrexate, phenytoin) or disease states that predispose to folate deficiency. Note that the US manufacturer of sulfadoxine with pyrimethamine recommended that the concurrent use of co-trimoxazole should be avoided. When high-dose pyrimethamine is used for the treatment of toxoplasmosis, the manufacturer recommends that all patients should receive a folate supplement.

Co-trimoxazole + **Rifampicin (Rifampin)**

Rifampicin reduces the AUCs of trimethoprim and sulfamethoxazole by 56% and 28%, respectively, in HIV-positive subjects, but apparently has no effect on trimethoprim in healthy subjects. Co-trimoxazole can increase rifampicin levels in patients with tuberculosis.

The efficacy of co-trimoxazole prophylaxis may be reduced in HIV-positive patients taking rifampicin. Bear this in mind when using the combination. The risk of hepatotoxicity may be increased due to raised rifampicin levels; however, liver function tests should already be closely monitored so no additional precautions seem necessary.

Co-trimoxazole + **Warfarin and related oral anticoagulants**

The anticoagulant effects of warfarin, acenocoumarol, and phenprocoumon are increased by co-trimoxazole. Bleeding may occur if the anticoagulant dose is not reduced appropriately.

The incidence of the interaction with co-trimoxazole appears to be high. If bleeding is to be avoided the INR should be well monitored and the warfarin, acenocoumarol, or phenprocoumon dose should be reduced accordingly. A pre-emptive warfarin dose reduction of about 10 to 20% has been suggested. However, others suggest that co-trimoxazole should be avoided. Consider using an alternative non-interacting antibacterial if appropriate.

Cyclophosphamide

Cyclophosphamide + **Digoxin**

Treatment with cyclophosphamide (as part of antineoplastic regimens) appears to damage the lining of the intestine so that digoxin is much less readily absorbed when given in tablet form.

In one of the studies this interaction was overcome by giving the digoxin in liquid or liquid-in-capsule form. Monitor carefully, adjusting dose, drug or preparation as appropriate.

Cyclophosphamide + **Prasugrel**

Prasugrel may slightly inhibit the metabolism of *bupropion* by CYP2B6 and decrease the levels of its metabolite by 23%. The manufacturers therefore suggest that the metabolism of other substrates of CYP2B6, such as cyclophosphamide, may also be affected.

A clinically significant interaction would seem unlikely. Consider an interaction if any increase in cyclophosphamide adverse effects, such as leucopenia and neutropenia, develop.

Cyclophosphamide + Vaccines ✗

The immune response of the body is suppressed by cytotoxic antineoplastics. The effectiveness of vaccines may be poor and generalised infection may occur in patients immunised with live vaccines. In one study the antibody response to pneumococcal vaccination was reduced by 60% in patients receiving antineoplastics including cyclophosphamide, and suboptimal responses to influenza and measles vaccines have been reported.

> Live vaccines should not be given to patients who are receiving cytotoxics or other immunosuppressant antineoplastics. In the UK, it is recommended that live vaccines should not be given during or within at least 6 months of such treatment. Monitor the immune response to other types of vaccine. Consider whether vaccination can be carried out before or after cyclophosphamide use.

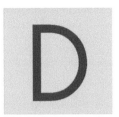

Dabigatran

Dabigatran + Dipyridamole

The concurrent use of antiplatelet drugs with dabigatran can theoretically increase the risk of bleeding.

The manufacturers do not recommend concurrent use. If both drugs are essential, patients should be closely monitored for signs and symptoms of bleeding.

Dabigatran + Dronedarone

Dronedarone, a P-glycoprotein inhibitor, increases the exposure to dabigatran.

The UK manufacturer of dabigatran contraindicates concurrent use with dronedarone. In moderate renal impairment, the US manufacturer states that the dabigatran dose should be reduced to 75 mg twice daily. Monitor for signs of bleeding or anaemia, and discontinue dabigatran if severe bleeding occurs.

Dabigatran + Heparin

The concurrent use of dabigatran with parenteral anticoagulants potentially increases the risk of haemorrhage.

Do not start parenteral anticoagulants until 12 hours (atrial fibrillation) or 24 hours (venous thromboembolism) after the last dabigatran dose. Do not start dabigatran until 0 to 2 hours before the next scheduled dose of the parenteral anticoagulant would have been due, or at the time of discontinuation of the parenteral anticoagulant in case of continuous treatment. However, heparin can be given concurrently with dabigatran at doses necessary to maintain a patent central venous or arterial catheter.

Dabigatran + Herbal medicines or Dietary supplements

St John's wort, a P-glycoprotein inducer, is predicted to decrease the exposure to dabigatran, which would be expected to affect its anticoagulant effects.

The UK and US manufacturers advise avoiding concurrent use. If this is unavoidable, monitor for efficacy.

D

Dabigatran + **Low-molecular-weight heparins**

The concurrent use of dabigatran with parenteral anticoagulants potentially increases the risk of haemorrhage.

Do not start parenteral anticoagulants until 12 hours (atrial fibrillation) or 24 hours (venous thromboembolism) after the last dabigatran dose. Do not start dabigatran until 0 to 2 hours before the next scheduled dose of the parenteral anticoagulant would have been due, or at the time of discontinuation of the parenteral anticoagulant in case of continuous treatment. However, heparin can be given concurrently with dabigatran at doses necessary to maintain a patent central venous or arterial catheter.

Dabigatran + **NNRTIs**

The UK manufacturer of rilpivirine predicts that it will increase dabigatran concentrations (by inhibiting P-glycoprotein).

Monitor for dabigatran adverse effects (such as bleeding or anaemia) and adjust the dabigatran dose if necessary.

Dabigatran + **NSAIDs**

The concurrent use of NSAIDs might theoretically increase the risk of bleeding with dabigatran.

Patients taking NSAIDs with dabigatran should be closely monitored for signs of bleeding, particularly with NSAIDs that have a half-life of greater than 12 hours.

Dabigatran + **Phenytoin**

Phenytoin is predicted to decrease the exposure to dabigatran, which would be expected to affect its anticoagulant effects. Fosphenytoin, a prodrug of phenytoin, might act similarly.

The UK and US manufacturers advise avoiding concurrent use. If this is unavoidable, monitor for efficacy.

Dabigatran + **Prasugrel**

The concurrent use of antiplatelet drugs with dabigatran might theoretically increase the risk of bleeding.

The UK manufacturer of dabigatran does not recommend concurrent use. If both drugs are essential, patients should be closely monitored for signs and symptoms of bleeding.

Dabigatran + **Quinidine**

Quinidine, a P-glycoprotein inhibitor, increases the exposure to dabigatran.

For thromboembolism prophylaxis, reduce the dabigatran dose to 150 mg daily and take both drugs at the same time. No dabigatran dose adjustment is necessary for stroke prophylaxis. Monitor for bleeding and anaemia and discontinue dabigatran if severe bleeding occurs.

Dabigatran + Rifampicin (Rifampin)

Rifampicin (rifampin), a P-glycoprotein inducer, decreases the exposure to single-dose dabigatran, which would be expected to affect its anticoagulant effects.

The UK and US manufacturers advise against concurrent use of dabigatran and rifampicin. If both drugs are given, monitor for dabigatran efficacy.

Dabigatran + Rivaroxaban

The concurrent use of rivaroxaban with dabigatran might theoretically increase the risk of bleeding.

The UK manufacturer of dabigatran contraindicates concurrent use unless switching between anticoagulants; monitor for signs of excessive bleeding.

Dabigatran + Sulfinpyrazone

The concurrent use of antiplatelet drugs with dabigatran might theoretically increase the risk of bleeding.

The UK manufacturer of dabigatran does not recommend concurrent use. If both drugs are essential, patients should be closely monitored for signs and symptoms of bleeding.

Dabigatran + Tacrolimus

Tacrolimus is predicted to increase the exposure to dabigatran.

The UK manufacturer contraindicates concurrent use. If it is unavoidable, monitor for signs of bleeding or anaemia, and discontinue dabigatran if severe bleeding occurs.

Dabigatran + Ticagrelor

Ticagrelor slightly increases dabigatran exposure, which might increase the risk of bleeding.

Monitor for signs and symptoms of bleeding.

Dabigatran + Ticlopidine

The concurrent use of antiplatelet drugs with dabigatran might theoretically increase the risk of bleeding.

The UK manufacturer of dabigatran does not recommend concurrent use. If both drugs are essential, patients should be closely monitored for signs and symptoms of bleeding.

Dabigatran + Ulipristal ⚠

The manufacturers of ulipristal predict that it will increase dabigatran concentrations by inhibiting P-glycoprotein.

Until more is known, monitor for dabigatran adverse effects (such as bleeding or anaemia), and adjust the dabigatran dose if necessary. The UK manufacturer of *low-dose* ulipristal recommends separating administration by at least 1.5 hours.

Dabigatran + Verapamil ⚠

Verapamil, a P-glycoprotein inhibitor, increases the exposure to dabigatran.

For venous thromboembolism prophylaxis, the UK manufacturer recommends that the dose of dabigatran should be reduced to 150 mg daily and both drugs should be taken at the same time, with a further dose reduction to 75 mg daily considered in those patients with moderate renal impairment. For stroke prophylaxis, the UK manufacturer states that the dose of dabigatran should be reduced to 110 mg twice daily, and both drugs should be taken at the same time, whereas the US manufacturer states that no dose adjustment is necessary. Monitor for bleeding and anaemia, and discontinue dabigatran if severe bleeding occurs.

Dabigatran + Warfarin and related oral anticoagulants ⚠

The concurrent use of coumarins and indanediones with dabigatran might theoretically increase the risk of bleeding.

Concurrent use is contraindicated unless switching between anticoagulants. When switching from dabigatran to a coumarin or indanedione for atrial fibrillation, the UK manufacturer states that the coumarin or indanedione should be started 3 days before stopping dabigatran in patients with a creatinine clearance greater than 50 mL/minute, or 2 days before stopping dabigatran in patients with a creatinine clearance of 30 to 50 mL/minute. When switching from a coumarin or indanedione to dabigatran for atrial fibrillation, the UK manufacturer states that dabigatran can be started when the patient's INR is less than 2.0.

Danazol

Danazol + Everolimus ⚠

Danazol is predicted to increase everolimus concentrations.

Monitor the concentrations and effects (e.g. on renal function) of everolimus more frequently if danazol is started or stopped, and adjust the everolimus dose as necessary.

Danazol + Sirolimus

The UK and US manufacturers predict that sirolimus concentrations will be increased by danazol.

Sirolimus concentrations and/or effects (e.g. on renal function) should be monitored as a matter of routine, but it might be prudent to increase monitoring if danazol is started or stopped, and adjust the sirolimus dose if necessary.

Danazol + Statins

Atorvastatin or Lovastatin

Cases of severe rhabdomyolysis and myoglobinuria have been reported in patients taking danazol with lovastatin. Atorvastatin might interact similarly as it is metabolised, at least in part, in the same way as lovastatin.

The US manufacturer of lovastatin suggests that the dose should be started at 10 mg daily, and should not exceed 20 mg daily in the presence of danazol. It would seem prudent to remind patients of the symptoms of myopathy if danazol is given to a patient taking atorvastatin or lovastatin, and advise them to report any unexplained muscle pain, tenderness, or weakness.

Simvastatin

Rhabdomyolysis has occurred in patients taking simvastatin and danazol.

The concurrent use of danazol with simvastatin is contraindicated. If both drugs are essential, monitor closely. Patients should be advised to report any unexplained muscle pain, tenderness, or weakness.

Danazol + Tacrolimus

There is one isolated report of an increase in tacrolimus concentrations in a patient also given danazol, however as danazol has also been seen to affect ciclosporin concentrations similarly (see Ciclosporin (Cyclosporine) + Danazol, page 252), it seems possible that an interaction with tacrolimus could be of more general importance.

Tacrolimus concentrations and/or effects (e.g. on renal function) should be monitored as a matter of routine. There is insufficient direct evidence to recommend increased monitoring in all patients given danazol and tacrolimus, but it would seem prudent to bear the possibility of an interaction in mind in cases of otherwise unexplained increases in tacrolimus concentrations or adverse effects

Danazol + Warfarin and related oral anticoagulants ⚠

Increased anticoagulant effects and bleeding have been seen when danazol was given to patients taking warfarin. Other coumarins may interact similarly.

It would seem prudent to increase the frequency of INR monitoring if danazol is started in a patient taking any coumarin. Some recommend reducing the dose of the anticoagulant (halved has been suggested) when danazol is started, but this has been disputed.

Dapoxetine

Dapoxetine + Duloxetine ⚠

The concurrent use of dapoxetine (an SSRI) with other drugs that have serotonergic effects (such as the SNRIs) may increase the risk of serious and possibly fatal adverse effects such as serotonin syndrome, page 580.

The manufacturer of dapoxetine advises avoiding concurrent use during and for 14 days after stopping duloxetine. Duloxetine should not be started for at least 7 days after stopping dapoxetine.

Dapoxetine + Herbal medicines or Dietary supplements ⚠

The concurrent use of dapoxetine (an SSRI) with other drugs that have serotonergic effects, such as St John's wort (*Hypericum perforatum*) may increase the risk of serious and possibly fatal adverse effects such as serotonin syndrome, page 580.

The manufacturer of dapoxetine advises avoiding concurrent use during and for 14 days after stopping St John's wort. St John's wort should not be started for at least 7 days after stopping dapoxetine.

Dapoxetine + HIV-protease inhibitors

Amprenavir or Fosamprenavir ⚠

The Swedish manufacturer of dapoxetine predicts that it will increase the exposure to amprenavir and fosamprenavir. As dapoxetine is also metabolised by CYP2D6, CYP2D6 metaboliser status is predicted to also affect this interaction.

The Swedish manufacturer recommends a maximum dose of dapoxetine 30 mg on the concurrent use of amprenavir or fosamprenavir. In CYP2D6 extensive metabolisers (which is generally unlikely to be known), the manufacturer advises a maximum dapoxetine dose of 60 mg.

Atazanavir, Nelfinavir, Ritonavir or Saquinavir

The Swedish manufacturer of dapoxetine predicts that atazanavir, nelfinavir, ritonavir and saquinavir might increase the exposure to dapoxetine.

An important adverse reaction of dapoxetine is syncope or orthostatic hypotension, and this is dose related. Therefore, the manufacturer contraindicates the use of dapoxetine with atazanavir, nelfinavir, ritonavir or saquinavir. Note that if the patient is known to be a CYP2D6 extensive metaboliser (which is generally unlikely), a 30-mg dose can be used.

Dapoxetine + Linezolid

The concurrent use of dapoxetine (an SSRI) with other drugs that have serotonergic effects (such as linezolid) may increase the risk of serious and possibly fatal adverse effects such as serotonin syndrome, page 580.

The manufacturer of dapoxetine advises avoiding concurrent use during and for 14 days after stopping linezolid. Linezolid should not be started for at least 7 days after stopping dapoxetine.

Dapoxetine + Lithium

The concurrent use of dapoxetine (an SSRI) with other drugs that have serotonergic effects (such as lithium) may increase the risk of serious and possibly fatal adverse effects such as serotonin syndrome, page 580.

The manufacturer of dapoxetine advises avoiding concurrent use during and for 14 days after stopping lithium. Lithium should not be started for at least 7 days after stopping dapoxetine.

Dapoxetine + Macrolides

Clarithromycin or Erythromycin

The Swedish manufacturer of dapoxetine predicts that clarithromycin and erythromycin might increase the exposure to dapoxetine. As dapoxetine is also metabolised by CYP2D6, CYP2D6 metaboliser status is predicted to also affect this interaction.

The Swedish manufacturer of dapoxetine recommends a maximum dose of dapoxetine 30 mg on the concurrent use of clarithromycin or erythromycin. In patients known to be CYP2D6 extensive metabolisers (which is generally unlikely), the manufacturer advises a maximum dapoxetine dose of 60 mg.

Telithromycin

Telithromycin is predicted to increase the exposure to dapoxetine.

An important adverse reaction of dapoxetine is syncope or orthostatic hypotension, and this is dose related. Therefore, the Swedish manufacturer of dapoxetine contraindicates the concurrent use of telithromycin. Note that dapoxetine is also metabolised by CYP2D6 and if the patient is known to be a CYP2D6 extensive metaboliser (which is generally unlikely), a 30-mg dose can be used.

Dapoxetine + MAOIs ✕

The concurrent use of dapoxetine (an SSRI) with other drugs that have serotonergic effects (such as the MAOIs) may increase the risk of serious and possibly fatal adverse effects such as serotonin syndrome, page 580.

> Concurrent use is contraindicated, during and for 14 days after stopping an MAOI, and an MAOI should not be started for at least 7 days after stopping dapoxetine.

Dapoxetine + Opioids ⚠

The concurrent use of dapoxetine (an SSRI) with other drugs that have serotonergic effects (such as tramadol) may increase the risk of serious and possibly fatal adverse effects such as serotonin syndrome, page 580.

> The manufacturer of dapoxetine advises avoiding concurrent use during and for 14 days after stopping tramadol. Tramadol should not be started for at least 7 days after stopping dapoxetine.

Dapoxetine + Triptans ⚠

The concurrent use of dapoxetine (an SSRI) with other drugs that have serotonergic effects (such as the triptans) might increase the risk of serious and possibly fatal adverse effects such as serotonin syndrome, page 580.

> The manufacturer of dapoxetine advises avoiding concurrent use during and for 14 days after stopping a triptan. A triptan should not be started for at least 7 days after stopping dapoxetine.

Dapoxetine + Tryptophan ⚠

The concurrent use of dapoxetine (an SSRI) with other drugs that have serotonergic effects (such as tryptophan) may increase the risk of serious and possibly fatal adverse effects such as serotonin syndrome, page 580.

> The manufacturer of dapoxetine advises avoiding concurrent use during and for 14 days after stopping tryptophan. Tryptophan should not be started for at least 7 days after stopping dapoxetine.

Dapoxetine + Venlafaxine ⚠

The concurrent use of dapoxetine (an SSRI) with other drugs that have serotonergic effects (such as the SNRIs) may increase the risk of serious and possibly fatal adverse effects such as serotonin syndrome, page 580.

> The manufacturer of dapoxetine advises avoiding concurrent use during and for 14 days after stopping venlafaxine. Venlafaxine should not be started for at least 7 days after stopping dapoxetine.

Dapoxetine + **Warfarin and related oral anticoagulants**

Dapoxetine had no effect on the pharmacokinetics or anticoagulant effect of a single dose of warfarin in one study. However, as dapoxetine has serotonergic effects, additive antiplatelet effects may theoretically occur: isolated cases of bleeding have been reported on the concurrent use of coumarin anticoagulants and the SSRIs, page 583.

> The manufacturer of dapoxetine advises caution on concurrent use: bear the possibility in mind in case of any unexplained bleeding or change in the INR.

Dapsone

Dapsone + **Probenecid**

Dapsone levels can be raised by about 50% by probenecid.

> The extent of the rise and evidence that the haematological toxicity of dapsone may be dose-related suggests that this interaction may be clinically important. Monitor concurrent use for dapsone adverse effects.

Dapsone + **Rifabutin**

Rifabutin increases the clearance of dapsone, but may also increase its toxicity (methaemoglobinaemia).

> Concurrent use should be well monitored to confirm that treatment is effective. It may be necessary to raise the dose of dapsone but note that this may increase its toxicity; therefore be alert for any evidence of methaemoglobinaemia.

Dapsone + **Rifampicin (Rifampin)**

Rifampicin increases the excretion of dapsone, lowers its serum levels, but increases the risk of toxicity (methaemoglobinaemia) by raising dapsone metabolite levels.

> Concurrent use should be well monitored to confirm that treatment is effective. It may be necessary to raise the dose of dapsone but note that this may increase its toxicity; therefore be alert for any evidence of dapsone toxicity (methaemoglobinaemia).

Dapsone + **Trimethoprim**

The levels of both dapsone and trimethoprim are possibly raised by concurrent use. Both increased efficacy and dapsone toxicity have been seen.

> Concurrent use appears to be an effective form of treatment, but be alert for evidence of apparently rare cases of increased dapsone toxicity (methaemoglobinaemia).

Darifenacin

Darifenacin + Digoxin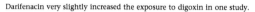

Darifenacin very slightly increased the exposure to digoxin in one study.

This increase would not be expected to be clinically relevant. Nevertheless, the UK manufacturer recommends monitoring digoxin concentrations if darifenacin is started or stopped, or when the dose is changed..

Darifenacin + Flecainide

Darifenacin increases the levels of CYP2D6 substrates such as the tricyclics (imipramine AUC increased by 70%). The manufacturers of darifenacin therefore advise caution with some other CYP2D6 substrates, and specifically name flecainide.

The clinical importance of this potential interaction does not appear to have been assessed, but be alert for the need to reduce the flecainide dose if darifenacin is added.

Darifenacin + Macrolides

Erythromycin causes a moderate increase in darifenacin exposure. Other macrolides, such as clarithromycin and telithromycin, are considered to be more potent CYP3A4 inhibitors and so they are predicted to have a greater effect on darifenacin concentrations.

Bear in mind the possibility of an interaction if antimuscarinic effects (dry mouth, constipation, drowsiness) are increased. The US manufacturer of darifenacin suggests that no dose adjustments are necessary with erythromycin, whereas the UK manufacturer suggests starting darifenacin at a dose of 7.5 mg daily, increasing to 15 mg daily according to tolerability. In addition, the UK manufacturer contraindicates the concurrent use of potent CYP3A4 inhibitors (which may be expected to include clarithromycin and telithromycin) whereas the US manufacturer recommends that the dose of darifenacin is limited to 7.5 mg daily.

Darifenacin + Phenobarbital

The manufacturers predict that CYP3A4 inducers, such as the phenobarbital, may decrease darifenacin levels. Primidone, which is in part metabolised to phenobarbital, would be expected to interact similarly.

Monitor the outcome of concurrent use to ensure that darifenacin is effective and adjust the dose if necessary.

Darifenacin + Phenytoin

The manufacturers predict that CYP3A4 inducers, such as phenytoin, may decrease darifenacin levels. Fosphenytoin, a prodrug of phenytoin, would be expected to interact similarly.

Monitor the outcome of concurrent use to ensure that darifenacin is effective.

Darifenacin + **Quinidine**

Paroxetine increases the AUC of darifenacin by a modest 33%. Quinidine is predicted to interact similarly (both paroxetine and quinidine are CYP2D6 inhibitors). However, changes of this magnitude seem unlikely to be clinically relevant.

No dose adjustments are recommended by the US manufacturer. The UK manufacturer recommends that the dose of darifenacin should be started at 7.5 mg daily and, if well tolerated, titrated to 15 mg daily. This seems a cautious approach. Bear in mind the possibility of an interaction if antimuscarinic effects (dry mouth, constipation, drowsiness) are increased.

Darifenacin + **Rifampicin (Rifampin)**

The manufacturers predict that CYP3A4 inducers, such as rifampicin, may decrease darifenacin levels.

Monitor the outcome of concurrent use to ensure that darifenacin is effective and adjust the dose if necessary.

Darifenacin + **SSRIs**

Paroxetine increases the AUC of darifenacin by a modest 33%, which is unlikely to be clinically relevant.

No dose adjustments are recommended by the US manufacturer. The UK manufacturer recommends that the dose of darifenacin should be started at 7.5 mg daily and, if well tolerated, titrated to 15 mg daily. This seems a cautious approach. Bear in mind the possibility of an interaction if antimuscarinic effects (dry mouth, constipation, drowsiness) are increased.

Darifenacin + **Terbinafine**

Paroxetine increases the AUC of darifenacin by a modest 33%. Terbinafine is predicted to interact similarly (both paroxetine and terbinafine are CYP2D6 inhibitors). However, changes of this magnitude seem unlikely to be clinically relevant.

No dose adjustments are recommended by the US manufacturer. The UK manufacturer recommends that the dose of darifenacin should be started at 7.5 mg daily and, if well tolerated, titrated to 15 mg daily. This seems a cautious approach. Bear in mind the possibility of an interaction if antimuscarinic effects (dry mouth, constipation, drowsiness) are increased.

Darifenacin + **Tricyclics**

Darifenacin increases the AUC of imipramine by about 70% and increases the AUC of its active metabolite 2.6-fold. Other tricyclics are similarly metabolised and therefore their levels may also be raised by darifenacin.

Monitor concurrent use for signs of tricyclic adverse effects (dry mouth, constipation, blurred vision).

D

Desmopressin

Desmopressin + Food

Food reduces the absorption of oral desmopressin; however, this does not appear to have a clinically relevant effect on the pharmacodynamic response to desmopressin (urine production and osmolality). Buccal desmopressin may interact similarly.

Despite the finding of a lack of pharmacodynamic effect, the UK manufacturer of desmopressin suggests considering an interaction if a patient fails to respond to desmopressin or a reduction in its efficacy occurs. Try taking desmopressin consistently with respect to food before increasing the desmopressin dose.

Desmopressin + Lamotrigine

Drugs that can cause water retention or hyponatraemia may have an additive effect with desmopressin: water overload and/or hyponatraemia may occur. Case reports suggest that lamotrigine may interact similarly, reducing desmopressin requirements.

The increased risk may be small, with severe complications being rare; however, it would be prudent to exercise caution on concurrent use, with more frequent monitoring of serum sodium.

Desmopressin + Loperamide

Loperamide may markedly increase the absorption of oral desmopressin. Sublingual desmopressin may also be similarly affected, but no interaction would be expected with intranasal or parenteral preparations.

Monitor the effects of oral or sublingual desmopressin in any patient given loperamide, reducing the desmopressin dose or dose frequency as necessary. Note that in primary nocturnal enuresis, the indication for loperamide (diarrhoea) is a reason to temporarily stop desmopressin.

Desmopressin + NSAIDs

Drugs that can cause water retention or hyponatraemia (e.g. NSAIDs) may have an additive effect with desmopressin: water overload and/or hyponatraemia may occur.

The increased risk may be small, with severe complications being rare; however, it would be prudent to exercise caution on concurrent use, with more frequent monitoring of serum sodium.

Desmopressin + SSRIs

Drugs that can cause water retention or hyponatraemia (e.g. SSRIs) may have an additive effect with desmopressin: water overload and/or hyponatraemia may occur.

The increased risk may be small, with severe complications being rare; however, it would be prudent to exercise caution on concurrent use, with more frequent monitoring of serum sodium.

Desmopressin + Tricyclics

Drugs that can cause water retention or hyponatraemia (e.g. tricyclics) may have an additive effect with desmopressin: water overload and/or hyponatraemia may occur.

The increased risk may be small, with severe complications being rare; however, it would be prudent to exercise caution on concurrent use, with more frequent monitoring of serum sodium.

Dextromethorphan

D

Dextromethorphan + Linezolid

Linezolid does not appear to affect the pharmacokinetics of dextromethorphan, but in one case concurrent use resulted in serotonin syndrome.

It would be prudent to monitor for symptoms of serotonin syndrome, page 580, if concurrent use is necessary.

Dextromethorphan + MAO-B inhibitors

Cases of serotonin syndrome, page 580, have been seen when dextromethorphan has been used with non-selective MAOIs. The likelihood of an interaction with MAO-B inhibitors would appear to be very small, but because of the potential severity of this syndrome, some caution would appear to be prudent.

The manufacturer of rasagiline contraindicates its use with dextromethorphan. Some consider that patients taking selegiline should also try to avoid dextromethorphan.

Dextromethorphan + MAOIs

Two fatal cases of hyperpyrexia and coma (symptoms similar to serotonin syndrome, page 580) have occurred in patients taking phenelzine with dextromethorphan (in overdosage in one case). Three other serious but non-fatal reactions occurred in patients taking dextromethorphan with isocarboxazid or phenelzine.

Concurrent use is generally contraindicated both with and within 14 days of taking an MAOI.

Dextromethorphan + Moclobemide

Moclobemide inhibits the metabolism of dextromethorphan, and isolated cases of severe CNS reactions have occurred in patients given the combination.

Moclobemide is contraindicated with dextromethorphan.

Dextromethorphan + **NSAIDs** ❓

The manufacturers say that valdecoxib (the pro-drug of parecoxib) caused a 3-fold increase in dextromethorphan levels.

> It seems unlikely that normal therapeutic doses of dextromethorphan will cause a problem in most patients taking parecoxib as dextromethorphan has a wide therapeutic range, but be aware that some patients may become more sensitive to its effects.

Dextromethorphan + **Opioids** ❓

Dextromethorphan-induced delirium has been attributed to an interaction with methadone.

> An interaction is not established and further study is needed. Concurrent use has been beneficial.

Dextromethorphan + **Quinidine** ⚠

Quinidine markedly increased dextromethorphan levels in one study. Some of the patients (given dextromethorphan 60 mg) experienced dextromethorphan toxicity (nervousness, tremors, restlessness, dizziness, shortness of breath, confusion etc.).

> It seems unlikely that normal therapeutic doses of dextromethorphan will cause a problem in most patients taking quinidine as dextromethorphan has a wide therapeutic range, but be aware that some patients may become more sensitive to its effects.

Dextromethorphan + **SSRIs** ❓

A serotonin-like syndrome has developed in several patients taking SSRIs with dextromethorphan, although in many of these cases the use of other drugs with serotonergic actions may have contributed. Paroxetine and fluoxetine moderately inhibit the metabolism of dextromethorphan.

> It would seem prudent for patients taking any SSRI to be cautious if using dextromethorphan-containing products because serotonin syndrome, page 580, can be serious. The pharmacokinetic interaction between dextromethorphan paroxetine and fluoxetine may increase the risks of this effect.

Digoxin

There is a relatively narrow gap between therapeutic and toxic digoxin levels. Normal therapeutic levels are about one-third of those that are fatal, and serious toxic arrhythmias begin at about two-thirds of the fatal levels. The normal range for digoxin levels is 0.8 to 2 nanograms/mL (or 1.02 to 2.56 nanomol/L). To convert nanograms/mL to nanomol/L multiply by 1.28, or to convert nanomol/L to nanograms/mL multiply by 0.781. Note that micrograms/L is the same as nanograms/mL. If a patient is over-digitalised, signs and symptoms of toxicity are likely to occur, which may include loss of appetite, nausea and vomiting, and bradycardia. These effects are often used as clinical indicators of toxicity, and a pulse rate of less than 60 bpm is usually considered to be an indication of over-treatment. Other symptoms include visual disturbances, headache, drowsiness and occasionally diarrhoea. Death may result from cardiac arrhythmias. Patients treated for cardiac arrhythmias can therefore demonstrate arrhythmias when they are both under- as well as over-digitalised.

Digoxin + **Diuretics**

Eplerenone

Digoxin exposure is negligibly increased by eplerenone.

> Changes of this magnitude are unlikely to cause problems in most patients and the US manufacturer states that the pharmacokinetic interaction is not clinically relevant. Nevertheless, the UK manufacturer of eplerenone advises caution in patients with digoxin plasma concentrations near the upper end of the therapeutic range.

Loop or Thiazide diuretics

Hypokalaemia, which can be caused by potassium-depleting diuretics, such as the loop or thiazide diuretics, increases the toxicity of digoxin.

> Plasma potassium concentrations should be routinely monitored during diuretic therapy. However, if symptoms of digoxin toxicity occur (see digoxin, page 326) it would be prudent to re-check potassium concentrations.

Spironolactone

Limited evidence suggests that digoxin levels might be increased up to 25% by spironolactone (greater increases can occur in some individuals), but because spironolactone or its metabolite, canrenone, can interfere with some digoxin assay methods, the evaluation of this interaction is difficult.

> Monitor concurrent use for digoxin adverse effects (see digoxin, page 326) and consider checking digoxin plasma concentrations. Adjust the dose as necessary. Measurement of free digoxin concentrations, or use of a chemiluminescent assay (CLIA) or turbidometric immunoassay for digoxin has been reported to mostly eliminate interference.

Digoxin + **Donepezil**

There is no pharmacokinetic interaction between digoxin and donepezil; however, the bradycardic effects of these drugs may possibly be additive.

> It may be prudent to be alert for bradycardia on concurrent use.

Digoxin + **Dronedarone**

Dronedarone increases digoxin exposure. The cardiac depressive effects of dronedarone, such as reduced AV-node conduction, can be increased by digoxin use, as can gastrointestinal adverse effects.

> The UK and US manufacturers of dronedarone advise that the need for digoxin

should be reviewed. If both drugs are considered necessary, the digoxin dose should be halved and its plasma concentrations monitored closely. The patient should also be monitored for any signs of digoxin toxicity (e.g. bradycardia, nausea, vomiting).

Digoxin + Galantamine 🔡

In a study galantamine had no pharmacokinetic effect on digoxin. However, the bradycardic effects of both drugs may possibly be additive and, in this study, one subject was hospitalised for second-and third-degree heart block and bradycardia.

It may be prudent to be alert for bradycardia on concurrent use.

Digoxin + Herbal medicines or Dietary supplements

Danshen ⚠

Danshen does not appear to interact with digoxin, but it can falsify the results of serum immunoassay methods.

These false readings could be eliminated by monitoring the free (i.e. unbound) digoxin concentrations or using another assay method (such as a chemiluminescent assay).

Ginkgo biloba ✅

A small study found that *Ginkgo biloba* leaf extract had no significant effects on the pharmacokinetics of a single dose of digoxin.

No dose adjustment would be expected to be necessary if patients taking digoxin also wish to take ginkgo.

Ginseng 🔡

Panax ginseng (Asian ginseng), *Panax quinquefolius* (American ginseng) and *Eleutherococcus senticosus* (Siberian ginseng) may interfere with the results of digoxin assays.

The general significance of this interaction is uncertain, but be aware that ginseng may possibly interfere with digoxin assays, particularly if an unexpected digoxin level is reported.

Liquorice (Kanzo) 🔡

An isolated case of digoxin toxicity has been reported in an elderly patient attributed to the use of a herbal laxative containing kanzo (liquorice). Excessive use of laxatives containing liquorice or anthraquinones may lead to hypokalaemia which increases the risk of digitalis toxicity.

An interaction is unlikely if these laxatives are used appropriately. However bear the potential for an interaction in mind in patients who regularly use or abuse liquorice or anthraquinone-containing laxatives.

St John's wort (Hypericum perforatum) ⚠

There is good evidence that St John's wort can reduce the levels of digoxin by roughly

30%. Digoxin toxicity has occurred in a patient taking digoxin when he stopped taking St John's wort.

> Digoxin levels should be well monitored if St John's wort is either started or stopped and appropriate digoxin dosage adjustments made if necessary. The recommendation of the CSM in the UK is that St John's wort should not be taken by patients taking digoxin.

Other herbal medicines

A digoxin level of 0.9 nanograms/mL was found in a patient taking an un-named herbal remedy, which contained black cohosh root (*Cimicifuga racemosa*), cayenne pepper fruit (*Capsicum annuum*), hops flowers (*Humulus lupulus*), skullcap herb (*Scutellaria lateriflora*), valerian root (*Valeriana officinalis*) and wood betony herb (*Pedicularis canadensis*), all of which contain digoxin-like compounds which are detected by digoxin antibody immunoassays. Three packaged teas (*Breathe Easy*, blackcurrant, and jasmine) and 3 herbs (pleurisy root, chaparral, peppermint) have been found, in theory, to provide a therapeutic daily dose of digoxin, if 5 cups a day are drunk.

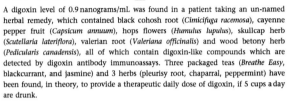

> It is apparent that if a patient taking digoxin also consumed these herbal remedies or teas they could develop symptoms of digoxin toxicity. However, theoretical interactions with herbal remedies are not always translated into practice. For example, hawthorn is used in cardiac disorders and the leaves and berries are reported to contain digoxin-like substances, but a study in healthy subjects found no pharmacokinetic or pharmacodynamic interaction between digoxin and an extract of hawthorn leaves and flowers (*Crataegus oxyacantha*). Therefore although these predicted interactions should be borne in mind when using digoxin and herbal remedies they cannot be taken as total proof that an interaction will occur.

Digoxin + HIV-protease inhibitors ⚠

A woman developed elevated digoxin concentrations and signs of toxicity after she was given ritonavir. Pharmacokinetic studies have shown that ritonavir, and saquinavir boosted with ritonavir, increase single-dose digoxin exposure. There appears to be a greater effect with intravenous digoxin than with oral digoxin.

> It would seem prudent to closely monitor patients taking digoxin when ritonavir and/or saquinavir are started or stopped, and adjust the digoxin dose as required. There do not appear to be any reports or studies of the interaction of digoxin with other HIV-protease inhibitors; however, most HIV-protease inhibitors are inhibitors of P-glycoprotein, so it would seem likely that they might all interact to a greater or lesser degree.

Digoxin + Levothyroxine ⚠

Hypothyroid subjects are relatively sensitive to the effects of digoxin and so need lower doses. As treatment with levothyroxine progresses, and they become euthyroid, the dose of digoxin will need to be increased.

> Monitor the outcome of resolving hypothyroidism, checking for to ensure that the effects of digoxin are adequate. Monitor digoxin levels as necessary.

Digoxin + Lithium ❓

No pharmacokinetic interaction seems to occur between digoxin and lithium. However, the addition of digoxin to lithium possibly has a short-term detrimental effect on the control of mania. An isolated report describes severe bradycardia in one patient given both drugs.

> The probability of a clinically significant interaction occurring seems low, but bear these cases in mind if both drugs are given.

Digoxin + Macrolides ⚠

Clarithromycin markedly increases digoxin levels, and numerous cases of digoxin toxicity have been reported. Increases in digoxin levels also occur with telithromycin. Cases of rapid and marked two- to fourfold increases in digoxin levels have also been reported for azithromycin, erythromycin, josamycin and roxithromycin.

> Monitor all patients well for signs of increased digoxin effects (see digoxin, page 326) when any macrolide is first given. Measure digoxin levels and reduce the dose as necessary.

Digoxin + Neomycin ⚠

The AUC of digoxin can be reduced by up to about 50% by the concurrent use of oral neomycin.

> Separating administration does not prevent this interaction. Monitor the response to digoxin treatment and adjust the dose as necessary.

Digoxin + NNRTIs ❓

Etravirine causes a very slight increase in digoxin exposure. Rilpivirine is predicted to increase digoxin exposure.

> The manufacturers of etravirine and rilpivirine recommend monitoring digoxin concentrations. If digoxin is started in a patient taking etravirine, the US manufacturer advises using the lowest possible dose of digoxin. However, not that the change in exposure seen would not generally be expected to be clinically relevant.

Digoxin + NSAIDs

Diclofenac and Ibuprofen ❓

Diclofenac might increase serum digoxin concentrations. Two studies found that ibuprofen raised serum digoxin concentrations, whereas another found no evidence of an interaction.

> Consider monitoring for digoxin adverse effects (e.g. bradycardia), and monitor digoxin concentrations if an interaction is suspected. Adjust the digoxin dose accordingly.

Indometacin

Rises in digoxin concentrations and digoxin toxicity have been reported in neonates given digoxin with indometacin. The picture is less clear in adults, as there are studies reporting either no change or increased digoxin levels and there seem to be no examples of a consistent interaction in practice.

In neonates, digoxin concentrations and urinary output should be monitored if concurrent use is necessary, and the dose reduced accordingly (a 50% reduction has been suggested). In adults, it is probably sufficient to monitor pulse rate (for bradycardia), and monitor digoxin concentrations if a problem is suspected.

Other NSAIDs

Etoricoxib, fenbufen, ketoprofen, meloxicam, nimesulide, piroxicam, and tiaprofenic acid appear to have small or no effect on the pharmacokinetics of digoxin.

No action needed. However, note that all NSAIDs can cause renal impairment, which would result in reduced renal elimination of digoxin and an increased risk of digoxin toxicity.

Digoxin + Opioids

Some UK manufacturers state that digoxin toxicity has occurred rarely during the concurrent use of digoxin and tramadol. There appear to be no published reports of an interaction.

In the absence of any more information, it is difficult to judge the general relevance of these cases.

Digoxin + Penicillamine

Digoxin levels can be reduced by up to about 60% by penicillamine.

The manufacturer of penicillamine advises that digoxin should not be taken within 2 hours of penicillamine. It is unclear whether separating the dose will be successful in managing this interaction. Patients should be monitored for signs of under-digitalisation. Consider checking digoxin levels if an interaction is suspected.

Digoxin + Phenytoin

Phenytoin moderately reduces digoxin levels, but the clinical significance of this is unknown. There are also isolated case reports of marked bradycardia in patients taking digoxin with phenytoin. Fatalities have been reported when phenytoin was used in cases of suspected digoxin toxicity.

It would seem sensible to monitor the effects of concurrent use and consider monitoring digoxin levels if an interaction is suspected. As fosphenytoin is a prodrug of phenytoin it would seem prudent to take similar precautions if it is given to patients taking digoxin. The use of phenytoin in digoxin toxicity appears to be obsolete.

Digoxin + **Propafenone** ⚠

Propafenone can increase digoxin levels by 30 to 90% or more (particularly in children).

> Most patients appear to be affected and dose reductions in the range of 15 to 70% were found necessary in one study. The extent of the rise may possibly depend on the propafenone level rather than on the propafenone dose. Monitor digoxin levels and adjust the dose accordingly.

Digoxin + **Proton pump inhibitors** ❓

The exposure to digoxin was negligibly to very slightly increased by omeprazole, pantoprazole, and rabeprazole. These changes are unlikely to be clinically important. However, one patient developed digoxin toxicity 3 months after starting to take omeprazole.

> No action needed. The isolated case of toxicity seems unlikely to be generally important. Nevertheless, some manufacturers advise caution on concurrent use, and suggests that digoxin concentrations should be monitored if a proton pump inhibitor is given, particularly in elderly patients given high doses.

Digoxin + **Quinidine** ⚠

The levels of digoxin in most patients are doubled on average within 5 days of quinidine being added; digoxin toxicity is likely to occur.

> Halve the digoxin dose, monitor digoxin levels and further adjust the dose as necessary. Patients with renal impairment may require larger dose reductions. Remember to increase the digoxin dose if quinidine is stopped.

Digoxin + **Quinine** ⚠

The digoxin levels of some but not all patients may rise by more than 60% if they are given quinine, and there is a report of digoxin toxicity in an elderly patient during concurrent use.

> Monitor the effects of concurrent use for digoxin adverse effects (see digoxin, page 326) and reduce the digoxin dose where necessary. Some patients may show a substantial increase in digoxin levels whereas others will show only a small or moderate rise.

Digoxin + **Ranolazine** ⚠

Ranolazine increases digoxin levels by 50%.

> It would seem prudent to monitor digoxin levels if ranolazine is started, anticipating the need to reduce the digoxin dose.

Digoxin + Rifampicin (Rifampin)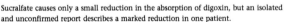

In general, digoxin levels may be modestly reduced by the concurrent use of rifampicin, although cases of greater reductions (up to 80%) have also been reported.

> It would seem sensible to monitor the outcome of concurrent use and monitor digoxin levels if an interaction is suspected. It may be that renal impairment increases the extent of this interaction.

Digoxin + Rivastigmine

There is no pharmacokinetic interaction between digoxin and rivastigmine; however, the bradycardic effects of both drugs may possibly be additive.

> It may be prudent to be alert for bradycardia on concurrent use.

Digoxin + Salbutamol (Albuterol) and related bronchodilators ⚠

In one study, oral salbutamol slightly reduced digoxin levels, by 0.3 nanomol/L. Note that all beta$_2$ agonists (oral and inhaled) can cause hypokalaemia, which could lead to the development of digitalis toxicity.

> It may be prudent to monitor potassium levels if beta$_2$ agonists are started, particularly nebulised, oral or intravenous beta$_2$ agonists. If symptoms of digoxin toxicity occur on concurrent use (see digoxin, page 326) it may be prudent to recheck potassium levels.

Digoxin + Statins ✅

Atorvastatin, fluvastatin and simvastatin cause minor increases in digoxin levels.

> The small changes seen in the digoxin levels with the statins seem unlikely to be clinically relevant in most patients.

Digoxin + Sucralfate ❓

Sucralfate causes only a small reduction in the absorption of digoxin, but an isolated and unconfirmed report describes a marked reduction in one patient.

> The reduction in digoxin levels is small and therefore normally unlikely to be clinically relevant. Nevertheless, consider an interaction if digoxin seems ineffective.

Digoxin + Sulfasalazine ⚠

Digoxin absorption can be reduced by up to 50% by sulfasalazine. Digoxin levels are reduced accordingly. This interaction appears to be dose related.

> Monitor to ensure that the effects of digoxin are adequate, and consider measuring digoxin levels if an interaction is suspected. Adjust the dose as necessary.

Digoxin + Tacrine

The pharmacokinetics of digoxin are unchanged by tacrine, but their bradycardic effects may possibly be additive.

It may be prudent to be alert for bradycardia on concurrent use.

Digoxin + Tizanidine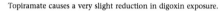

The manufacturers state that the concurrent use of digoxin and tizanidine may potentiate bradycardia, but there do not appear to be any reports of problems with concurrent use.

Monitor heart rate and adjust the digoxin dose accordingly.

Digoxin + Topiramate

Topiramate causes a very slight reduction in digoxin exposure.

The UK manufacturer suggests good monitoring of digoxin if topiramate is added or withdrawn, but changes of this magnitude are unlikely to be clinically relevant in most patients. Note that the US manufacturer makes no suggestion that monitoring is necessary.

Digoxin + Trimethoprim

Digoxin levels can be increased by about 22% by trimethoprim, but some individuals may show a much greater rise.

Monitor the effects of digoxin (see digoxin, page 326) if trimethoprim is given, and consider measuring digoxin levels, particularly in the elderly. Adjust the dose as necessary.

Digoxin + Ulipristal

The manufacturers of ulipristal predict that it will increase digoxin concentrations by inhibiting P-glycoprotein.

Until more is known, monitor for digoxin adverse effects (such as bradycardia), and adjust the digoxin dose if necessary. One UK manufacturer of *low-dose* ulipristal recommends separating administration by at least 1.5 hours.

Dipyridamole

Dipyridamole + Duloxetine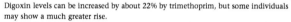

The bleeding risk associated with antiplatelet drugs such as dipyridamole might be further increased by the concurrent use of an SSRI, although the data appears to be conflicting. SNRIs (e.g. duloxetine) are expected to interact similarly.

The UK manufacturers of duloxetine advise caution on concurrent use in patients taking antiplatelet drugs (such as dipyridamole). Consider giving gastroprotective drugs to those at high risk of gastrointestinal bleeding (e.g. the elderly, those with a history of gastrointestinal bleeding, patients taking multiple antiplatelet drugs). Advise patients to report any signs of excessive bleeding.

Dipyridamole + Herbal medicines or Dietary supplements ⚠

Ginkgo biloba has been associated with platelet, bleeding and clotting disorders and there are isolated reports of serious adverse reactions after its concurrent use with antiplatelet drugs. Dipyridamole would be expected to interact similarly.

The evidence is too slim to advise patients against taking dipyridamole with *Ginkgo biloba*. However, caution should be exercised if *Ginkgo biloba* is used with any drug that affects platelet aggregation as bleeding has been seen with the use of *Ginkgo biloba* alone. Patients should be told to seek professional advice if any bleeding problems arise.

Dipyridamole + H₂-receptor antagonists ❓

The effective disintegration, dissolution and eventual absorption of dipyridamole in tablet or suspension form depends upon having a low pH in the stomach. Drugs that significantly raise the gastric pH (such as the H₂-receptor antagonists) are expected to reduce the bioavailability of immediate-release formulations of dipyridamole such as the tablets and suspension. This effect has been seen with famotidine.

The clinical significance of this interaction is unknown; however, bear it in mind if should any unexpected reduction in immediate-release dipyridamole efficacy occur. Note that modified-release preparations of dipyridamole (that are buffered) do not appear to be affected, and may be a suitable alternative.

Dipyridamole + Prasugrel ❓

The concurrent use of dipyridamole and prasugrel might theoretically increase the risk of bleeding.

Although combinations of antiplatelet drugs are commonly used and can be clinically beneficial in some conditions, be aware of the increased risk of bleeding.

Dipyridamole + Proton pump inhibitors ❓

The effective disintegration, dissolution and eventual absorption of dipyridamole in tablet or suspension form depends upon having a low pH in the stomach. Drugs that significantly raise the gastric pH (such as the proton pump inhibitors) are expected to reduce the bioavailability of immediate-release formulations of dipyridamole such as the tablets or suspension. This effect has been seen with lansoprazole.

The clinical significance of this interaction is unknown; however, bear it in mind should any unexpected reduction in dipyridamole efficacy occur. Note that modified-release preparations of dipyridamole (that are buffered) do not appear to be affected and may be a suitable alternative.

Dipyridamole + **Riociguat** ✕

The US manufacturer of riociguat predicts that the concurrent use with dipyridamole will lead to hypotension.

Dipyridamole is a non-specific phosphodiesterase inhibitor, which together with riociguat can affect vascular tone resulting in hypotension. Concurrent use is therefore contraindicated.

Dipyridamole + **Rivaroxaban** ❓

The concurrent use of rivaroxaban and dipyridamole might increase the risk of bleeding.

Advise patients to be aware of increased bruising or prolonged bleeding, and to seek medical advice if this occurs.

Dipyridamole + **SSRIs** ❓

The bleeding risk associated with antiplatelet drugs such as dipyridamole might be further increased by the concurrent use of an SSRI, although the data appears to be conflicting.

In general, the manufacturers of the SSRIs advise caution on the concurrent use of drugs that affect platelet function, such as dipyridamole. Consider giving gastroprotective drugs to those at high risk of gastrointestinal bleeding (e.g. the elderly, those with a history of gastrointestinal bleeding, patients taking multiple antiplatelet drugs). Advise patients to report any signs of excessive bleeding.

Dipyridamole + **Ticagrelor** ❓

The concurrent use of dipyridamole and ticagrelor might theoretically increase the risk of bleeding.

Although combinations of antiplatelet drugs are commonly used and can be clinically beneficial in some indications, be aware of the increased risk of bleeding.

Dipyridamole + **Ticlopidine** ❓

The concurrent use of dipyridamole and ticlopidine might theoretically increase the risk of bleeding.

Although combinations of antiplatelet drugs are commonly used and can be clinically beneficial in some conditions, be aware of the increased risk of bleeding.

Dipyridamole + **Venlafaxine** ❓

The bleeding risk associated with antiplatelet drugs such as dipyridamole might be further increased by the concurrent use of an SSRI, although the data appears to be conflicting. SNRIs (e.g. venlafaxine) are expected to interact similarly.

The UK manufacturer of venlafaxine advises caution on concurrent use in patients taking antiplatelet drugs (such as dipyridamole). Consider giving gastroprotective drugs to those at high risk of gastrointestinal bleeding (e.g. the elderly, those with a history of gastrointestinal bleeding, patients taking multiple antiplatelet drugs). Advise patients to report any signs of excessive bleeding.

Dipyridamole + Warfarin and related oral anticoagulants

Mild bleeding (epistaxis, bruising, haematuria) can sometimes occur if anticoagulants are given with dipyridamole. Note that prothrombin times remain stable and well within the therapeutic range.

D

These effects would not be unexpected if an antiplatelet and an anticoagulant are used concurrently. Bear them in mind when considering the combination. There is some evidence that maintaining anticoagulant control at the lower end of the therapeutic range minimises possible bleeding complications.

Disopyramide

Disopyramide + HIV-protease inhibitors

Saquinavir

Saquinavir may prolong the QT interval and this may be additive with other drugs that prolong the QT interval such as disopyramide. Dangerous QT prolongation may occur if they are used together.

Concurrent use is generally considered to be contraindicated. For more information on QT prolongation, see drugs that prolong the QT interval, page 352.

Other HIV-protease inhibitors

Disopyramide levels may be increased by ritonavir, which may increase the risk arrhythmias and other adverse effects. Other HIV-protease inhibitors are predicted to interact similarly.

Monitor concurrent use closely for adverse effects, and decrease the disopyramide dose as necessary.

Disopyramide + Lacosamide

Dose-dependent prolongation of the PR interval may occur with lacosamide. The UK manufacturer therefore advises that lacosamide should be used with caution in patients taking class I antiarrhythmics, such as disopyramide.

Be aware that ECG changes may occur on concurrent use.

Disopyramide + Macrolides ⚠️

Erythromycin appears to raise disopyramide levels; concurrent use has led to QT prolongation, cardiac arrhythmias and heart block. The concurrent use of clarithromycin and disopyramide has led to torsade de pointes, ventricular fibrillation and severe hypoglycaemia, and the concurrent use of azithromycin and disopyramide has led to ventricular fibrillation. Disopyramide and some macrolides can prolong the QT interval. See drugs that prolong the QT interval, page 352.

Some of the manufacturers of disopyramide recommend avoiding the combination of disopyramide and macrolides that inhibit CYP3A, and this would certainly be prudent in situations where close monitoring is not possible. If concurrent use of any macrolide is essential, monitor closely for signs of disopyramide toxicity and QT prolongation.

Disopyramide + NNRTIs ⚠️

The manufacturers predict that etravirine may decrease the levels of disopyramide.

The manufacturers recommend caution on concurrent use and state that disopyramide levels should be monitored, if this is possible.

Disopyramide + Phenobarbital ⚠️

Disopyramide exposure is reduced by about 35% by phenobarbital. Note that primidone is metabolised to phenobarbital and therefore may interact similarly.

The extent to which this interaction would reduce the antiarrhythmic effects of disopyramide is unknown, but monitor disopyramide efficacy and levels (if possible) if phenobarbital is added or withdrawn. One manufacturer suggests avoiding the combination.

Disopyramide + Phenytoin ⚠️

Disopyramide levels are reduced by phenytoin and may fall below therapeutic levels. Loss of arrhythmic control may occur. Fosphenytoin, a prodrug of phenytoin, may interact similarly.

Monitor disopyramide efficacy and levels (where possible). Adjust the disopyramide dose as necessary. Disopyramide levels appear to return to normal within 2 weeks of withdrawing the phenytoin. Note that one manufacturer of disopyramide recommends avoiding the combination.

Disopyramide + Rifampicin (Rifampin) ⚠️

Disopyramide levels can be reduced by rifampicin.

It seems likely that the dose of disopyramide will need to be increased in most patients taking rifampicin. Monitor the effects of concurrent use and adjust the dose as necessary.

Disopyramide + **Warfarin and related oral anticoagulants**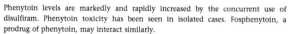

Limited data suggests that warfarin requirements can be increased or decreased by disopyramide.

> There is insufficient evidence to recommend monitoring all patients, but bear this interaction in mind if any unexplained change in anticoagulant control occurs in patients taking warfarin who are given disopyramide.

Disulfiram

D

Disulfiram + Isoniazid

In most patients the use of isoniazid with disulfiram is uneventful, but a small number of patients have developed difficulties in co-ordination, changes in affect and behaviour, and drowsiness.

> Concurrent use need not be avoided, but if marked changes in mental status occur, or if there is unsteady gait, the manufacturers recommend that the disulfiram should be withdrawn.

Disulfiram + Metronidazole

Acute psychoses and confusion can be caused by the concurrent use of metronidazole and disulfiram.

> Concurrent use should be avoided or very well monitored. Withdrawing the drugs appears to resolve any adverse effects.

Disulfiram + Phenytoin

Phenytoin levels are markedly and rapidly increased by the concurrent use of disulfiram. Phenytoin toxicity has been seen in isolated cases. Fosphenytoin, a prodrug of phenytoin, may interact similarly.

> This interaction seems to occur in most patients and develops rapidly. Monitor phenytoin levels and adverse effects (e.g. blurred vision, nystagmus, ataxia or drowsiness) carefully during concurrent use. Phenytoin dose reductions may be needed, but it may be difficult to maintain the balance required. Recovery may take 2 to 3 weeks after the disulfiram is withdrawn.

Disulfiram + Theophylline

Disulfiram causes a negligible to slight decrease in the clearance of theophylline. Aminophylline would be expected to interact similarly.

> Be alert for theophylline adverse effects (such as headache, nausea, and tremor) on concurrent use, particularly where the metabolism of theophylline might already

be reduced (other drugs or diseases), and monitor theophylline concentrations accordingly.

Disulfiram + Tizanidine ⚠

Disulfiram is predicted to increase the exposure to tizanidine, increasing its hypotensive and sedative effects.

The UK and US manufacturers suggest that concurrent use should be avoided. Until more is known be alert for adverse effects such as bradycardia, hypotension, and drowsiness.

Disulfiram + Warfarin and related oral anticoagulants ⚠

The anticoagulant effects of warfarin are increased by disulfiram, and in some cases bleeding has occurred.

It seems likely that most individuals will demonstrate this interaction. Monitor the INR in response to warfarin and adjust the dose accordingly when adding or withdrawing disulfiram. In patients taking disulfiram consideration should be given to using a smaller warfarin loading dose.

Diuretics

Diuretics + Herbal medicines or Dietary supplements

Germanium ❓

On two occasions severe oedema (12 to 13 kg weight gain) developed over 10 to 14 days in a patient taking furosemide after he also took a preparation containing ginseng and germanium. The effects were attributed to the germanium.

This is an isolated report, and its general significance is unclear. However, note that it has been said that the use of germanium should be discouraged due to its potential to cause renal toxicity.

Liquorice ❓

A patient developed hypokalaemia after taking liquorice and hydrochlorothiazide. This interaction seems possible with liquorice (which can lower potassium levels) and any potassium-depleting diuretic (i.e. thiazides or loop diuretics).

The additive effects of these drugs may result in clinically significant hypokalaemia, but evidence is extremely sparse. Consider this interaction in a case of otherwise unexplained hypokalaemia.

St John's wort (Hypericum perforatum)

St John's wort decreases the AUC of eplerenone by 30%.

Concurrent use is not recommended by the manufacturers because of the possibility of decreased efficacy.

Diuretics + HIV-protease inhibitors ⊗

Saquinavir increases the AUC of eplerenone 2.1-fold. The manufacturer predicts that nelfinavir and ritonavir will interact to a greater extent.

In the UK, the manufacturer recommends that the dose of eplerenone should not exceed 25 mg daily in patients taking saquinavir. In the US, the manufacturer recommends that the starting dose of eplerenone for hypertension should be reduced to 25 mg daily for patients taking these drugs. This seems a sensible precaution. It seems likely that most HIV-protease inhibitors will interact similarly; however, because the manufacturers predict a greater effect with nelfinavir and ritonavir they contraindicate the concurrent use of these HIV-protease inhibitors.

Diuretics + HRT

Drospirenone, which is given as the progestogen component in some HRT formulations, might increase the risk of hyperkalaemia when given with other drugs that can cause hyperkalaemia such as potassium-sparing diuretics and aldosterone antagonists. The UK manufacturer of drospirenone-containing HRT notes that the increase in potassium levels may be more pronounced in diabetic women.

The risk of hyperkalaemia appears to be low, especially if renal function is normal. In the US, it is recommended that consideration be given to monitoring potassium levels during the first cycle in women [with normal renal function] who regularly take a potassium-sparing diuretic or an aldosterone antagonist, whereas the UK manufacturer recommends that the potassium level is measured during the first cycle or month of treatment only in women with mild or moderate renal impairment. In patients at higher risk of developing hyperkalaemia (e.g. in renal impairment) it is generally recommended that potassium levels are measured during the first cycle of treatment with drospirenone.

Diuretics + Lithium

Amiloride

Some manufacturers suggest that amiloride reduces the renal clearance of lithium, thereby increasing the risk of lithium toxicity. There appears to be no evidence to confirm this alleged interaction and several studies suggesting that no interaction occurs.

No additional monitoring of lithium levels appears to be necessary, but as an interaction has been reported with other potassium-sparing diuretics, it would be prudent to reinforce the symptoms of lithium toxicity (see lithium, page 468) and tell patients to report them if they should occur.

Eplerenone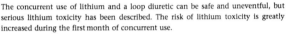

The concurrent use of eplerenone and lithium has not been studied, but the manufacturers predict that eplerenone may raise lithium levels.

The UK manufacturers state that concurrent use should be avoided or lithium levels closely monitored. Patients taking lithium should be aware of the symptoms of lithium toxicity (see lithium, page 468) and told to report them immediately should they occur.

Loop diuretics

The concurrent use of lithium and a loop diuretic can be safe and uneventful, but serious lithium toxicity has been described. The risk of lithium toxicity is greatly increased during the first month of concurrent use.

Patients taking lithium should be aware of the symptoms of lithium toxicity (see lithium, page 468) and told to report them immediately should they occur. Consider increased monitoring of lithium levels in patients newly started on this combination. Note that, in rare cases lithium has been associated with QT prolongation. In theory, this may be exacerbated by hypokalaemia caused by loop diuretics. For more information, see Drugs that prolong the QT interval, page 352.

Spironolactone

One study found that spironolactone caused the lithium levels to rise from 0.63 to 0.9 mmol/L. However, another study found no interaction.

Evidence for this interaction is sparse, no additional monitoring is necessary, but patients taking lithium should be aware of the symptoms of lithium toxicity (see lithium, page 468) and told to report them immediately should they occur.

Thiazides

The thiazide and related diuretics can cause a rapid rise in lithium concentrations, which can lead to lithium toxicity.

The rise in serum lithium concentrations and the accompanying toxicity develops most commonly within about one week to 10 days, although it has been seen after 3 months. None of the thiazides should be given to patients taking lithium unless the serum lithium concentrations can be closely monitored and appropriate downward dose adjustments made. Patients taking lithium should be aware of the symptoms of lithium toxicity (see lithium, page 468) and told to report them immediately should they occur. Note that, in rare cases lithium has been associated with QT prolongation. In theory, this may be exacerbated by hypokalaemia caused by thiazides. For more information, see Drugs that prolong the QT interval, page 352.

Triamterene

Triamterene appears to increase lithium excretion.

Information is sparse. The reports available do not give a clear indication of the outcome of concurrent use, but some monitoring would seem prudent. Patients taking lithium should be aware of the symptoms of lithium toxicity (see lithium, page 468) and told to report them immediately should they occur.

Diuretics + **Macrolides**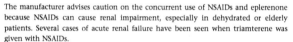

Erythromycin increases the AUC of eplerenone 2.9-fold. The manufacturer predicts that clarithromycin and telithromycin will interact to a greater extent. Eplerenone reduced the AUC of erythromycin by 14%, which was not considered clinically relevant.

> The manufacturers recommend a maximum eplerenone dose of 25 mg daily in those taking erythromycin. Because they predict a greater effect with clarithromycin and telithromycin they contraindicate the concurrent use of these macrolides. Other macrolides seem less likely to interact, see macrolides, page 474.

Diuretics + **NSAIDs**

Potassium-sparing diuretics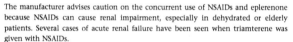

The manufacturer advises caution on the concurrent use of NSAIDs and eplerenone because NSAIDs can cause renal impairment, especially in dehydrated or elderly patients. Several cases of acute renal failure have been seen when triamterene was given with NSAIDs.

> Patients should be well hydrated and have their renal function checked before starting this combination.

Loop diuretics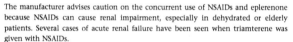

The antihypertensive and diuretic effects of loop diuretics appear to be reduced by NSAIDs, although the extent of this interaction largely depends on the individual NSAID. Indometacin appears to cause the most clinically relevant effect. The concurrent use of NSAIDs with loop diuretics can exacerbate congestive heart failure and increase the risk of hospitalisation.

> Concurrent use need not be avoided but the effects should be checked and the diuretic dose raised as necessary. Not all patients are affected. Patients at greatest risk are likely to be the elderly with cirrhosis, cardiac failure and/or renal impairment, and they might need to avoid NSAIDs.

Thiazides

There is evidence that most NSAIDs can increase blood pressure in patients taking antihypertensives, including diuretics, although some studies have not found the increase to be clinically relevant. The concurrent use of NSAIDs with thiazide diuretics can exacerbate congestive heart failure and increase the risk of hospitalisation. Diuretics might increase the risk of NSAID-induced acute renal failure.

> Only some patients are affected. Nevertheless, some have suggested that the use of NSAIDs should be kept to a minimum in patients taking antihypertensives, whereas, others suggest that the interaction is, generally, not clinically relevant. Consider monitoring blood pressure if an NSAID is started or stopped. Note that NSAIDs should generally be avoided in those with heart failure.

Diuretics + **Phenobarbital**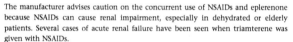

St John's wort (Hypericum perforatum) decreases the AUC of eplerenone by 30%. The manufacturers therefore predict that more potent enzyme inducers, such as phenobarbital, may have a greater effect. Note that primidone is metabolised to phenobarbital and therefore may interact similarly.

Concurrent use is not recommended by the manufacturers.

Diuretics + **Phenytoin**

Eplerenone ⚠

St John's wort (*Hypericum perforatum*) slightly decreases the eplerenone exposure. The manufacturers therefore predict that more potent enzyme inducers, such as phenytoin, might have a greater effect. Fosphenytoin, a prodrug of phenytoin, might interact similarly.

Concurrent use is not recommended by the manufacturers.

Furosemide ⚠

The diuretic effects of furosemide can be reduced as much as 50% if phenytoin is taken concurrently.

The clinical relevance of this finding is unclear. However, it would be prudent to consider monitoring the diuretic effects of furosemide if phenytoin is started. Fosphenytoin, a prodrug of phenytoin, might interact similarly.

Diuretics + **Potassium** ⚠

The concurrent use of spironolactone or triamterene with potassium supplements can result in severe and even life-threatening hyperkalaemia. Amiloride and eplerenone are expected to interact similarly. Potassium-containing salt substitutes can be as hazardous as potassium supplements.

The manufacturers of eplerenone contraindicate the concurrent use of potassium supplements, but in the US, this contraindication is only in patients given eplerenone for hypertension. If a potassium supplement is given to a patient taking a potassium-sparing diuretic close monitoring of plasma potassium concentrations, both before and during treatment, is necessary.

Diuretics + **Proton pump inhibitors** ❓

Proton pump inhibitors can cause hypomagnesaemia, which might be additive with the magnesium-lowering effects of diuretics.

Hypomagnesaemia can develop after more than one year of concurrent use, so consider monitoring magnesium concentrations before and annually during proton pump inhibitor use, or in response to symptoms of hypomagnesaemia (e.g. muscle twitching or cramps, tremors, vomiting, tiredness, or loss of appetite). In those patients who develop hypomagnesaemia, oral and parenteral magnesium supplements might not be as effective as anticipated. Stopping the proton pump inhibitor (where possible) might be necessary.

Diuretics + **Reboxetine**

Reboxetine may reduce potassium levels. Hypokalaemia is therefore possible if reboxetine is used with potassium-depleting diuretics (e.g. loop or thiazide diuretics).

Monitor potassium levels on concurrent use.

Diuretics + **Rifampicin (Rifampin)**

St John's wort (*Hypericum perforatum*) decreases the AUC of eplerenone by 30%. The manufacturers therefore predict that more potent enzyme inducers, such as rifampicin, may have a greater effect.

Concurrent use is not recommended by the manufacturers.

D

Diuretics + **Salbutamol (Albuterol) and related bronchodilators**

Beta$_2$ agonists, such as salbutamol and terbutaline, can cause hypokalaemia. This can be increased by other potassium-depleting drugs such as the loop or thiazide diuretics. In severe cases the risk of serious cardiac arrhythmias could be increased.

The CSM in the UK advises monitoring potassium in severe asthma, because of the probability of multiple potassium-depleting drugs being used, and because some conditions predispose these patients to hypokalaemia (e.g. hypoxia). Consider monitoring based on the severity of the patient's condition, and the number of potassium-depleting drugs used.

Diuretics + **Sevelamer**

Sevelamer abolished the diuretic effect of furosemide 250 mg twice daily in a haemodialysis patient. Urine output returned to the patient's normal levels 24 hours after sevelamer was stopped, and the reduction in urine output was not seen when the dosing frequency was altered so that furosemide was taken in the morning and sevelamer was taken at lunch and dinnertime.

If the effect of furosemide seems less than expected, give the furosemide at least 1 hour before or 3 hours after sevelamer.

Diuretics + **Tacrolimus**

The concurrent use of tacrolimus and potassium-sparing diuretics might cause hyperkalaemia.

The UK and US manufacturers of tacrolimus suggest that concurrent use should be avoided. If concurrent use is essential, potassium concentrations should be monitored closely.

Diuretics + **Theophylline**

Furosemide is reported to increase, decrease, or to have no effect on theophylline concentrations. Both theophylline and loop or thiazide diuretics can cause hypokalaemia, which may be additive. Aminophylline is expected to interact similarly.

> Be aware for the potential for changes in theophylline concentrations if furosemide is also given. Consider measuring theophylline concentrations, and make appropriate dose adjustments as necessary. It may be prudent to monitor potassium concentrations in any patient given theophylline or aminophylline and a thiazide or loop diuretic.

Diuretics + Toremifene

Hypercalcaemia is a recognised adverse effect of toremifene, and the manufacturers suggest that drugs such as the thiazides, which decrease renal calcium excretion, might increase the risk of hypercalcaemia.

> This warning is based on theoretical considerations, and its clinical importance awaits confirmation.

Domperidone

Domperidone + Dopamine agonists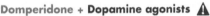

Domperidone may reduce the prolactin-lowering effect of bromocriptine. Other dopamine agonists may be similarly affected.

> Consider alternatives to domperidone wherever possible if prolactin levels are to be reduced. Note that domperidone is the antiemetic of choice in Parkinson's disease.

Domperidone + Drugs that prolong the QT interval

The MHRA in the UK and the European Medicines Agency state that domperidone has a higher risk of serious cardiac drug reactions, including QTc prolongation. For more general information about this effect, see Drugs that prolong the QT interval, page 352.

> The MHRA and the European Medicines Agency contraindicate the concurrent use of domperidone with other drugs that prolong the QT interval

Domperidone + HIV-protease inhibitors

Potent CYP3A4 inhibitors, such as nelfinavir, ritonavir, saquinavir, and other HIV-protease inhibitors boosted with ritonavir, are predicted to increase the exposure to domperidone, which might increase the risk of QT-interval prolongation, possibly leading to the potentially fatal torsade de pointes arrhythmia.

> The MHRA in the UK and the European Medicines Agency contraindicate the concurrent use of domperidone with potent CYP3A4 inhibitors or with other

drugs that prolong the QT interval (such as saquinavir boosted with ritonavir, see Drugs that prolong the QT interval, page 352).

Domperidone + Macrolides ✕

Erythromycin increases the exposure to domperidone about 3-fold by inhibiting CYP3A4, and further increases the QT-interval prolongation seen with domperidone alone.

Evidence for an interaction between domperidone and the macrolides is limited to that with erythromycin. The increase in the QT interval due to increased domperidone exposure caused by CYP3A4 inhibition alone would probably not be clinically relevant, however when added to the increase in QT interval seen with erythromycin alone, the overall increase might reach a level at which some concern is warranted. Due to a higher risk of serious cardiac drug reactions, including QTc prolongation, the MHRA in the UK and the European Medicines Agency contraindicate the concurrent use of domperidone with other drugs that prolong the QT interval (see Drugs that prolong the QT interval, page 352) or with potent CYP3A4 inhibitors (which would include clarithromycin, erythromycin, and telithromycin).

D

Donepezil

Donepezil + SSRIs ❓

Two case reports suggest that paroxetine may increase donepezil levels and adverse effects. The manufacturers predict that fluoxetine will also interact, as, like paroxetine, it inhibits CYP2D6.

The general importance of this interaction is unknown, but consider this interaction if adverse effects are troublesome.

Dopamine agonists

Dopamine agonists + Ergot derivatives ⚠

Bromocriptine and cabergoline are ergot dopamine agonists and although the manufacturers have no evidence of an interaction with other ergot derivatives, they do not recommend concurrent use, presumably because of the risks of additive adverse effects. It would seem prudent to use similar caution with other dopamine agonists that are ergot derivatives (e.g. lisuride, pergolide), although there appears to be no information available.

Avoid concurrent use.

Dopamine agonists + Everolimus

Bromocriptine is predicted to increase everolimus concentrations.

A clinically relevant interaction is unlikely. However, consider an interaction if should an increase in everolimus adverse effects (such as stomatitis, blood dyscrasias, renal impairment) occur.

Dopamine agonists + H₂-receptor antagonists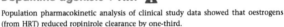

Cimetidine may reduce the clearance of pramipexole by 35%. *Ciprofloxacin* increases the AUC of ropinirole by 84%. The manufacturers therefore predict that other CYP1A2 inhibitors (they name cimetidine) will interact similarly.

The clinical relevance of these interactions do not appear to have been assessed but it would be prudent to be alert for adverse effects (such as nausea, hypotension, drowsiness). Consider reducing the dose of the dopamine agonist if these become troublesome.

Dopamine agonists + HRT

Population pharmacokinetic analysis of clinical study data showed that oestrogens (from HRT) reduced ropinirole clearance by one-third.

In women already receiving HRT, ropinirole treatment may be started using the usual dose titration. However, a reduction in the ropinirole dose may be needed if HRT is started, and an increase if it is withdrawn.

Dopamine agonists + Macrolides

Erythromycin markedly increases bromocriptine levels (up to 4.6-fold), and a case of toxicity has been reported. Bromocriptine toxicity has also occurred in a patient given josamycin. Clarithromycin increases the bioavailability of cabergoline about 2- to 4-fold.

Concurrent use should be well monitored if macrolides that affect CYP3A4 are given (e.g. clarithromycin, erythromycin, telithromycin, see macrolides, page 474, for further details). It has been suggested that the bromocriptine dose may need to be reduced by 50% to avoid toxicity. One manufacturer of cabergoline advises avoiding the concurrent use of macrolides, and specifically names erythromycin.

Dopamine agonists + Metoclopramide

Centrally-acting dopamine antagonists (such as metoclopramide) are expected to oppose the effects of the dopamine agonists (reduction in clinical response seen). Metoclopramide would also be expected to reduce the prolactin-lowering effect of bromocriptine.

Concurrent use should be avoided, or monitored closely to ensure that the dopamine agonist remains effective. Domperidone is the antiemetic of choice in Parkinson's disease.

Dopamine agonists + **Nasal decongestants**

Post-partum women taking bromocriptine have developed symptoms such as severe headache, marked hypertension, psychosis, or seizures with cerebral vasospasm after also taking phenylpropanolamine or pseudoephedrine.

Direct information seems to be limited to these cases, but the severity of the reactions suggests that it might be prudent for postpartum patients to avoid these and related drugs while taking bromocriptine. Advise patients to also avoid non-prescription products containing these drugs (often cough and cold remedies). Note that bromocriptine is not recommended for the routine suppression of lactation postpartum.

Dopamine agonists + **Quinolones**

Ciprofloxacin increases the AUC of ropinirole by 84%.

The clinical relevance of this pharmacokinetic interaction has not been assessed, but it may be prudent to monitor for an increase in ropinirole adverse effects (such as nausea, hypotension, drowsiness). The manufacturers suggest that an adjust-ment of the ropinirole dose may be required in the presence of ciprofloxacin. Other quinolones may also interact, see quinolones, page 564.

Dopamine agonists + **SSRIs**

Ciprofloxacin increases the AUC of ropinirole by 84%. The manufacturers therefore predict that other CYP1A2 inhibitors (they name fluvoxamine) will interact similarly.

The clinical relevance of this pharmacokinetic interaction has not been assessed but it may be prudent to monitor for an increase in ropinirole adverse effects (such as nausea, hypotension, drowsiness). The manufacturers suggest that the ropinirole dose may need to be adjusted in patients taking fluvoxamine.

Doripenem

Doripenem + **Probenecid**

Probenecid increases the AUC of doripenem by 75%.

The manufacturers do not recommend concurrent use.

Doripenem + **Valproate**

Doripenem can dramatically reduce the serum concentration of valproate. Seizures have occurred in some patients taking valproate with a carbapenem.

Avoid concurrent use if possible. If it is essential, consider using intravenous valproate (which has been successfully substituted in some cases) and monitor valproate serum concentrations closely, adjusting the valproate dose if necessary. Consider using another antibacterial, or an alternative to valproate: limited evidence suggests that carbamazepine and phenytoin are not affected.

Doxapram

Doxapram + Theophylline

No pharmacokinetic interaction appears to occur between theophylline and doxapram in neonates. However, the UK manufacturer of doxapram states that agitation and increased muscle activity might occur in adults. Aminophylline would be expected to interact similarly.

> Although this reaction seems rare, it would be prudent to monitor concurrent use for any adverse outcome.

D

Dronedarone

Dronedarone + Everolimus

Dronedarone is predicted to increase the plasma concentration of everolimus.

> Everolimus concentrations and effects should be closely monitored, and the dose adjusted as needed.

Dronedarone + Grapefruit juice ✗

Grapefruit juice moderately increases dronedarone exposure.

> The UK and US manufacturers of dronedarone state that grapefruit juice should be avoided in patients taking dronedarone.

Dronedarone + Herbal medicines or Dietary supplements

St John's wort is predicted to reduce dronedarone exposure.

> The UK & US manufacturers of dronedarone advise that the concurrent use of St John's wort should be avoided.

Dronedarone + HIV-protease inhibitors ✗

HIV-protease inhibitors boosted with ritonavir, or ritonavir or saquinavir alone, are predicted to increase dronedarone exposure. Saquinavir has QT-prolonging effects, which might be additive with those of other drugs with such effects, such as dronedarone, see drugs that prolong the QT interval, page 352.

> The UK and US manufacturers of dronedarone contraindicate the concurrent use of ritonavir. It would appear prudent to avoid the concurrent use of saquinavir.

Dronedarone + Macrolides ✗

Clarithromycin and telithromycin are predicted to increase dronedarone exposure. In addition, the concurrent use of dronedarone with some macrolides might result in additive QT-prolonging effects, see drugs that prolong the QT interval, page 352

The UK and US manufacturers of dronedarone contraindicate the concurrent use of clarithromycin or telithromycin.

Dronedarone + Phenobarbital

Phenobarbital is predicted to reduce dronedarone exposure. Primidone is metabolised to phenobarbital and would be expected to interact similarly.

The UK and US manufacturers of dronedarone advise that the concurrent use of phenobarbital (and therefore, probably primidone) should be avoided.

Dronedarone + Phenytoin

Phenytoin is predicted to reduce dronedarone exposure. Fosphenytoin, a prodrug of phenytoin, would be expected to interact similarly.

The UK and US manufacturers of dronedarone advise that the concurrent use of phenytoin (and therefore, probably fosphenytoin) should be avoided.

Dronedarone + Rifampicin (Rifampin)

Rifampicin markedly reduces dronedarone exposure.

The UK and US manufacturers of dronedarone advise that the concurrent use of rifampicin should be avoided.

Dronedarone + Sirolimus

Dronedarone increased the sirolimus concentration of a patient.

Sirolimus concentrations and effects should be closely monitored as a matter of routine, however it would be prudent to increase the frequency of monitoring the concentration of sirolimus if dronedarone is started, and the dose adjusted as needed.

Dronedarone + Statins

Dronedarone moderately increases simvastatin exposure and slightly increases that of atorvastatin and rosuvastatin. Other statins metabolised similarly are predicted to interact in the same way when given with dronedarone.

The moderate increase in simvastatin exposure is likely to be clinically important, and as such the US manufacturer of dronedarone advises avoiding simvastatin doses greater than 10 mg daily in patients taking dronedarone, and the UK manufacturer states that lower starting and maintenance doses of the statin should be considered. The slight increases in atorvastatin and rosuvastatin exposure are unlikely to be clinically important, but until more is known some caution on their concurrent use with dronedarone would seem prudent. Likewise, similar precautions would seem warranted for lovastatin, which is metabolised in the same way as simvastatin. If dronedarone is given with any statin, monitor for signs of muscle toxicity and adjust the statin dose if necessary. Counsel patients regarding myopathy (e.g. report any unexplained muscle pain, tenderness or weakness).

Dronedarone + Tacrolimus ⚠

Tacrolimus plasma concentrations are predicted to be increased by dronedarone,.

Tacrolimus concentrations and effects should be closely monitored, and the dose adjusted as needed.

Drugs that prolong the QT interval

The consensus of opinion is that the concurrent use of two or more drugs that prolong the QT interval should generally be avoided because of the risk of additive effects, leading to the possible development of serious and potentially life-threatening torsade de pointes arrhythmias. It is thought that torsade de pointes is unlikely to develop until the corrected QT (QTc) interval exceeds 500 milliseconds, but this is not an exact figure and the risks are uncertain and unpredictable. Because of these uncertainties, many drug manufacturers and regulatory agencies now contraindicate the concurrent use of drugs known to prolong the QT interval, and a 'blanket' warning is often issued because the QT-prolonging effects of the drugs are expected to be additive. The extent of the drug-induced prolongation usually depends on the dose of the drug and the particular drugs in question. Note also that some conditions (increasing age, female sex, cardiac disease, bradycardia and some metabolic disturbances (particularly hypokalaemia) predispose to QT prolongation and may further increase the risk of QT prolongation: greater caution is therefore warranted in their presence. For some drugs QT prolongation is a fairly frequent effect when the drug is used alone, and it is well accepted that use of these drugs requires careful monitoring (e.g. a number of the antiarrhythmics). Pairs of antiarrhythmics should therefore be avoided where possible. For other drugs, QT prolongation is rare, but because of the relatively benign indications for these drugs, the risk-benefit ratio is considered poor, and use of these drugs has been severely restricted or discontinued (e.g. astemizole, terfenadine, cisapride). For others there is less clear evidence of the risk of QT prolongation and therefore the associated risks of combinations of these types of drug are much lower. Drugs known to have a high risk of causing QT-prolongation include:

- Antiarrhythmics (class Ia: disopyramide, procainamide, quinidine)
- Antiarrhythmics (class III: amiodarone, dronedarone, sotalol)
- Antipsychotics (haloperidol (high dose and intravenous use), pimozide, sertindole, thioridazine)
- Arsenic trioxide
- Artemether

Drugs known to be associated with some risk of causing QT-prolongation include:

- Antipsychotics (amisulpride, chlorpromazine, droperidol, levomepromazine, pali-peridone, ziprasidone)
- Antidepressants (citalopram, escitalopram, clomipramine; risk with other tricyclics appears to be mainly in overdose)
- 5-HT_3-receptor antagonists (dolasetron and ondansetron, although all 5-HT_3-receptor antagonists have been associated with QT-interval prolongation, but the evidence is variable—see Drugs that prolong the QT interval + 5-HT_3-receptor antagonists, page 353)

- Methadone (doses greater than 100 mg)
- Pasireotide
- Quinolones (gatifloxacin, moxifloxacin, sparfloxacin)
- Quinine
- Ranolazine
- Saquinavir boosted with ritonavir
- Sildenafil
- Tolterodine
- Vardenafil

In some instances drugs have been associated with QT prolongation and the risk is difficult to categorize. For some drugs there appears to be a strong likelihood of QT prolongation whereas for others warnings appear to represent a cautious approach on the part of the manufacturers. Such drugs include:

- Atomoxetine, post-marketing reports of QT prolongation
- Clarithromycin, post-marketing reports of QT prolongation
- Clozapine, post-marketing reports of QT prolongation
- Erythromycin (greater risk with intravenous use)
- Lithium, particularly if concentrations increased
- Lofexidine; post-marketing reports of QT prolongation
- Olanzapine, based on the effect seen with other antipsychotics
- Pentamidine (intravenous use)
- Quetiapine, data inconclusive
- Risperidone, based on a possible effect with paliperidone
- Solifenacin, post-marketing reports of QT prolongation
- Spiramycin
- Tizanidine, based on chronic toxicity studies in *animals*
- Trazodone, post-marketing reports of QT prolongation
- Zuclopenthixol, QT prolongation seen in overdose

Further, hypokalaemia increases the risks of torsade de pointes arrhythmias and so potassium concentrations should be closely monitored when drugs that can cause hypokalaemia are used with drugs that prolong the QT interval. However, there appear to be very few reports of this interaction. Drugs known to lower potassium concentrations include:

- Amphotericin B
- Corticosteroids
- Loop diuretics
- Salbutamol (Albuterol) and related bronchodilators
- Stimulant laxatives (in abuse or overuse)
- Theophylline
- Thiazide diuretics

Drugs that prolong the QT interval + 5-HT₃-receptor antagonists ⊗

It is generally considered that the 5-HT₃-receptor antagonists as a class have the propensity to increase the QT interval, which could theoretically be additive with the effects of other drugs that also prolong the QT interval, but the evidence is variable. Dolasetron and ondansetron are both known to prolong the QT interval (see Drugs that prolong the QT interval, page 352) however studies have found that granisetron, palonosetron, and tropisteron did not increase the QT interval. Nevertheless, the manufacturers of the 5-HT₃-receptor antagonists note that they have been associated with QT prolongation, either specifically or as a class, and they give differing guidance about the concurrent use of the 5-HT$_3$-receptor antagonists together with other drugs that prolong the QT interval. For more general information about this effect, see Drugs that prolong the QT interval, page 352.

Both the UK and US manufacturers of granisetron advise caution with other drugs known to cause QT prolongation. The UK manufacturer of palonosetron recommends caution with antiarrhythmics and other drugs that prolong the QT interval, or cause electrolyte abnormalities. The Australian manufacturer of tropisetron recommends care when it is used with other drugs that are likely to prolong the QT interval.

D

Duloxetine

Duloxetine + Flecainide ▲

Duloxetine (a moderate inhibitor of CYP2D6) may inhibit the metabolism of flecainide (a substrate for CYP2D6), increasing the risk of flecainide adverse effects.

The manufacturer advises caution. It would seem prudent to closely monitor for flecainide adverse effects.

Duloxetine + Herbal medicines or Dietary supplements ▲

Concurrent use of duloxetine and St John's wort (*Hypericum perforatum*) may lead to serotonin syndrome, page 580. One possible case has been reported.

The manufacturers advise caution. Monitor concurrent use carefully for symptoms including agitation, confusion and tremor.

Duloxetine + Linezolid ▲

In theory the use of duloxetine and linezolid might result in serotonin syndrome. A case report describes a patient who developed symptoms similar to serotonin syndrome while taking these drugs.

The interaction is probably rare. The UK manufacturer contraindicates concurrent use unless patients are closely observed for signs and symptoms of serotonin syndrome, and have their blood pressure monitored.

Duloxetine + Lithium ▲

The concurrent use of duloxetine with lithium may lead to serotonin syndrome, page 580.

The manufacturers advise caution. Monitor concurrent use carefully for symptoms including agitation, confusion and tremor.

Duloxetine + MAOIs

The concurrent use of MAOIs and duloxetine may lead to serotonin syndrome, page 580.

The manufacturers contraindicate the use of duloxetine with non-selective irreversible MAOIs, during and for 14 days after discontinuing an MAOI. At least 5 days should be allowed after stopping duloxetine before starting an MAOI.

Duloxetine + MAO-B inhibitors

Rasagiline

Cases of serotonin syndrome, page 580 have been reported when rasagiline was given with antidepressants (such as duloxetine).

The UK manufacturer of rasagiline advises caution, whereas the US manufacturer advises against the concurrent use of antidepressants, including the SNRIs, and for 14 days after stopping rasagiline. Patients should be monitored for signs and symptoms of serotonin syndrome (such as flushing, ataxia, tremor, hyperthermia, agitation and confusion).

Selegiline

Cases of serotonin syndrome, page 580 have been reported when selegiline was given with antidepressants (such as duloxetine).

The manufacturers of selegiline contraindicate the concurrent use of the SNRIs. A 2-week washout period would seem appropriate when switching from one of these drugs to the other.

Duloxetine + Moclobemide

There is a possible risk of serotonin syndrome, page 580, if duloxetine is used with moclobemide; one case has been reported.

The manufacturers advise against concurrent use but give no specific advice about a washout period, but, based on other interactions, it would seem prudent to wait for 5 days after duloxetine is stopped before starting the other drug. It has been suggested that no washout is needed after moclobemide, but others consider a 24-hour washout a prudent measure.

Duloxetine + Opioids

The concurrent use of duloxetine with tramadol or pethidine (meperidine) may lead to serotonin syndrome, page 580.

The manufacturers advise caution. Monitor concurrent use carefully for symptoms including agitation, confusion and tremor.

Duloxetine + Prasugrel

The bleeding risk associated with antiplatelet drugs such as prasugrel might be further increased by the concurrent use of an SSRI, although the data appears to be conflicting. SNRIs (e.g. duloxetine) are expected to interact similarly.

The manufacturer of duloxetine advises caution on concurrent use in patients taking antiplatelet drugs (such as prasugrel). Consider giving gastroprotective drugs to those at high risk of gastrointestinal bleeding (e.g. the elderly, those with a history of gastrointestinal bleeding, patients taking multiple antiplatelet drugs). Advise patients to report any signs of excessive bleeding.

Duloxetine + Propafenone

Duloxetine (a moderate inhibitor of CYP2D6) may inhibit the metabolism of propafenone (a substrate for CYP2D6), increasing the risk of propafenone adverse effects.

If the combination is used it would be prudent to closely monitor for propafenone adverse effects (such as postural hypotension, bradycardia, urinary retention, etc.).

Duloxetine + Quinidine

Inhibitors of CYP2D6 are expected to increase duloxetine levels. This has been seen with *fluoxetine* and is predicted to occur with quinidine.

The manufacturer advises caution on concurrent use. Monitor for duloxetine adverse effects, which include nausea, dry mouth, and hot flushes.

Duloxetine + Quinolones

Potent inhibitors of CYP1A2 are expected to increase duloxetine levels. A 6-fold increase has been seen with *fluvoxamine* and is predicted to occur with quinolones (e.g. ciprofloxacin and enoxacin).

The manufacturer advises that concurrent use should be avoided. Note that the quinolones may interact to varying extents, see quinolones, page 564.

Duloxetine + SSRIs

Fluvoxamine

The concurrent use of duloxetine and an SSRI may result in serotonin syndrome, page 580. Fluvoxamine increases duloxetine exposure 6-fold.

The manufacturers contraindicate concurrent use.

Other SSRIs

The concurrent use of duloxetine and an SSRI may result in serotonin syndrome, page 580. Low-dose paroxetine caused a modest increase in the AUC of duloxetine, and fluoxetine is predicted to interact similarly.

The manufacturers of duloxetine advise caution on the concurrent use of SSRIs. Monitor concurrent use carefully for symptoms including agitation, confusion and tremor.

Duloxetine + Ticagrelor ❓

The bleeding risk associated with antiplatelet drugs might be further increased by the concurrent use of an SNRI, such as duloxetine.

> The manufacturer of duloxetine advises caution on concurrent use in patients taking antiplatelet drugs (such as ticagrelor). Consider giving gastroprotective drugs to those at high risk of gastrointestinal bleeding (e.g. the elderly, those with a history of gastrointestinal bleeding, patients taking multiple antiplatelet drugs). Advise patients to report any signs of excessive bleeding.

Duloxetine + Ticlopidine ❓

The bleeding risk associated with antiplatelet drugs such as ticlopidine might be further increased by the concurrent use of an SSRI, although the data appears to be conflicting. SNRIs (e.g. duloxetine) are expected to interact similarly.

> The manufacturer of duloxetine advises caution on concurrent use in patients taking antiplatelet drugs (such as ticlopidine). Consider giving gastroprotective drugs to those at high risk of gastrointestinal bleeding (e.g. the elderly, those with a history of gastrointestinal bleeding, patients taking multiple antiplatelet drugs). Advise patients to report any signs of excessive bleeding.

Duloxetine + Tricyclics ⚠

Duloxetine markedly increases the AUC of desipramine. Other tricyclics metabolised by CYP2D6, such as nortriptyline, amitriptyline and imipramine, may interact similarly. The use of duloxetine with other serotonergic drugs, such as the tricyclics, may increase the risk of serotonin syndrome, page 580.

> The manufacturer advises caution on concurrent use. Monitor for tricyclic adverse effects (blurred vision, dry mouth, confusion), and for signs of serotonin syndrome. Patients should report symptoms including agitation, confusion and tremor.

Duloxetine + Triptans ⚠

Concurrent use of duloxetine and the triptans (e.g. sumatriptan) might lead to serotonin syndrome, page 580: cases have been reported to the FDA in the US.

> The combination need not be avoided, but monitor carefully for signs of serotonin syndrome (such as weakness, hyperreflexia, and incoordination), especially during treatment initiation and dose increases, and if other serotonergic drugs are used.

Duloxetine + Tryptophan ⚠

Concurrent use of duloxetine and tryptophan may lead to serotonin syndrome, page 580.

> The UK manufacturers advise caution with concurrent use (e.g. be alert for symptoms including agitation, confusion and tremor); however, the US manufacturer advises avoiding concurrent use.

Duloxetine + **Warfarin and related oral anticoagulants**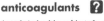

A study in healthy subjects found no clinically relevant interaction on the concurrent use of duloxetine and warfarin; however, a case report describes a markedly raised INR in a patient taking warfarin when duloxetine was also given, and another case report describes a decrease in INR with acenocoumarol when duloxetine was given. Note that SNRIs alone have, rarely, been associated with bleeding, and there is the theoretical possibility that the risk might be increased when used with warfarin and related drugs.

> The general relevance of the isolated case reports is uncertain. Consider increasing INR monitoring if duloxetine is added or withdrawn from treatment with warfarin or any coumarin. Also bear in mind the possibility of increased bleeding risk in the absence of alterations in INR.

D

Dutasteride

Dutasteride + **HIV-protease inhibitors**

Moderate CYP3A4 inhibitors increase dutasteride levels by 60 to 80%, which, due to the wide safety margin of dutasteride, is not thought to be clinically significant. However, potent CYP3A4 inhibitors, such as the HIV-protease inhibitors (particularly indinavir and ritonavir), would be expected to have a larger effect, which may cause a clinically significant rise in dutasteride levels.

> The manufacturers suggest reducing the dosing frequency if increased dutasteride adverse effects occur.

Dutasteride + **Testosterone**

Testosterone is poorly bioavailable by the oral route, and is rapidly metabolised to dihydrotestosterone by 5-alpha reductase. By inhibiting this enzyme, dutasteride reduces the formation of dihydrotestosterone and increases the exposure to oral testosterone.

> Dutasteride might be useful in increasing testosterone oral bioavailability for oral replacement therapy. No action needed.

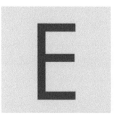

Elvitegravir

Elvitegravir + Herbal medicines or Dietary supplements

St John's wort (*Hypericum perforatum*) is predicted to decrease elvitegravir plasma concentrations, which might reduce its efficacy.

The US manufacturer of elvitegravir boosted with cobicistat (in a fixed-dose combination also including emtricitabine and tenofovir) contraindicates concurrent use.

Elvitegravir + HIV-protease inhibitors

Low-dose ritonavir very markedly increases elvitegravir exposure.

The US manufacturer of elvitegravir boosted with cobicistat (in a fixed-dose combination also including emtricitabine and tenofovir disoproxil fumarate) states that this product should not be given with ritonavir or other products containing ritonavir because of the similar action of cobicistat and ritonavir on CYP3A4. They also state that it should not be given with HIV-protease inhibitors.

Elvitegravir + Maraviroc

Elvitegravir boosted with ritonavir moderately increases maraviroc exposure.

When elvitegravir, boosted with either ritonavir or cobicistat, is given to a patient taking maraviroc, the maraviroc dose should be reduced to 150 mg daily.

Elvitegravir + Orlistat

Orlistat might reduce the absorption of antiretroviral drugs, such as elvitegravir, resulting in reduced efficacy.

Monitoring of antiretroviral drug concentrations, if concurrent use is considered essential, would seem sensible. Further, the MHRA in the UK advises that orlistat should only be started after careful consideration of the possible impact it might have on the efficacy of antiretroviral medicines.

Elvitegravir + **Oxcarbazepine**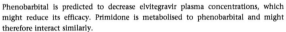

Oxcarbazepine is predicted to decrease elvitegravir plasma concentrations, which might reduce its efficacy.

The UK manufacturer of elvitegravir with cobicistat (in a fixed-dose combination also including emtricitabine and tenofovir) contraindicates concurrent use. Consider an alternative to oxcarbazepine.

Elvitegravir + **Phenobarbital** ⊗

Phenobarbital is predicted to decrease elvitegravir plasma concentrations, which might reduce its efficacy. Primidone is metabolised to phenobarbital and might therefore interact similarly.

The UK manufacturer of elvitegravir with cobicistat (in a fixed-dose combination also including emtricitabine and tenofovir) contraindicates concurrent use. Consider an alternative to phenobarbital.

Elvitegravir + **Phenytoin** ⊗

Phenytoin is predicted to decrease elvitegravir plasma concentrations, which might reduce its efficacy. Fosphenytoin, a prodrug of phenytoin, might interact similarly.

The UK manufacturer of elvitegravir with cobicistat (in a fixed-dose combination also including emtricitabine and tenofovir) contraindicates concurrent use. Consider an alternative to phenytoin.

Elvitegravir + **Rifabutin** ⚠

Elvitegravir exposure is reduced by rifabutin, and rifabutin exposure is increased by elvitegravir with cobicistat.

If both drugs are given, monitor for reduced elvitegravir efficacy and an increase in rifabutin adverse effects (such as leucopenia, uveitis, and arthralgia). The US manufacturer of a combination preparation containing elvitegravir and cobicistat (with emtricitabine and tenofovir) advises that concurrent use of rifabutin with elvitegravir boosted with cobicistat is not recommended due to the risk of reduced antiviral efficacy.

Elvitegravir + **Rifampicin (Rifampin)** ⊗

Rifampicin is predicted to decrease elvitegravir concentrations.

The US manufacturer of a combination preparation containing elvitegravir and cobicistat (with emtricitabine and tenofovir) contraindicates concurrent use.

Elvitegravir + **Warfarin and related oral anticoagulants**

Elvitegravir is predicted to increase warfarin concentrations.

Monitor the INR to ensure warfarin remains effective, adjusting the warfarin dose as necessary.

Endothelin receptor antagonists

Endothelin receptor antagonists + **Gestrinone**

The manufacturers warn that *rifampicin (rifampin)* might increase the metabolism of gestrinone and thereby reduce its effects. Other enzyme inducers, such as bosentan, might interact similarly.

The clinical significance of this warning is unclear and there appear to be no reports of an interaction in practice; however, be aware that gestrinone might be less effective if bosentan is given concurrently.

Endothelin receptor antagonists + **HIV-protease inhibitors**

Lopinavir boosted with ritonavir markedly increases bosentan exposure. Other HIV-protease inhibitors boosted with ritonavir, and saquinavir alone, are predicted to interact similarly. A case of subtherapeutic indinavir concentrations has been reported in a patient after he started to take bosentan. .

Concurrent use should be closely monitored for antiviral efficacy and bosentan adverse effects (e.g. oedema, liver function test abnormalities), adjusting the bosentan dose as necessary. For indinavir or nelfinavir, reduce the bosentan dose to 62.5 mg daily or on alternate days. For patients already established on other HIV-protease inhibitors for at least 10 days, a similar bosentan starting dose is advised. In those already taking bosentan, the bosentan should be stopped for 36 hours before starting an HIV-protease inhibitor, and restarted after the HIV-protease inhibitors has been given for at least 10 days at this reduced dose.

Endothelin receptor antagonists + **HRT**

The hormones in HRT are similar to those used in hormonal contraceptives, page 291, and so may be affected by enzyme-inducing drugs, such as bosentan, in the same way.

The clinical significance of any interaction is unclear; however, consider the possibility of reduced HRT efficacy on concurrent use. This effect is most noticeable where HRT is prescribed for menopausal vasomotor symptoms, but might be difficult to detect where the indication is osteoporosis. The interaction is not relevant to HRT applied locally for menopausal vaginitis.

Endothelin receptor antagonists + **Phosphodiesterase type-5 inhibitors**

Bosentan markedly reduces the exposure to sildenafil (by about 70%) and modestly reduces the exposure to tadalafil (by about 40%). Bosentan exposure is modestly reduced by sildenafil, but are not affected to a clinically relevant extent by tadalafil. Bosentan is predicted to reduce the exposure to avanafil.

> The efficacy of sildenafil and tadalafil might be reduced in patients taking bosentan, and should be closely monitored. Sildenafil might increase the effects of bosentan, therefore patients should be monitored for signs of bosentan adverse effects such as flushing, headache and oedema. Tadalafil is unlikely to have this effect. The UK manufacturer of avanafil contraindicates concurrent use with bosentan due to the potential loss of efficacy.

Endothelin receptor antagonists + **Rifampicin (Rifampin)**

Ambrisentan

When rifampicin is initially given simultaneously with ambrisentan, ambrisentan exposure is slightly increased, whereas at steady-state rifampicin has no effect on ambrisentan exposure.

> Be alert for an increase in ambrisentan adverse effects (such as headache and peripheral oedema) on the initial concurrent use of rifampicin. Any increase in adverse effects would be expected to resolve after the first week.

Bosentan

Rifampicin might cause transient increases in the minimum concentrations of bosentan, but at steady-state rifampicin, bosentan exposure is decreased. The UK manufacturer warns that the risk of liver impairment might be increased on concurrent use.

> The UK manufacturer of bosentan does not recommend that concurrent use. The US manufacturer of bosentan recommends weekly monitoring of hepatic function for the first 4 weeks after starting rifampicin.

Endothelin receptor antagonists + **Sirolimus**

The concurrent use of sirolimus with bosentan has not been studied. Based on the information available for ciclosporin, page 253 the manufacturers suggest that an interaction is possible.

> The UK manufacturer of bosentan advises against concurrent use, but if this is required, close monitoring of bosentan adverse effects and immunosuppressant levels is recommended.

Endothelin receptor antagonists + **Statins**

Bosentan slightly reduces the exposure to simvastatin and its active metabolite, which could lead to a reduction in simvastatin efficacy. Lovastatin might be similarly affected by bosentan, but any effect on atorvastatin is likely to be smaller.

Monitor the outcome of concurrent use to ensure that these statins are effective.

Endothelin receptor antagonists + Tacrolimus

The concurrent use of tacrolimus with bosentan has not been studied. Based on the information available for ciclosporin, page 253 the manufacturers suggest that an interaction is possible.

The UK manufacturer of bosentan advises against concurrent use, but if this is required, close monitoring of bosentan adverse effects and immunosuppressant levels is recommended.

Endothelin receptor antagonists + Ulipristal

The UK and US manufacturers of ulipristal predict that CYP3A4 inducers might reduce the plasma concentration of ulipristal and reduce its efficacy. Bosentan would be expected to interact in this way.

The US manufacturer of ulipristal gives no specific advice about how to manage this potential interaction, whereas the UK manufacturer advises that ulipristal should not be used for emergency contraception in women taking CYP3A4 inducers (such as bosentan), or who have stopped taking an enzyme inducer within the last 2 to 3 weeks. Until more is known, this advice seems prudent.

Endothelin receptor antagonists + Warfarin and related oral anticoagulants

Bosentan appears to cause a modest reduction in warfarin levels, which may result in an increase in warfarin requirements in some patients.

It is recommended that the INR should be closely monitored in any patient taking warfarin during the period that bosentan is started or stopped, or if the dose is altered. Other coumarins should be similarly monitored until further information is available.

Entacapone or Tolcapone

Entacapone or Tolcapone + Inotropes and Vasopressors

Entacapone potentiated the increase in heart rate and arrhythmogenic effects of isoprenaline (isoproterenol) and adrenaline (epinephrine) in a study in healthy subjects. Tolcapone would be expected to interact similarly.

The manufacturers of entacapone and tolcapone suggest caution on the concur-

E

rent use of drugs such as adrenaline (epinephrine), dobutamine, dopamine, isoprenaline (isoproterenol) and noradrenaline (norepinephrine). The use of these drugs is usually closely monitored, but be aware that drug levels and effects may be greater than expected.

Entacapone or Tolcapone + Iron

Entacapone forms chelates with iron *in vitro*.

The manufacturer recommends that iron preparations and entacapone are given 2 to 3 hours apart.

Entacapone or Tolcapone + MAOIs

In theory, the concurrent use of entacapone or tolcapone and an MAOI may result in hypertension.

Concurrent use is contraindicated.

Entacapone or Tolcapone + Mirtazapine

Both COMT inhibitors and drugs with noradrenaline re-uptake inhibitory activity (the manufacturers of tolcapone name mirtazapine) can impair the inactivation of catecholamines, so in theory the effects of catecholamines may be increased by concurrent use. This may lead to increases in blood pressure.

The manufacturers advise caution on concurrent use, but note that studies with the tricyclics, which were predicted to interact similarly, suggest that no adverse interaction occurs.

Entacapone or Tolcapone + Moclobemide

In a single dose study, there was no adverse effect on heart rate or blood pressure when entacapone was given with moclobemide.

The manufacturers of entacapone and tolcapone recommend caution until further clinical experience is gained.

Entacapone or Tolcapone + Tricyclics

Studies suggest that no important interaction occurs between entacapone and imipramine or between tolcapone and desipramine.

Despite these studies, the manufacturer of entacapone recommends caution as there is limited clinical experience of the use of entacapone with a tricyclic antidepressant. Similarly, the manufacturers of tolcapone suggest that caution should be exercised if desipramine is taken concurrently.

E

Entacapone or Tolcapone + **Venlafaxine**

Both COMT inhibitors and drugs with noradrenaline re-uptake inhibitory activity (the manufacturers of tolcapone name venlafaxine) can impair the inactivation of catecholamines, so in theory the effects of catecholamines may be increased by concurrent use. This may lead to increases in blood pressure.

The manufacturers advise caution on concurrent use, but note that studies with the tricyclics, which were predicted to interact similarly, suggest that no adverse interaction occurs.

Entacapone or Tolcapone + **Warfarin and related oral anticoagulants**

Entacapone slightly increases *R*-warfarin levels and causes a slight increase in INR of 13%, which is unlikely to be generally relevant. Tolcapone is not expected to interact with warfarin, but this needs confirmation.

The manufacturer of entacapone advises monitoring the INR if patients taking warfarin are given entacapone. Similar advice is given for tolcapone (due to the lack of clinical data).

E

Enteral feeds

Consider also the interactions of food.

Enteral feeds + **Phenytoin**

A 70% reduction in phenytoin absorption has been described when it is given with enteral feeds (e.g. *Isocal, Jevity*) administered via nasogastric or jejunostomy tubes.

This interaction has been managed by giving the phenytoin diluted in water 2 hours after stopping the feed, flushing with 60 mL of water, and waiting another 2 hours before restarting the feed. However, one study found this method unsuccessful. Other suggestions include waiting 6 hours after the phenytoin dose before restarting the feed, stopping continuous feed 1 hour rather than 2 hours before and after phenytoin administration, the use of twice daily phenytoin or the use of intravenous phenytoin. Monitor the outcome carefully. The same problem can also occur when enteral feeds are given by a jejunostomy tube but methods to manage this are not established.

Enteral feeds + **Quinolones**

The absorption of ciprofloxacin can be as much as halved by enteral feeds such as *Ensure, Jevity, Osmolite, Pulmocare* and *Sustacal*.

No treatment failures have been reported but this interaction is expected to be clinically important. Monitor the outcome of concurrent use carefully.

Enteral feeds + **Sucralfate**

Sucralfate can interact with the protein component of enteral feeds within the oesophagus to produce an obstructive plug (a bezoar).

The manufacturers recommend separating the administration of sucralfate suspension and enteral feeds given by nasogastric tube by one hour.

Enteral feeds + **Theophylline**

Clinically relevant reductions in theophylline concentration have been seen in some patients given enteral feeds (a reduction of 50% was seen in one case).

Avoiding giving enteral feeds for one hour either side of theophylline seems to be an effective way of managing this interaction, but it would still be prudent to monitor the outcome on theophylline concentrations and adjust the dose as necessary. Not all preparations of theophylline are necessarily affected, but there is insufficient evidence to identify those that may be a problem.

E

Enteral feeds + **Warfarin and related oral anticoagulants**

Enteral feeds might contain sufficient vitamin K_1 (commonly about 4 to 10 micrograms per 100 mL) to antagonise the effects of warfarin and other vitamin K antagonists.

Starting, stopping, or changing between different enteral feeds might affect dose requirements of vitamin K antagonists (coumarins and indanediones). It is also possible that there is a local interaction in the gut, as in one case separating the administration of the warfarin and an enteral feed by 3 hours or more was effective. Limited evidence suggests that withholding the enteral feed for an hour before and after warfarin administration might slightly reduce the effect of any interaction. Nevertheless, patients should be advised not to add or substitute dietary supplements such as *Ensure* without increased monitoring of their coagulation status.

Ergot derivatives

Ergot derivatives + **Grapefruit juice**

Grapefruit juice is predicted to increase the exposure to ergot derivatives (by inhibiting CYP3A4), which could lead to ergot toxicity.

If concurrent use is unavoidable advise patients to report any coldness, numbness or tingling of the hands and feet.

Ergot derivatives + H₂-receptor antagonists

Cimetidine is predicted to increase the exposure to ergot derivatives (by inhibiting CYP3A4), which could lead to ergot toxicity.

> If concurrent use is unavoidable advise patients to report any coldness, numbness or tingling of the hands and feet.

Ergot derivatives + HIV-protease inhibitors

A patient taking indinavir rapidly developed ergotism after taking usual doses of ergotamine. Several other patients taking ritonavir with ergotamine have had the same reaction. A patient taking nelfinavir developed peripheral arterial vasoconstriction after taking ergotamine. Other ergot derivatives and HIV-protease inhibitors are predicted to interact similarly.

> Concurrent use is generally contraindicated.

Ergot derivatives + Macrolides

Ergot toxicity can develop rapidly in patients taking ergotamine or dihydroergotamine if they are given erythromycin, clarithromycin, and probably telithromycin. Cases of toxicity have also been reported with josamycin and toxicity is predicted to occur with midecamycin. No cases of toxicity appear to have been reported with azithromycin; nevertheless, the manufacturers suggest an interaction could occur.

> The combination of ergot derivatives and macrolides that inhibit CYP3A4 is best avoided. Note that the macrolides differ in their ability to inhibit CYP3A4, see macrolides, page 474.

Ergot derivatives + NNRTIs

Delavirdine, a CYP3A4 inhibitor, is predicted to inhibit the metabolism of ergot derivatives, which might result in the development of ergotism. Efavirenz is usually considered to be a CYP3A4 *inducer*, and therefore would be expected to increase the metabolism of the ergot derivatives; however, some have predicted that it might have the opposite effect.

> The concurrent use of ergot derivatives with delavirdine or efavirenz is contraindicated; however, the clinical relevance of the predicted interaction with efavirenz is unclear.

Ergot derivatives + Reboxetine

The UK manufacturer of reboxetine suggests that concurrent use with ergot derivatives might result in increased blood pressure, although no clinical data are quoted.

> The general significance of this interaction is unclear; however, bear it in mind should a patient develop an increase in blood pressure, particularly when either the ergot derivative or reboxetine is newly started.

Ergot derivatives + **Rifampicin (Rifampin)**

Rifampicin is predicted to increase the metabolism of ergot derivatives, and might therefore be expected to reduce their efficacy. Note that rifampicin has been used as a potent enzyme inducer to reduce ergotamine levels in a patient with ergotism.

It might be prudent to consider an alternative antimigraine treatment, such as one of the triptans not metabolised by CYP3A4. However, if concurrent use is necessary, monitor the efficacy of the ergot derivative.

Ergot derivatives + **SSRIs**

Isolated cases of serotonin syndrome have been seen in patients taking paroxetine (with imipramine), or sertraline, when they were also given dihydroergotamine. Fluoxetine and fluvoxamine are predicted to decrease the metabolism of the ergot derivatives, possibly by inhibiting CYP3A4, which might result in ergot toxicity.

These cases of serotonin syndrome appear to be isolated and not of general importance. Nevertheless, they illustrate the potential for the development of serotonin syndrome, page 580 in patients given multiple drugs that affect serotonin receptors. Patients should be advised to report signs of ergot toxicity (such as coldness, numbness or tingling of the hands and feet) on concurrent use with fluoxetine and fluvoxamine.

Ergot derivatives + **Tetracyclines**

Several patients taking ergotamine or dihydroergotamine developed ergotism when they were also given doxycycline or tetracycline. In some patients concurrent illnesses, including liver impairment might have been a contributory factor.

An interaction is not established; however, consider an interaction if signs of ergotism (such as nausea, vomiting, diarrhoea, cold hands or feet) develop. Note that one UK manufacturer of ergotamine recommends that the concurrent use of tetracycline should be avoided.

Ergot derivatives + **Ticagrelor**

Ticagrelor might increase the exposure to the ergot derivatives.

If concurrent use is unavoidable, be alert for symptoms of ergotism (such as numb, cold or tingling extremities).

Ergot derivatives + **Triptans**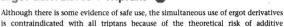

Although there is some evidence of safe use, the simultaneous use of ergot derivatives is contraindicated with all triptans because of the theoretical risk of additive vasoconstriction.

In the UK, the manufacturers of sumatriptan state that ergotamine should not be given less than 6 hours after taking sumatriptan, and recommend that sumatriptan should not be taken less than 24 hours after taking ergotamine. Similar recommendations are made by the UK manufacturers of almotriptan, rizatriptan, and zolmitriptan, whereas the UK manufacturers of eletriptan, frovatriptan and naratriptan recommend that ergot derivatives are not given for a minimum of 24 hours (not just 6 hours) after these triptans. In general, in the US, it is recommended that triptans and ergotamine or ergot-type medication should not be taken within 24 hours of each other.

Ergot derivatives + Zileuton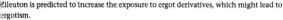

Zileuton is predicted to increase the exposure to ergot derivatives, which might lead to ergotism.

If concurrent use is unavoidable, advise patients to report coldness, numbness or tingling of the hands and feet.

Ertapenem

E

Ertapenem + Valproate

Ertapenem appears to dramatically and rapidly reduce valproate serum concentrations, resulting in increased seizure frequency.

Avoid concurrent use if possible. If it is essential, consider using intravenous valproate (which has been successfully substituted in some cases) and monitor valproate serum concentrations closely, adjusting the valproate dose if necessary. Consider using another antibacterial, or an alternative to valproate; limited evidence suggests that carbamazepine and phenytoin do not interact. Note that ertapenem should be used with caution in patients with a history of seizures.

Eslicarbazepine

Eslicarbazepine + MAOIs

The use of *tricyclics*, page 491 and MAOIs results in a serious potentially fatal adverse reaction. Eslicarbazepine is structurally related to the tricyclics and may therefore interact similarly.

Avoid concurrent use. It is usual to wait until 2 weeks after an MAOI is stopped before starting a potentially interacting drug.

Eslicarbazepine + Phenobarbital ?

Eslicarbazepine does not appear to affect phenobarbital concentrations, but barbiturates might increase eslicarbazepine clearance.

Be aware of the possible need to increase the eslicarbazepine dose if phenobarbital is also given.

Eslicarbazepine + Phenytoin ⚠

Exposure to phenytoin is increased by eslicarbazepine and exposure to eslicarbazepin is reduced by phenytoin. Fosphenytoin, a prodrug of phenytoin, might interac similarly.

> Monitor the plasma concentration of both drugs on concurrent use, and adjust the doses as necessary.

Eslicarbazepine + Statins ⚠

Eslicarbazepine moderately reduces simvastatin exposure. Other statins metabolised i the same way as simvastatin (lovastatin, and to a lesser extent, atorvastatin) might b similarly affected.

> A simvastatin dose increase seems likely to be necessary. Monitor concurrent use to check that simvastatin is effective. Until more is known it would seem prudent to follow the same advice for lovastatin and probably atorvastatin.

Eslicarbazepine + Ulipristal ⚠

The UK and US manufacturers of ulipristal predict that CYP3A4 inducers, such a eslicarbazepine, might reduce the plasma concentration of ulipristal and reduce i efficacy.

> The US manufacturer of ulipristal gives no specific advice about how to manage this potential interaction, whereas the UK manufacturer advises that ulipristal should not be used for emergency contraception in women taking CYP3A4 inducers (such as eslicarbazepine), or who have stopped taking an enzyme inducer within the last 2 to 3 weeks. Until more is known, this advice seems prudent.

Eslicarbazepine + Warfarin and related oral anticoagulants

Eslicarbazepine appears to cause a small decrease in exposure to S-warfarin but no R-warfarin.

> It would seem prudent to increase monitoring of the INR when starting or stopping eslicarbazepine, and this is recommended by the UK manufacturer of eslicarbazepine.

Ethosuximide

Ethosuximide + HIV-protease inhibitors ⚠

Ritonavir is predicted to increase ethosuximide concentrations.

> The US manufacturer of ritonavir advises that a dose reduction of ethosuximide may be needed and monitoring of ethosuximide concentrations is recommended, if available.

Ethosuximide + Isoniazid

A single report describes a patient who developed psychotic behaviour and signs of ethosuximide toxicity when concurrently treated with isoniazid.

> The clinical importance of this interaction is unknown, but bear it in mind in case of an unexpected response to treatment. Indicators of ethosuximide toxicity include nausea, vomiting, anorexia and insomnia.

Ethosuximide + Orlistat

The MHRA in the UK suggests that the absorption of antiepileptics might be decreased by orlistat, leading to a loss of seizure control.

> Although an interaction has not been established, the MHRA advises that patients should be monitored for changes in the severity or frequency of convulsions, and consideration given to separating the administration of orlistat and the antiepileptic.

E

Ethosuximide + Phenobarbital

Primidone modestly lowers ethosuximide levels and possibly shortens its half-life. Similarly, phenobarbital has been reported both to reduce and not affect the half-life of ethosuximide. Phenobarbital levels (derived from primidone) do not appear to be affected by ethosuximide.

> A clinically relevant interaction seems unlikely in most patients; however, consider monitoring the effect of concurrent use and increase the dose of ethosuximide if necessary.

Ethosuximide + Phenytoin

Three cases have occurred in which ethosuximide appeared to have been responsible for increasing phenytoin levels, leading to the development of phenytoin toxicity in 2 patients. Phenytoin may reduce the half-life of ethosuximide but not all studies have found this. Fosphenytoin, a prodrug of phenytoin, may interact similarly.

> Warn the patient to monitor for indicators of phenytoin toxicity (blurred vision, nystagmus, ataxia or drowsiness). Take phenytoin levels as necessary, and monitor the effectiveness of ethosuximide treatment.

Ethosuximide + Sodium oxybate

The UK manufacturer of sodium oxybate predicts that ethosuximide might affect its metabolism, however there are no clinical studies to confirm this prediction.

> Monitor concurrent use, and adjust the dose of sodium oxybate as needed.

Ethosuximide + Valproate

Sodium valproate has increased the levels of ethosuximide by about 50%. Sedation occurred and ethosuximide dose reductions were necessary. However, other studies have described no changes or even reduced ethosuximide levels when valproate was also given. Ethosuximide may also lower valproate levels.

Monitor the effects of concurrent use for adverse effects such as sedation, and efficacy, adjusting the ethosuximide dose and increasing the valproate dose accordingly. Valproate levels may be helpful.

Etoposide

Etoposide + Phenobarbital ⚠

Etoposide clearance appears to be increased by almost 80% by phenobarbital, and this may result in reduced efficacy. Note that primidone is metabolised to phenobarbital and therefore may interact similarly.

Monitor the outcome of concurrent use and be alert for the possible need to give larger doses of etoposide.

Etoposide + Phenytoin ⚠

Etoposide clearance appears to be increased by almost 80% by phenytoin, and this may result in reduced efficacy. Fosphenytoin, a prodrug of phenytoin, may interact similarly.

Monitor the outcome of concurrent use and be alert for the possible need to give larger doses of etoposide.

Etoposide + Warfarin and related oral anticoagulants ❓

Etoposide, as part of several different antineoplastic regimens, has been seen to increase the INR of patients taking warfarin.

These are isolated cases, and no specific drug interaction is established. Nevertheless, other factors due to the disease or patient might alter the response to anticoagulants. Therefore, the anticoagulant doses might need adjustment. Note that, from a disease perspective, when treating venous thromboembolic disease in patients with cancer, warfarin is generally inferior (higher risk of major bleeds and recurrent thrombosis) to low-molecular-weight heparins.

Everolimus

Everolimus + Grapefruit juice ⚠

Grapefruit juice is predicted to increase everolimus concentrations.

The concurrent use of grapefruit juice is not recommended with everolimus because the effect of the expected increases in everolimus exposure varies widely. The US manufacturers also extend this recommendation to patients eating whole grapefruit.

Everolimus + H₂-receptor antagonists

Cimetidine is predicted to increase the concentration of everolimus.

Monitor the concentrations and effects (e.g. on renal function) of everolimus more frequently if cimetidine is started or stopped, and adjust the everolimus dose as necessary.

Everolimus + Herbal medicines or Dietary supplements

St John's wort is predicted to reduce the bioavailability and increases the clearance of everolimus.

The UK and US manufacturers recommend avoiding concurrent use. If it is essential, increase the everolimus dose according to the indication for use, and monitor everolimus concentrations closely.

Everolimus + HIV-protease inhibitors

The HIV-protease inhibitors are predicted to increase everolimus concentrations.

Some UK and US manufacturers advise against concurrent use. If it is essential, monitor everolimus concentrations and adverse effects (stomatitis, blood dyscrasias, renal impairment): an everolimus dose reduction is likely to be necessary.

Everolimus + Macrolides

Erythromycin increased everolimus concentrations in one study. Other macrolides probably interact similarly, to varying extents (see macrolides, page 474).

If concurrent use of a macrolide with everolimus is considered necessary, monitor everolimus concentrations and adverse effects (e.g. stomatitis, blood dyscrasias, renal impairment), adjusting the everolimus dose as necessary. Several manufacturers recommend initial everolimus dose reductions.

Everolimus + Metoclopramide ❓

The UK and US manufacturers predict that metoclopramide might increase everolimus concentrations.

The extent of any change in everolimus concentrations is uncertain, and the clinical relevance of any effect is therefore unclear. Bear this potential interactions in mind should an increase in everolimus adverse effects (such as stomatitis, blood dyscrasias, renal impairment) occur.

Everolimus + NNRTIs ⚠

Efavirenz, etravirine, and nevirapine are predicted to increase the metabolism of everolimus.

> If concurrent use is unavoidable, increase the everolimus dose according to the indication for use, and monitor everolimus concentrations closely.

Everolimus + Phenobarbital ⚠

Phenobarbital and primidone are predicted to reduce the bioavailability and increase the clearance of everolimus.

> If concurrent use is unavoidable, increase the everolimus dose according to the indication for use, and monitor everolimus concentrations closely.

Everolimus + Phenytoin ⚠

Phenytoin and its prodrug, fosphenytoin, are predicted to reduce the bioavailability and increase the clearance of everolimus.

> If concurrent use is unavoidable, increase the everolimus dose according to the indication for use, and monitor everolimus concentrations closely.

Everolimus + Rifabutin ⚠

Rifabutin is predicted to reduces the bioavailability and increase the clearance of everolimus.

> If concurrent use is unavoidable, increase the everolimus dose according to the indication for use, and monitor everolimus concentrations closely.

Everolimus + Rifampicin (Rifampin) ⚠

Rifampicin moderately reduces the bioavailability and increases the clearance of everolimus.

> If concurrent use is unavoidable, increase the everolimus dose according to the indication for use, and monitor everolimus concentrations closely.

Everolimus + Vaccines

The body's immune response is suppressed by everolimus. The antibody response to vaccines might be reduced and the use of live attenuated vaccines might result in generalised infection.

> For many inactivated vaccines even the reduced response seen is considered clinically useful and, in the case of renal transplant patients, influenza vaccination is actively recommended. If a vaccine is given, it would be prudent to monitor the response, so that alternative prophylactic measures can be considered where the response is inadequate. Note that even where effective antibody titres are produced, these might not persist as long as in healthy subjects, and more

frequent booster doses might be required. The use of live vaccines is generally considered to be contraindicated. Ideally, vaccines should be given before immunosuppressive treatment is started, and live vaccines should not be given for up to 6 months after treatment has stopped.

Exemestane

Exemestane + Food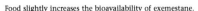

Food slightly increases the bioavailability of exemestane.

The effect of food on the absorption of exemestane is small. Nevertheless, the UK and US manufacturers recommend that exemestane is taken after a meal, presumably to maximise its absorption.

E

Exemestane + Herbal medicines or Dietary supplements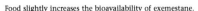

Rifampicin (rifampin) reduces the exposure to exemestane. St John's wort (*Hypericum perforatum*) is predicted to interact similarly.

Monitor concurrent use for reduced exemestane efficacy. The US manufacturer recommends doubling the dose of exemestane to 50 mg daily in patients taking *phenytoin* or *rifampicin*. Similar dose adjustments might be necessary with St John's wort.

Exemestane + HRT

HRT would be expected to oppose the effects of anti-oestrogens such as exemestane.

Oestrogen-containing HRT is generally considered contraindicated in patients with current or a history of breast cancer: the manufacturers of exemestane contraindicate concurrent use. If it is essential, use the lowest HRT dose for the shortest duration: the patient should be fully aware of the potential risks.

Exemestane + Phenobarbital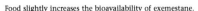

Rifampicin (rifampin) reduces the exposure to exemestane. Phenobarbital (and therefore probably primidone) is predicted to interact similarly.

Monitor concurrent use for reduced exemestane efficacy. The US manufacturer recommends doubling the dose of exemestane to 50 mg daily in patients taking *phenytoin* or *rifampicin*. Similar dose adjustments might be necessary with phenobarbital and primidone.

Exemestane + Phenytoin

Rifampicin (rifampin) reduces the exposure to exemestane. Phenytoin (and therefore probably fosphenytoin) is predicted to interact similarly.

Monitor concurrent use for reduced exemestane efficacy. The US manufacturer suggests doubling the exemestane dose to 50 mg daily in patients taking phenytoin.

Exemestane + Rifampicin (Rifampin)

Rifampicin reduces the exposure to exemestane.

It would seem prudent to monitor concurrent use for reduced exemestane efficacy. The US manufacturer suggests doubling the exemestane dose to 50 mg daily in patients also taking rifampicin.

E

Exemestane + Tibolone

Tibolone appears to increase the risk of recurrent breast cancer in women taking an aromatase inhibitor (such as exemestane).

Concurrent use is not recommended.

Ezetimibe

Ezetimibe + Fibrates

Fenofibrate and gemfibrozil might slightly increase the exposure to ezetimibe, but ezetimibe does not alter fenofibrate or gemfibrozil pharmacokinetics. The concurrent use of ezetimibe and a fibrate is predicted to increase cholesterol excretion into the bile, which increases the risk of gallstone formation.

The pharmacokinetic changes are unlikely to be clinically relevant. The UK and US manufacturers of ezetimibe state that the safety of concurrent use with fibrates is not yet established. In the US the concurrent use of fibrates is not recommended, except fenofibrate, where longer-term safety studies have been undertaken. If gallstones or gall bladder disease is suspected in a patient receiving ezetimibe and fenofibrate then the combination should be discontinued.

Ezetimibe + Rifampicin (Rifampin)

Simultaneous single-doses of rifampicin increase ezetimibe concentrations without altering its overall effects on sterols, whereas multiple doses of rifampicin decrease single-dose ezetimibe concentrations and almost totally abolish its effects when administration is separated.

It would be prudent to monitor concurrent use to ensure that ezetimibe is effective.

Ezetimibe + Statins

Ezetimibe does not appear to have adverse pharmacokinetic interactions with atorvastatin, fluvastatin, lovastatin, pitavastatin, rosuvastatin, or simvastatin, and the available evidence suggests that there is no increase in the risk of myopathy when ezetimibe is given with a statin, when compared with statins given alone. Nevertheless, isolated reports describe myopathy on the concurrent use of ezetimibe with atorvastatin, and raised creatine kinase on the concurrent use of ezetimibe with fluvastatin.

Patients taking statins should be counselled regarding myopathy (e.g. report any unexplained muscle pain, tenderness, or weakness). This should be reinforced if they are also given ezetimibe. Note that the use of ezetimibe and a statin results in additive lipid-lowering effects, and combination preparations are available.

Ezetimibe + Warfarin and related oral anticoagulants ⚠

No clinically significant interaction occurred between ezetimibe and warfarin in one study. However, the manufacturers have received post-marketing reports of raised INRs in patients taking warfarin or fluindione after they were also given ezetimibe.

An interaction is not established. The manufacturers advise monitoring the prothrombin time in any patients taking a coumarin or indanedione and adjusting the dose as necessary.

E

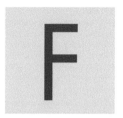

F

Famciclovir

Famciclovir + Probenecid ⚠

Probenecid is predicted to increase the exposure to penciclovir, the active metabolite of famciclovir, possibly resulting in increased adverse effects.

> Evidence is limited and an interaction is not established. Consider an interaction as a possible cause if famciclovir adverse effects (such as diarrhoea, nausea, sweating and pruritus) occur.

Febuxostat

Febuxostat + Theophylline ⚠

Febuxostat is predicted to increase the exposure to theophylline, however febuxostat 80 mg daily had no effect on the pharmacokinetics of single-dose theophylline.

> If both drugs are considered essential, check for signs of theophylline adverse effects (headache, nausea, tremor), monitoring theophylline concentrations and adjusting the dose accordingly. The UK manufacturer states that no special precautions are necessary when febuxostat 80 mg is given with theophylline

Felbamate

Felbamate + Gabapentin ❓

There is some evidence to suggest that the half-life of felbamate may be prolonged by gabapentin.

> The clinical importance of this interaction is unknown, but be alert for the need to reduce the felbamate dose.

Felbamate + **Perampanel**

Felbamate possibly decreases perampanel concentrations.

Until more is known, monitor perampanel efficacy and increase the dose if necessary.

Felbamate + **Phenobarbital**

Felbamate normally causes a moderate increase of about 25 to 30% in phenobarbital levels (derived from phenobarbital or primidone). Phenobarbital toxicity has occurred in one patient when felbamate was added.

Warn the patient to monitor for indicators of phenobarbital toxicity (drowsiness, ataxia or dysarthria), and take levels if necessary.

Felbamate + **Phenytoin**

Felbamate causes a moderate increase in phenytoin levels. Felbamate levels are reduced by phenytoin but the importance of this is uncertain. It seems possible that fosphenytoin, which is a prodrug of phenytoin, will interact similarly.

Warn the patient to monitor for indicators of phenytoin toxicity (blurred vision, nystagmus, ataxia or drowsiness). Take phenytoin levels and adjust the dose as necessary. The phenytoin dose may need to be reduced by up to 40%.

Felbamate + **Ulipristal**

The US manufacturer of ulipristal predicts that CYP3A4 inducers (they name felbamate) might decrease the exposure to ulipristal and reduce its efficacy.

Felbamate is not an established CYP3A4 inducer and so a clinically relevant interaction with ulipristal would not be expected.

Felbamate + **Valproate**

Felbamate can raise valproate levels (by about 50% with a 2.4 g dose of felbamate), which may cause toxicity. Valproate may slightly decrease the clearance of felbamate.

Monitor valproate levels if toxicity is suspected (indicators of valproate toxicity include nausea, vomiting and dizziness); some have suggested a 30 to 50% dose reduction may be needed. Be aware that the felbamate dose may need to be decreased.

Fesoterodine

Fesoterodine + **HIV-protease inhibitors**

Ketoconazole increases fesoterodine exposure about 2.5-fold by inhibiting CYP3A4. The

HIV-protease inhibitors inhibit CYP3A4 to varying extents, but are generally considered to be potent CYP3A4 inhibitors, and therefore they may be expected to interact similarly.

> The manufacturers state that the dose of fesoterodine should be restricted to 4 mg daily with potent CYP3A4 inhibitors; however, note that they contraindicate the concurrent use of potent CYP3A4 inhibitors in patients with moderate to severe hepatic or renal impairment, and advise avoiding concurrent use in those with mild renal or hepatic impairment. Monitor for an increase in fesoterodine adverse effects (e.g. dry mouth, dizziness, insomnia), and consider reducing the fesoterodine dose if these become troublesome.

Fesoterodine + Macrolides

Clarithromycin or Telithromycin

Ketoconazole increases fesoterodine exposure up to about 2.5-fold by inhibiting CYP3A4. Other potent CYP3A4 inhibitors (e.g. clarithromycin or telithromycin) are predicted to interact similarly.

> The manufacturers state that the dose of fesoterodine should be restricted to 4 mg daily on concurrent use with potent CYP3A4 inhibitors such as clarithromycin or telithromycin; however, note that they contraindicate the concurrent use of potent CYP3A4 inhibitors in those with moderate to severe hepatic or renal impairment, and advise avoiding concurrent use in those with mild renal or hepatic impairment. It may be prudent to monitor for an increase in fesoterodine adverse effects (e.g. dry mouth, dizziness, insomnia), and consider reducing the fesoterodine dose if these become troublesome.

Other macrolides

Fluconazole, a moderate CYP3A4 inhibitor, slightly increases the exposure to the active metabolite of fesoterodine, although an increase in some minor adverse effects, such as nausea and dizziness, occurred. Erythromycin would be expected to interact similarly.

> No fesoterodine dose adjustment is necessary on concurrent use. Bear in mind the possibility of an interaction should an increase in adverse effects occur (e.g. dry mouth, dizziness, insomnia). Concurrent use should be avoided in patients with severe renal impairment, and a maximum fesoterodine dose of 4 mg daily given to those with mild to moderate renal impairment. Concurrent use should also be avoided in patients with moderate or severe hepatic impairment, and a maximum dose of fesoterodine 4 mg daily given to those with mild hepatic impairment.

Fesoterodine + Phenobarbital

Rifampicin reduces the levels of the active metabolite of fesoterodine by about 75%. Phenobarbital, and primidone, which is in part metabolised to phenobarbital, would be expected to interact similarly.

> Concurrent use is not recommended by the UK manufacturer. However, the US manufacturer states that no fesoterodine dose adjustments are recommended. If both drugs are given it would be prudent to monitor for fesoterodine efficacy.

Fesoterodine + Phenytoin

Rifampicin reduces the levels of the active metabolite of fesoterodine by about 75%. Phenytoin, and fosphenytoin, a prodrug of phenytoin, would be expected to interact similarly.

Concurrent use is not recommended by the UK manufacturer. However, the US manufacturer states that no fesoterodine dose adjustments are recommended. If both drugs are given it would be prudent to monitor for fesoterodine efficacy.

Fesoterodine + Rifampicin (Rifampin)

Rifampicin reduces the levels of the active metabolite of fesoterodine by about 75%.

Concurrent use is not recommended by the UK manufacturer. However, the US manufacturer states that no fesoterodine dose adjustments are recommended. If both drugs are given it would be prudent to monitor for fesoterodine efficacy.

Fibrates

F

Fibrates + HIV-protease inhibitors

Lopinavir boosted with ritonavir slightly decreases gemfibrozil exposure.

It seems possible that gemfibrozil efficacy will be decreased. Bear this possibility in mind on the concurrent use of these drugs.

Fibrates + Montelukast

Gemfibrozil moderately increases the exposure to montelukast

Monitor concurrent use for an increase in montelukast adverse effects (such as abdominal pain, headache; and hyperkinesia in young children) and reduce the montelukast dose, if necessary. Some have suggested that a dose reduction of 50 to 80% might be required.

Fibrates + Statins

The concurrent use of a statin and a fibrate increases the risks of muscle toxicity (e.g. myopathy or rhabdomyolysis). Clinically relevant pharmacokinetic interactions appear to occur between some statins and gemfibrozil, with gemfibrozil moderately increasing the exposure to lovastatin, pravastatin, and simvastatin. This increases the risk of muscle toxicity.

In general, the concurrent use of a statin and a fibrate should only be undertaken if the benefits of treatment outweigh the risks, with the lowest necessary doses of each drug given. Patients taking statins should be counselled regarding myopathy (e.g. report any unexplained muscle pain, tenderness, or weakness). This should be reinforced if they are also given a fibrate. Various dose adjustments are recommended on the concurrent use of certain statins and fibrates, as follows:

- Atorvastatin – starting dose of 10 mg daily with a fibrate (UK advice), with alternatives to gemfibrozil considered.
- Lovastatin – avoid gemfibrozil where possible, particularly in patients with compromised liver or renal function, unless the benefits outweigh the risks. A maximum of 20 mg daily with a starting dose of 5 mg daily is recommended with a fibrate (US advice).
- Rosuvastatin – avoid gemfibrozil where possible, unless the benefits outweigh the risks. A starting dose of 5 mg daily (UK advice) and a maximum dose of 10 mg daily (US advice) is advised with gemfibrozil. Avoid 40 mg daily with any fibrate (UK advice).
- Simvastatin – concurrent use with gemfibrozil is contraindicated. A maximum 10 mg daily is recommended with a fibrate (UK advice), except for fenofibrate, where no dose restrictions are deemed necessary.

In addition, the manufacturer of bezafibrate contraindicates the use of any statin if a number of conditions considered to be risk factors for myopathy (such as renal impairment and hypothyroidism) are present.

Fibrates + Ursodeoxycholic acid (Ursodiol)

The concurrent use of fibrates is predicted to decrease the efficacy of ursodeoxycholic acid by increasing cholesterol elimination in the bile and thus encouraging gallstone formation.

The manufacturers do not recommend concurrent use.

Fibrates + Warfarin and related oral anticoagulants

The fibrates increase the effects of the coumarins and fatalities have resulted from this interaction. Most data is with the coumarins, although case reports suggest the indanediones may interact similarly. Gemfibrozil did not interact in a controlled study, although two cases of an interaction have been reported.

Evidence is not available for all combinations of fibrates and coumarins or indanediones, but it would seem prudent to expect them all to interact, to a greater or lesser extent. Coumarin and indanedione dose reductions may be needed to avoid the risk of bleeding. Monitor the INR and adjust the dose accordingly.

Finasteride

Finasteride + Herbal medicines or Dietary supplements

St John's wort moderately reduces the exposure to finasteride.

It is possible that finasteride will be less effective in those taking St John's wort. Therefore it would seem prudent to bear the potential for reduced efficacy in mind, especially in patients taking finasteride for benign prostatic hyperplasia.

Finasteride + **Testosterone**

Testosterone is poorly bioavailable by the oral route, and is rapidly metabolised to dihydrotestosterone by 5-alpha reductase. By inhibiting this enzyme, finasteride reduces the formation of dihydrotestosterone and increases the exposure to oral testosterone.

Finasteride might be useful in increasing testosterone oral bioavailability for oral replacement therapy. No action needed.

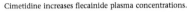

Flecainide

Flecainide + **H$_2$-receptor antagonists**

Cimetidine increases flecainide plasma concentrations.

The clinical importance of this interaction does not appear to have been assessed, but be alert for flecainide adverse effects (such as dizziness, nausea and tremor) and consider the need to reduce the flecainide dose, if cimetidine is added. The interaction is likely to be enhanced in the presence of renal impairment.

Flecainide + **HIV-protease inhibitors**

Ritonavir and tipranavir might increase the plasma concentration of flecainide. This increases the risk of arrhythmias and other adverse effects. Other HIV-protease inhibitors boosted with ritonavir are expected to interact similarly.

Concurrent use is generally contraindicated. If concurrent use is necessary, monitor carefully for flecainide adverse effects (such as dizziness, nausea or tremors) and adjust the flecainide dose if required.

Flecainide + **Lacosamide**

Dose-dependent prolongation of the PR interval may occur with lacosamide. The UK manufacturer therefore advises that lacosamide should be used with caution in patients taking class I antiarrhythmics, such as flecainide.

Be aware that ECG changes may occur on concurrent use.

Flecainide + **Lumefantrine**

The manufacturer of a preparation containing artemether and lumefantrine notes that *in vitro* lumefantrine significantly inhibits CYP2D6. They therefore contraindicate any drug that is metabolised by CYP2D6, and specifically name flecainide.

These contraindications seem unnecessarily restrictive, especially as flecainide is not contraindicated with other established inhibitors of CYP2D6. Until more is known, it would be prudent to closely monitor the effects of any CYP2D6 substrate in patients given lumefantrine.

F

Flecainide + NNRTIs

The manufacturers predict that etravirine may decrease the levels of flecainide. However, note that flecainide is more usually affected by CYP2D6 inhibitors or inducers, effects that etravirine does not appear to have.

> The manufacturers recommend caution on concurrent use and state that flecainide levels should be monitored, if this is possible.

Flecainide + NSAIDs

Because valdecoxib (the metabolite of parecoxib) increases *dextromethorphan* levels about 3-fold and celecoxib increases *dextromethorphan* levels about 2.4-fold, the manufacturers predict that the levels of flecainide (which is similarly metabolised) will also be raised by these coxibs.

> The general importance of this interaction is unclear. Monitor concurrent use for adverse effects, and consider reducing the dose of the antiarrhythmic if these become troublesome.

Flecainide + Quinidine

Quinidine slightly increases the exposure to flecainide.

> The clinical importance of this interaction is uncertain, but it is probably minor. However, note that one UK manufacturer of flecainide states that concurrent use is not recommended because both drugs block sodium channels.

Flecainide + Ranolazine

Ranolazine increases the levels of *metoprolol* by about 80% (by inhibiting CYP2D6). The manufacturers predict that flecainide will be similarly affected.

> Be aware of a possible interaction if flecainide adverse effects (such as abdominal pain, dizziness, hypotension, bradycardia) occur. The manufacturer of ranolazine suggests a dose reduction of flecainide may be needed.

Flecainide + SSRIs

Paroxetine, a potent inhibitor of CYP2D6, slightly increases the exposure to flecainide and an isolated case report describes increased flecainide concentrations and adverse effects in a patient taking paroxetine. Fluoxetine would be expected to interact similarly. The manufacturers of escitalopram predict that it could also interact in this way (although any effect is likely to be modest).

> The slight increase in flecainide exposure would not generally be expected to be of clinical relevance; however, any interaction might be of clinical importance in some patients, such as those with renal impairment. There appear to be no reported interactions, but, given that fluoxetine interacts this way with other CYP2D6 substrates (such as propafenone, page 559), it would seem prudent to be alert for an increase in flecainide adverse effects (such as dizziness, nausea, and tremor) and consider a flecainide dose reduction if necessary.

Flecainide + Terbinafine

In vitro studies suggest that terbinafine is an inhibitor of CYP2D6. It might therefore be expected to increase the plasma concentration of drugs that are substrates of this isoenzyme, such as flecainide.

Until more is known it would seem wise to be aware of the possibility of an increase in flecainide adverse effects if flecainide is given with terbinafine and consider a dose reduction if necessary.

Flutamide

Flutamide + Theophylline ❓

The UK manufacturer of flutamide notes that cases of increased theophylline plasma concentrations have been reported in patients taking these two drugs concurrently. Aminophylline is predicted to interact similarly.

The manufacturer suggests the reason for this is that flutamide and theophylline are both metabolised by CYP1A2; however, note that interactions by this mechanism are rarely clinically relevant.

Flutamide + Warfarin and related oral anticoagulants

Case reports suggest that in some patients flutamide may increase the effects of warfarin. The interaction developed over 2 months in some cases but developed within 4 days in another.

An interaction is not established. Nevertheless, the manufacturer of flutamide recommends that the prothrombin time be carefully monitored when these drugs are given with coumarins, adjusting the dose when necessary.

Folates

Folates + Methotrexate

Folic acid or folinic acid are sometimes added if low-dose methotrexate is given for rheumatoid arthritis or psoriasis to reduce adverse effects. Folinic acid is frequently used to minimise toxicity with high-dose methotrexate.

Patients taking methotrexate should avoid the inadvertent use of folates in multivitamin preparations.

Folates + Phenobarbital

If folic acid supplements are given to treat folate deficiency, which can be caused by the use of phenobarbital or primidone, the antiepileptic levels may fall, leading to decreased seizure control in some patients.

Monitor phenobarbital levels and adjust the dose of phenobarbital or primidone accordingly.

Folates + **Phenytoin** ⚠

If folic acid supplements are given to treat folate deficiency, which can be caused by the use of phenytoin, phenytoin levels may fall, leading to decreased seizure control in some patients. Reductions in phenytoin levels of 16 to 50% have been described with folic acid doses between 5 mg and 15 mg; doses as low as folic acid 1 mg may interact.

Monitor phenytoin levels and adjust the dose accordingly. Fosphenytoin is a prodrug of phenytoin. Although it does not appear to have been studied, it may interact similarly.

Folates + **Sulfasalazine** ❓

Sulfasalazine can reduce the absorption of folic acid by about 30%.

The clinical significance of this interaction is unclear. Note that sulfasalazine is itself associated with blood dyscrasias due to folate deficiency, and this may be treated with folic acid or folinic acid.

Food

Food + **Furazolidone** ❌

After 5 to 10 days of use furazolidone has MAO-inhibitory activity about equivalent to that of the antidepressant MAOIs. It might therefore be expected to interact with tyramine-rich foods.

It would seem prudent to warn patients given furazolidone not to take any of the foods or drinks that are prohibited with non-selective MAOIs. See MAOIs, page 389.

Food + **Griseofulvin** ❓

The rate and probably extent of griseofulvin absorption is increased by food, especially high-fat meals.

Griseofulvin should be taken with or after food to ensure adequate absorption.

Food + **HIV-protease inhibitors**

Atazanavir ❓

Food increases the bioavailability of atazanavir (boosted with ritonavir).

Atazanavir should be taken with food to enhance bioavailability and minimise variability in its absorption.

Darunavir ⚠

Food increases the bioavailability of darunavir boosted with ritonavir.

The UK and US manufacturers advise that tablets of darunavir (boosted with ritonavir) should be taken with food.

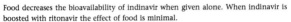

Fosamprenavir

Food slightly decreases the bioavailability of fosamprenavir suspension.

Adults should take the oral suspension without food and on an empty stomach. However, in order to improve palatability and ensure compliance, children may take the suspension with food.

Indinavir

Food decreases the bioavailability of indinavir when given alone. When indinavir is boosted with ritonavir the effect of food is minimal.

Indinavir should be taken one hour before or 2 hours after meals, or with low-fat light meals only (such as dry toast with jam, juice, and coffee with skimmed milk and sugar; or corn flakes, skimmed milk, and sugar). Indinavir boosted with ritonavir may be given without regard to meals.

Lopinavir

Food increases the bioavailability of lopinavir boosted with ritonavir when it is given as a solution, but has little effects on the tablet formulation.

The oral solution of lopinavir boosted with ritonavir should be taken with food, whereas the tablets may be taken without regard to meals.

Nelfinavir

Food increases the absorption of nelfinavir.

Nelfinavir should be given with food.

Ritonavir

Food has little effect on ritonavir bioavailability.

The UK and US manufacturers advise that ritonavir is taken with food.

Saquinavir

Food increases the bioavailability of saquinavir (boosted with ritonavir).

Saquinavir boosted with ritonavir should be given with, or up to 2 hours after, a meal.

Tipranavir

Food minimally affects the pharmacokinetics of tipranavir boosted with ritonavir, when given as capsules.

The US manufacturer states that tipranavir boosted with ritonavir capsules can be taken with, or without food, when given as capsules or the oral solution, but the tablets should be taken with meals. The UK manufacturer states that food improves the tolerability of tipranavir boosted with ritonavir, and recommends that it should be taken with food.

F

Food + Isoniazid

The absorption of isoniazid is reduced by food. Patients taking isoniazid who eat some foods, particularly fish from the scombroid family (e.g. tuna, mackerel, salmon) that are not fresh, may experience an exaggerated histamine poisoning reaction e.g. chills, diarrhoea, flushing and itching of the skin, headache, tachycardia, vomiting, wheeze. Cheese has also been implicated in this reaction, but the adverse effects may be due to the weak MAOI effects of isoniazid rather than histamine poisoning.

> For maximal absorption isoniazid should be taken without food, hence the manufacturer's guidance to take it at least 30 minutes before or 2 hours after food. There is no need to introduce general dietary restrictions, but if any of these reactions is experienced, examine the patient's diet and advise the avoidance of any probable offending foodstuffs.

Food + Levodopa ❓

The timing of meals and the type of diet, particularly high-protein diets, may affect the absorption of levodopa possibly leading to fluctuations in disease control.

> If problems occur, a change in the pattern of drug and food administration on a trial-and-error basis may be helpful. Multiple small doses of levodopa and spreading out the intake of proteins may also diminish the effects of these interactions. Taking levodopa with food may help to minimise adverse effects such as anorexia, nausea, vomiting, and diarrhoea.

Food + Linezolid

Linezolid has some MAOI activity and therefore has the potential to cause potentially life-threatening hypertensive crisis when taken with tyramine-rich food (e.g. cheeses, salami, yeast extracts, pickled herrings). A severe hypertensive reaction crisis of the proportions possible with the antidepressant MAOIs seems unlikely as linezolid only modestly increases the blood pressure in response to tyramine.

> Patients taking linezolid should not consume excessive amounts of tyramine-rich foods and drinks (100 mg of tyramine per meal is recommended by the manufacturers).

Food + Lumefantrine ❓

Food, especially high-fat food (including soya milk), markedly increases the bioavailability of lumefantrine.

> As soon as patients can tolerate food, lumefantrine should be taken with food to increase absorption. Patients who remain averse to food during treatment should be closely monitored since they might be at greater risk of recrudescence (reappearance of the disease after a period of inactivity).

Food + Macrolides ⚠

Food reduces the absorption of azithromycin from capsules but does not affect the AUC of azithromycin from tablets or suspension.

> Azithromycin capsules should be taken at least one hour before or 2 hours after a meal. Azithromycin suspension and tablets may be taken without regard to food.

Food + MAOIs

A potentially life-threatening hypertensive crisis can develop in patients taking non-selective MAOIs who eat tyramine-rich food (e.g. cheeses, salami, yeast extracts, pickled herrings) and drinks (e.g. some beers and wines) or young broad bean pods, which contain dopa. Fatalities have occurred.

As little as 20 mg of tyramine can raise the blood pressure by 30 mmHg in patients taking tranylcypromine. However, because tyramine levels vary so much it is impossible to guess the amount of tyramine present in any food or drink. Fermented or aged foods, such as cheeses (particularly over-ripe or strong smelling cheeses), sausages and beer, or smoked meats tend to be the most common tyramine-rich foods. There is no guarantee that patients who have uneventfully eaten these hazardous foodstuffs on many occasions may not eventually experience a full-scale hypertensive crisis, if all the possible variables conspire together. Therefore tyramine-rich foods should be avoided. In addition, avoidance of the prohibited foods should be continued for 2 to 3 weeks after stopping the MAOI to allow full recovery of the enzymes.

Food + Moclobemide

Tyramine 150 mg has been found to cause a 30 mmHg rise in systolic blood pressure when given with moclobemide. No reports of the potentially life-threatening hypertensive reactions seen with non-selective MAOIs appear to have been published for moclobemide.

Note that 150 mg of tyramine is equivalent to that found in about 200 g of Stilton cheese or 300 g of Gorgonzola cheese, which are really excessive amounts of cheese to be eaten in a few minutes. Most patients therefore do not need to follow the special dietary restrictions required with the non-selective MAOIs, but, to be on the safe side, the manufacturers of moclobemide advise all patients to avoid large amounts of tyramine-rich foods, because a few individuals may be particularly sensitive to its effects.

Food + NRTIs

Didanosine or Entecavir A

Food moderately decreases the extent of absorption of buffered didanosine, and slightly reduces the extent of absorption of enteric-coated didanosine. Food can slightly decrease entecavir exposure.

Buffered didanosine should be taken at least 30 minutes before, or 2 hours after, food. Enteric coated didanosine should be taken 2 hours before, or after, food. The UK manufacturer of entecavir states that patients with lamivudine-resistant, or decompensated, disease should take entecavir on an empty stomach, at least 2 hours before, or 2 hours after, meals. In the US, the advice is always to take entecavir on an empty stomach, at least 2 hours before, or 2 hours after, meals.

Tenofovir

Tenofovir absorption is increased by high-fat food.

The UK manufacturer recommends that tenofovir is taken with food, whereas the US manufacturer states that tenofovir tablets can be taken without regard to food. The combination preparation containing tenofovir, emtricitabine, and efavirenz should be taken on an empty stomach.

Food + NSAIDs

Food reduces the rate of absorption but has little or no clinically relevant effect on the extent of absorption of most NSAIDs.

> The small changes seen will have no clinical relevance if these drugs are being used regularly to treat chronic pain and inflammation. However, if they are being used for the treatment of acute pain, administration on an empty stomach would be preferable in terms of onset of effect. However, it is usually recommended that NSAIDs are given with or after food, in an attempt to minimise their gastrointestinal adverse effects.

Food + Penicillamine

Food can reduce the absorption of penicillamine by about 50%.

> If maximal effects are required penicillamine should be taken at least 30 minutes before food.

Food + Penicillins ⚠

Food can reduce the absorption of ampicillin by about 30%, and the peak levels and AUC of phenoxymethylpenicillin by about 50%. Limited evidence suggests that food has no significant effect on the bioavailability of flucloxacillin.

> Ampicillin and phenoxymethylpenicillin should be taken one hour before food or on an empty stomach. Despite the apparent lack of interaction with flucloxacillin, it is recommended that it should be taken one hour before food or on an empty stomach to optimise absorption.

Food + Praziquantel ❓

Food increases the bioavailability of praziquantel.

> If praziquantel is used for systemic worm infections, administration with food is advisable. Note that this interaction is of no importance when praziquantel is used for intestinal worm infections (where its action is a local effect on the worms in the gut).

Food + Proton pump inhibitors ⚠

Food reduces the bioavailability of esomeprazole and lansoprazole by up to 70%.

> The US manufacturer recommends that esomeprazole capsules and suspension should be taken one hour before meals. The manufacturers recommend that, to achieve optimal efficacy, lansoprazole should be given in the morning at least 30 minutes before food.

Food + Quinolones

Dairy products reduce the bioavailability of ciprofloxacin (AUC reduced by about 30%) and norfloxacin (peak plasma levels reduced by about 50%).

> The effect of these changes on the control of infection is uncertain but it would seem prudent to advise patients not to take these dairy products within one to 2 hours of either ciprofloxacin or norfloxacin. Enoxacin, lomefloxacin, and ofloxacin do not appear to interact significantly with food. They therefore may provide a useful alternative to the interacting quinolones. Consider also enteral feeds, page 365.

Food + Retinoids

Fatty foods increase the absorption of acitretin, etretinate and isotretinoin.

> Acitretin, etretinate and isotretinoin should be taken with food to maximise absorption. On the basis of these interactions, the UK manufacturers of oral alitretinoin and oral tretinoin also recommend administration with food.

Food + Rifampicin (Rifampin)

Food delays and reduces the absorption of rifampicin.

> Rifampicin should be taken on an empty stomach, 30 minutes before a meal, or 2 hours after a meal to ensure rapid and complete absorption.

Food + Rivaroxaban

The absorption of rivaroxaban is dose-dependent and can be affected by food.

> The UK and US manufacturers state that rivaroxaban can be taken with or without food when given at a dose of 10 mg, but must be taken with food when given at a dose of 15 or 20 mg.

Food + Sodium oxybate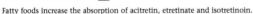

Food delays and reduces the absorption of sodium oxybate.

> The first dose of sodium oxybate should be taken at least 2 to 3 hours after the evening meal, and patients should always try to keep the same timing of dosing in relation to meals.

Food + Strontium

The manufacturer notes that food, milk and dairy products reduce the bioavailability of strontium by about 60 to 70%, when compared with administration 3 hours after a meal.

> Strontium should not be taken within 2 hours of eating. The manufacturer recommends that it should be taken at bedtime, at least 2 hours after eating.

Food + Tetracyclines

The absorption of most tetracyclines can be markedly reduced (by up to 80%) by milk or other dairy products. Doxycycline and minocycline are less affected by dairy products (25 to 30% reduction).

> It is usual to recommend that tetracyclines are taken one hour before food or 2 hours after food to avoid an interaction with all forms of dietary calcium. Note that lymecycline appears not to interact.

Food + Warfarin and related oral anticoagulants

Cranberry juice ❓

A number of case reports suggest that cranberry juice can increase the INR of patients taking warfarin, and one patient has died as a result of this interaction. Other patients have developed unstable INRs, or, in one isolated case, a reduced INR. However, in several controlled studies, cranberry juice or concentrate did not alter the anticoagulant effect or the pharmacokinetics of warfarin, or had only very minor effects on the INR.

> An interaction is not established. It could be that there is no specific interaction, and that the case reports just represent idiosyncratic reactions in which other unknown factors (e.g. altered diet) were more important. In 2004, on the basis of the then available case reports and lack of controlled studies, the CSM/MHRA in the UK advised that patients taking warfarin should avoid drinking cranberry juice unless the health benefits are considered to outweigh any risks. They recommended increased INR monitoring for any patient taking warfarin and who has a regular intake of cranberry juice (and cranberry capsules or concentrates). These might still be prudent precautions, although the controlled studies now available do provide some reassurance that, in otherwise healthy individuals, moderate amounts of cranberry juice are unlikely to have an important impact on anticoagulation.

Foods, general ❓

A number of foodstuffs have been implicated in interactions with warfarin. Some of these were not thought to be related to their vitamin K content. These include:

- antagonism of the effects of warfarin by ice cream, avocado, soybean protein, and soybean oil and other intravenous lipids
- an increase in warfarin requirements and/or prothrombin time with the use of aspartame, following the consumption of mango fruit or after starting high-protein, low-carbohydrate diets.

The rate of absorption of dicoumarol can be increased by food.

> These reactions seem unlikely to be of general importance, although bear them in mind in case of an unexpected response to oral anticoagulants. Note that any big changes in diet have the potential to alter the effects of warfarin on the INR, and it would therefore be prudent to increase monitoring in patients wishing to start a diet.

Foods containing vitamin K ❓

The effects of warfarin can be reduced or abolished by vitamin K, including that found in health foods, food supplements, enteral feeds or exceptionally large amounts of some green vegetables or green tea.

Patients should be counselled about the effects of dietary supplements or dramatic dietary alterations when they start taking vitamin K antagonist anticoagulants (coumarins and indanediones). Patients taking anticoagulants should be advised to eat a normal balanced diet, maintaining a relatively consistent amount of vitamin-K rich foods. They should be told to avoid making major changes to their diet, including starting a weight-loss diet, without increased monitoring of their INR. Consider also enteral feeds, page 366.

Natto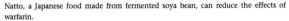

Natto, a Japanese food made from fermented soya bean, can reduce the effects of warfarin.

Patients taking warfarin, and probably indanedione anticoagulants, should be advised to avoid natto unless they want to consume a regular, constant amount.

Pomegranate juice

Case reports suggest that pomegranate juice increases the INR in response to warfarin. Other coumarins could potentially interact similarly.

There is currently insufficient evidence to suggest that patients taking warfarin should avoid pomegranate juice, but it may be prudent to consider pomegranate juice consumption in a patient with otherwise unexplained fluctuations in INR, or unexpectedly raised INRs.

Furazolidone

Furazolidone + Nasal decongestants

After 5 to 10 days of use, furazolidone has MAO-inhibitory activity about equivalent to that of the non-selective MAOIs. Concurrent use with drugs such as phenylpropanolamine or ephedrine, might be expected to result in a potentially serious rise in blood pressure.

Although reports of hypertensive crises with furazolidone appear lacking it would still seem prudent to warn patients to avoid any of the nasal decongestants with indirect sympathomimetic activity (e.g. ephedrine, pseudoephedrine, phenylpropanolamine). Note that a few UK manufacturers of pseudoephedrine-containing cold and influenza preparations contraindicate their use with furazolidone.

Fusidate

Fusidate + HIV-protease inhibitors

A patient taking fusidate with saquinavir and ritonavir developed elevated fusidate concentrations with toxicity, and elevated saquinavir and ritonavir concentrations (roughly 4-fold increases).

The clinical significance of this case is unclear. It has been suggested that fusidate be avoided in patients taking these HIV-protease inhibitors. However, if the combination is needed it would seem sensible to monitor concurrent use carefully so any elevation in concentrations is detected before they become problematic.

Fusidate + Statins ⚠

Isolated cases of rhabdomyolysis have been described in patients given atorvastatin or simvastatin with fusidate. The possibility of an interaction with other statins cannot be excluded.

An interaction is not established, and all the cases described had other risk factors for myopathy or rhabdomyolysis. However, the MHRA in the UK advise against the concurrent use of all statins, and for 7 days after fusidate is stopped. If concurrent use is essential, patients should be closely monitored and counselled regarding the risk of myopathy (e.g. report any unexplained muscle pain, tenderness or weakness). This guidance would not apply to topical use of fusidic acid as creams and eye drops.

F

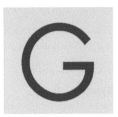

Gabapentin

Gabapentin + Orlistat

The MHRA in the UK suggests that the absorption of antiepileptics might be decreased by orlistat, leading to a loss of seizure control.

Although an interaction has not been established, the MHRA advises that patients should be monitored for changes in the severity or frequency of convulsions, and consideration given to separating the administration of orlistat and the antiepileptic.

Galantamine

Galantamine + Quinidine

Paroxetine increases the risk of galantamine adverse effects (in particular nausea and vomiting) probably by inhibiting the metabolism of galantamine by CYP2D6. The manufacturers therefore predict that other CYP2D6 inhibitors (such as quinidine) will interact similarly.

If the adverse effects of galantamine (e.g. nausea and vomiting) develop or worsen, consider reducing its dose.

Galantamine + SSRIs

Paroxetine increases the risk of galantamine adverse effects probably by inhibiting the metabolism of galantamine by CYP2D6. The manufacturers therefore predict that other CYP2D6 inhibitors (such as fluoxetine) will interact similarly. They also name fluvoxamine but note that fluvoxamine is usually considered to be a *weak* inhibitor of this isoenzyme.

If the adverse effects of galantamine (e.g. nausea and vomiting) develop or worsen, consider reducing its dose.

Ganciclovir

Valganciclovir is a prodrug of ganciclovir and therefore has the potential to interact similarly.

Ganciclovir + Imipenem

The manufacturer notes that generalised seizures have been reported in patients who received ganciclovir and imipenem with cilastatin. Note that both ganciclovir and imipenem alone can cause seizures. Valganciclovir is a prodrug of ganciclovir and would therefore be expected to interact similarly.

The UK and US manufacturers recommend that ganciclovir or valganciclovir should not be used with imipenem, unless the benefits outweigh the risks.

Ganciclovir + Mycophenolate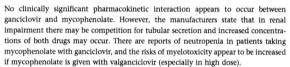

No clinically significant pharmacokinetic interaction appears to occur between ganciclovir and mycophenolate. However, the manufacturers state that in renal impairment there may be competition for tubular secretion and increased concentrations of both drugs may occur. There are reports of neutropenia in patients taking mycophenolate with ganciclovir, and the risks of myelotoxicity appear to be increased if mycophenolate is given with valganciclovir (especially in high dose).

No action is needed, but increased monitoring may be prudent in patients with reduced renal function. Both mycophenolate mofetil and ganciclovir and its prodrug, valganciclovir, have the potential to cause neutropenia and leucopenia, therefore patients should be closely monitored for additive toxicity.

Ganciclovir + NRTIs

Didanosine

Ganciclovir increases the exposure to didanosine, even when the drugs are given 2 hours apart, but there is limited evidence suggesting that the efficacy of ganciclovir might be reduced by didanosine. Valganciclovir is a prodrug of ganciclovir and would therefore be expected to interact similarly.

Monitor concurrent use for didanosine toxicity and ganciclovir efficacy.

Tenofovir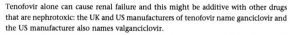

Tenofovir alone can cause renal failure and this might be additive with other drugs that are nephrotoxic: the UK and US manufacturers of tenofovir name ganciclovir and the US manufacturer also names valganciclovir.

Avoid concurrent use. If this is not possible, the UK and US manufacturers of tenofovir advise that renal function should be monitored at least weekly.

Zidovudine

Anaemia, neutropenia, leucopenia, and gastrointestinal disturbances were seen when

G

zidovudine and ganciclovir were used concurrently. The dose of zidovudine had to be reduced to 300 mg daily in many patients. Valganciclovir is a prodrug of ganciclovir and would therefore be expected to interact similarly.

Monitor for zidovudine toxicity (such as neutropenia) on concurrent use.

Ganciclovir + Probenecid ⚠

Probenecid reduces the renal excretion of ganciclovir and increases its exposure.

The clinical importance of this interaction is uncertain. Be alert for increased ganciclovir adverse effects (such as diarrhoea, nausea, neutropenia and thrombocytopenia) if probenecid is given with ganciclovir or its prodrug, valganciclovir.

Gestrinone

Gestrinone + Herbal medicines or Dietary supplements ❓

The manufacturers warn that *rifampicin (rifampin)* might increase the metabolism of gestrinone and thereby reduce its effects. Other enzyme inducers, such as St John's wort (*Hypericum perforatum*) might interact similarly.

The clinical significance of this warning is unclear and there appear to be no reports of an interaction in practice; however, be aware that gestrinone might be less effective if St John's wort is also given.

Gestrinone + NNRTIs ❓

The manufacturers warn that *rifampicin (rifampin)* might increase the metabolism of gestrinone and thereby reduce its effects. Other enzyme inducers, such as efavirenz and nevirapine, might interact similarly.

The clinical significance of this warning is unclear and there appear to be no reports of an interaction in practice; however, be aware that gestrinone might be less effective if efavirenz or nevirapine are given concurrently.

Gestrinone + Phenobarbital ❓

The manufacturers state that phenobarbital (and therefore probably primidone, which is metabolised to phenobarbital) may increase the metabolism of gestrinone and thereby reduce its effects.

The clinical significance of this warning is unclear and there appear to be no reports of an interaction in practice; however, be aware that gestrinone may not be as effective if phenobarbital or primidone are given concurrently.

G

Gestrinone + Phenytoin ?

The manufacturers state that phenytoin (and therefore probably fosphenytoin, a pro-drug of phenytoin) may increase the metabolism of gestrinone and thereby reduce its effects.

> The clinical significance of this warning is unclear and there appear to be no reports of an interaction in practice; however, be aware that gestrinone may not be as effective if phenytoin or fosphenytoin are given concurrently.

Gestrinone + Rifabutin ?

The manufacturers warn that *rifampicin (rifampin)* might increase the metabolism of gestrinone and thereby reduce its effects. Rifabutin might interact similarly, although to a lesser extent than rifampicin.

> The clinical significance of this warning is unclear and there appear to be no reports of an interaction in practice; however, be aware that gestrinone might be less effective if rifabutin is also given.

Gestrinone + Rifampicin (Rifampin) ?

The manufacturers state that rifampicin may increase the metabolism of gestrinone and thereby reduce its effects.

> The clinical significance of this warning is unclear and there appear to be no reports of an interaction in practice; however, be aware that gestrinone may not be as effective if rifampicin is also given.

G

Gestrinone + Topiramate ?

The manufacturers warn that *rifampicin (rifampin)* might increase the metabolism of gestrinone and thereby reduce its effects. Other enzyme inducers, such as high-dose topiramate, might interact similarly.

> The clinical significance of this warning is unclear and there appear to be no reports of an interaction in practice; however, be aware that gestrinone might be less effective if high-dose topiramate (doses greater than 200 mg daily) are given concurrently.

Glucagon

Glucagon + Warfarin and related oral anticoagulants

The anticoagulant effects of warfarin are rapidly and markedly increased by glucagon in large doses (total dose exceeding 50 mg over 2 days), and bleeding can occur. This interaction did not occur in patients given, in total, less than 30 mg of glucagon over 1 to 2 days.

> It has been suggested that if glucagon 25 mg per day or more is given for two or

more days, the dose of warfarin should be reduced in anticipation of the interaction, and prothrombin times closely monitored. Information about other anticoagulants is lacking, but it would be prudent to assume that all coumarins will interact similarly.

Gold

Gold + Leflunomide

The manufacturers state that the concurrent use of leflunomide and gold has not yet been studied but it would be expected to increase the risk of serious adverse reactions (haematological toxicity or hepatotoxicity).

The manufacturers advise avoiding concurrent use. As the active metabolite of leflunomide has a long half-life of 1 to 4 weeks a washout with colestyramine or activated charcoal may decrease the risks of toxicity if patients are to be switched to other DMARDs.

Gold + Penicillamine

Gold appears to increase the risk of penicillamine toxicity.

Avoid concurrent use. Increased penicillamine monitoring should be considered in those with previous adverse effects to gold, as these patients are likely to experience increased adverse effects to penicillamine.

G

Grapefruit juice

In general, grapefruit juice inhibits intestinal CYP3A4, and only slightly affects hepatic CYP3A4. This is demonstrated by the fact that intravenous preparations of drugs that are metabolised by CYP3A4 are not much affected, whereas oral preparations of the same drugs are, and their levels are increased by grapefruit juice. Some drugs that are not metabolised by CYP3A4 show decreased levels with grapefruit juice. This is probably because grapefruit juice is an inhibitor of some drug transporters. The active constituent of grapefruit juice is uncertain. However, grapefruit contains naringin, which degrades during processing to naringenin, a substance known to inhibit CYP3A4. Because of this, it has been assumed that whole grapefruit will not interact, but that processed grapefruit juice will. However, subsequently some reports have implicated the whole fruit. Other possible active constituents in the whole fruit include bergamottin and dihydroxybergamottin.

Grapefruit juice + Ivabradine

Grapefruit juice increases ivabradine levels 2-fold.

The manufacturers advise restricting the intake of grapefruit juice in patients taking ivabradine, but note that its enzyme inhibiting effects are variable so caution is needed. Note that this increase is similar to that seen with moderate inhibitors of CYP3A4, for which a lower starting dose of 2.5 mg twice daily of ivabradine has been suggested.

Grapefruit juice + Phosphodiesterase type-5 inhibitors ⚠

Grapefruit juice slightly increases the AUC of sildenafil. Avanafil, tadalafil, and vardenafil are predicted to interact similarly.

It has been suggested that although the pharmacokinetic changes are unlikely to be clinically significant, the combination is best avoided because concurrent use results in an increased variability in sildenafil pharmacokinetics. However, this seems over-cautious, as reduced doses of sildenafil can be given with more potent CYP3A4 inhibitors. The manufacturers of tadalafil and vardenafil advise caution and avoidance, respectively, in those who drink grapefruit juice. The UK manufacturer of avanafil advises that the patient avoids grapefruit juice for 24 hours before taking avanafil.

Grapefruit juice + Praziquantel ❓

Grapefruit juice nearly doubles the exposure to praziquantel.

Until more is known about the clinical relevance of this interaction it might be prudent to be alert for an increase in praziquantel adverse effects (e.g. headache, diarrhoea, dizziness, or drowsiness) in patients who drink grapefruit juice.

Grapefruit juice + Ranolazine ✗

Ketoconazole increases ranolazine levels, which increases the risk of QT prolongation and potentially life-threatening arrhythmias. Although not specifically studied grapefruit juice would be expected to interact similarly.

The manufacturer contraindicates concurrent use.

Grapefruit juice + Sirolimus ✗

Grapefruit juice appears to increase the exposure to oral sirolimus.

Avoid concurrent use. Grapefruit juice should not be used for the dilution of sirolimus oral solution.

Grapefruit juice + SSRIs ❓

Grapefruit juice slightly increases the exposure to fluvoxamine, and there is a case report of adverse effects attributed to this pharmacokinetic interaction. Sertraline exposure appears to be moderately increased by grapefruit juice. Excessive consumption of grapefruit caused symptoms similar to serotonin syndrome in a patient taking fluoxetine and trazodone.

Bear an interaction in mind in case of increased SSRI adverse effects. The UK manufacturer of sertraline advises avoiding concurrent use.

G

Grapefruit juice + **Statins**

Atorvastatin

Grapefruit juice, in large amounts, moderately increases the exposure to atorvastatin.

> In general, the occasional glass of grapefruit juice would not appear to be a problem: the UK manufacturer suggests that large quantities (greater than 1.2 litres daily) should be avoided. Remember, any patient taking a statin should be told to report any unexplained muscle pain, tenderness, or weakness.

Lovastatin or Simvastatin

When taken at the same time, large amounts of grapefruit juice (200 mL of double-strength grapefruit juice three times daily) very markedly increase the exposure to lovastatin and simvastatin. Smaller amounts of grapefruit juice and separating administration by 12 hours results in a smaller effect.

> Large increases in the exposure to lovastatin and simvastatin are potentially hazardous because they carry the risk of toxicity (muscle damage and the possible development of rhabdomyolysis). As even small quantities of grapefruit juice can affect simvastatin exposure, the UK manufacturer states that concurrent use should be avoided, whereas the US manufacturers of simvastatin and lovastatin recommend restricting intake to less than 1 litre daily.

Grapefruit juice + **Tacrolimus**

Grapefruit juice can greatly increase the concentrations of tacrolimus.

> The UK and US manufacturers of tacrolimus advise avoiding concurrent use. Note that the US manufacturer includes whole grapefruit as well as the juice. This would appear prudent. Patients should be informed of the potential risk of this interaction.

Griseofulvin

Griseofulvin + **Phenobarbital**

The antifungal effects of griseofulvin can be reduced (concentrations reduced by about one-third) or even abolished by the concurrent use of phenobarbital. Note that primidone is metabolised to phenobarbital and might therefore interact similarly.

> Concurrent use should be well monitored to confirm that griseofulvin is effective. If appropriate, a non-interacting antiepileptic such as valproate might be a suitable alternative.

Griseofulvin + **Ulipristal** [?]

The US manufacturer of ulipristal predicts that CYP3A4 inducers (they name griseofulvin) might decrease the exposure to ulipristal and reduce its efficacy.

> Griseofulvin is not an established CYP3A4 inducer and so a clinically relevant interaction with ulipristal would not be expected.

Griseofulvin + **Warfarin and related oral anticoagulants**

The anticoagulant effects of warfarin can be reduced by griseofulvin in some patients. In one patient a 41% increase in the dose of warfarin was needed. Other coumarins may interact similarly.

> Monitor the anticoagulant effect if griseofulvin is added or withdrawn in patients taking a coumarin, and adjust the dose as necessary. Note that in one patient the interaction took 12 weeks to develop.

Guanethidine

Guanethidine + **Inotropes and Vasopressors**

The pressor effects of noradrenaline (norepinephrine), phenylephrine, metaraminol and other related drugs can be increased in the presence of guanethidine. In addition the incidence and severity of cardiac arrhythmias is increased. Dopamine would be expected to interact similarly. Some of these drugs can also be used as eye drops, and in this situation their mydriatic effects are similarly enhanced and prolonged by guanethidine.

G

> The doses of these inotropes or vasopressors should be reduced appropriately in patients taking guanethidine; monitor the outcome of concurrent use carefully. Consider also the possibility of an arrhythmogenic effect.

Guanethidine + **Methylphenidate**

The antihypertensive effects of guanethidine can be reduced or abolished by methylphenidate. The blood pressure may even rise higher than before treatment with the antihypertensive.

> The concurrent use of guanethidine and methylphenidate should be avoided.

Guanethidine + **Nasal decongestants**

The antihypertensive effects of guanethidine can be reduced or abolished by ephedrine. The blood pressure may even rise higher than before treatment with the antihypertensive. Other related drugs, such as pseudoephedrine and phenylpropanolamine, that are used as cough and cold remedies, may also interact in this way.

> Concurrent use should be avoided. Warn patients about the use of non-prescription nasal decongestants containing any of these drugs to relieve the nasal stuffiness commonly associated with the use of guanethidine and related drugs.

Guanethidine + Pizotifen

Pizotifen may antagonise the blood pressure-lowering effects of guanethidine, but evidence for this appears sparse.

> If both drugs are given be aware that the hypotensive effects of guanethidine may be reduced.

Guanethidine + Tricyclics ⚠

The antihypertensive effects of guanethidine are reduced or abolished by amitriptyline, desipramine, imipramine, nortriptyline and protriptyline. Doxepin in doses of 300 mg or more daily interacts similarly, but in smaller doses it may not interact, although one case is reported with doxepin 100 mg daily.

> Not every combination of guanethidine and a tricyclic antidepressant has been studied but all are expected to interact similarly. Concurrent use should be avoided unless the effects are very closely monitored and the interaction balanced by raising the dose of the antihypertensive.

G

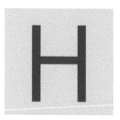

H₂-receptor antagonists

Cimetidine is a non-specific enzyme inhibitor and therefore interacts with a number of cytochrome P450 substrates. Other H₂-receptor antagonists do not have enzyme-inhibitory effects and therefore do not interact in this way. They may therefore provide useful alternatives to cimetidine. However, note that if an interaction occurs due to an alteration in gastric pH, all H₂-receptor antagonists would be expected to interact similarly.

H₂-receptor antagonists + HIV-protease inhibitors

Atazanavir and fosamprenavir exposure is reduced by H₂-receptor antagonists such as ranitidine, probably by affecting gastric acidity. Amprenavir is predicted to be similarly affected. Not all H₂-receptor antagonists have been studied, but they would be expected to interact similarly. Saquinavir exposure appears to be increased by ranitidine and cimetidine.

The manufacturers suggest that atazanavir boosted with ritonavir should be given once daily with food, at the same time or at least 10 hours after famotidine 20 mg twice daily (or the comparable dose of another H₂-receptor antagonist). In the US, famotidine up to 40 mg twice daily may be given to treatment-naive patients, with the same dose and dose interval as the lower famotidine dose. In the UK, if famotidine 40 mg twice daily or more is required, then the manufacturers suggest considering increasing the dose of atazanavir boosted with ritonavir to 400/100 mg. For unboosted atazanavir in treatment-naive patients, the US manufacturer recommends a dose of 400 mg should be given once daily with food; the maximum dose of famotidine should not exceed 20 mg as a single dose or 40 mg daily. If tenofovir is also given, the combination should preferably be avoided. The UK manufacturer suggests that no fosamprenavir dose adjustment is needed with ranitidine or other H₂-receptor antagonists; however, the US manufacturer states the combination should be used with caution because fosamprenavir might become less effective. US guidelines recommend that fosamprenavir should be given at least 2 hours before the H₂-receptor antagonist, and that consideration be given to boosting fosamprenavir with ritonavir. The clinical relevance of the effect on saquinavir is unclear as it is more usually given boosted with ritonavir. Consider monitoring for saquinavir adverse effects if an H₂-receptor antagonist is given.

H₂-receptor antagonists + 5-HT₃-receptor antagonists

The US manufacturer of alosetron predicts that cimetidine might increase alosetron concentrations.

The effects of cimetidine seem likely to be slight. Monitor for alosetron adverse effects (e.g. constipation, abdominal discomfort, nausea) and reduce the dose if necessary. Note that, because of a lack of data, the US manufacturer of alosetron suggest that concurrent use should be avoided.

H₂-receptor antagonists + Lidocaine

Cimetidine slightly reduces the clearance of intravenous and possibly oral lidocaine, and raises its serum concentrations in some patients. Lidocaine toxicity can occur if the dose is not reduced. However, not all patients are affected.

Monitor all patients closely for evidence of lidocaine toxicity (e.g. bradycardia, hypotension, pins and needles) and, if possible, consider checking lidocaine concentrations regularly. A reduced infusion rate may be needed. Ranitidine does not interact and so would appear to be a suitable alternative to cimetidine.

H₂-receptor antagonists + Macrolides

Cimetidine can almost double the levels of erythromycin, although this has only been seen in a single dose study. A single case report describes reversible deafness attributed to this interaction.

Evidence for this interaction is very limited and its general importance is uncertain. If deafness occurs, stop the erythromycin. Ranitidine is a possible non-interacting alternative, as are azithromycin and clarithromycin.

H

H₂-receptor antagonists + Mirtazapine

Cimetidine increases the AUC and peak levels of mirtazapine by 54% and 22%, respectively. Mirtazapine does not appear to affect the pharmacokinetics of cimetidine.

The manufacturers advise that the mirtazapine dose may need to be reduced during concurrent use and increased if cimetidine is stopped. Monitor for an increase in adverse effects (e.g. oedema, drowsiness, headache) when starting cimetidine.

H₂-receptor antagonists + Moclobemide

Cimetidine increases the levels of moclobemide by almost 40%.

Some consider no dose adjustment to be necessary. One manufacturer recommends that moclobemide should be started at the lowest therapeutic dose in patients taking cimetidine, with the dose of moclobemide titrated as required. If cimetidine is given to a patient taking stable doses of moclobemide, the dose of the moclobemide should initially be reduced by 50% and later adjusted as necessary.

H₂-receptor antagonists + **NNRTIs**

Delavirdine

H₂-receptor antagonists are predicted to reduce delavirdine exposure. The efficacy of delavirdine seems likely to be decreased.

> The long-term concurrent use of H₂-receptor antagonists with delavirdine is not recommended.

Rilpivirine

Famotidine moderately reduces rilpivirine exposure. Other H₂-receptor antagonists would be expected to interact similarly and the efficacy of rilpivirine seems likely to be decreased.

> The UK and US manufacturers advise that H₂-receptor antagonists should be taken at least 12 hours before, or 4 hours after, rilpivirine. They also advise that only H₂-receptor antagonists that can be taken once daily are given with rilpivirine.

H₂-receptor antagonists + **Opioids**

Cimetidine increases the levels of alfentanil, and some preliminary observations suggest that cimetidine may increase the half-life of fentanyl. Isolated reports describe adverse reactions in patients taking methadone, morphine, or mixed opium alkaloids when cimetidine was also given, or morphine when ranitidine was also given.

> The clinical relevance of these effects on alfentanil and fentanyl are unknown. However, the UK manufacturer of alfentanil warns that cimetidine could increase the risk of respiratory depression, and that it may be necessary to lower the dose of alfentanil; monitor concurrent use carefully, or consider using ranitidine, which does not appear to interact. The case reports are not expected to be of general significance, although some manufacturers advise caution on concurrent use.

H₂-receptor antagonists + **Pentoxifylline**

Cimetidine moderately increases pentoxifylline levels and adverse effects, such as headache and nausea, are more common.

> Be aware that the adverse effects of pentoxifylline may be increased, and if necessary decrease its dose.

H₂-receptor antagonists + **Phenytoin**

Phenytoin levels are raised by cimetidine (maximum rise of 280% over 3 weeks). Very rarely bone marrow depression develops on concurrent use. Limited evidence suggests that low (non-prescription) doses of cimetidine may not interact. Fosphenytoin, a prodrug of phenytoin, may interact similarly.

> Monitor phenytoin levels and adjust the dose accordingly. Alternatively other H₂-receptor antagonists (ranitidine, famotidine, nizatidine) do not usually interact, although isolated cases have been reported. Be alert for signs of phenytoin toxicity (e.g. blurred vision, nystagmus, ataxia or drowsiness) when these H₂-receptor antagonists are first given.

H₂-receptor antagonists + **Phosphodiesterase type-5 inhibitors**

Cimetidine increases the AUC of sildenafil by 56%.

Both increased efficacy and adverse effects may occur. For erectile dysfunction, the UK manufacturer of sildenafil suggests that a low starting dose of 25 mg should be used if cimetidine is given, although the modest increase in levels seems unlikely to cause particular problems. For pulmonary hypertension, no dose adjustment of sildenafil is necessary. The US manufacturers do not recommend any additional precautions.

H₂-receptor antagonists + **Procainamide**

Cimetidine can increase procainamide levels by more than 50%, which may lead to procainamide toxicity.

Patients, particularly the elderly and those with renal impairment, should be closely monitored for signs of procainamide toxicity, and a dose reduction should be considered. Ranitidine and famotidine appear to interact only minimally or not at all.

H₂-receptor antagonists + **Propafenone**

Cimetidine appears to interact minimally with propafenone.

The UK manufacturer of propafenone advises that all patients are closely monitored and the dose adjusted accordingly on concurrent use with cimetidine. Until more is known, it would seem prudent to monitor all patients for an increase in propafenone adverse effects (such as hypotension, bradycardia, dizziness, dry mouth), and adjust the propafenone dose if necessary.

H

H₂-receptor antagonists + **Quinidine**

Cimetidine can raise quinidine levels and toxicity may develop in some patients.

Be alert for changes in the response to quinidine if cimetidine is started or stopped. Ideally quinidine levels should be monitored and the dose reduced as necessary. Reductions of 25% (oral) to 35% (intravenous) have been suggested.

H₂-receptor antagonists + **Quinine**

The clearance of quinine is reduced by cimetidine.

The clinical importance of this is uncertain, but be particularly alert for any evidence of quinine adverse effects on concurrent use. Note that ranitidine does not appear to interact.

H₂-receptor antagonists + Roflumilast

Cimetidine increases the exposure to roflumilast and its active metabolite, roflumilast N-oxide, and also increases its phosphodiesterase type-4 inhibitory effect.

Some patients might develop roflumilast adverse effects (such as nausea, diarrhoea, headache). Be alert for these and, if possible, adjust the roflumilast dose as necessary.

H₂-receptor antagonists + Sirolimus

The UK and US manufacturers of sirolimus predict that its concentrations will be increased by cimetidine. However, cimetidine is a moderate non-specific inhibitor of cytochrome P450, and would be expected to cause only a minor interaction via this mechanism.

Sirolimus concentrations and/or effects (e.g. on renal function) should be monitored as a matter of routine, but until more is known, it may be prudent to increase monitoring if cimetidine is started or stopped.

H₂-receptor antagonists + SSRIs

The exposure to citalopram, escitalopram, paroxetine, and sertraline is slightly increased by cimetidine.

Initial dose reductions are not needed, but be aware that some patients might have an increase in SSRI adverse effects (such as dry mouth, nausea, diarrhoea, dyspepsia, tremor), in which case dose reductions would be appropriate. As citalopram has been reported to cause small dose-related increases in the QT interval, the FDA in the US advise that the citalopram dose is limited to 20 mg daily in those patients also taking cimetidine. See also Drugs that prolong the QT interval, page 352.

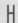

H₂-receptor antagonists + Sucralfate

Sucralfate does not appear to have a clinically relevant effect on the absorption of cimetidine, roxatidine or ranitidine. On this basis, other H₂–receptor antagonists, such as famotidine, would also not be expected to interact.

There appears to be no clear reason for avoiding the concurrent use of sucralfate and H₂-receptor antagonists. Nevertheless, the UK manufacturer of famotidine states that sucralfate should not be given within 2 hours of famotidine.

H₂-receptor antagonists + Tacrine

Cimetidine increases the levels of tacrine by up to about 50%, possibly increasing tacrine beneficial and adverse effects.

Monitor concurrent use for an increase in tacrine adverse effects (nausea, vomiting, diarrhoea).

H₂-receptor antagonists + **Theophylline**

Cimetidine increases theophylline concentrations (by about one-third) and toxicity has been seen. The interaction is unlikely to be clinically relevant in most patients with low-dose cimetidine (200 mg twice daily) . Aminophylline would be expected to interact similarly.

> Monitor theophylline concentrations if cimetidine is added or withdrawn: initial theophylline dose reductions of 30 to 50% have been suggested. The peak effect appears to occur after 3 days. Alternatively, use ranitidine or famotidine, which appear not to interact.

H₂-receptor antagonists + **Tizanidine**

Ciprofloxacin, a CYP1A2 inhibitor, markedly increases tizanidine exposure, which increases the hypotensive and sedative effects of tizanidine. Other CYP1A2 inhibitors (the UK and US manufacturers name cimetidine) are expected to interact similarly.

> The effects of cimetidine on CYP1A2 are less potent than those of ciprofloxacin; nevertheless, the manufacturers suggest that concurrent use should be avoided. Until more is known be alert for tizanidine adverse effects such as bradycardia, hypotension, and drowsiness.

H₂-receptor antagonists + **Tricyclics**

The concurrent use of cimetidine can raise the levels of amitriptyline, desipramine, doxepin, imipramine and nortriptyline. Severe adverse effects have occurred in a few patients. Other tricyclic antidepressants are expected to interact similarly.

> Patients taking tricyclics and cimetidine should be monitored for evidence of increased toxicity (dry mouth, urinary retention, blurred vision, constipation, tachycardia, postural hypotension). Reduce the tricyclic dose if necessary. Ranitidine does not appear to interact.

H

H₂-receptor antagonists + **Triptans** ⚠

Cimetidine slightly increases the exposure to zolmitriptan by about 2-fold.

> The UK manufacturer recommends a zolmitriptan dose reduction to a maximum of 5 mg in 24 hours if patients are also taking cimetidine. The US manufacturer does not suggest a dose adjustment.

H₂-receptor antagonists + **Warfarin and related oral anticoagulants** ⚠

The anticoagulant effects of warfarin can be increased by cimetidine. Severe bleeding has occurred in a few patients but some show no interaction at all. Acenocoumarol and phenindione seem to interact similarly.

> Monitor the INR if cimetidine is added or withdrawn. The interaction is rapid and may occur within days and even as early as after 24 hours. Famotidine, nizatidine

and ranitidine usually appear to be non-interacting alternatives, although isolated cases of bleeding have been seen.

Heparin

Heparin + HRT

Drospirenone, which is given as the progestogen component in some HRT formulations, might increase the risk of hyperkalaemia when given with other drugs that can cause hyperkalaemia such as heparin. The UK manufacturer of drospirenone-containing HRT notes that the increase in potassium levels may be more pronounced in diabetic women.

The risk of hyperkalaemia appears to be low, especially if renal function is normal. In the US, it is recommended that consideration be given to monitoring potassium levels during the first cycle in women [with normal renal function] who regularly take heparin, whereas the UK manufacturer recommends that the potassium level is measured during the first cycle or month of treatment only in women with mild or moderate renal impairment. In patients at higher risk of developing hyperkalaemia (e.g. in renal impairment) it is generally recommended that potassium levels are measured during the first cycle of treatment with drospirenone.

Heparin + Nitrates

Some studies claim that the effects of heparin are reduced by the concurrent infusion of nitrates, but others have not confirmed this interaction.

On balance it appears that a clinically relevant interaction is generally unlikely to be seen. Furthermore, given that heparin is routinely monitored, it is likely that if an interaction did occur, it would be rapidly detected.

Heparin + NSAIDs

Ketorolac

The risk of bleeding is said to be particularly high if ketorolac is used with anticoagulants including heparin. However, one study found no increase in bleeding time when ketorolac was given with heparin.

The CSM in the UK and the manufacturer of ketorolac state that the concurrent use of anticoagulants is contraindicated, and they include low doses of heparin. Conversely, the US manufacturers of ketorolac advise that physicians should carefully weigh the benefits against the risks and use heparin with ketorolac only extremely cautiously.

NSAIDs, general

An increased risk of bleeding occurs when NSAIDs (that have antiplatelet actions) are given with heparin. Anticoagulants can exacerbate gastrointestinal bleeding caused by NSAIDs. Cases of spinal haematomas after epidural anaesthesia have been reported with the concurrent use of heparin and NSAIDs.

> Concurrent use is not uncommon, but prescribers should be aware that there is an increased risk of bleeding and monitor appropriately. Extreme caution is needed if concurrent use is considered appropriate in patients undergoing epidural anaesthesia.

Heparin + Prasugrel ❓

No significant interaction was reported between prasugrel and a single intravenous bolus of heparin; however, the manufacturers advise that there is a possible increased risk of bleeding on concurrent use. The use of prasugrel and heparin may contribute to the development of epidural or spinal haematoma after epidural anaesthesia.

> Concurrent use need not be avoided, but be aware of the potential for this interaction if bleeding occurs. If they are used together, the manufacturers of the LMWHs recommend caution or careful clinical and laboratory monitoring. Extreme caution is needed if concurrent use is considered appropriate in patients undergoing epidural anaesthesia.

Heparin + Rivaroxaban ⚠

The concurrent use of rivaroxaban and anticoagulants increases the risk of bleeding.

> Monitor for signs of bleeding. The US manufacturer of rivaroxaban advises avoiding rivaroxaban for prophylaxis of deep vein thrombosis in patients taking other anticoagulants. The UK manufacturer of rivaroxaban contraindicates concurrent use unless switching between anticoagulants.

H

Heparin + Ticagrelor ⚠

The antiplatelet effects of ticagrelor are not altered by heparin. However, the UK manufacturer of ticagrelor states that the concurrent use of other drugs that affect coagulation might theoretically increase the risk of bleeding.

> Concurrent use might be clinically beneficial; however, it would seem prudent to monitor the outcome of concurrent use, being aware that the risk of bleeding might be increased.

Heparin + Ticlopidine ⚠

Concurrent use of ticlopidine with heparin increases haemorrhagic risk, and may contribute to the development of epidural or spinal haematoma after epidural anaesthesia.

> If concurrent use is undertaken, there should be close clinical and laboratory monitoring. Extreme caution is needed if concurrent use is considered appropriate in patients undergoing epidural anaesthesia.

Herbal medicines or Dietary supplements

There seem to be few clinical reports of interactions between herbal medicines (with the exception of St John's wort) or dietary supplements and so recommendations regarding the interactions are often difficult to make. An additional problem in interpreting these interactions, is that the interacting constituent of the herb is usually not known and is therefore not standardised for. It could vary widely between different products, and batches of the same product. Bear this in mind.

Herbal medicines or Dietary supplements + HIV-protease inhibitors

Garlic

A garlic supplement reduced saquinavir exposure in one study, but had little effect in another.

> All garlic supplements should probably be avoided if saquinavir is ever given as the sole HIV-protease inhibitor (not recommended). The clinical relevance of this interaction with saquinavir boosted with ritonavir is unclear, but note that no appreciable interaction appears to occur with single-dose ritonavir.

St John's wort (Hypericum perforatum) ⊗

St John's wort reduces indinavir exposure, which might result in HIV treatment failure. Other HIV-protease inhibitors, whether used alone or boosted with ritonavir, are predicted to interact similarly.

> In general concurrent use is either contraindicated or not recommended. The CSM in the UK advise that patients taking HIV-protease inhibitors with St John's wort should stop the St John's wort and have their HIV RNA viral load measured. The UK manufacturer also notes that the exposure to HIV-protease inhibitors might increase in the 2 weeks after stopping St John's wort, and the dose could need adjusting.

Herbal medicines or Dietary supplements + HRT

The hormones in HRT are similar to those used in hormonal contraceptives, and so may be affected by enzyme-inducing drugs, such as St John's wort (*Hypericum perforatum*), in the same way as contraceptives, page 293. Reduced effects are therefore possible if St John's wort is also given.

> The clinical significance of any interaction is unclear; however, consider the possibility of reduced HRT efficacy on concurrent use. The effect is most likely to be noticed where HRT is prescribed for menopausal vasomotor symptoms, but might be difficult to detect where the indication is osteoporosis. The interaction is not relevant to HRT applied locally for menopausal vaginitis.

H

Herbal medicines or Dietary supplements +
Ivabradine

St John's wort (*Hypericum perforatum*) reduces the exposure to ivabradine by about 50%.

Monitor concurrent use for ivabradine efficacy and adjust the dose as necessary. Remember to re-adjust the dose of ivabradine if the concurrent use of these drugs is stopped. The UK manufacturer suggests that the use of St John's wort should be restricted in patients taking ivabradine.

Herbal medicines or Dietary supplements +
Lacosamide

The manufacturer predicts that St John's wort (*Hypericum perforatum*) may moderately decrease lacosamide exposure.

The clinical significance of this is unknown; however, be aware that starting or stopping St John's wort may alter lacosamide levels.

Herbal medicines or Dietary supplements + Lithium

Herbal diuretic

A woman developed lithium toxicity after taking a herbal diuretic containing corn silk, *Equisetum hyemale*, juniper, ovate buchu, parsley and bearberry.

This interaction is similar to that seen with prescription diuretics, page 341. Concurrent use needs monitoring, and patients should be encouraged to seek advice before self-medicating.

St John's wort (*Hypericum perforatum*)

A case report describes mania in a patient taking St John's wort and lithium.

The general importance of this interaction is unclear. Bear it in mind in case of an unexpected response to treatment.

Herbal medicines or Dietary supplements + MAOIs

Two patients developed headache, insomnia, and in one case hallucinations, when they took phenelzine with ginseng.

The general importance of these poorly documented early cases is unclear. Nevertheless, consider the possibility of an interaction in case of an unexpected response to treatment with phenelzine (or potentially any MAOI) in a patient taking any type of ginseng.

Herbal medicines or Dietary supplements +

Maraviroc ✗

St John's wort is predicted to reduce maraviroc exposure and reduce its antiviral efficacy.

The UK and US manufacturers of maraviroc and the US HIV guidelines recommend avoiding concurrent use.

Herbal medicines or Dietary supplements +

NNRTIs ✗

There is evidence to suggest that St John's wort (*Hypericum perforatum*) might decrease nevirapine concentrations. Delavirdine, efavirenz, etravirine, and rilpivirine would be expected to interact similarly.

It is generally recommended that the concurrent use of St John's wort and NNRTIs should be avoided.

Herbal medicines or Dietary supplements + **NSAIDs**

Ginkgo biloba ❓

Case reports describe fatal intracerebral bleeding in a patient taking *Ginkgo biloba* with ibuprofen, and prolonged bleeding and subdural haematomas in a patient taking *Ginkgo biloba* with rofecoxib. Studies with diclofenac and flurbiprofen showed that *Ginkgo biloba* had no effect on the pharmacokinetics of these drugs.

The evidence from these reports is too slim to advise patients against taking NSAIDs and *Ginkgo biloba* concurrently, but some do recommend caution. Medical professionals should be aware of the possibility of increased bleeding tendency with *Ginkgo biloba* and monitor patients appropriately.

Tamarindus indica ⚠

Tamarindus indica (tamarind) fruit extract caused a 2-fold increase in the AUC of ibuprofen.

The clinical relevance of this interaction is unknown, but large rises in the ibuprofen levels may result in toxicity.

Herbal medicines or Dietary supplements + **Opioids**

Alfentanil, Buprenorphine, Fentanyl, or Methadone ⚠

St John's wort (*Hypericum perforatum*) reduces the plasma concentrations of methadone, and withdrawal symptoms have been reported. Buprenorphine, fentanyl, and alfentanil are predicted to interact similarly.

Advise patients taking these opioids to avoid St John's wort.

Oxycodone or Tapentadol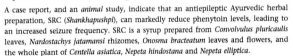

St John's wort reduces the exposure to oxycodone but its analgesic effects do not appear to be notably altered. St John's wort is predicted to induce the metabolism of tapentadol.

Consider an interaction in the case of any unexpected reduction in analgesic effect, and adjust the opioid dose accordingly.

Herbal medicines or Dietary supplements + Penicillins ⚠

Chewing khat reduces the absorption of ampicillin, and to a lesser extent amoxicillin, but the effects are minimal 2 hours after khat chewing stops.

The authors of one of the studies concluded that both ampicillin and amoxicillin should be taken 2 hours after khat chewing to ensure that maximum absorption occurs.

Herbal medicines or Dietary supplements + Perampanel ⚠

St John's wort is predicted to decrease perampanel exposure.

Monitor for perampanel efficacy and increase the perampanel dose if necessary.

Herbal medicines or Dietary supplements + Phenobarbital ⚠

St John's wort (*Hypericum perforatum*) is predicted to reduce the levels of phenobarbital (and therefore possibly primidone-derived phenobarbital).

Until more is known, it would probably be prudent to avoid concurrent use. The CSM in the UK advise that St John's wort should be stopped and that the phenobarbital dose should be adjusted.

H

Herbal medicines or Dietary supplements + Phenytoin

Ayurvedic medicines ✕

A case report, and an *animal* study, indicate that an antiepileptic Ayurvedic herbal preparation, SRC (*Shankhapushpi*), can markedly reduce phenytoin levels, leading to an increased seizure frequency. SRC is a syrup prepared from *Convolvulus pluricaulis* leaves, *Nardostachys jatamansi* rhizomes, *Onosma bracteatum* leaves and flowers, and the whole plant of *Centella asiatica*, *Nepeta hindostana* and *Nepeta elliptica*.

Shankhapushpi (SRC) is given because it has some antiepileptic activity but there is little point in combining it with phenytoin if the outcome is a fall in phenytoin levels, accompanied by an increase in seizure frequency. For this reason concurrent use should be avoided. It would seem prudent to be similarly cautious with the use of fosphenytoin, a prodrug of phenytoin.

St John's wort (*Hypericum perforatum*)

St John's wort is predicted to reduce the levels of phenytoin. Fosphenytoin, a prodrug of phenytoin, may interact similarly.

> Until more is known, it would probably be prudent to avoid concurrent use in patients taking phenytoin, especially as phenytoin is a substrate of CYP2C19, which St John's wort appears to induce. The CSM in the UK advise that St John's wort should be stopped and that the phenytoin dose should be adjusted.

Herbal medicines or Dietary supplements + Phosphodiesterase type-5 inhibitors

St John's wort is predicted to reduce the exposure to the phosphodiesterase type-5 inhibitors, because other inducers of CYP3A4 have been shown to do so.

> If standard doses of these phosphodiesterase type-5 inhibitors are not effective for erectile dysfunction in patients taking St John's wort, consider reviewing the need for concurrent use. If concurrent use is necessary, a dose increase in the phosphodiesterase type-5 inhibitor might be required. For pulmonary hypertension, it might be prudent to follow the same advice for rifampicin: the UK manufacturer of sildenafil states that sildenafil efficacy should be closely monitored, with the sildenafil dose increased as necessary, whereas the manufacturers of tadalafil for pulmonary hypertension do not recommend the concurrent use of St John's wort. The UK and US manufacturers of avanafil contraindicate concurrent use with all CYP3A4 inducers.

Herbal medicines or Dietary supplements + Prasugrel

Ginkgo biloba has been associated with platelet, bleeding and clotting disorders and there are isolated reports of serious adverse reactions after its concurrent use with antiplatelet drugs. Prasugrel would be expected to interact similarly.

> The evidence is too slim to advise patients against taking prasugrel with *Ginkgo biloba*. However, caution should be exercised if *Ginkgo biloba* is used with any drug that affects platelet aggregation as bleeding has been seen with the use of *Ginkgo biloba* alone. Patients should be told to seek professional advice if any bleeding problems arise.

Herbal medicines or Dietary supplements + Proton pump inhibitors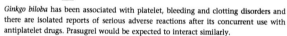

Both *Gingko biloba* and St John's wort (*Hypericum perforatum*) induce the metabolism of omeprazole, and this might result in reduced efficacy. Other proton pump inhibitors are likely to be similarly affected.

> There is insufficient evidence to suggest that these herbs should be avoided in patients taking proton pump inhibitors. However, the potential reduction in their efficacy should be borne in mind, particular where the consequences may be serious, such as in patients with healing ulcers.

Herbal medicines or Dietary supplements +

Ranolazine

Rifampicin (rifampin) reduces ranolazine levels by 95%, and loss of efficacy is expected. St John's wort is predicted to interact in the same way as rifampicin.

The manufacturers recommend avoiding concurrent use. In the absence of any information on the magnitude of the effect of St John's wort on ranolazine levels, this seems prudent.

Herbal medicines or Dietary supplements +

Rivaroxaban

St John's wort is predicted to decrease the exposure to rivaroxaban, and therefore decrease its anticoagulant effects.

Given the likely clinical risk of reduced rivaroxaban efficacy, it would seem prudent to consider using an alternative drug; however, if this is not possible, consider closely monitoring the prothrombin time to ensure the anticoagulant effect of rivaroxaban is maintained. The US manufacturer of rivaroxaban advises avoiding concurrent use.

Herbal medicines or Dietary supplements +

Sirolimus

St John's wort (*Hypericum perforatum*) is predicted to decrease sirolimus concentrations.

If concurrent use cannot be avoided, increase the frequency of monitoring of sirolimus concentrations, and adjust the dose as necessary.

Herbal medicines or Dietary supplements + SSRIs

Ayahuasca ❓

A man taking fluoxetine experienced symptoms of serotonin syndrome after drinking the psychoactive beverage ayahuasca (also known as caapi, daime, hoasca, natema, yage), which is characteristically derived from the vine *Banisteriopsis caapi*.

This appears to be the only report of an interaction. However, as ayahuasca contains monoamine oxidase-inhibiting harmala alkaloids concurrent use with any SSRIs may potentially cause serotonin syndrome, page 580.

St John's wort (*Hypericum perforatum*)

Cases of severe sedation, mania and serotonin syndrome, page 580, have been reported in patients taking St John's wort with SSRIs.

The incidence of an interaction is probably small, but because of the potential severity of the reaction it would seem prudent to avoid the concurrent use of any SSRI and St John's wort. The CSM in the UK advise that St John's wort should be stopped if patients are taking an SSRI.

H

Herbal medicines or Dietary supplements + Statins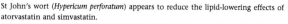

St John's wort (*Hypericum perforatum*) appears to reduce the lipid-lowering effects of atorvastatin and simvastatin.

> The clinical importance of this interaction is unclear but it might be prudent to consider an interaction if lipid-lowering targets are not met, and advise the patient to stop taking St John's wort or adjust the dose of atorvastatin or simvastatin if needed. Pravastatin does not appear to interact.

Herbal medicines or Dietary supplements + Tacrolimus ✕

St John's wort (*Hypericum perforatum*) has been found, on average, to decrease tacrolimus maximum levels by 65% and its AUC by 32%. However, the decrease in AUC ranged from 15% to 64%, with one patient having a 31% *increase* in AUC.

> Given the unpredictability of the interaction (and the variability in content of St John's wort products) it would seem prudent to avoid St John's wort in transplant patients, and possibly patients taking tacrolimus for other indications. If St John's wort is withdrawn monitor tacrolimus levels and adjust the dose accordingly.

Herbal medicines or Dietary supplements + Ticlopidine ⚠

Ginkgo biloba has been associated with platelet, bleeding and clotting disorders and there are isolated reports of serious adverse reactions after its concurrent use with antiplatelet drugs including ticlopidine.

> The evidence is too slim to advise patients against taking ticlopidine with *Ginkgo biloba*. However, caution should be exercised if *Ginkgo biloba* is used with any drug that affects platelet aggregation as bleeding has been seen with the use of *Ginkgo biloba* alone. Patients should be told to seek professional advice if any bleeding problems arise.

Herbal medicines or Dietary supplements + Trazodone ❓

Coma developed in an elderly patient with Alzheimer's disease after she took trazodone with *Ginkgo biloba*. She later recovered.

> This appears to be an isolated case, from which no general conclusions can be drawn.

Herbal medicines or Dietary supplements + Tricyclics ✅

The levels of amitriptyline and its metabolite nortriptyline are modestly reduced by St John's wort (*Hypericum perforatum*). Other tricyclics would be expected to interact similarly.

> The clinical significance of this interaction is unknown, although it is likely to be

small. However, bear it in mind should an unexpected reduction in tricyclic efficacy occur. Both the tricyclics and St John's wort are antidepressants, but whether concurrent use is beneficial or safe is not known. Further study is needed.

Herbal medicines or Dietary supplements +
Triptans

Serotonin syndrome (see serotonin syndrome, page 580) has been reported in a patient taking eletriptan and St John's wort (*Hypericum perforatum*). This reaction is possible with any triptan and St John's wort.

.Monitor carefully for signs of serotonin syndrome (such as weakness, hyperreflexia, and incoordination).

Herbal medicines or Dietary supplements +
Ulipristal

The UK and US manufacturers of ulipristal predict that CYP3A4 inducers such as St John's wort (*Hypericum perforatum*) might reduce the plasma concentration of ulipristal and reduce its efficacy.

The US manufacturer of ulipristal gives no specific advice about how to manage this potential interaction, whereas the UK manufacturer advises that ulipristal should not be used for emergency contraception or the symptomatic management of fibroids in women taking CYP3A4 inducers (such as St John's wort), or who have stopped taking an enzyme inducer within the last 2 to 3 weeks. Note that the MHRA in the UK specifically advises that women taking hormonal contraceptives for pregnancy prevention (except IUDs, but probably including emergency hormonal contraceptives) should not take herbal products containing St John's wort.

H

Herbal medicines or Dietary supplements +
Venlafaxine

Jujube ❓

An isolated report describes an acute serotonin reaction when venlafaxine was given with a Chinese herbal remedy, jujube (sour date nut; suanzaoren; *Ziziphus jujuba*).

Patients should be asked about the use of herbal remedies and advised to discontinue them before prescribing antidepressant drugs if there is any possibility of an interaction.

St John's wort (*Hypericum perforatum*)

A possible case of serotonin syndrome has been reported in a patient taking venlafaxine and St John's wort.

Caution is advised if venlafaxine is given with other drugs that affect the serotonergic neurotransmitter systems, such as St John's wort. See serotonin syndrome, page 580, for further monitoring advice.

Herbal medicines or Dietary supplements + Warfarin and related oral anticoagulants

Boldo

A report describes a woman on warfarin whose INR rose modestly when she began to take boldo and fenugreek. She was eventually restabilised with a 15% dose reduction.

> Evidence is limited to one isolated case. Because of the many other factors influencing anticoagulant control, it is not possible to reliably ascribe a change in INR specifically to a drug interaction in a single case report without other supporting evidence. Advise patients to discuss the use of any herbal products they wish to try, and to increase monitoring if this is thought advisable.

Chamomile

A single case describes a woman taking warfarin who developed a marked increase in her INR with bleeding complications 5 days after she started drinking chamomile tea (an infusion of *Matricaria chamomilla* (German chamomile)) and using a chamomile-based skin lotion.

> Note that there appear to be no reports of German chamomile alone causing anticoagulation, which might suggest that the risk of an additive effect is small. Because of the many other factors influencing anticoagulant control, it is not possible to reliably ascribe a change in INR specifically to a drug interaction in a single case report without other supporting evidence. Advise patients to discuss the use of any herbal products they wish to try, and to increase monitoring if this is thought advisable.

Chinese angelica (Angelica sinensis)

Two case reports describe a very marked increase in the anticoagulant effects of warfarin when Chinese angelica was added.

> Patients taking warfarin and related anticoagulants should be warned of the potential risks of also taking Chinese angelica. Until more information is available, Chinese angelica should be avoided unless the effects on anticoagulation can be monitored.

Cucurbita

The INR of a patient taking warfarin increased from 2.4 to 3.5 after he took curbicin, which contains saw palmetto (*Serenoa repens*) and *Cucurbita pepo*.

> Evidence is limited to one isolated case. Because of the many other factors influencing anticoagulant control, it is not possible to reliably ascribe a change in INR specifically to a drug interaction in a single case report without other supporting evidence. Advise patients to discuss the use of any herbal products they wish to try, and to increase monitoring if this is thought advisable.

Danshen

Several case reports indicate that danshen (the root of *Salvia miltiorrhiza*), a Chinese herbal remedy, can increase the effects of warfarin resulting in bleeding. There seems to be no evidence about other related anticoagulants, but it seems possible that they may be similarly affected.

> Avoid concurrent use where possible. However, if concurrent use is felt desirable it

H

would seem sensible to warn patients to be alert for any signs of bruising or bleeding, and report these immediately, should they occur.

Fenugreek 🛈

A report describes a woman taking warfarin whose INR rose modestly when she began to take boldo and fenugreek. She was eventually restabilised with a 15% dose reduction.

Evidence is limited to one isolated case. Because of the many other factors influencing anticoagulant control, it is not possible to reliably ascribe a change in INR specifically to a drug interaction in a single case report without other supporting evidence. Advise patients to discuss the use of any herbal products they wish to try, and to increase monitoring if this is thought advisable.

Fish oils ⚠

The use of warfarin with fish oils did not alter warfarin efficacy in two studies, nor the incidence of bleeding episodes in another. However, there are a couple of reports of an increased INR in patients taking warfarin and fish oils, and one of a life-threatening bleed without an increase in INR in a patient taking high-dose fish oils with aspirin and warfarin.

This interaction is not established. Based on the possible modest increase in bleeding times with high-dose fish oils, the manufacturers of one product state that patients receiving anticoagulants should be monitored (e.g. for bruising or bleeding), and the dose of anticoagulant adjusted as necessary. Note that monitoring the INR would not pick up this pharmacodynamic interaction.

Garlic 🛈

Two patients taking warfarin and one taking fluindione developed increased INRs after the addition of garlic capsules. One patient developed haematuria. However, a controlled study with warfarin suggests no interaction occurs.

This interaction seems rare, but bear it in mind in case of unexpected bleeding. It is worth noting that there have been cases of spontaneous bleeding attributed to garlic alone. In addition, garlic may have some antiplatelet effects, and although there appear to be no clinical reports of an adverse interaction, it may be prudent to consider the potential for an increase in the severity of bleeding if garlic is given with anticoagulants.

Ginkgo biloba 🛈

Evidence from studies suggests that *Ginkgo biloba* does not interact with warfarin. However, an isolated report describes intracerebral haemorrhage associated with the use of *Ginkgo biloba* and warfarin

There is insufficient evidence to justify telling patients taking warfarin to avoid *Ginkgo biloba* but, because bleeding has been reported with *Ginkgo biloba* alone, they should be told to monitor for early signs of bruising or bleeding and seek informed professional advice if any bleeding problems arise.

Ginseng ⚠

One pharmacological study found that *Panax quinquefolius* (American ginseng) modestly decreased the effect of warfarin, whereas another study found that *Panax*

H

ginseng (Asian ginseng) did not alter the effect of warfarin. Two case reports describe decreased warfarin effects, one with thrombosis, attributed to the use of ginseng (probably *Panax ginseng*). Note that there have been reports of spontaneous bleeding with ginseng alone, and *Panax ginseng* has been found to contain antiplatelet components.

> Be alert for a possible decrease in the effects of warfarin and related drugs in patients using ginseng, particularly *Panax quinquefolius*.Patients should be warned to monitor for early signs of bruising or bleeding and seek informed professional advice if any bleeding problems arise.

Glucosamine +/- Chondroitin

A couple of reports suggest that glucosamine with or without chondroitin may increase the INR in patients taking warfarin. In contrast, one case of a *decreased* INR has been reported when glucosamine was taken with acenocoumarol.

> An interaction would seem to be rare, and there do not appear to have been any controlled studies of this interaction. The cases described suggest it would be prudent to monitor the INR more closely if glucosamine is started. If a patient shows an unexpected change in INR, bear in mind the possibility of self-medication with supplements such as glucosamine.

Lycium barbarum

One patient developed a raised INR after taking a tea made from the fruits of *Lycium barbarum* L. (also known as Chinese wolfberry, gou qi zi, Fructus Lycii Chinensis, or *Lycium chinense*).

> Evidence is limited to one isolated case. Because of the many other factors influencing anticoagulant control, it is not possible to reliably ascribe a change in INR specifically to a drug interaction in a single case report without other supporting evidence. Advise patients to discuss the use of any herbal products they wish to try, and to increase monitoring if this is thought advisable.

Quilinggao ❓

A single case report describes a man taking warfarin who had a marked increase in his INR with bleeding complications, 9 days after he switched the brand of quilinggao (a Chinese herbal product made from a mixture of herbs) he was using.

> The general importance of this isolated case report is unknown, but bear it in mind in case of an increased response to anticoagulant treatment.

Saw palmetto ❓

The INR of a patient taking warfarin increased from 2.4 to 3.5 after he took curbicin, which contains saw palmetto and cucurbita. Excessive bleeding during surgery has been reported in another patient who had been taking saw palmetto.

> Because of the many other factors influencing anticoagulant control, it is not possible to reliably ascribe a change in INR specifically to a drug interaction in a single case report without other supporting evidence. Advise patients to discuss the use of any herbal products they wish to try, and to increase monitoring if this is thought advisable.

St John's wort (Hypericum perforatum) ❌

St John's wort can reduce the anticoagulant effects of phenprocoumon and warfarin.

It would be prudent to monitor the INRs of patients taking any coumarin if they start taking St John's wort, increasing the anticoagulant dose if needed. However, note that the CSM in the UK advise against the concurrent use of St John's wort with warfarin: if St John's wort is being taken by patients also taking anticoagulants the herb should be stopped and the anticoagulant dose adjusted as necessary.

Ubidecarenone (Coenzyme Q10) ⚠

Coenzyme Q10 did not alter the INR or required warfarin dose in a controlled study in patients stabilised on warfarin. However, cases of either reduced, or transiently increased anticoagulant effects have been reported in patients taking warfarin and ubidecarenone.

The general importance of this interaction is unknown. Until more is known it would seem prudent to increase the frequency of INR monitoring in patients taking warfarin if coenzyme Q10 is started.

HIV-protease inhibitors

The HIV-protease inhibitors are extensively metabolised by cytochrome P450, particularly CYP3A4. All of the HIV-protease inhibitors inhibit CYP3A4, with ritonavir being the most potent inhibitor, followed by indinavir, nelfinavir, amprenavir, and saquinavir. The HIV-protease inhibitors therefore have the potential to interact with other drugs metabolised by CYP3A4, and may also be affected by CYP3A4 inhibitors and inducers. Ritonavir and tipranavir also affect some other cytochrome P450 isoenzymes, particularly CYP2D6. In addition, HIV-protease inhibitors are substrates as well as inhibitors of P-glycoprotein. The plasma level of HIV-protease inhibitors is thought to be critical in maintaining efficacy and minimising the potential for development of viral resistance. Therefore even modest reductions in concentrations are potentially clinically important.

HIV-protease inhibitors + HRT ❓

The hormones in HRT are similar to those used in hormonal contraceptives, and so may be affected by the HIV-protease inhibitors in the same way as contraceptives, page 294. Reduced effects are therefore theoretically possible if a HIV-protease inhibitor is also given; however, note that some HIV-protease inhibitors have actually *increased* hormone levels.

Any interaction resulting in reduced effect would be most likely to be noticed where HRT is prescribed for menopausal vasomotor symptoms, but might be difficult to detect where the indication is osteoporosis. Further study is needed to confirm the clinical significance of this possible interaction but it may be prudent to use the lowest possible dose of HRT and gradually titrate to effect. The interaction is not relevant to HRT applied locally for menopausal vaginitis.

HIV-protease inhibitors + **Ivabradine**

Ketoconazole, a potent inhibitor of CYP3A4, increases ivabradine levels up to 8-fold. The manufacturer predicts that other CYP3A4 inhibitors, such as the HIV-protease inhibitors, will interact similarly.

> The manufacturer contraindicates the concurrent use of ivabradine with the HIV-protease inhibitors (they name nelfinavir and ritonavir).

HIV-protease inhibitors + **Lamotrigine**

Atazanavir and lopinavir boosted with ritonavir and possibly saquinavir boosted with ritonavir might moderately reduce lamotrigine concentrations, whereas the HIV-protease inhibitor concentrations do not appear to be altered. Reduced lamotrigine concentrations should be anticipated with any ritonavir-boosted regimen.

> Lamotrigine efficacy should be monitored in patients taking any ritonavir-boosted regimen (seizures have occurred as a result of this interaction). Anticipate the need to increase the lamotrigine dose.

HIV-protease inhibitors + **Lidocaine**

Ritonavir appears to increase lidocaine concentrations more than 3-fold, which would be expected to increase the risk of lidocaine adverse effects, including arrhythmias. Other HIV-protease inhibitors might interact similarly.

> The UK manufacturers of darunavir and saquinavir contraindicate concurrent use. The manufacturers of fosamprenavir, indinavir, nelfinavir, and tipranavir contraindicate the concurrent use of drugs with a narrow therapeutic range that are metabolised by CYP3A4, which could reasonably be expected to include lidocaine. If concurrent use cannot be avoided, it would seem prudent to monitor closely for lidocaine adverse effects (such as bradycardia, hypotension, pins and needles), monitoring lidocaine concentrations if possible. Reduce the lidocaine dose as necessary.

HIV-protease inhibitors + **Levothyroxine**

Case reports suggest that HIV-protease inhibitors boosted with ritonavir increase levothyroxine dose requirements. Nelfinavir might interact similarly. The situation with indinavir is less clear, with no effect, a reduction and an increase in levothyroxine requirements reported in different cases; the outcome seems likely to depend on the other antiretrovirals given.

> Direct information is limited and the presence of an interaction seems to depend on the individual HIV-protease inhibitor, how it affects glucuronidation, and how much remaining thyroid function a patient has. Until more is known about this interaction it would seem prudent to monitor thyroid function more closely if a HIV-protease inhibitor is given to a patient with pre-existing thyroid dysfunction.

HIV-protease inhibitors + **Loperamide**

Ritonavir

Ritonavir increases the levels of loperamide without increasing its CNS adverse effects.

> The increase in loperamide bioavailability is not expected to be clinically relevant.

Saquinavir

Loperamide reduces the bioavailability of unboosted saquinavir by about 50%. Unboosted saquinavir modestly increases the bioavailability of loperamide.

> Evidence for an interaction between loperamide and unboosted saquinavir is limited, but until more is known, it would seem prudent to monitor patients to ensure that saquinavir remains effective. The increase in loperamide bioavailability is not expected to be clinically relevant.

Tipranavir

Tipranavir, both alone and boosted with ritonavir, *reduces* the exposure to loperamide and its metabolites.

> The clinical relevance of the decrease in loperamide exposure with tipranavir, alone or boosted with ritonavir, is unknown, but might not be important as loperamide is thought to have a local action in the gut.

HIV-protease inhibitors + **Macrolides**

Azithromycin with Nelfinavir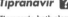

The pharmacokinetics of nelfinavir are minimally affected by azithromycin, but azithromycin exposure is roughly doubled by nelfinavir.

> The clinical significance of this interaction has not been established. Monitor for increased azithromycin adverse effects.

Clarithromycin with HIV-protease inhibitors

Most HIV-protease inhibitors (atazanavir, indinavir, ritonavir, saquinavir, and darunavir, and tipranavir boosted with ritonavir) increase clarithromycin exposure and reduce exposure to the 14-hydroxyclarithromycin metabolite, with the possible exception of unboosted amprenavir. Clarithromycin has no effect on the pharmacokinetics of amprenavir, darunavir boosted with ritonavir, indinavir, and ritonavir, but it slightly increases the exposure to atazanavir and tipranavir boosted with ritonavir, and might moderately increase saquinavir exposure (from soft capsules).

> Patients with **normal renal function**: although most manufacturers suggest that no dose adjustment is necessary the UK manufacturer of tipranavir advises monitoring clarithromycin adverse effects in those taking a dose of clarithromycin of more than 500 mg twice daily and the US manufacturer of atazanavir suggests that the clarithromycin dose should be reduced by 50%. As the levels of 14-hydroxyclarithromycin are significantly reduced it is generally advised that for most infections an alternative to clarithromycin should be considered with the exception of *Mycobacterium avium* complex infections, where this metabolite is less active. If concurrent use is undertaken, some dose adjustments of the clarithromycin may

H

be needed. Patients with **renal impairment**: the manufacturers of ritonavir and clarithromycin recommend a 50% reduction in the dose of clarithromycin for those with a creatinine clearance of 30 to 60 mL/minute and a 75% reduction for clearances of less than 30 mL/minute. Some advise avoiding clarithromycin in doses exceeding 1 g daily. Similar clarithromycin dose reductions in renal impairment are recommended for a number of HIV-protease inhibitors boosted with ritonavir. Note that clarithromycin has been associated with QT prolongation, and rises in its concentrations might increase this risk. In addition, saquinavir might prolong the QT interval and the manufacturers contraindicate its concurrent use with other drugs that prolong the QT interval. See Drugs that prolong the QT interval, page 352, for a general discussion of QT prolongation.

Erythromycin with Saquinavir

Erythromycin might increase saquinavir exposure from soft capsules. Saquinavir boosted with ritonavir is associated with a high risk of prolonging the QT interval; erythromycin (particularly intravenous erythromycin) can also prolong the QT interval. The UK and US manufacturers suggest that a serious prolongation is possible if they are used together.

Because of the potential risks of QT prolongation, the UK manufacturer contra-indicates the concurrent use of erythromycin and saquinavir boosted with ritonavir. See Drugs that prolong the QT interval, page 352, for a general discussion of QT prolongation.

Erythromycin with Other HIV-protease inhibitors

The concurrent use of fosamprenavir or amprenavir with erythromycin is predicted to increase the concentrations of both the HIV-protease inhibitor and erythromycin. The manufacturers predict that ritonavir (including ritonavir used to boost other HIV-protease inhibitors) will greatly elevate erythromycin concentrations.

Carefully monitor the outcome of giving erythromycin with amprenavir or fosamprenavir. Advise patients to be alert for erythromycin and amprenavir or fosamprenavir adverse effects (such as gastrointestinal effects, tremors). The concurrent use of erythromycin and ritonavir should not be undertaken unless the benefits outweigh the risks. Monitor for erythromycin adverse effects (e.g. gastrointestinal effects). Note that high levels of erythromycin can cause temporary hearing loss.

Telithromycin with HIV-protease inhibitors

Ketoconazole increases the exposure to telithromycin. The manufacturers therefore predict that the exposure to telithromycin moderately increased in the presence of ritonavir, which is a more potent inhibitor of telithromycin metabolism than ketoconazole. Other HIV-protease inhibitors might also inhibit telithromycin metabolism.

The UK manufacturer of telithromycin advises caution on concurrent use. Monitor for telithromycin adverse effects (such as diarrhoea, dizziness, and headache). Note that concurrent use is contraindicated in severe hepatic or renal impairment. Note that saquinavir boosted with ritonavir and telithromycin have been associated with QT prolongation, see Drugs that prolong the QT interval, page 352 for more information.

HIV-protease inhibitors + **Mebendazole**

Ritonavir reduces the exposure to mebendazole.

It might be necessary to increase the mebendazole dose when treating systemic worm infections in patients also taking ritonavir. Monitor the outcome of concurrent use. The interaction is of no importance when mebendazole is used for intestinal worm infections.

HIV-protease inhibitors + **Mexiletine**

Ritonavir appears to increase the concentrations of mexiletine, probably by inhibiting CYP2D6. Tipranavir, and any other HIV-protease inhibitor boosted with ritonavir, would be expected to interact similarly.

Until more is known, it would seem prudent to monitor any patient taking mexiletine with ritonavir, tipranavir, or any HIV-protease inhibitor boosted with ritonavir, for an increase in mexiletine adverse effects (such as nausea, tremor, hypotension), and titrate the mexiletine dose slowly, according to clinical response.

HIV-protease inhibitors + **Mirtazapine**

Ketoconazole increases the exposure to mirtazapine (by inhibiting CYP3A4). The HIV-protease inhibitors are predicted to interact similarly.

The manufacturers advise caution on concurrent use and that a decrease in the dose of mirtazapine may be needed. Monitor for adverse effects (most commonly sedation, fatigue, headache) and adjust the mirtazapine dose as needed.

H

HIV-protease inhibitors + **Opioids**

Alfentanil and Fentanyl

Ritonavir very markedly increases the concentrations of intravenous and oral alfentanil and intravenous fentanyl, and increases alfentanil-induced miosis. Concurrent use is expected to increase the risk of prolonged or delayed respiratory depression. Indinavir (boosted and unboosted with ritonavir) increases the concentrations of oral and intravenous alfentanil. Similarly, nelfinavir reduces alfentanil clearance. Other HIV-protease inhibitors are expected to interact similarly.

If alfentanil is given with an HIV-protease inhibitor, it would be prudent to consider reducing the dose of alfentanil and monitoring closely for increased and prolonged sedation. Similarly, caution is required in patients taking a HIV-protease inhibitor who are given fentanyl by any route (oral, parenteral, or transdermal) and similar precautions are advisable.

Buprenorphine

Ritonavir and atazanavir (boosted and unboosted) increase buprenorphine concentrations, and increase its adverse effects, such as sedation. In contrast, darunavir, fosamprenavir, lopinavir, and tipranavir (all boosted with ritonavir) and nelfinavir do not affect buprenorphine concentrations, but appear to affect those of its active metabolite.

Some suggest halving the starting dose of buprenorphine in patients taking HIV-protease inhibitors when it is used for opioid dependence, although note that the interaction might not be of significance with low-dose ritonavir alone in patients who are opioid-tolerant. If buprenorphine is given with any HIV-protease inhibitor it would seem prudent to monitor the outcome of concurrent use and adjust the dose of buprenorphine accordingly. Note that one manufacturer of sublingual and injectable buprenorphine states that concurrent use should be avoided. There appears to be less likelihood of an interaction with buprenorphine used transdermally.

Dextropropoxyphene (Propoxyphene)

Ritonavir is predicted to increase the effects of dextropropoxyphene. Other HIV-protease inhibitors might also be expected to interact similarly, but there seems little documented about these effects in practice.

The UK manufacturer of ritonavir contraindicates its use with dextropropoxyphene as extremely raised dextropropoxyphene concentrations might occur, which would increase the risk of serious adverse events (e.g. respiratory depression). However, the US manufacturer only suggests that a dose decrease might be needed. If both drugs are given it would seem prudent to monitor for adverse effects, such as sedation, and decrease the dextropropoxyphene dose accordingly.

Methadone ⚠

Methadone concentrations can be reduced by amprenavir, nelfinavir, and high-dose ritonavir; as well as darunavir, lopinavir, saquinavir, and tipranavir, all boosted with ritonavir. Some, but not all, patients might experience opioid withdrawal. Isolated cases of QT prolongation have been reported in patients taking HIV-protease inhibitors and methadone. Saquinavir has QT-prolonging effects, which might be additive with those of other drugs with such effects, such as high-dose methadone, see drugs that prolong the QT interval, page 352.

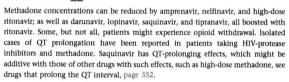

Some suggest screening for opioid withdrawal 4 days after starting an HIV-protease inhibitor. If withdrawal symptoms develop, increase the methadone dose by 10 mg every 2 to 7 days until symptoms abate. If the HIV-protease inhibitor is stopped the methadone dose should be gradually reduced to pretreatment amounts over the course of one to 2 weeks. Patients taking methadone in doses greater than 100 mg and with additional risk factors for QT prolongation should be carefully monitored. Note that the UK manufacturer of saquinavir contraindicates the concurrent use of methadone because of the possible risk of QT prolongation.

Morphine ⚠

Ritonavir is predicted to decrease morphine concentrations.

The clinical significance of this prediction is unclear however it would be prudent to monitor concurrent use to ensure morphine is effective and pain control is adequate.

Oxycodone

Ritonavir and lopinavir boosted with ritonavir appear to increase the exposure to oxycodone, and increase its adverse effects (such as drowsiness).

> Monitor concurrent use for an increase in oxycodone adverse effects and consider an oxycodone dose reduction, if necessary.

Pethidine (Meperidine)

Ritonavir decreased pethidine concentrations but increased those of its metabolite, norpethidine, which might increase toxicity on long-term use.

> The manufacturers of pethidine oral preparations and injection contraindicate, or advise against, its use with ritonavir because of the risk of norpethidine toxicity. Long-term use of pethidine with other HIV-protease inhibitors that are given with low-dose ritonavir is also not recommended.

Other opioids

Ritonavir is predicted to increase the effects of dihydrocodeine and tramadol. Although, there is no clinical evidence that this occurs it is in line with the known metabolism of these drugs. Ritonavir might also *decrease* the effects of codeine by inhibiting its metabolism to an active metabolite.

> Caution and careful monitoring of effects is warranted with dihydrocodeine and tramadol as high concentrations might lead to CNS depression. Smaller initial doses might be appropriate. In contrast, codeine might be less effective than expected. Low-dose ritonavir would be expected to have a less potent effect on the metabolism of these opioids and dose adjustments would not generally be required.

HIV-protease inhibitors + Orlistat

Orlistat might reduce the absorption of antiretroviral drugs, such as the HIV-protease inhibitors, resulting in reduced efficacy.

> Monitoring of antiretroviral drug concentrations, if concurrent use is considered essential, would seem sensible. Further, the MHRA in the UK advises that orlistat should only be started after careful consideration of the possible impact it might have on the efficacy of antiretroviral medicines.

HIV-protease inhibitors + Perampanel

HIV-protease inhibitors boosted with ritonavir, and also ritonavir or saquinavir alone, are predicted to increase perampanel exposure.

> Until more is known, monitor for perampanel adverse effects (dizziness, blurred vision, gait disturbances) and reduce the dose of perampanel according to clinical need.

HIV-protease inhibitors + Phenobarbital

Phenobarbital and other barbiturates are predicted to increase the metabolism of the

HIV-protease inhibitors, thereby reducing their concentrations and possibly resulting in therapeutic failure. However, a small number of case reports suggest that this might not always occur. Furthermore, the US manufacturer states that the concentrations of darunavir boosted with ritonavir are not affected by phenobarbital, but phenobarbital concentrations might be decreased by darunavir boosted with ritonavir.

> The combination of HIV-protease inhibitors and barbiturates should be used with caution, with increased monitoring for antiviral and/or barbiturate efficacy. Note that some advise against concurrent use.

HIV-protease inhibitors + Phenytoin ⚠

Nelfinavir, and fosamprenavir and lopinavir boosted with ritonavir appear to slightly reduce phenytoin exposure. In case reports, ritonavir has decreased, increased, or not altered phenytoin concentrations. Phenytoin appears to reduce the concentrations of a number of HIV-protease inhibitors, although the effect on amprenavir (from fosamprenavir boosted with ritonavir) and nelfinavir appears minimal.

> Phenytoin should be used with caution in combination with any HIV-protease inhibitor, with close monitoring of antiviral efficacy and phenytoin concentrations. Consider using an alternative antiepileptic where possible. Some advise against concurrent use. Note that fosphenytoin, a prodrug of phenytoin, might interact in the same way as phenytoin and similar precautions might be prudent.

HIV-protease inhibitors + Phosphodiesterase type-5 inhibitors

Ritonavir ⚠

Ritonavir very markedly increases vardenafil exposure, and moderately increases sildenafil and tadalafil exposure. A fatal heart attack occurred in a man taking ritonavir and saquinavir when he also took sildenafil.

> The concurrent use of ritonavir with sildenafil for pulmonary hypertension is not advised by the US manufacturer, and is contraindicated by the UK manufacturer. This would include ritonavir used with other HIV-protease inhibitors as a pharmacokinetic enhancer, as the FDA in the US contraindicates all HIV-protease inhibitors with sildenafil for this indication. When single doses of sildenafil are used for erectile dysfunction, the UK manufacturer states that concurrent use with ritonavir is not advised. However, if sildenafil is given, the dose should not exceed 25 mg in 48 hours, with close monitoring for an increase in sildenafil adverse effects (such as headache, flushing, hypotension). The US manufacturer advises that, for erectile dysfunction, the 'as needed' tadalafil dose should not exceed 10 mg every 72 hours and the daily dose should not exceed 2.5 mg, whereas the UK manufacturer simply advises caution. For pulmonary hypertension, the UK manufacturer does not recommend concurrent use. However, the US manufacturer advises that tadalafil can be started at a lower dose of 20 mg daily in those taking ritonavir for at least one week, and increased to 40 mg daily, if tolerated. In those already taking tadalafil and starting ritonavir, they recommend stopping tadalafil at least 24 hours before starting ritonavir, and then restarting tadalafil at least one week later, at a dose of 20 mg daily, increasing to 40 mg daily, if tolerated. For benign prostatic hyperplasia, the US manufacturer recommends that the daily dose of tadalafil should not exceed 2.5 mg daily in patients taking ritonavir. The

UK manufacturer of vardenafil contraindicates concurrent use, whereas the US manufacturer recommends that the dose of vardenafil should not exceed 2.5 mg in 72 hours when used with ritonavir. The UK and US manufacturers of avanafil contraindicate concurrent use with potent CYP3A4 inhibitors, such as ritonavir and other HIV-protease inhibitors boosted with ritonavir.

Saquinavir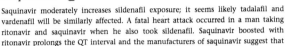

Saquinavir moderately increases sildenafil exposure; it seems likely tadalafil and vardenafil will be similarly affected. A fatal heart attack occurred in a man taking ritonavir and saquinavir when he also took sildenafil. Saquinavir boosted with ritonavir prolongs the QT interval and the manufacturers of saquinavir suggest that this effect might be potentiated in the presence of sildenafil.

If saquinavir is given with sildenafil for erectile dysfunction, the UK and US manufacturers recommend that a low starting dose of 25 mg should be considered. Concurrent use of saquinavir and sildenafil given for pulmonary hypertension is contraindicated by the FDA in the US, whereas the UK manufacturer suggests considering reducing the sildenafil dose to 20 mg twice daily (oral) or 10 mg twice daily (intravenous). Monitor the outcome of concurrent use closely for sildenafil adverse effects (such as headache, flushing, hypotension). Note that the UK manufacturer of saquinavir contraindicates the concurrent use of saquinavir boosted with ritonavir with sildenafil because of a possible risk of QT prolongation, see drugs that prolong the QT interval, page 352. In the absence of specific information, it is probably prudent to exercise caution in patients taking saquinavir and tadalafil. However, note that the UK manufacturer of saquinavir specifically contraindicates the concurrent use of saquinavir boosted with ritonavir with tadalafil because of a possible risk of QT prolongation, see drugs that prolong the QT interval, page 352. The US manufacturer recommends that the dose of vardenafil should not exceed 2.5 mg in 24 hours when used with saquinavir. Note that the UK manufacturer of saquinavir contraindicates the concurrent use of saquinavir boosted with ritonavir with vardenafil because of a possible risk of QT prolongation, see drugs that prolong the QT interval, page 352. The UK and US manufacturers of avanafil contraindicate concurrent use with potent CYP3A4 inhibitors, such as saquinavir. For HIV-protease inhibitors boosted with ritonavir, it would be prudent to also consider the dosing advice under *Ritonavir*, above.

Other HIV-protease inhibitors ▲

Indinavir markedly increases vardenafil exposure, and moderately increases sildenafil exposure; tadalafil would be expected to be similarly affected. Darunavir boosted with ritonavir moderately increase sildenafil exposure and tipranavir boosted with ritonavir moderately increases tadalafil exposure. Increases in the concentrations of these phosphodiesterase type-5 inhibitors are predicted to occur with other HIV-protease inhibitors .

If sildenafil is given for erectile dysfunction a low starting dose (25 mg) should be considered, although some suggest that a starting dose of 12.5 mg might be more appropriate in those taking indinavir, with a maximum dose frequency of once or twice weekly. If sildenafil is given for pulmonary hypertension, consider reducing the sildenafil dose to 20 mg twice daily. Similar dose adjustments are recommended for the concurrent use of tadalafil and tipranavir boosted with ritonavir as with tadalafil and ritonavir (see above), and might be expected to apply to all HIV-protease inhibitors boosted with ritonavir. Until more is known, it might be prudent to use the precautions advised for ritonavir (see above) and titrate to

H

effect. The UK manufacturer of vardenafil contraindicates the concurrent use of indinavir, whereas the US manufacturer recommends that the dose of vardenafil should not exceed 2.5 mg in 24 hours. The US manufacturers of nelfinavir advise that the dose of vardenafil should not exceed 2.5 mg in 72 hours. The US manufacturer of fosamprenavir recommends that the dose of vardenafil should not exceed 2.5 mg in 24 hours. Similarly, the US manufacturer of vardenafil recommends that the dose should not exceed 2.5 mg in 24 hours when used with atazanavir. For other HIV-protease inhibitors, it would seem prudent to start with a low dose and titrate to effect. The UK and US manufacturers of avanafil contraindicate concurrent use with potent CYP3A4 inhibitors, such as nelfinavir and other HIV-protease inhibitors boosted with ritonavir. For HIV-protease inhibitors boosted with ritonavir, it might be prudent to also consider the dosing advice under *Ritonavir*, above.

HIV-protease inhibitors + **Proguanil**

Atazanavir and lopinavir, both boosted with ritonavir, appear to decrease proguanil exposure. Ritonavir alone and when used to boost other HIV-protease inhibitors, is predicted to interact similarly.

> The UK manufacturer of atovaquone with proguanil advises avoiding concurrent use with [ritonavir-] boosted HIV-protease inhibitors where possible. Similarly, the US HIV guidelines recommend that patients taking atazanavir, or lopinavir, boosted with ritonavir, use an alternative drug to atovaquone with proguanil for malaria prophylaxis if possible.

HIV-protease inhibitors + **Propafenone**

Ritonavir is expected to increase the plasma concentration of propafenone, which could lead to life-threatening arrhythmias. Other HIV-protease inhibitors, alone or boosted with ritonavir, are expected to interact similarly.

> It would seem prudent to avoid the concurrent use of propafenone with HIV-protease inhibitors, alone or boosted with ritonavir, if possible. However if concurrent use is necessary, closely monitor for an increase in propafenone adverse effects (such as hypotension, bradycardia, dizziness, dry mouth) and monitor propafenone concentrations wherever possible. Note that some manufacturers contraindicate concurrent use.

HIV-protease inhibitors + **Proton pump inhibitors**

Atazanavir, Nelfinavir, or Saquinavir

Proton pump inhibitors reduce atazanavir exposure given alone or boosted with ritonavir; nelfinavir is similarly affected by omeprazole. In contrast, omeprazole has been shown to increase the exposure to saquinavir.

> Atazanavir should not be given with omeprazole or other proton pump inhibitors even if boosted with ritonavir. One UK manufacturer states that if concurrent use is necessary, the dose of atazanavir boosted with ritonavir should be increased to 400/100 mg daily, and both UK and US manufacturers advise a maximum dose of 20 mg of omeprazole (or the equivalent in other proton pump inhibitors). The US

manufacturers limit this advice to treatment-naive patients, and advise that the dose of the proton pump inhibitor should be taken 12 hours before atazanavir. The US manufacturer contraindicates the concurrent use of nelfinavir and a proton pump inhibitor whereas the UK manufacturers contraindicate omeprazole and esomeprazole, and advise caution with other proton pump inhibitors. If omeprazole or other proton pump inhibitors are taken with saquinavir monitor for potential saquinavir toxicity. However, the UK manufacturers note that because saquinavir might prolong the QT interval, this increase in exposure is clinically important, and concurrent use is not recommended.

Indinavir or Tipranavir

Omeprazole appears to reduce indinavir exposure (by about 50% in one study) but not all patients seem to be affected. Ritonavir appears to negate the effects of any interaction. Omeprazole does not appear to affect the concentration of tipranavir boosted with ritonavir, whereas tipranavir boosted with ritonavir reduces omeprazole exposure by about 70%. Esomeprazole is similarly affected.

Omeprazole should probably not be used with indinavir unless ritonavir is also given. This would be likely to apply to other proton pump inhibitors given with indinavir. The use of tipranavir with omeprazole or esomeprazole is not recommended by the UK manufacturer. If both drugs are given, consider increasing the dose of the proton pump inhibitor according to response.

HIV-protease inhibitors + Quinidine

The HIV-protease inhibitors are generally expected to increase quinidine concentrations, which might increase the risk of arrhythmias and other adverse effects such as nausea, diarrhoea, and tinnitus. Saquinavir has QT-prolonging effects, which might be additive with those of other drugs with such effects, such as quinidine, see drugs that prolong the QT interval, page 352.

The manufacturers of ritonavir contraindicate concurrent use with quinidine, and for this reason, in general, the UK manufacturers of other HIV-protease inhibitors also contraindicate concurrent use, the exceptions being lopinavir, where caution is advised: quinidine concentrations should be monitored, where possible. In contrast, in the US, most manufacturers advise caution and close monitoring of quinidine concentrations, with the exception of the manufacturers of nelfinavir, saquinavir and tipranavir, who contraindicate the concurrent use of quinidine.

HIV-protease inhibitors + Quinine

Ritonavir moderately increases the exposure to quinine, whereas quinine has only very slight effects on ritonavir pharmacokinetics. Lopinavir boosted with ritonavir moderately reduces the exposure to quinine.

It would be prudent to avoid the concurrent use of HIV-protease inhibitors with quinine, where possible. If it is essential, monitor both for reduced quinine efficacy and for increased quinine adverse effects (e.g. tinnitus, headache, vomiting and vertigo) and adjust the dose of quinine as necessary. Note that increased quinine concentrations are likely to increase the risk of QT prolongation, see Drugs that prolong the QT interval, page 352 for more information. Note particularly that saquinavir boosted with ritonavir has been reported to cause QT prolongation and therefore additive QT-prolonging effects are also a possibility.

H

HIV-protease inhibitors + **Raltegravir**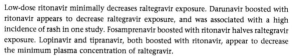

Low-dose ritonavir minimally decreases raltegravir exposure. Darunavir boosted with ritonavir appears to decrease raltegravir exposure, and was associated with a high incidence of rash in one study. Fosamprenavir boosted with ritonavir halves raltegravir exposure. Lopinavir and tipranavir, both boosted with ritonavir, appear to decrease the minimum plasma concentration of raltegravir.

> Monitor virological efficacy on concurrent use of higher doses of ritonavir and darunavir boosted with ritonavir. The pharmacokinetic interaction between raltegravir and fosamprenavir boosted with ritonavir could be clinically important, and might result in virological failure: concurrent use is not recommended. Similar precautions would seem prudent with amprenavir. Consider monitoring plasma drug concentrations, if possible, and virological efficacy in patients taking lopinavir, or tipranavir, boosted with ritonavir..

HIV-protease inhibitors + **Ranolazine**

Ketoconazole increases the AUC, maximum and minimum concentrations, and half-life of ranolazine 2.5- to 4.5-fold. The dose-related adverse effects of ranolazine such as nausea and dizziness were increased by *ketoconazole*. Further, increases in plasma concentrations of ranolazine might cause significant QT prolongation and increase the risk of arrhythmias. The HIV-protease inhibitors are expected to interact in the same way as ketoconazole. Saquinavir has QT-prolonging effects, which might be additive with those of other drugs with such effects, such as ranolazine, see drugs that prolong the QT interval, page 352.

> The manufacturers of ranolazine contraindicate its use with potent CYP3A4 inhibitors. They specifically name indinavir, nelfinavir, ritonavir and saquinavir.

HIV-protease inhibitors + **Retinoids**

The UK manufacturer of alitretinoin predicts that the HIV-protease inhibitors will increase alitretinoin concentrations.

> Monitor concurrent use and be alert for an increase in the adverse effects of alitretinoin (such as flushing and headaches) if HIV-protease inhibitors are also being taken.

HIV-protease inhibitors + **Rifabutin**

Rifabutin exposure is moderately increased, and that of its partially active 25-O-desacetylrifabutin metabolite greatly increased, by the HIV-protease inhibitors, and this is associated with an increased risk of toxicity. Rifabutin slightly decreases the exposure to indinavir, nelfinavir, and particularly saquinavir (with an increased risk of therapeutic failure), and appears to increase the bioavailability of darunavir and fosamprenavir (both boosted with ritonavir).

> The combination of rifabutin with HIV-protease inhibitors can be used, but large dose reductions of rifabutin (of 50 to 75%) and/or increases in the doses of the HIV-protease inhibitors are often necessary. The treatment of tuberculosis in patients taking antiretrovirals is complex and up-to-date guidelines should be consulted.

HIV-protease inhibitors + **Rifampicin (Rifampin)**

Rifampicin moderately to markedly reduces the exposure to most HIV-protease inhibitors, with the exception of ritonavir, which is only slightly affected. Some HIV-protease inhibitors increase rifampicin concentrations.

The use of many of the HIV-protease inhibitors (particularly those boosted with ritonavir) with rifampicin is contraindicated because of the risk of reduced antiviral efficacy and the emergence of resistance. Increasing the doses of the HIV-protease inhibitors appears to increase toxicity, notably hepatotoxicity. The treatment of tuberculosis in patients taking antiretrovirals is complex and up-to-date guidelines should be consulted.

HIV-protease inhibitors + **Riociguat**

Potent CYP3A4 inhibitors, such as nelfinavir, ritonavir, saquinavir, and other HIV-protease inhibitors boosted with ritonavir, are predicted to increase the exposure to riociguat.

The US manufacturer suggests considering a riociguat starting dose of 0.5 mg three times a day, while the UK manufacturer advises avoiding concurrent use with potent CYP3A4 inhibitors. If the HIV-protease inhibitors and riociguat are used together, monitor for any riociguat adverse effects such as hypotension, peripheral oedema, and headache.

HIV-protease inhibitors + **Rivaroxaban**

Ritonavir increases the exposure to rivaroxaban, increasing its effects. Other HIV-protease inhibitors are predicted to interact similarly.

Concurrent use is not recommended because of the increased bleeding risk. If both drugs are given, monitor closely for signs of bleeding.

HIV-protease inhibitors + **Salbutamol (Albuterol) and related bronchodilators**

The HIV-protease inhibitors are predicted to increase the systemic exposure to inhaled salmeterol, increasing the risk of cardiovascular adverse effects of salmeterol (such as QT prolongation, palpitations, and sinus tachycardia).

Concurrent use of the HIV-protease inhibitors and salmeterol should be avoided.

HIV-protease inhibitors + **Sirolimus**

Nelfinavir greatly increased the sirolimus concentrations in one patient. The concurrent use of sirolimus with fosamprenavir boosted with ritonavir resulted in a lower sirolimus dose being necessary to maintain therapeutic sirolimus concentrations. Other HIV-protease inhibitors are predicted to raise sirolimus concentrations.

Sirolimus concentrations and effects (e.g. on renal function) should be monitored closely on concurrent use. Consider a pre-emptive sirolimus dose reduction or an increased dosing interval. Note that the UK and US manufacturers of sirolimus advise against the concurrent use of potent inhibitors of CYP3A4.

HIV-protease inhibitors + Solifenacin

Ketoconazole increases solifenacin exposure 2- to 3-fold by inhibiting CYP3A4. The manufacturers state that other potent CYP3A4 inhibitors (such as the HIV-protease inhibitors) will have the same effect. Solifenacin might slightly increase the risk of QT prolongation, and this effect may be additive with the QT-prolonging effects of saquinavir, see Drugs that prolong the QT interval, page 352 for further information.

It is recommended that the daily dose of solifenacin is limited to 5 mg daily in patients taking potent CYP3A4 inhibitors. The concurrent use of solifenacin is contraindicated in patients with severe renal impairment or moderate hepatic impairment who are taking potent CYP3A4 inhibitors.

HIV-protease inhibitors + SSRIs

Protease inhibitors boosted with ritonavir appear to reduce paroxetine and sertraline concentrations. Fluoxetine would be expected to be similarly affected. However, the UK manufacturer of ritonavir, and the US manufacturer of tipranavir (boosted with ritonavir) predict that they will*increase* the concentrations of fluoxetine, paroxetine, and sertraline.. Two cases of serotonin syndrome have been attributed to the use of fluoxetine and ritonavir.

It would be prudent to anticipate some reduction in efficacy when starting HIV-protease inhibitors boosted with ritonavir in patients taking fluoxetine, sertraline, or paroxetine. Monitor the clinical effect and increase the SSRI dose as necessary. The general relevance of the few cases of serotonin syndrome, page 580 is uncertain. Note that saquinavir boosted with ritonavir and some SSRIs can prolong the QT interval, see Drugs that prolong the QT interval, page 352 for further information.

HIV-protease inhibitors + Statins

Atorvastatin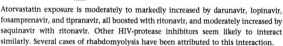

Atorvastatin exposure is moderately to markedly increased by darunavir, lopinavir, fosamprenavir, and tipranavir, all boosted with ritonavir, and moderately increased by saquinavir with ritonavir. Other HIV-protease inhibitors seem likely to interact similarly. Several cases of rhabdomyolysis have been attributed to this interaction.

It is generally recommended that the concurrent use of atorvastatin in patients taking HIV-protease inhibitors should only be undertaken if the benefits outweigh the risks and that atorvastatin is used at low initial doses (i.e. 10 mg). If atorvastatin is used in the presence of any HIV-protease inhibitor, patients should be counselled regarding myopathy (e.g. report any unexplained muscle pain, tenderness, or weakness). If myopathy does occur, the statin should be stopped immediately. The UK manufacturers of atorvastatin give specific dose advice if concurrent use is necessary as follows: for tipranavir, the maximum dose of atorvastatin should not exceed 10 mg daily; for lopinavir, it should only exceed

20 mg daily with clinical monitoring; and for darunavir, fosamprenavir, fosamprenavir boosted with ritonavir, and saquinavir, it should only exceed 40 mg daily with clinical monitoring. The US manufacturer of atorvastatin recommends a maximum dose of 20 mg daily with concurrent use of darunavir, fosamprenavir, or saquinavir, all boosted with ritonavir.

Fluvastatin or Pravastatin

Pravastatin pharmacokinetics are usually only modestly affected by the HIV-protease inhibitors, although there can be large interindividual variations in effect. There do not appear to be any reports of interactions with fluvastatin and the HIV-protease inhibitors.

Pravastatin and fluvastatin can probably be used without dose adjustments with most HIV-protease inhibitors, but monitoring is needed to confirm this. Until more is known, it would seem prudent to initiate the concurrent use of these statins in patients taking HIV-protease inhibitors at the lowest dose. Patients should be counselled regarding myopathy (e.g. report any unexplained muscle pain, tenderness, or weakness). If myopathy does occur, the statin should be stopped immediately.

Pitavastatin

Unboosted atazanavir slightly increases the steady-state exposure of pitavastatin, whereas lopinavir boosted with ritonavir very slightly decreases it.

These alterations are not expected to be clinically relevant.

Rosuvastatin

HIV-protease inhibitors boosted with ritonavir have variable effects on rosuvastatin exposure: fosamprenavir has no effect, tipranavir slightly increases exposure, and atazanavir and lopinavir increase exposure 3-fold and 2-fold, respectively.

The US manufacturer of rosuvastatin states that the dose should be limited to 10 mg daily in patients taking atazanavir or lopinavir, both boosted with ritonavir, or started at 5 mg daily with fosamprenavir or tipranavir, both boosted with ritonavir. However, the UK manufacturer of rosuvastatin states that the concurrent use of an HIV-protease inhibitor is not recommended. If concurrent use is undertaken, patients should be advised to report any unexplained muscle pain, tenderness, or weakness. If myopathy does occur, the statin should be stopped immediately.

Simvastatin or Lovastatin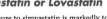

The exposure to simvastatin is markedly to very markedly increased by nelfinavir and saquinavir with ritonavir. Other HIV-protease inhibitors seem likely to interact similarly. Several cases of rhabdomyolysis have been attributed to this interaction. Lovastatin is metabolised in the same way as simvastatin, and is therefore likely to be similarly affected by the HIV-protease inhibitors.

The concurrent use of simvastatin and lovastatin with any HIV-protease inhibitor is contraindicated.

H

HIV-protease inhibitors + Tacrolimus

HIV-protease inhibitors markedly inhibit the metabolism of tacrolimus and increase its concentrations. The effect is most apparent with ritonavir boosted regimens.

When HIV-protease inhibitors are given to patients taking tacrolimus, careful monitoring of tacrolimus concentrations and probably a marked reduction in the dose of tacrolimus is required. Note that in some cases tacrolimus was dosed just once weekly to achieve appropriate concentrations.

HIV-protease inhibitors + Theophylline

Ritonavir slightly reduces the exposure to theophylline. Aminophylline would be expected to interact similarly.

Monitor the effect of concurrent use on theophylline concentration and increase the theophylline or aminophylline dose if necessary.

HIV-protease inhibitors + Ticagrelor

The HIV-protease inhibitors boosted with ritonavir are predicted to markedly increase the exposure to ticagrelor.

Because the marked increase in exposure increases the risk of bleeding, concurrent use is contraindicated.

HIV-protease inhibitors + Tolterodine

Ketoconazole raises the exposure to tolterodine more than 2-fold in some patients. Other potent inhibitors of CYP3A4, such as the HIV-protease inhibitors, are predicted to interact similarly. Tolterodine may slightly increase the risk of QT prolongation, and this effect may be additive with the QT-prolonging effects of saquinavir, see Drugs that prolong the QT interval, page 352 for further information.

The UK manufacturers advise avoiding concurrent use. The US manufacturers suggest reducing the tolterodine dose to 1 mg twice daily, which seems practical. It may be prudent to assess experience of adverse effects (such as dry mouth, constipation and drowsiness) in these patients, and to reduce the dose further or withdraw the drug if it is not tolerated.

HIV-protease inhibitors + Trazodone

Ritonavir increases the AUC of trazodone more than 2-fold and sedation and fatigue were increased. Cases of serotonin syndrome, page 580 have been reported in patients taking trazodone and ritonavir or indinavir. Other HIV-protease inhibitors might interact similarly.

A lower dose of trazodone should be considered if it is given with potent CYP3A4 inhibitors such as ritonavir and indinavir, although note that in the UK it has been suggested that the combination should be avoided where possible. Note that, because saquinavir might prolong the QT interval, in the UK, its concurrent use with trazodone is contraindicated.

HIV-protease inhibitors + Tricyclics ⚠️

Ritonavir increases desipramine concentrations and is predicted to also increase the concentrations of other tricyclic antidepressants. Theoretically, tipranavir might interact similarly.

> Monitor for increased tricyclic adverse effects (e.g. dry mouth, urinary retention, constipation). Consider starting desipramine at a low dose in patients taking ritonavir 500 mg twice daily, increasing the dose slowly. When ritonavir is given as a pharmacokinetic booster (i.e. at a dose of 100 mg twice daily) a dose adjustment of the tricyclic is unlikely to be necessary. There seems to be little information regarding other tricyclics, but similar precautions to those suggested for desipramine would seem prudent. Note that, because saquinavir (boosted with ritonavir) might prolong the QT interval, in the UK, its concurrent use with tricyclics is contraindicated. See drugs that prolong the QT interval, page 352, for a general discussion on QT prolongation.

HIV-protease inhibitors + Triptans

Almotriptan ⚠️

HIV-protease inhibitors, such as ritonavir, indinavir, or nelfinavir, would be expected to increase the plasma concentration of almotriptan.

> The US manufacturer of almotriptan recommends a starting dose of almotriptan 6.25 mg on concurrent use.

Eletriptan ⊗

HIV-protease inhibitors, such as ritonavir, indinavir, or nelfinavir, are predicted to increase the plasma concentration of eletriptan.

> The UK and US manufacturers of eletriptan state that the concurrent use of indinavir, nelfinavir and ritonavir should be avoided. In addition, the US manufacturer recommends that eletriptan should not be given within 72 hours of ritonavir and nelfinavir.

H

HIV-protease inhibitors + Ulipristal ⚠️

Potent inhibitors of CYP3A4, such as nelfinavir, ritonavir, saquinavir, and other HIV-protease inhibitors boosted with ritonavir, are predicted to markedly increase the exposure to ulipristal.

> The UK manufacturer of low-dose ulipristal for the symptomatic management of uterine fibroids does not recommend its concurrent use with potent CYP3A4 inhibitors. If low-dose ulipristal is given with an HIV-protease inhibitor, monitor for an increase in the adverse effects of ulipristal (for example nausea, abdominal pain, and breast tenderness) or any unexpected outcome occurring during concurrent use. The UK manufacturer of ulipristal for emergency contraception states that CYP3A4 inhibitors are unlikely to have any clinically relevant effects.

HIV-protease inhibitors + **Valproate**

Lopinavir concentrations appeared to be raised by valproate in one study in HIV-positive patients. Valproate concentrations did not appear to be affected; however, a case report describes a reduction in valproate concentrations, which resulted in an exacerbation of mania. Ritonavir is predicted to reduce valproate concentrations.

Monitor valproate concentrations when any antiretroviral regimen that includes ritonavir is used. Note that there has been some concern about using valproate in HIV infection, but there seems to be no established reason to avoid or specifically promote the use of valproate in HIV-infection *per se*.

HIV-protease inhibitors + **Venlafaxine**

Indinavir

Venlafaxine appears to decrease single-dose indinavir concentrations, and indinavir is predicted to increase venlafaxine concentrations.

Monitor concurrent use to confirm that the effects of indinavir remain adequate and that adverse effects of venlafaxine are not increased.

Other HIV-protease inhibitors

The HIV-protease inhibitors are predicted to increase venlafaxine exposure.

Monitor concurrent use to ensure that the adverse effects of venlafaxine are not increased.

HIV-protease inhibitors + **Warfarin and related oral anticoagulants** ⚠

In pharmacokinetic studies, ritonavir did not affect exposure to *S*-warfarin but slightly decreased *R*-warfarin exposure, while lopinavir boosted with ritonavir decreased exposure to both *R*- and *S*-warfarin. Most case reports describe a decrease in warfarin or acenocoumarol effects with HIV-protease inhibitors, although a few describe an increase in warfarin effects.

It would seem prudent to monitor for an alteration in anticoagulant effect, and adjust the dose as necessary.

HRT

As HRT contains many of the same hormones as the contraceptives, studies with contraceptives, page 288, may be applicable to HRT and *vice versa*, although the relative doses should be borne in mind.

HRT + **Lasofoxifene** ⚠

HRT and other drugs with oestrogenic effects might be expected to oppose the effects of oestrogen antagonists such as lasofoxifene.

Oestrogen-containing HRT is generally considered contraindicated in patients with current or a history of breast cancer. If it is essential, use the lowest HRT dose for the shortest duration: the patient should be fully aware of the potential risks.

HRT + Letrozole

HRT would be expected to diminish the effects of letrozole (which has anti-oestrogenic effects).

Oestrogen-containing HRT is generally considered contraindicated in patients with current or a history of breast cancer. If it is essential, use the lowest HRT dose for the shortest duration: the patient should be fully aware of the potential risks.

HRT + Levothyroxine

Oral oestrogens appear to increase the requirement for levothyroxine in some patients.

It would be prudent to monitor thyroid function several months after starting or stopping oral oestrogens to check levothyroxine requirements. Transdermal HRT would not be expected to interact, but this needs confirmation.

HRT + MAO-B inhibitors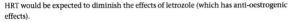

In a controlled study, the AUC of selegiline was modestly increased by estradiol-containing HRT (60%), but this was not considered to be clinically significant.

The UK manufacturers of selegiline advise that the concurrent use of HRT should be avoided. If concurrent use is necessary, monitor for increased selegiline adverse effects (such as nausea, constipation, hypotension and diarrhoea).

HRT + Modafinil

The hormones in HRT are similar to those used in hormonal contraceptives, and so may be affected by enzyme-inducing drugs, such as modafinil, in the same way as contraceptives, page 296. Armodafinil, the R-isomer of modafinil, would be expected to interact similarly.

The clinical significance of any interaction is unclear; however, consider the possibility of reduced HRT efficacy on concurrent use. The effect is most likely to be noticed where HRT is prescribed for menopausal vasomotor symptoms, but might be difficult to detect where the indication is osteoporosis. The interaction is not relevant to HRT applied locally for menopausal vaginitis.

HRT + NSAIDs

High-dose etoricoxib appears to increase the exposure to conjugated oestrogens from HRT; however, this increased oestrogen exposure is less than half that seen with twice the dose of conjugated oestrogens (1.25 mg) taken alone. Drospirenone may increase the risk of hyperkalaemia if it is given to patients with other drugs which increase potassium levels such as NSAIDs (although this is rare).

There would appear to be no reason for avoiding concurrent use but the manufacturers suggest that this increase in oestrogen levels should be considered when choosing an HRT preparation. It is generally recommended that potassium levels are measured during the first cycle of treatment with drospirenone.

HRT + NNRTIs ❓

The hormones in HRT are similar to those used in oral hormonal contraceptives, and so may be affected by enzyme-inducing drugs, such as nevirapine and efavirenz, in the same way as contraceptives, page 297. Reduced effects are therefore possible if either of these drugs is also given.

The clinical significance of any interaction is unclear; however, consider the possibility of reduced HRT efficacy on concurrent use. Any interaction would be most likely to be noticed where HRT is prescribed for menopausal vasomotor symptoms, but might be difficult to detect where the indication is osteoporosis. The interaction is not relevant to HRT applied locally for menopausal vaginitis.

HRT + Phenobarbital ❓

The hormones in HRT are similar to those used in hormonal contraceptives, and so may be affected by enzyme-inducing drugs, such as phenobarbital, in the same way as contraceptives, page 299. Reduced effects are therefore possible if phenobarbital is also given. Primidone is metabolised to phenobarbital and may interact similarly.

The clinical significance of any interaction is unclear; however, consider the possibility of reduced HRT efficacy on concurrent use. The effect is most likely to be noticed where HRT is prescribed for menopausal vasomotor symptoms, but might be difficult to detect where the indication is osteoporosis. The interaction is not relevant to HRT applied locally for menopausal vaginitis.

HRT + Phenytoin ❓

The hormones in HRT are similar to those used in hormonal contraceptives, and so may be affected by enzyme-inducing drugs, such as phenytoin, in the same way as contraceptives, page 299. Reduced effects are therefore possible if phenytoin is also given. Fosphenytoin is a prodrug of phenytoin and would be expected to interact similarly.

The clinical significance of any interaction is unclear; however, consider the possibility of reduced HRT efficacy on concurrent use. The effect is most likely to be noticed where HRT is prescribed for menopausal vasomotor symptoms, but might be difficult to detect where the indication is osteoporosis. The interaction is not relevant to HRT applied locally for menopausal vaginitis.

HRT + Potassium ❓

Drospirenone, which is given as the progestogen component in some HRT formulations, might increase the risk of hyperkalaemia when given with other drugs that can cause hyperkalaemia such as potassium supplements. The UK manufacturer of drospirenone-containing HRT notes that the increase in potassium levels may be more pronounced in diabetic women.

The risk of hyperkalaemia appears to be low, especially if renal function is normal. In the US, it is recommended that consideration be given to monitoring potassium levels during the first cycle in women [with normal renal function] who regularly take potassium supplements, whereas the UK manufacturer recommends that the potassium level is measured during the first cycle or month of treatment only in women with mild or moderate renal impairment. In patients at higher risk of developing hyperkalaemia (e.g. in renal impairment) it is generally recommended that potassium levels are measured during the first cycle of treatment with drospirenone.

HRT + Rifabutin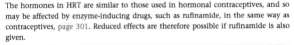

The hormones in HRT are similar to those used in hormonal contraceptives, and so may be affected by enzyme-inducing drugs, such as rifabutin, in the same way as contraceptives, page 300. Reduced effects are therefore possible if rifabutin is also given.

> The clinical significance of any interaction is unclear; however, consider the possibility of reduced HRT efficacy on concurrent use. The effect is most likely to be noticed where HRT is prescribed for menopausal vasomotor symptoms, but might be difficult to detect where the indication is osteoporosis. The interaction is not relevant to HRT applied locally for menopausal vaginitis.

HRT + Rifampicin (Rifampin)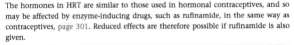

The hormones in HRT are similar to those used in hormonal contraceptives, and so may be affected by enzyme-inducing drugs, such as rifampicin, in the same way as contraceptives, page 301. Reduced effects are therefore possible if rifampicin is also given.

> The clinical significance of any interaction is unclear; however, consider the possibility of reduced HRT efficacy on concurrent use. The effect is most likely to be noticed where HRT is prescribed for menopausal vasomotor symptoms, but might be difficult to detect where the indication is osteoporosis. The interaction is not relevant to HRT applied locally for menopausal vaginitis.

HRT + Rufinamide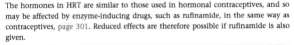

The hormones in HRT are similar to those used in hormonal contraceptives, and so may be affected by enzyme-inducing drugs, such as rufinamide, in the same way as contraceptives, page 301. Reduced effects are therefore possible if rufinamide is also given.

> The clinical significance of any interaction is unclear; however, consider the possibility of reduced HRT efficacy on concurrent use. The effect is most likely to be noticed where HRT is prescribed for menopausal vasomotor symptoms, but might be difficult to detect where the indication is osteoporosis. The interaction is not relevant to HRT applied locally for menopausal vaginitis.

HRT + Tacrine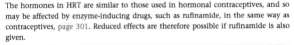

HRT (conjugated oestrogens, estradiol or estrone sulfate) increases the AUC of tacrine by 60% (and even up to 3-fold in one individual) and reduces its clearance by about 30%.

> The importance of this interaction is unclear. Increased tacrine levels may increase

both the efficacy and adverse effects of tacrine. Monitor patients for signs of tacrine toxicity and consider a tacrine dose reduction if indicated.

HRT + Tamoxifen

HRT would be expected to diminish the effects of tamoxifen and other anti-oestrogens. This effect has been seen in one study, but in another study, no increased risk of breast cancer was seen.

> Oestrogen-containing HRT is generally considered contraindicated in patients with current or a history of breast cancer. If it is essential, use the lowest HRT dose for the shortest duration: the patient should be fully aware of the potential risks.

HRT + Topiramate

The hormones in HRT are similar to those used in hormonal contraceptives, and so may be affected by enzyme-inducing drugs, such as high-dose topiramate, in the same way as contraceptives, page 302. Reduced effects are therefore possible if high-dose topiramate is also given.

> The clinical significance of any interaction is unclear; however, consider the possibility of reduced HRT efficacy on concurrent use. Any interaction would be most likely to be noticed where HRT is prescribed for menopausal vasomotor symptoms, but might be difficult to detect where the indication is osteoporosis. The interaction is not relevant to HRT applied locally for menopausal vaginitis.

HRT + Toremifene

HRT would be expected to diminish the effects of toremifene (which has anti-oestrogenic effects).

> Oestrogen-containing HRT is generally considered contraindicated in patients with current or a history of breast cancer. If it is essential, use the lowest HRT dose for the shortest duration: the patient should be fully aware of the potential risks.

HRT + Ursodeoxycholic acid (Ursodiol)

Ursodeoxycholic acid does not affect the bioavailability of ethinylestradiol. However, oestrogens may decrease the effectiveness of ursodeoxycholic acid by increasing the elimination of cholesterol in bile.

> The manufacturers suggest that concurrent use should be avoided.

HRT + Warfarin and related oral anticoagulants

There is conflicting data on whether or not the use of HRT (oral or topical) affects warfarin or phenindione dosing. In one case, the acenocoumarol dose was increased by 75% when oral conjugated oestrogens were changed to transdermal estradiol. Tibolone may increase the INR in some patients taking warfarin or phenindione.

> Direct information is limited. Note that, because of the increased risk of developing venous thromboembolism with HRT, the use of HRT in women already receiving an anticoagulant requires careful consideration of the risks and

benefits. If the combination is used be aware that the anticoagulant response may be affected. Increased INR monitoring is advised when starting tibolone in patients stabilised on warfarin, other coumarins, or indanediones.

5-HT₃-receptor antagonists

5-HT₃-receptor antagonists + Opioids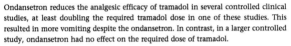

Ondansetron reduces the analgesic efficacy of tramadol in several controlled clinical studies, at least doubling the required tramadol dose in one of these studies. This resulted in more vomiting despite the ondansetron. In contrast, in a larger controlled study, ondansetron had no effect on the required dose of tramadol.

Monitor for an adequate analgesic response and adjust the tramadol dose accordingly.

5-HT₃-receptor antagonists + Phenobarbital

Rifampicin (rifampin) appears to reduce ondansetron exposure: phenobarbital would be expected to interact similarly. The Australian manufacturer of tropisetron states that drugs known to induce hepatic enzymes might lower tropisetron concentrations: they name phenobarbital. Note that as primidone is metabolised to phenobarbital it would be expected to interact similarly.

The US manufacturer of ondansetron states that no ondansetron dose adjustment is necessary on concurrent use with phenobarbital; however, it may be prudent to monitor the outcome of concurrent use to assess ondansetron efficacy, increasing the ondansetron dose if necessary. Until more is known, it would seem prudent to use similar caution with tropisetron and phenobarbital.

5-HT₃-receptor antagonists + Phenytoin

A preliminary report of a controlled study reported a marked reduction in ondansetron exposure in patients taking long-term phenytoin, when compared with control subjects. The Australian manufacturer of tropisetron states that drugs known to induce hepatic enzymes might lower tropisetron concentrations: phenytoin would be expected to interact in this way. Fosphenytoin, a prodrug of phenytoin, may interact similarly.

The US manufacturer of ondansetron states that no ondansetron dose adjustment is necessary on concurrent use with phenytoin; however, it may be prudent to monitor the outcome of concurrent use to assess ondansetron efficacy, increasing the ondansetron dose if necessary. Until more is known, it would seem prudent to use similar caution with the concurrent use of tropisetron and phenytoin.

5-HT₃-receptor antagonists + **Rifampicin (Rifampin)**

Rifampicin causes a modest to marked reduction in the exposure to ondansetron. The Australian manufacturer of tropisetron states that drugs known to induce hepatic enzymes (they name rifampicin) might lower tropisetron concentrations.

> The US manufacturer of ondansetron states that no ondansetron dose adjustment is necessary on concurrent use with rifampicin; however, it may be prudent to monitor the outcome of concurrent use to assess ondansetron efficacy, increasing the ondansetron dose if necessary. Until more is known, it would seem prudent to use similar caution with the concurrent use of tropisetron and rifampicin.

5-HT₃-receptor antagonists + **SSRIs**

Fluvoxamine

Fluvoxamine markedly increases the exposure to alosetron.

> If concurrent use of fluvoxamine and alosetron is unavoidable, monitor for alosetron adverse effects (constipation, abdominal discomfort, nausea). Concurrent use is contraindicated by the US manufacturer of alosetron.

Paroxetine or Sertraline

Symptoms similar to serotonin syndrome have been reported in two patients receiving paroxetine and ondansetron or sertraline and dolasetron.

> Bear the possibility of serotonin syndrome in mind if similar adverse effects occur, including agitation, confusion, and tremor.

Hydralazine

Hydralazine + **NSAIDs**

Indometacin abolished the hypotensive effects of intravenous hydralazine in one study, but did not affect it in another.

> Although information is limited, various NSAIDs have been reported to reduce the efficacy of other antihypertensive drug classes. It would be prudent to monitor the concurrent use of hydralazine and NSAIDs.

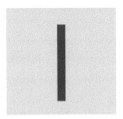

Imipenem

Imipenem + Valproate

Imipenem can dramatically reduce the serum concentration of valproate, and seizures have been reported.

Avoid concurrent use if possible. If it is essential, consider using intravenous valproate (which has been successfully substituted in some cases) and monitor valproate serum concentrations closely, adjusting the valproate dose if needed. Consider using another antibacterial, or an alternative to valproate; limited evidence suggests that carbamazepine and phenytoin are not affected. Note that imipenem should be used with caution in patients with a history of seizures.

Inotropes and Vasopressors

Inotropes and Vasopressors + Linezolid

Because of its weak MAO-inhibitory properties, the manufacturers of linezolid suggest that it may interact with adrenaline (epinephrine), dopamine, dobutamine, and noradrenaline (norepinephrine) in the same way as the non-selective MAOIs. However, the evidence available suggests that blood pressure rises are only very moderate and certainly unlikely to be of the hypertensive crisis proportions seen with the non-selective MAOIs.

The manufacturers contraindicate the use of sympathomimetics with linezolid unless there are facilities available for close observation of the patient and monitoring of blood pressure.

Inotropes and Vasopressors + MAO-B inhibitors

A case report describes a hypertensive reaction attributed to the concurrent use of dopamine and selegiline.

The manufacturers of selegiline recommend that dopamine should be used cautiously, if at all, in patients who are receiving selegiline long-term or who have received selegiline in the 2 weeks before needing dopamine.

Inotropes and Vasopressors + **MAOIs**

Dopamine, Dopexamine, Metaraminol or Phenylephrine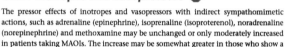

Metaraminol and phenylephrine are vasopressors with both direct and indirect sympathomimetic actions. This means that it may cause serious and potentially fatal hypertensive reactions in patients taking MAOIs. Dopamine and dopexamine may possibly interact similarly.

Avoid the use of these vasopressors in patients who are either taking MAOIs or who have stopped taking them in the previous 2 weeks. One UK manufacturer of dopamine suggests that patients who have been taking an MAOI should be given a starting dose of dopamine that is one-tenth of the usual dose.

Other inotropes and vasopressors

The pressor effects of inotropes and vasopressors with indirect sympathomimetic actions, such as adrenaline (epinephrine), isoprenaline (isoproterenol), noradrenaline (norepinephrine) and methoxamine may be unchanged or only moderately increased in patients taking MAOIs. The increase may be somewhat greater in those who show a significant hypotensive response to the MAOI. Dobutamine would be expected to interact similarly.

Although this interaction is unlikely to be important in most patients, some may experience greater effects. The manufacturers of the MAOIs contraindicate concurrent use, although some consider this overly cautious.

Inotropes and Vasopressors + Phenytoin

There is some limited evidence that patients needing dopamine to support their blood pressure can become severely hypotensive if phenytoin is added to their treatment.

Blood pressure is doubtless being monitored in patients receiving dopamine, and should be measured when phenytoin is given intravenously. However, more frequent monitoring may be necessary as this interaction appears to develop rapidly.

Inotropes and Vasopressors + Tricyclics

Patients taking tricyclic antidepressants show a grossly exaggerated response (hypertension, cardiac arrhythmias, etc.) to parenteral noradrenaline (norepinephrine), adrenaline (epinephrine), and to a lesser extent, to phenylephrine.

The parenteral use of these inotropes should, where possible, be avoided in patients taking tricyclic antidepressants. If they must be used, the rate and amount injected must be very much reduced. The risk is probably lower when drugs such as adrenaline (epinephrine) are used with a local anaesthetic for surface or infiltration anaesthesia, or nerve block and anecdotal evidence suggests that concurrent use is common; however, it would still seem advisable to be aware of the potential for interaction. The effects of phenylephrine given orally or as nasal drops does not appear to have been studied. Nevertheless, one manufacturer of an eye drop preparation contraindicates concurrent use.

Iron

Iron + Levodopa ❓

The absorption of levodopa can be reduced by 30 to 50% by ferrous sulfate due to levodopa chelation. Therefore all iron compounds are expected to act similarly. Carbidopa levels are also reduced by iron. There is some evidence that this interaction causes a decrease in symptom control.

Be alert for any signs of reduced levodopa efficacy. If this occurs, separating the administration of the iron as much as possible seems likely to be an effective way of managing this interaction.

Iron + Levothyroxine ❓

Ferrous sulfate (and therefore probably other iron compounds) causes a reduction in the effects of levothyroxine.

Be alert for this effect if both drugs are given, and monitor thyroid function if an interaction is suspected: adjust the levothyroxine dose accordingly. The same precautions would seem appropriate with any other iron compound.

Iron + Methyldopa ⚠

The antihypertensive effects of methyldopa can be reduced by ferrous sulfate or ferrous gluconate. Most other iron compounds are expected to interact similarly.

Monitor the effects of concurrent use and increase the methyldopa dose as necessary. Separating the dosages by up to 2 hours apparently only partially reduces the effects of this interaction.

Iron + Mycophenolate

One study found that oral iron compounds markedly reduced the absorption of mycophenolate. However, four subsequent studies, including one of identical design to the first study, found that oral iron compounds had no significant effect on the absorption of mycophenolate.

On balance, it would appear that oral iron compounds do not alter the pharmacokinetics of mycophenolate, and that no special precautions are required on concurrent use.

Iron + Penicillamine

The absorption of penicillamine can be reduced as much as two-thirds by oral iron.

For maximal absorption give the iron at least 2 hours after the penicillamine. Do not stop iron suddenly in a patient stabilised on penicillamine as the marked increase in absorption that follows may precipitate penicillamine toxicity.

Iron + Proton pump inhibitors

Omeprazole may impair the absorption of oral iron preparations and vegetable sources of iron. Other proton pump inhibitors may interact similarly.

Many factors and disease states can affect oral iron absorption. However bear these reports in mind should a patient taking any proton pump inhibitor fail to respond to treatment with oral iron.

Iron + Quinolones

Iron compounds reduce the absorption of many of the quinolones. In descending order the extent of the interaction appears to be: norfloxacin, levofloxacin, ciprofloxacin, moxifloxacin, gatifloxacin, ofloxacin/sparfloxacin. Serum levels of the antibacterial may become subtherapeutic as a result.

Most quinolones should not be taken at the same time as iron. As the quinolones are rapidly absorbed, taking them 2 hours before the iron should largely avoid this interaction. The exceptions are fleroxacin, which appears not to interact, and lomefloxacin, which seems to interact only minimally.

Iron + Tetracyclines

The absorption of the tetracyclines is markedly reduced by concurrent use. Tetracycline levels are reduced by 30 to 90% and their therapeutic effectiveness may be reduced or even abolished. The absorption of iron may also be reduced.

The extent of the reductions depends on a number of factors.

- the particular tetracycline used: tetracycline and oxytetracycline were affected the least in one study.
- the time interval between the administration of the two drugs: giving the iron 3 hours before or 2 to 3 hours after the antibacterial is satisfactory with tetracycline, but one study found that even 11 hours was inadequate for doxycycline.
- the particular iron compound used: the reduction in tetracycline levels with ferrous sulfate was 80 to 90%; with ferrous fumarate, succinate and gluconate, 70 to 80%; with ferrous tartrate, 50%; and with ferrous sodium edetate, 30%. This was with doses containing equivalent amounts of elemental iron.

The interaction can therefore be accommodated by separating the doses as much as possible. It would also seem logical to choose one of the iron preparations causing minimal interference, but it seems unlikely that there will be a clinically significant difference between those that are commonly available (i.e. sulfate, fumarate and gluconate).

Isoniazid

Isoniazid + Levodopa

Levodopa-induced dyskinesias are improved by isoniazid, but the control of Parkinson's disease is worsened. This may take several weeks to develop.

> The combination need not be avoided, but be aware that an adjustment in treatment may be needed if parkinsonism deteriorates.

Isoniazid + NRTIs

The risk of peripheral neuropathy appears to be increased if isoniazid is given with stavudine, and is predicted to be increased by didanosine.

> The 2011 British HIV Association (BHIVA) guidelines, and the 2012 US guidelines, advise that stavudine should not be given with isoniazid because of the risk of peripheral neuropathy. Similarly the US and BHIVA guidelines also state that alternatives to didanosine should be given to patients taking isoniazid.

Isoniazid + Paracetamol (Acetaminophen) ❓

A number of reports suggest that the toxicity of paracetamol might be increased by isoniazid so that normal analgesic doses (4 g daily) might not be safe in some individuals. Pharmacokinetic studies suggest that isoniazid usually inhibits the metabolism of paracetamol, but that metabolism to toxic metabolites might be induced shortly after stopping isoniazid, or late in the isoniazid dose-interval in fast acetylators of isoniazid.

> It would seem prudent to consider warning patients taking isoniazid to limit their use of paracetamol, as some individuals risk possible paracetamol-induced liver toxicity, even with normal recommended doses of paracetamol. It is possible that the risk is greatest shortly after stopping isoniazid. The risk might also be higher if paracetamol is taken late in the isoniazid dosing interval, particularly in fast acetylators of isoniazid.

Isoniazid + Phenytoin

Phenytoin levels can be raised by isoniazid and some patients may develop toxicity. If both rifampicin (rifampin) and isoniazid are given, phenytoin levels may fall in patients who are fast acetylators of isoniazid, but may occasionally rise in those who are slow acetylators (said to be about 50% of the population).

> It is unlikely that the acetylator status of the patient will be known. Therefore monitor phenytoin adverse effects (e.g. blurred vision, nystagmus, ataxia or drowsiness) and phenytoin levels and adjust the dose accordingly. In some patients the interaction has taken several weeks to develop.

Isoniazid + Theophylline

Isoniazid has been reported to slightly increase and decrease theophylline clearance (given either as aminophylline or theophylline). An isolated case of theophylline toxicity has also been reported with concurrent use.

> The outcome of concurrent use is uncertain but it would be prudent to be alert for any evidence of increased theophylline concentrations and adverse effects (such as headache, nausea, tremor) if isoniazid is given concurrently. It may take 3 to 4 weeks for a clinically significant increase in theophylline concentration to develop.

Ivabradine

Ivabradine + Macrolides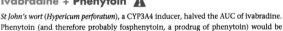

Ketoconazole, a potent inhibitor of CYP3A4, increases ivabradine levels up to 8-fold. The manufacturers predict that other potent CYP3A4 inhibitors, such as clarithromycin, telithromycin and oral erythromycin, will interact similarly.

> The manufacturer contraindicates the concurrent use of ivabradine with clarithromycin, telithromycin and oral erythromycin. The use of intravenous erythromycin is also not recommended.

Ivabradine + Phenobarbital

St John's wort (Hypericum perforatum), a CYP3A4 inducer, halved the AUC of ivabradine. The manufacturers predict that the barbiturates will interact similarly.

> Monitor the concurrent use of barbiturates for ivabradine efficacy and adjust the ivabradine dose as necessary.

Ivabradine + Phenytoin

St John's wort (Hypericum perforatum), a CYP3A4 inducer, halved the AUC of ivabradine. Phenytoin (and therefore probably fosphenytoin, a prodrug of phenytoin) would be expected to interact similarly.

> Monitor concurrent use of phenytoin for ivabradine efficacy and adjust the ivabradine dose as necessary.

Ivabradine + Rifampicin (Rifampin)

St John's wort (Hypericum perforatum), a CYP3A4 inducer, halved the AUC of ivabradine. Rifampicin would be expected to interact similarly.

> Monitor concurrent use of rifampicin for ivabradine efficacy and adjust the ivabradine dose as necessary.

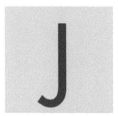

No interactions monographs have been included for drugs beginning with the letter J.

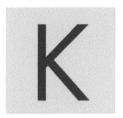

K

Kaolin

Kaolin + Quinidine ⚠

Limited evidence from single-dose studies suggests that kaolin-pectin may reduce the absorption of quinidine and lower its levels (salivary concentration reduced by about 50%; which correlates with serum levels).

Be alert for the need to increase the quinidine dose if kaolin-pectin is used concurrently.

Kaolin + Tetracyclines ⚠

Kaolin-pectin reduces the absorption of tetracycline by about 50%.

If these two drugs are given together, consider separating the doses by at least 2 hours to minimise admixture in the gut. Information about other tetracyclines is lacking, but be alert for them to interact similarly.

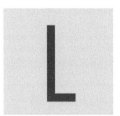

Lacosamide

Lacosamide + Lamotrigine ❓

Lacosamide does not appear to affect lamotrigine levels.

A clinically relevant interaction is not expected. Note that the manufacturers advise caution if lacosamide is given with drugs known to be associated with PR prolongation, and they name lamotrigine; however, the UK manufacturer reports that one study did not find an increase in PR prolongation on concurrent use.

Lacosamide + Lidocaine ❓

Dose-dependent prolongation of the PR interval may occur with lacosamide. The UK manufacturer therefore advises that lacosamide should be used with caution in patients taking class I antiarrhythmics, such as lidocaine.

Be aware that ECG changes may occur on concurrent use.

Lacosamide + Mexiletine ❓

Dose-dependent prolongation of the PR interval may occur with lacosamide. The UK manufacturer therefore advises that lacosamide should be used with caution in patients taking class I antiarrhythmics, such as mexiletine.

Be aware that ECG changes may occur on concurrent use.

Lacosamide + Pregabalin ❓

Dose-dependent prolongation of the PR interval may occur with lacosamide. The UK manufacturer therefore advises that lacosamide should be used with caution in patients taking pregabalin, which they suggest may also cause PR prolongation.

Be aware that ECG changes may occur on concurrent use.

Lacosamide + **Procainamide**

Dose-dependent prolongation of the PR interval may occur with lacosamide. The UK manufacturer therefore advises that lacosamide should be used with caution in patients taking class I antiarrhythmics, such as procainamide.

Be aware that ECG changes may occur on concurrent use.

Lacosamide + **Propafenone**

Dose-dependent prolongation of the PR interval may occur with lacosamide. The UK manufacturer therefore advises that lacosamide should be used with caution in patients taking class I antiarrhythmics, such as propafenone.

Be aware that ECG changes may occur on concurrent use.

Lacosamide + **Quinidine**

Dose-dependent prolongation of the PR interval may occur with lacosamide. The UK manufacturer therefore advises that lacosamide should be used with caution in patients taking class I antiarrhythmics, such as quinidine.

Be aware that ECG changes may occur on concurrent use.

Lacosamide + **Rifampicin (Rifampin)**

The manufacturer predicts that rifampicin may moderately decrease lacosamide exposure.

The clinical significance of this is unknown; however, be aware that starting or stopping rifampicin may alter lacosamide levels.

Lamotrigine

Lamotrigine + **Orlistat**

Orlistat might reduce the absorption of lamotrigine.

The MHRA in the UK advises that patients should be monitored for changes in the severity or frequency of convulsions, and consideration given to separating the administration of orlistat and the antiepileptic.

Lamotrigine + **Oxcarbazepine**

Oxcarbazepine appears to lower lamotrigine levels by about 15 to 75%. Lamotrigine appears to increase the levels of the active metabolite of oxcarbazepine. Not all studies have found these effects.

The clinical relevance of any interaction is uncertain, but it seems possible that

L

some patients will have significantly reduced lamotrigine levels. Monitor concurrent use carefully, being aware that dose adjustments may be necessary. The importance of the increase in oxcarbazepine metabolite levels is less clear.

Lamotrigine + Phenobarbital

Phenobarbital has been associated with reduced lamotrigine concentrations. Primidone is expected to interact similarly. Lamotrigine does not appear to affect phenobarbital or primidone concentrations.

Phenobarbital induces the metabolism of lamotrigine, and the recommended starting dose and long-term maintenance dose of lamotrigine in patients already taking phenobarbital or primidone is twice that of patients receiving lamotrigine monotherapy. However, note that if they are also taking valproate in addition to phenobarbital, the lamotrigine dose should be reduced.

Lamotrigine + Phenytoin

Phenytoin has been associated with reduced lamotrigine serum concentrations. Fosphenytoin, a pro-drug of phenytoin, is expected to interact similarly. Lamotrigine has no effect on phenytoin concentrations.

Phenytoin (and therefore probably fosphenytoin) induces the metabolism of lamotrigine, and the recommended starting dose and long-term maintenance dose of lamotrigine in patients already taking phenytoin is twice that of patients receiving lamotrigine monotherapy. However, note that if they are also taking valproate in addition to phenytoin, the lamotrigine dose should be reduced.

Lamotrigine + Rifampicin (Rifampin)

Rifampicin increases the clearance of lamotrigine and reduces its AUC by 97% and 44%, respectively. A lamotrigine dose increase was required in one case report.

Information is limited but rifampicin could reduce the efficacy of lamotrigine. Monitor the patient and increase the lamotrigine dose if required.

Lamotrigine + Valproate

The serum concentrations of lamotrigine can be increased by valproate. Small increases, decreases, or no changes in valproate concentrations have been seen with lamotrigine. Concurrent use has been associated with skin rashes, tremor, and other toxic reactions.

The lamotrigine dose should be reduced by about half when valproate is added to avoid possible toxicity (sedation, tremor, ataxia, fatigue, rash). In patients already taking valproate, the UK manufacturer of lamotrigine recommends a lamotrigine starting dose that is half that of lamotrigine monotherapy, irrespective of whether they are also receiving enzyme-inducing antiepileptics, and a very gradual dose titration. The development of rashes should be investigated promptly.

L

Lanthanum

Lanthanum + **Levothyroxine**

Lanthanum carbonate decreases levothyroxine absorption and the reduced thyroxine concentrations that result seem likely to be of clinical importance.

The UK and US manufacturers of lanthanum carbonate advise that thyroid replacement therapy should not be taken within 2 hours of lanthanum and that closer monitoring of TSH concentrations is recommended during concurrent use, so that any necessary thyroid hormone dose adjustments can be made.

Lanthanum + **Quinolones**

Lanthanum markedly decreases the bioavailability of ciprofloxacin. Other quinolones are expected to be similarly affected.

It is recommended that quinolones are not taken for 2 hours before or 4 hours after lanthanum.

Lanthanum + **Tetracyclines**

The bioavailability of tetracyclines is expected to be reduced by lanthanum, as concurrent use may result in the formation of insoluble chelates (as with other polyvalent cations).

It is recommended that tetracycline are not taken within 2 hours of a dose of lanthanum.

Lasofoxifene

Lasofoxifene + **Proton pump inhibitors**

Lasofoxifene solubility is pH-dependent. Proton pump inhibitors might decrease lasofoxifene absorption and theoretically decrease efficacy.

The extent of this effect is unknown. Be alert for reduced lasofoxifene efficacy.

Lasofoxifene + **Warfarin and related oral anticoagulants**

In a study, lasofoxifene caused a minor decrease in the prothrombin time in response to warfarin without changing warfarin pharmacokinetics.

This effect might not be clinically relevant. However, until more is known, it is recommended that prothrombin times should be monitored (with any coumarin) when starting or stopping lasofoxifene.

L

Laropiprant

Laropiprant + NRTIs

The UK manufacturer of laropiprant predicts that it might increase the concentrations of zidovudine by inhibiting its metabolism by glucuronidation.

There appear to be no reports of an interaction, however until more is known, bear the possibility in mind should an unexpected increase in zidovudine adverse effects occur (such as blood dyscrasias).

Leflunomide

Leflunomide + Methotrexate

Although no pharmacokinetic interaction appears to occur between methotrexate and leflunomide, elevated liver enzyme levels have been seen.

The UK manufacturers state that concurrent use is not advisable. The US manufacturers state that if concurrent use is undertaken, monitoring should be increased to monthly intervals. Close liver enzyme monitoring is also recommended if switching between these drugs, and colestyramine or activated charcoal washout recommended as it may reduce the risk of toxicity when switching from leflunomide to methotrexate.

Leflunomide + Penicillamine

The manufacturers state that the concurrent use of leflunomide and penicillamine has not yet been studied but it would be expected to increase the risk of serious adverse reactions (haematological toxicity or hepatotoxicity).

The manufacturers advise avoiding concurrent use. As the active metabolite of leflunomide has a long half-life of 1 to 4 weeks, a washout of colestyramine or activated charcoal is recommended if patients are to be switched to other DMARDs as this may reduce the risk of toxicity.

Leflunomide + Phenytoin ▲

In vitro studies have found that the active metabolite of leflunomide is an inhibitor of CYP2C9, the isoenzyme concerned with the metabolism of phenytoin and fosphenytoin.

Although no cases of phenytoin toxicity appear to have been reported as a result of this interaction, caution is advisable, especially as leflunomide has, in practice, been seen to inhibit the metabolism of other CYP2C9 substrates. Monitor for phenytoin toxicity (e.g. blurred vision, nystagmus, ataxia or drowsiness) and take levels as necessary. Adjust the phenytoin dose accordingly.

L

Leflunomide + Rifampicin (Rifampin)

Rifampicin increases the levels of the active metabolite of leflunomide by 40%.

There would seem to be no reason for avoiding concurrent use, but the manufacturers advise caution as levels may build up over time. It may be prudent to increase the frequency of leflunomide monitoring if these two drugs are used together.

Leflunomide + Vaccines

The body's immune response is suppressed by leflunomide. The antibody response to vaccines may be reduced and the use of live attenuated vaccines may result in generalised infection.

For many inactivated vaccines even the reduced response seen is considered clinically useful and, in the case of renal transplant patients, influenza vaccination is actively recommended. If a vaccine is given, it may be prudent to monitor the response, so that alternative prophylactic measures can be considered where the response is inadequate. Note that even where effective antibody titres are produced, these may not persist as long as in healthy subjects, and more frequent booster doses may be required. The use of live vaccines is generally considered to be contraindicated. Ideally vaccines should take place before immunosuppressive treatment is started, and live vaccines should not be given for up to 6 months after treatment has stopped.

Leflunomide + Warfarin and related oral anticoagulants

Leflunomide appears to raise the INR of patients taking warfarin. Case reports describe bleeding, and INRs as high as 6 and 11. Other coumarins may be similarly affected.

It would seem prudent to closely monitor the INR of any patient taking a coumarin who starts taking leflunomide.

Letrozole

Letrozole + Tibolone

Tibolone appears to increase the risk of recurrent breast cancer in women taking an aromatase inhibitor (such as letrozole).

Concurrent use is not recommended.

Levetiracetam

Levetiracetam + Orlistat

The MHRA in the UK suggests that the absorption of antiepileptics might be decreased by orlistat, leading to a loss of seizure control.

Although an interaction has not been established, the MHRA advises that patients should be monitored for changes in the severity or frequency of convulsions, and consideration given to separating the administration of orlistat and the antiepileptic.

Levodopa

Levodopa + MAOIs

A rapid, serious and potentially life-threatening hypertensive reaction can occur in patients taking MAOIs if they are also given levodopa.

An interaction with levodopa given with carbidopa or benserazide is less likely. Even so, the manufacturers continue to list the MAOIs among their contraindications and say that patients should not be given levodopa during treatment with MAOIs, nor for 14 days after an MAOI has been stopped.

Levodopa + Methyldopa

Methyldopa can increase the effects of levodopa. This has allowed a dose reduction of about 30 to 70% in some patients taking levodopa alone, but the benefit may only be temporary and dyskinesias may be worsened in some patients. A small increase in the hypotensive actions of methyldopa may also occur, see also Antihypertensives, page 97.

This interaction is expected to be minimised in the presence of carbidopa or benserazide and so it seems unlikely that a dose reduction of levodopa would usually be required. The increased hypotensive effects seem to be small, but be aware they are possible.

Levodopa + Metoclopramide

Metoclopramide is a centrally-acting dopamine antagonist, which can oppose the effects of levodopa and worsen Parkinson's disease. It also stimulates gastric emptying and this may lead to a small increase in the bioavailability of levodopa.

Concurrent use should generally be avoided. However if concurrent use of metoclopramide is essential, monitor the outcome closely. Note that domperidone is the antiemetic of choice in Parkinson's disease.

L

Levodopa + **Penicillamine**

Penicillamine can raise levodopa levels in some patients. This may improve the control of the parkinsonism but the adverse effects of levodopa may also be increased.

Concurrent use need not be avoided, but monitor for an increase in the adverse effects of levodopa.

Levodopa + **Phenytoin**

The therapeutic effects of levodopa can be reduced or abolished by phenytoin.

Evidence is limited (effects in 5 patients only). If concurrent use is necessary, it would seem prudent to monitor concurrent use for any evidence of reduced levodopa efficacy. It seems possible that fosphenytoin, a prodrug of phenytoin, could have similar effects.

Levodopa + **Pyridoxine**

The effects of levodopa are reduced or abolished by pyridoxine, but this interaction does not occur when levodopa is given with the dopa-decarboxylase inhibitors carbidopa or benserazide, as is usual clinical practice.

In the rare cases that levodopa is used alone, pyridoxine in doses as low as 5 mg daily can reduce the effects of levodopa and should therefore be avoided. Warn patients about proprietary pyridoxine-containing preparations such as multivitamins and supplements. There is no evidence to suggest that a low-pyridoxine diet is desirable.

Levodopa + **SSRIs**

The use of an SSRI is often beneficial in patients with Parkinson's disease taking levodopa. However, sometimes parkinsonian symptoms are worsened.

In some cases parkinsonism can, rarely, be worsened by SSRIs. Concurrent use is valuable and need not be avoided, but monitor the outcome and withdraw the SSRI if necessary.

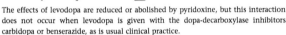

Levothyroxine

Levothyroxine + **Orlistat**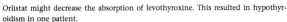

Orlistat might decrease the absorption of levothyroxine. This resulted in hypothyroidism in one patient.

One US manufacturer of levothyroxine recommends that the administration of levothyroxine and orlistat should be separated by 4 hours. It would be prudent to monitor the response to concurrent use, to ensure that this is effective.

Levothyroxine + Phenobarbital

An isolated report describes thyrotoxicosis in a patient taking levothyroxine when she reduced her dose of secobarbital with amobarbital. It seems possible that all barbiturates might interact in this way. Note that phenobarbital has been shown to reduce the concentrations of endogenous thyroid hormones in some studies.

The general importance of this interaction is almost certainly small, but be alert for any evidence of changes in thyroid status if barbiturates are added or withdrawn from patients taking levothyroxine. Monitor thyroid function if an interaction is suspected, and adjust the levothyroxine dose accordingly.

Levothyroxine + Phenytoin

Clinical hypothyroidism can occur when patients taking a stable dose of levothyroxine start to take phenytoin. Phenytoin can reduce endogenous thyroid hormone concentrations, but clinical hypothyroidism caused by an interaction seems to be rare.

The general importance of this interaction seems small, but be alert for any evidence of changes in thyroid status if phenytoin is added or withdrawn from patients taking levothyroxine. Monitor thyroid hormone concentrations if an interaction is suspected and adjust the levothyroxine dose accordingly.

Levothyroxine + Raloxifene

Two patients developed increased levothyroxine requirements after taking raloxifene for a number of months.

Consider monitoring thyroid function if both drugs are given, especially if symptoms of hypothyroidism develop, and try separating administration by 12 hours before increasing the levothyroxine dose.

Levothyroxine + Rifampicin (Rifampin)

Two case reports suggest that rifampicin might possibly reduce the effects of thyroid hormones.

The evidence for this interaction is by no means conclusive. Bear this interaction in mind if rifampicin is given to a patient taking levothyroxine. If symptoms of hypothyroidism develop, monitor thyroid function and adjust the dose of levothyroxine accordingly.

Levothyroxine + Sevelamer ⚠

Sevelamer decreases levothyroxine absorption and appears to increase levothyroxine requirements.

It would be prudent to monitor levothyroxine requirements in patients requiring sevelamer. Whether separation of administration would minimise any interaction remains to be demonstrated, but, where absorption is a problem, it is generally recommend avoiding giving other drugs at least 1 hour before, or 3 hours after, sevelamer.

L

Levothyroxine + SSRIs ❓

A study suggests that the effects of levothyroxine can be opposed by sertraline in some patients, but another study suggests that sertraline does not affect thyroid function in patients taking levothyroxine.

Evidence for an interaction between levothyroxine and sertraline is conflicting. If an interaction is suspected, monitor thyroid function and adjust the levothyroxine dose accordingly. However, note that this interaction seems relatively rare.

Levothyroxine + Sucralfate ❓

Sucralfate might reduce levothyroxine absorption, but not all studies have found this effect.

An interaction is not established; however, it might be prudent to avoid taking sucralfate until a few hours after levothyroxine. If an interaction is suspected, monitor thyroid function and adjust the levothyroxine dose accordingly.

Levothyroxine + Theophylline ⚠️

Thyroid function affects theophylline metabolism: in hypothyroidism it is decreased. Correction of thyroid function (e.g. with levothyroxine) is likely to increase theophylline metabolism (including that derived from aminophylline,) and so larger doses of theophylline are needed.

Monitor the outcome of adjusting thyroid status on the theophylline concentration (this may take weeks or months to stabilise) and adjust the theophylline or aminophylline dose as necessary.

Levothyroxine + Tricyclics ❓

The antidepressant response to imipramine, amitriptyline and possibly other tricyclics can be accelerated by the use of thyroid hormones. Isolated cases of paroxysmal atrial tachycardia, thyrotoxicosis and hypothyroidism have been attributed to concurrent use.

These apparent interactions remain unexplained and concurrent use seems generally advantageous. Unless problems arise there would seem to be no good reason for avoiding concurrent use.

Levothyroxine + Warfarin and related oral anticoagulants ⚠️

The anticoagulant effects of acenocoumarol, phenindione, and warfarin are increased by thyroid hormones and bleeding has been seen. This is largely due to alteration of thyroid function, rather than a direct drug-drug interaction.

Hypothyroid patients taking an anticoagulant who are subsequently given thyroid hormones as replacement therapy will need a downward adjustment of the anticoagulant dose as treatment proceeds. Monitor the INR (weekly has been suggested) until patients are euthyroid, and adjust the coumarin or indanedione dose as necessary.

Lidocaine

Lidocaine + NNRTIs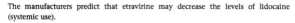

The manufacturers predict that etravirine may decrease the levels of lidocaine (systemic use).

The manufacturers recommend caution on concurrent use and state that lidocaine levels should be monitored, if this is possible.

Lidocaine + Phenobarbital

Plasma lidocaine concentrations, following slow intravenous injection, might be slightly reduced in patients who are taking phenobarbital. It seems likely that other barbiturates will interact similarly.

It might be necessary to increase the dose of lidocaine to achieve the desired therapeutic response in patients taking phenobarbital or other barbiturates.

Lidocaine + Phenytoin

The incidence of central adverse effects might be increased following the concurrent intravenous infusion of lidocaine and phenytoin. Sinoatrial arrest has been reported in one patient receiving the combination. Lidocaine concentrations might be reduced by phenytoin. Fosphenytoin, a prodrug of phenytoin, might interact similarly.

The clinical importance of this interaction is most likely to be small. However, the sinoatrial arrest emphasises the need to exercise caution when giving two drugs that have cardiodepressant actions.

Linezolid

Linezolid is a non-selective, reversible inhibitor of MAO, and it therefore shares some of the interactions of the MAOIs. However, its effects are weak, and serious adverse interactions of the magnitude seen with the MAOIs do not seem to occur. However, some caution is prudent if linezolid is given with drugs that interact with MAOIs.

Linezolid + MAO-B inhibitors

Linezolid is a is a weak, reversible, non-selective inhibitor of MAO and the manufacturers state that its effects are likely to be additive with any other drug that inhibits MAO-B.

The use of linezolid is contraindicated with and within 2 weeks of the use of any drug with MAO-inhibitory effects.

L

Linezolid + MAOIs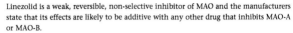

Linezolid is a weak, reversible, non-selective inhibitor of MAO and the manufacturers state that its effects are likely to be additive with any other drug that inhibits MAO-A or MAO-B.

> The use of linezolid is contraindicated with and within 2 weeks of the use of any drug with MAO-inhibitory effects.

Linezolid + Mirtazapine ⚠

In theory, the use of mirtazapine and linezolid might result in serotonin syndrome. One patient developed symptoms similar to serotonin syndrome, page 580 while taking these drugs.

> The UK manufacturer of linezolid contraindicates the concurrent use of serotonergic drugs (which would include mirtazapine) unless it is essential. If concurrent use is necessary, patients should have their blood pressure monitored and be closely observed for symptoms of serotonin syndrome, page 580, which can take several weeks to manifest.

Linezolid + Moclobemide ✗

Linezolid is a weak, reversible, non-selective inhibitor of MAO and the manufacturers state that its effects are likely to be additive with any other drug that inhibits MAO-A.

> The use of linezolid is contraindicated with and within 2 weeks of the use of any drug with MAO-inhibitory effects.

Linezolid + Nasal decongestants ⚠

Because of its weak MAO-inhibitory properties, the manufacturers of linezolid predict its use with drugs such as phenylpropanolamine and pseudoephedrine will result in raised blood pressure. However, the evidence available suggests that blood pressure rises are only very moderate and certainly unlikely to be of the hypertensive crisis proportions seen with the antidepressant MAOIs.

> The manufacturers contraindicate the use of pseudoephedrine and phenylpropanolamine with linezolid unless there are facilities available for close observation of the patient and monitoring of blood pressure. In addition, they advise careful dose titration. Patients should be warned about cough and cold remedies containing these and related drugs.

Linezolid + Opioids ⚠

The use of pethidine (meperidine) with MAOIs has resulted in a potentially life-threatening reaction in a few patients. Excitement, muscle rigidity, hyperpyrexia, flushing, sweating and unconsciousness occur very rapidly. Respiratory depression and hypotension have also been seen. Because linezolid has weak MAOI properties the manufacturers predict it may interact similarly. A case report supports this prediction.

> Avoid concurrent use unless facilities are available for close observation and monitoring of blood pressure.

Linezolid + Salbutamol (Albuterol) and related bronchodilators

Linezolid has weak, reversible MAO-inhibitory properties and, on this basis, the manufacturer predicts that it may interact with the beta-$_2$ agonists in the same way as the non-selective MAOIs, although to a much lesser extent. However, note that an interaction between beta-$_2$ agonists and MAOIs is not established, see MAOIs + Salbutamol (Albuterol) and related bronchodilators, page 490.

The manufacturers of linezolid contraindicate its use with sympathomimetics, unless facilities are available for close observation and monitoring of blood pressure: the UK manufacturer specifically names the beta$_2$-agonist bronchodilators.

Linezolid + SSRIs

Several case reports describe the development of serotonin syndrome in patients given linezolid with SSRIs (citalopram, escitalopram, fluoxetine, paroxetine and sertraline are implicated).

The interaction is probably rare. The manufacturers of linezolid contraindicate concurrent use unless patients are closely observed for serotonin syndrome and have their blood pressure monitored. See serotonin syndrome, page 580 for more information.

Linezolid + Tricyclics

Serotonin syndrome, page 580, is predicted to occur when linezolid is used with tricyclics.

The UK manufacturer contraindicates concurrent use unless patients are closely observed for serotonin syndrome and have their blood pressure monitored.

Linezolid + Triptans

As both the triptans and linezolid can affect serotonin transmission, their concurrent use may, in theory, lead to serotonin syndrome.

The manufacturers of linezolid contraindicate its use with the triptans, unless concurrent use is essential. If both drugs are given, patients should be closely monitored for signs of serotonin syndrome, page 580.

Linezolid + Venlafaxine

In theory the use of venlafaxine and linezolid may result in serotonin syndrome, page 580. Case reports describe a number of patients who developed symptoms similar to serotonin syndrome while taking these drugs.

The interaction is probably rare. The UK manufacturer contraindicates concurrent use unless patients are closely observed for signs and symptoms of serotonin syndrome, and have their blood pressure monitored.

L

Lithium

Lithium is given under close supervision with regular monitoring of serum concentrations because there is a narrow margin between therapeutic concentrations and those that are toxic. The dose of lithium is adjusted to give levels of 0.4 to 1 mmol/L, although it should be noted that this is the range used in the UK, and other ranges have been quoted. Initially weekly monitoring is advised, dropping to every 3 months for those on stable regimens. It is usual to take lithium samples about 10 to 12 hours after the last oral dose. Adverse effects that are not usually considered serious include nausea, weakness, fine tremor, mild polydipsia and polyuria. If levels rise into the 1.5 to 2 mmol/L range, toxicity usually occurs, and may present as lethargy, drowsiness, coarse hand tremor, lack of coordination, muscular weakness, increased nausea and vomiting, or diarrhoea. Higher levels result in neurotoxicity, which manifests as ataxia, giddiness, tinnitus, confusion, dysarthria, muscle twitching, nystagmus, and even coma or seizures. Cardiovascular symptoms may also develop and include ECG changes and circulatory problems, and there may be a worsening of polyuria. Virtually all of the reports are concerned with the carbonate, but sometimes lithium is given as other compounds. There is no reason to believe that these lithium compounds will interact any differently to lithium carbonate.

Lithium + Maprotiline ⚠

The concurrent use of *tricyclic antidepressants* and lithium has been successful but some patients may develop adverse effects. Serotonin syndrome, page 580, and neuroleptic malignant syndrome have been reported. One study suggests that maprotiline interacts similarly.

If both drugs are used monitor for any evidence of neurotoxicity.

Lithium + Methyldopa ⚠

Symptoms of lithium toxicity, not always associated with raised lithium levels, have been described in patients and healthy subjects when they were also given methyldopa.

If both drugs are given, the effects should be closely monitored (see lithium, above). Monitoring lithium levels may be unreliable because symptoms of toxicity can occur even though the levels remain within the normally accepted therapeutic range.

Lithium + Metronidazole ⚠

The lithium levels of 3 patients were raised following the use of metronidazole. However, 2 of these patients had evidence of renal impairment, and one other report describes safe concurrent use.

Some have recommended that a reduction in the lithium dose should be considered, especially in patients maintained at relatively high lithium levels. Patients taking lithium should be aware of the symptoms of lithium toxicity (see lithium, above) and told to report them immediately should they occur. This should be reinforced when they are given metronidazole.

Lithium + NSAIDs ⚠

NSAIDs may increase lithium levels leading to toxicity, but there is great variability between different NSAIDs and also between individuals taking the same NSAID. For example, studies have found that celecoxib causes a modest 17% increase in lithium levels, yet case reports describe increases of up to about 350%. Similar effects occur with other NSAIDs, and it seems likely that all NSAIDs will interact similarly. However, note that sulindac seems unique in that it is the only NSAID that has been reported to also cause a *decrease* in lithium levels.

> NSAIDs should be avoided, especially if other risk factors for lithium toxicity (such as advanced age, impaired renal function, decreased sodium intake, volume depletion, renal artery stenosis, and heart failure) are present, unless lithium levels can be very well monitored (initially every few days) and the lithium dose reduced appropriately. Patients taking lithium should be aware of the symptoms of lithium toxicity (see lithium, page 468) and told to report them immediately should they occur. This should be reinforced when they are given an NSAID.

Lithium + Oxcarbazepine ⚠

Neurotoxicity (with therapeutic lithium concentrations) has developed in some patients given carbamazepine and lithium. The manufacturers of oxcarbazepine predict it will interact similarly with lithium.

> If severe neurotoxicity develops, stop lithium. Risk factors include a history of neurotoxicity with lithium and compromised medical or neurological functioning.

Lithium + Phenytoin ❓

Lithium toxicity has been seen in patients also taking phenytoin.

> The interaction is not well established. Patients taking lithium should be aware of the symptoms of lithium toxicity (see lithium, page 468) and told to immediately report them should they occur. This should be reinforced when they are given phenytoin. Increased lithium monitoring does not appear to be of value in this situation as the interaction occurred in patients with lithium levels within the normally accepted range.

Lithium + SSRIs ⚠

The concurrent use of lithium and SSRIs can be advantageous and uneventful, but various kinds of neurotoxicities have occurred. Isolated reports describe the development of symptoms similar to those of serotonin syndrome in patients taking lithium with fluoxetine, fluvoxamine, paroxetine and possibly citalopram. In addition, fluoxetine appears to have caused increases and decreases in lithium levels.

> If lithium is used with an SSRI be alert for any evidence of toxicity (see serotonin syndrome, page 580). If these symptoms occur treatment should be withdrawn. Note that lithium and some SSRIs (escitalopram and citalopram) have been associated with QT prolongation, see Drugs that prolong the QT interval, page 352 for more information.

L

Lithium + Theophylline ⚠

Lithium levels are reduced by 20 to 30% by theophylline, which in some cases has caused patients to relapse. However, these fluctuations are generally considered small. Aminophylline may interact similarly.

> Monitor lithium levels if theophylline or aminophylline is also given, and adjust the lithium dose if necessary. Note that, in rare cases lithium has been associated with QT prolongation. In theory, this may be exacerbated by hypokalaemia caused by the xanthines. For more information, see Drugs that prolong the QT interval, page 352.

Lithium + Tricyclics ⚠

The concurrent use of a tricyclic antidepressant and lithium can be beneficial in some patients. However, some patients may rarely develop adverse effects, a few of them severe. Cases of neurotoxicity, serotonin syndrome, and neuroleptic malignant syndrome have been reported.

> If both drugs are used be alert for any evidence of neurotoxicity (see under serotonin syndrome, page 580). Note that lithium and some tricyclics might prolong the QT interval, see Drugs that prolong the QT interval, page 352 for further information.

Lithium + Triptans ❓

Case reports describe the development of serotonin syndrome in patients taking sumatriptan and lithium. This is in line with the known effects of lithium and the triptans.

> If lithium is used with any triptan be alert for any evidence of toxicity (see serotonin syndrome, page 580). If these symptoms occur treatment should be withdrawn.

Lithium + Venlafaxine ⚠

Studies suggest that no clinical pharmacokinetic interaction appears to occur if venlafaxine is given with lithium. However, serotonin syndrome has been reported in some patients on concurrent use.

> If both drugs are used, monitor for any evidence of neurotoxicity (see under serotonin syndrome, page 580).

Lofexidine

Lofexidine + Opioids ⚠

The concurrent use of methadone and low-dose lofexidine can cause clinically important hypotension and additional CNS depression.

> Monitor for adverse effects, particularly hypotension and cognitive changes. Note

that both lofexidine and high-dose methadone might prolong the QT interval, see Drugs that prolong the QT interval, page 352.

Loperamide

Loperamide + **Quinidine**

Quinidine increases absorption of loperamide into the brain resulting in respiratory depression.

Be alert for the CNS adverse effects of loperamide (such as drowsiness) if quinidine is given. If adverse effects are troublesome consider reducing the dose of loperamide.

Low-molecular-weight heparins

Low-molecular-weight heparins + **NSAIDs**

Ketorolac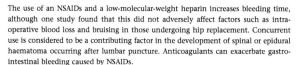

The effects of low-molecular-weight-heparins can be increased by other drugs that affect anticoagulation, platelet function or increase the risks of bleeding, such as NSAIDs. Cases of severe bleeding and prolonged bleeding times have been reported with ketorolac. Concurrent use is considered to be a contributing factor in the development of spinal or epidural haematoma occurring after lumbar puncture.

The CSM in the UK and the UK manufacturers say that ketorolac is contraindicated with anticoagulants. Conversely, the US manufacturers of ketorolac advise that physicians should carefully weigh the benefits against the risks and use heparins with ketorolac only extremely cautiously. Extreme caution is needed if concurrent use is considered appropriate in patients undergoing epidural anaesthesia.

Other NSAIDs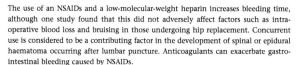

The use of an NSAIDs and a low-molecular-weight heparin increases bleeding time, although one study found that this did not adversely affect factors such as intra-operative blood loss and bruising in those undergoing hip replacement. Concurrent use is considered to be a contributing factor in the development of spinal or epidural haematoma occurring after lumbar puncture. Anticoagulants can exacerbate gastro-intestinal bleeding caused by NSAIDs.

Concurrent use is not uncommon, but prescribers should be aware that there is an increased risk of bleeding and monitor appropriately. Extreme caution is needed if concurrent use is considered appropriate in patients undergoing epidural anaes-thesia.

L

Low-molecular-weight heparins + **Prasugrel**

In phase III studies, no clinically significant interaction was reported when low-molecular-weight heparins were given with prasugrel. Nevertheless, due to the actions of both drugs there is a possible increased risk of bleeding on concurrent use. Furthermore, the use of prasugrel and heparin may contribute to the development of epidural or spinal haematoma after epidural anaesthesia.

> Be aware of the potential for this interaction if bleeding occurs. If they are used together, the manufacturers of the LMWHs recommend caution or careful clinical and laboratory monitoring. Extreme caution is needed if concurrent use is considered appropriate in patients undergoing epidural anaesthesia.

Low-molecular-weight heparins + Rivaroxaban

The concurrent use of rivaroxaban and enoxaparin increases the risk of bleeding. Other low-molecular-weight heparins would be expected to interact similarly.

> Monitor for signs of bleeding. The US manufacturer of rivaroxaban advises avoiding rivaroxaban for prophylaxis of deep vein thrombosis in patients taking other anticoagulants. The UK manufacturer of rivaroxaban contraindicates concurrent use unless switching between anticoagulants.

Low-molecular-weight heparins + Ticagrelor

The manufacturer of ticagrelor states that the concurrent use of other drugs (e.g. low-molecular-weight heparins) that affect coagulation might theoretically increase the risk of bleeding. However, one clinical study found no increase in bleeding with the concurrent use of enoxaparin.

> Concurrent use might be clinically beneficial; however, it would seem prudent to monitor the outcome of concurrent use, being aware that the risk of bleeding might be increased.

Low-molecular-weight heparins + Ticlopidine

Concurrent use of ticlopidine with a low-molecular-weight heparin increases haemorrhagic risk. The risk of epidural or spinal haematomas with a low-molecular-weight heparin may be increased if they are used concurrently with other drugs affecting haemostasis, such as antiplatelet drugs.

> If concurrent use is undertaken, there should be close clinical and laboratory monitoring. Extreme caution is needed if concurrent use is considered appropriate in patients undergoing epidural or spinal anaesthesia.

L

Lumefantrine

Lumefantrine + Tricyclics

The manufacturer of a preparation containing artemether with lumefantrine notes that *in vitro* data indicate that lumefantrine significantly inhibits CYP2D6. As a consequence, they contraindicate the use of artemether with lumefantrine in patients taking any drug that is metabolised by CYP2D6 (they include imipramine, amitriptyline, and clomipramine as examples).

These contraindications seem unnecessarily restrictive, especially as the tricyclics are not contraindicated with other established inhibitors of CYP2D6. Until more is known, it would be prudent to closely monitor the effects of any CYP2D6 substrate in patients given lumefantrine. However, more seriously, note that additive QT-prolonging effects are possible with some tricyclics and the artemether component, see drugs that prolong the QT interval, page 352.

L

Macrolides

The macrolides are generally considered to be inhibitors of CYP3A4; however, it should be noted that they vary in the strength of their effect. Macrolides that are more potent inhibitors of CYP3A4 are likely to have greater effects on substrates of this isoenzyme, and therefore their use seems more likely to be associated with greater clinical consequences. Clinically, clarithromycin and telithromycin have the greatest effects, and are considered potent CYP3A4 inhibitors, while erythromycin is a moderate inhibitor of CYP3A4. Roxithromycin is a weak inhibitor of CYP3A4, while azithromycin, dirithromycin, josamycin, midecamycin, and spiramycin do not appear to inhibit CYP3A4 to a clinically irrelevant extent.

Macrolides + Maraviroc

Clarithromycin and telithromycin are predicted to increase the exposure to maraviroc.

> The UK and US manufacturers of maraviroc recommend reducing the maraviroc dose to 150 mg twice daily if these macrolides are also given.

Macrolides + Mirtazapine

Ketoconazole increases the exposure to mirtazapine (by inhibiting CYP3A4). The manufacturers predict that erythromycin may interact in this way. Other macrolides (such as clarithromycin) may interact similarly; however, note that the macrolides differ in their ability to inhibit CYP3A4, see macrolides, above.

> The manufacturers advise caution on concurrent use and that a decrease in the dose of mirtazapine may be needed. Monitor for adverse effects (e.g. sedation, fatigue, headache) and adjust the mirtazapine dose if needed.

Macrolides + NNRTIs

Delavirdine increases clarithromycin exposure, whereas efavirenz, etravirine, and nevirapine reduce clarithromycin exposure and increase the exposure to the active hydroxy metabolite of clarithromycin. Clarithromycin and erythromycin are predicted to increase rilpivirine concentrations.

> The US manufacturer of delavirdine recommends that the dose of clarithromycin need only be reduced in patients with renal impairment. The clinical significance of the reduction in clarithromycin exposure with efavirenz, etravirine, and

nevirapine is unknown and further experience of the use of these NNRTIs with clarithromycin is needed. Until then, caution is warranted. Alternatives to clarithromycin should be considered, in particular for the treatment of *Mycobacterium avium* complex (MAC) infection. The UK manufacturer advises monitoring liver function tests if nevirapine is given with clarithromycin. The UK and US manufacturers of rilpivirine advise that, where possible, alternatives to clarithromycin and erythromycin (they name azithromycin) should be used. Note that rilpivirine and some macrolides have been associated with QT prolongation, see Drugs that prolong the QT interval, page 352 for more information.

Macrolides + Opioids

Clarithromycin and telithromycin decrease the metabolism of oxycodone, leading to an increase in oxycodone concentrations and effects. Erythromycin might interact similarly. Erythromycin, clarithromycin, and telithromycin are predicted to increase the concentrations of buprenorphine and methadone. Some patients might experience prolonged and increased alfentanil effects if they are given erythromycin. Clarithromycin and telithromycin are predicted to interact similarly. A case of serious respiratory depression has been described in a patient receiving transdermal fentanyl, after clarithromycin was added.

> Monitor for an increase in oxycodone adverse effects. An oxycodone dose decrease of 25 to 50% might be necessary, with further titration according to response. It has been suggested that the macrolides that are potent CYP3A4 inhibitors (see macrolides, page 474) should be avoided when buprenorphine is used parenterally or sublingually as an analgesic. If concurrent use is essential in opioid addiction, the manufacturers suggest that the buprenorphine dose should be halved. Monitor concurrent use for increased and prolonged sedation if erythromycin, clarithromycin, or telithromycin are given with methadone, and adjust the dose of methadone accordingly. Consider avoiding or giving smaller doses of alfentanil in patients taking, or who have recently taken, erythromycin, clarithromycin, or telithromycin. If concurrent use is necessary, be alert for evidence of prolonged alfentanil effects and respiratory depression. Fentanyl by any route of administration should probably be used with caution with clarithromycin and telithromycin. If fentanyl is given with these macrolides, and, until more is known if erythromycin is given with oral transmucosal fentanyl, monitor for increased and prolonged effects, particularly sedation, and adjust the fentanyl dose accordingly. Note that additive QT-prolonging effects might occur in predisposed individuals taking macrolides and high-dose methadone, see drugs that prolong the QT interval, page 352.

Macrolides + Oxybutynin

Ketoconazole a potent CYP3A4 inhibitor moderately increased oxybutynin concentrations, however the pharmacokinetics of its active metabolite were unchanged. Clarithromycin and telithromycin are potent CYP3A4 inhibitors, and are expected to interact similarly; erythromycin is a moderate inhibitor of CYP3A4, and is predicted to also increase oxybutynin exposure, but to a lesser extent. Further evidence suggests interactions between oxybutynin and CYP3A4 inhibitors are not clinically relevant, however manufacturers advise an increase in oxybutynin concentrations cannot be ruled out.

> It would be prudent to bear in mind the possibility of an interaction should any

M

oxybutynin adverse effects occur, such as dry mouth, constipation, and drowsiness.

Macrolides + Perampanel [?]

Clarithromycin and telithromycin are predicted to increase perampanel exposure.

Until more is known, monitor for perampanel adverse effects (dizziness, blurred vision, gait disturbances) and reduce the dose of perampanel according to clinical need.

Macrolides + Phenytoin

Clarithromycin [?]

Limited evidence suggests that clarithromycin may raise phenytoin levels. Fosphenytoin, a prodrug of phenytoin, may interact similarly.

The clinical importance of this interaction is unknown, but bear it in mind in case of an unexpected response to treatment. Indicators of phenytoin toxicity include blurred vision, nystagmus, ataxia or drowsiness. Note that erythromycin does not appear to interact.

Telithromycin [!]

As *rifampicin (rifampin)* reduces telithromycin levels by about 80%, and reduces its efficacy, the manufacturers predict that phenytoin (and therefore probably fosphenytoin, a prodrug of phenytoin) will interact similarly.

The manufacturers state that telithromycin should be avoided during and for up to 2 weeks after phenytoin has been taken. Note that erythromycin does not appear to interact.

Macrolides + Phosphodiesterase type-5 inhibitors

Sildenafil or Vardenafil [!]

Erythromycin and clarithromycin increase the exposure to sildenafil up to 3-fold. It seems likely that telithromycin will interact similarly. Erythromycin increases the exposure to vardenafil 4-fold; it seems likely that clarithromycin and telithromycin will interact similarly. Other macrolides have less effect on CYP3A4, see macrolides, page 474, and therefore seem less likely to interact.

Dosing guidance is given as follows: Sildenafil for erectile dysfunction – consider a starting dose of 25 mg. Sildenafil for pulmonary hypertension – with erythromycin consider reducing the oral sildenafil dose to 20 mg twice daily and the intravenous sildenafil dose to 10 mg twice daily. With clarithromycin or telithromycin consider reducing the oral sildenafil dose to 20 mg daily and the intravenous sildenafil dose to 10 mg daily. Vardenafil – the dose of vardenafil should not exceed 5 mg in 24 hours with erythromycin. The dose of vardenafil should not exceed 5 mg in 24 hours (UK) or 2.5 mg in 24 hours with clarithromycin (US). It would seem prudent to follow this advice for telithromycin. Note that vardenafil can cause QT prolongation, and this effect might be additive with those of other drugs with QT-prolonging effects, such as some macrolides. For more information of the concurrent use of two or more drugs that prolong the QT interval see Drugs that prolong the QT interval, page 352.

Tadalafil

Erythromycin, clarithromycin, and therefore probably telithromycin, are expected to raise tadalafil levels by inhibiting its metabolism by CYP3A4. This effect has been seen with other inhibitors of CYP3A4 (up to 4-fold rise with ketoconazole). Other macrolides have less effect on CYP3A4, see macrolides, page 474, and therefore seem less likely to interact.

Monitor the outcome of concurrent use, and decrease the dose of tadalafil if adverse effects (such as headache, flushing or dyspepsia) become troublesome.

Avanafil

The manufacturers note that the moderate CYP3A4 inhibitor erythromycin, increases avanafil exposure and prolongs its half life. Clarithromycin and telithromycin are predicted to increase avanafil exposure to a greater extent, due to the fact that they are potent CYP3A4 inhibitors.

The UK and US manufacturers of avanafil contraindicate concurrent use with potent CYP3A4 inhibitors. The US manufacturer advises that a maximum dose of 50 mg avanafil every 24 hours should not be exceeded with moderate CYP3A4 inhibitors, such as erythromycin. The UK manufacturer however, advises a maximum dose of 100 mg once every 48 hours with moderate CYP3A4 inhibitors.

Macrolides + Proton pump inhibitors

Clarithromycin almost doubles the levels of esomeprazole, lansoprazole and omeprazole. A small rise in the levels of clarithromycin also occurs, which may be therapeutically useful. Some very limited evidence indicates that erythromycin raises omeprazole levels, without altering its gastric acid lowering effect.

Given the wide use of *Helicobacter pylori* eradication regimens containing these drugs it seems unlikely that this interaction is detrimental.

Macrolides + Ranolazine

Ketoconazole increases the AUC, peak and trough levels, and half-life of ranolazine 2.5- to 4.5-fold. The dose-related adverse effects of ranolazine such as nausea and dizziness were increased by *ketoconazole*. Further, increases in plasma levels of ranolazine may cause significant QT prolongation and increase the risk of arrhythmias. Clarithromycin and telithromycin are expected to interact in the same way as ketoconazole, and erythromycin may also interact, but to a lesser extent.

The manufacturers of ranolazine contraindicate the concurrent use of clarithromycin, and the UK manufacturer also contraindicates telithromycin. The US manufacturer recommends that the dose of ranolazine should be limited to 500 mg twice daily when given to patients taking erythromycin, whereas the UK manufacturer recommends careful dose titration of ranolazine in patients taking erythromycin. Note that additive QT-prolonging effects may occur in some individuals taking macrolides and ranolazine, see Drugs that prolong the QT interval, page 352.

M

Macrolides + **Reboxetine** ⚠

The manufacturers predict that macrolides will decrease the clearance of reboxetine by inhibiting CYP3A4. Other CYP3A4 inhibitors have been shown to have this effect.

The manufacturers recommend that macrolides (they specifically name erythromycin) should not be given with reboxetine. Note that the macrolides differ in their ability to inhibit CYP3A4, see macrolides, page 474.

Macrolides + **Rifabutin**

Azithromycin ⚠

The concurrent use of rifabutin and azithromycin does not appear to alter the levels of either drug, but in one study a very high incidence of neutropenia and leucopenia was seen.

Until more information is available it would seem wise to monitor white cell counts during concurrent use.

Clarithromycin ⚠

Rifabutin markedly reduces clarithromycin levels, and clarithromycin increases rifabutin levels. There is an increased risk of uveitis and neutropenia with the combination.

Monitor the outcome of concurrent use to ensure treatment with the macrolide is effective. Because of the increased risk of uveitis the CSM in the UK says that consideration should be given to reducing the dose of rifabutin to 300 mg daily. If uveitis occurs the CSM recommends that rifabutin should be stopped and the patient should be referred to an ophthalmologist. Full blood counts should also be monitored with concurrent use.

Macrolides + **Rifampicin (Rifampin)**

Clarithromycin ⚠

Limited evidence suggests that rifampicin markedly reduces the clarithromycin levels (90% in one study).

Monitor the outcome of concurrent use to ensure clarithromycin treatment is effective.

Telithromycin ⚠

Rifampicin reduces the AUC and maximum levels of telithromycin by 86% and 79% respectively.

The UK manufacturers recommend that telithromycin should not be given during and for 2 weeks after the use of rifampicin.

Macrolides + **Riociguat** ⚠

Potent CYP3A4 inhibitors such as clarithromycin and telithromycin are predicted to increase the exposure to riociguat.

The US manufacturer suggests considering a riociguat starting dose of 0.5 mg three times a day, while the UK manufacturer advises avoiding concurrent use with potent CYP3A4 inhibitors. If these macrolides and riociguat are used together, monitor for any riociguat adverse effects, such as hypotension, peripheral oedema, and headache.

Macrolides + Rivaroxaban

Both clarithromycin and erythromycin increase the exposure to rivaroxaban, potentially increasing its effects. Telithromycin is predicted to interact similarly.

> The increase in exposure is not expected to be clinically relevant. However, if both drugs are given, monitor for signs of bleeding, advising patients to seek medical advice if bleeding occurs. Patients with renal impairment might have increased rivaroxaban plasma concentrations and therefore could have a greater risk of increased bleeding or prolonged bleeding on the concurrent use with these macrolides.

Macrolides + Roflumilast

Erythromycin inhibits the metabolism of roflumilast to its active *N*-oxide metabolite, but this does not appear to affect the total phosphodiesterase type-4 inhibitory effects to a clinically relevant extent.

> No roflumilast dose adjustments are expected to be necessary on concurrent use.

Macrolides + Salbutamol (Albuterol) and related bronchodilators

Clarithromycin and telithromycin are predicted to increase the systemic concentrations of inhaled salmeterol, increasing the risk of cardiovascular adverse events (such as QT prolongation, palpitations, and sinus tachycardia). Erythromycin does not appear to have a clinically relevant effect on salmeterol metabolism.

> Concurrent use of clarithromycin or telithromycin with salmeterol should be avoided. Consider giving erythromycin as an alternative, as this does not appear to interact.

Macrolides + Sirolimus

Erythromycin greatly increases sirolimus concentrations. A case of a sizeable increase in sirolimus concentrations and renal impairment has also been reported with clarithromycin. Telithromycin would be expected to interact similarly.

> The US manufacturer of sirolimus advises avoiding concurrent use of sirolimus with erythromycin, whereas the UK manufacturers advise monitoring sirolimus concentrations and decreasing the dose of both drugs as appropriate. They both state that concurrent use with clarithromycin or telithromycin should be avoided. If any macrolide is considered essential in a patient taking sirolimus, it would be prudent to closely monitor sirolimus concentrations and decrease the dose accordingly. Note that the macrolides differ in their ability to inhibit CYP3A4, see macrolides, page 474; other macrolides seem less likely to interact.

M

Macrolides + Solifenacin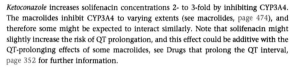

Ketoconazole increases solifenacin concentrations 2- to 3-fold by inhibiting CYP3A4. The macrolides inhibit CYP3A4 to varying extents (see macrolides, page 474), and therefore some might be expected to interact similarly. Note that solifenacin might slightly increase the risk of QT prolongation, and this effect could be additive with the QT-prolonging effects of some macrolides, see Drugs that prolong the QT interval, page 352 for further information.

It is recommended that the daily dose of solifenacin is limited to 5 mg daily in patients taking potent CYP3A4 inhibitors, such as clarithromycin or telithromycin. Bear in mind the possibility of an interaction should an increase in solifenacin adverse effects occur (e.g. dry mouth, constipation, dizziness), and consider reducing the solifenacin dose if these become troublesome. The concurrent use of solifenacin is contraindicated in patients with severe renal impairment or moderate hepatic impairment who are taking potent CYP3A4 inhibitors.

Macrolides + Statins

Atorvastatin

Clarithromycin, erythromycin, and/or telithromycin slightly to moderately increase atorvastatin exposure.

The UK manufacturer of atorvastatin states that the concurrent use of clarithromycin or telithromycin should be avoided, if possible. If concurrent use of these macrolides, or erythromycin is necessary, it should only be undertaken if the benefits outweigh the risks: lower doses of atorvastatin are recommended. Close monitoring is specifically advised when atorvastatin doses greater than 20 mg daily are given with clarithromycin. Advise patients to report promptly symptoms of myopathy (e.g. muscle pain or weakness). Note that the UK and US manufacturers of telithromycin contraindicate concurrent use.

Fluvastatin or Rosuvastatin

Erythromycin has little effect on fluvastatin or rosuvastatin exposure. Other macrolides would be expected to behave similarly.

Although no interaction would generally be expected to occur, note that there have been case reports of rhabdomyolysis in patients taking statin/macrolide combinations that have been predicted not to interact. Any patient taking a statin should be advised to report promptly symptoms of myopathy (e.g. muscle pain or weakness). It would be prudent to reinforce this when macrolides are given.

Pitavastatin

Erythromycin moderately increases the exposure to pitavastatin.

The US manufacturer recommends limiting the dose of pitavastatin to 1 mg daily (the lowest available dose). It would be prudent to extend this caution to any macrolide. Any patient taking a statin should be advised to report promptly symptoms of myopathy (e.g. muscle pain or weakness). It would be prudent to reinforce this if pitavastatin is given with a macrolide.

M

Pravastatin

Pravastatin exposure is moderately increased by clarithromycin and possibly slightly increased by erythromycin, and in adverse event databases, some potential cases of muscle toxicity were attributed to the use of pravastatin with a macrolide.

> Any patient taking a statin should be advised to report promptly symptoms of myopathy (e.g. muscle pain or weakness). It would be prudent to reinforce this when pravastatin is given with any macrolide. The US manufacturer specifically recommends that the dose of pravastatin be limited to 40 mg daily when given with clarithromycin.

Simvastatin or Lovastatin

The exposure to simvastatin and lovastatin is markedly increased by clarithromycin, erythromycin, and telithromycin. Rhabdomyolysis has been reported.

> Concurrent use is contraindicated: simvastatin and lovastatin should be temporarily withdrawn during short courses of clarithromycin, erythromycin, or telithromycin.

Macrolides + Tacrolimus

Several patients have had large increases in tacrolimus concentrations, accompanied by evidence of renal toxicity or haemolytic uraemic syndrome, when they also took erythromycin. The same interaction has been seen in patients given clarithromycin, and is predicted with josamycin. A case of increased tacrolimus concentrations has been reported with concurrent use of azithromycin.

> Tacrolimus concentrations and/or effects (e.g. on renal function) should be monitored as a matter of routine, but it would be prudent to increase monitoring, adjusting the tacrolimus dose as necessary, if clarithromycin, erythromycin, or telithromycin are started or stopped. Note that the macrolides differ in their ability to inhibit CYP3A4, see macrolides, page 474.

Macrolides + Theophylline

Erythromycin

Theophylline clearance can be reduced by erythromycin and toxicity might develop. The onset can be delayed for 2 to 7 days. Erythromycin exposure might be modestly reduced by theophylline. Aminophylline would be expected to interact similarly.

> Monitor the theophylline concentration after 48 hours and adjust the dose accordingly. Monitor the effects of oral erythromycin to ensure that they are adequate. Intravenous erythromycin appears not to be affected.

Other macrolides

Azithromycin, clarithromycin, dirithromycin, josamycin, midecamycin, roxithromycin, spiramycin, and telithromycin normally only cause small changes in theophylline concentrations, or do not interact at all. However, there are unexplained and isolated case reports of theophylline toxicity with josamycin and clarithromycin. Aminophylline would be expected to interact similarly.

> A clinically relevant interaction seems unlikely; however, consider an interaction

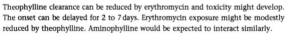

if any unexplained reduction in efficacy or theophylline adverse effects (such as headache, nausea, or tremor) occur, and monitor theophylline concentrations accordingly.

Macrolides + Ticagrelor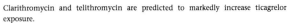

Clarithromycin and telithromycin are predicted to markedly increase ticagrelor exposure.

Because the marked increase in exposure can increase the risk of bleeding, concurrent use of clarithromycin or telithromycin with ticagrelor is contra-indicated. The UK and US manufacturers of ticagrelor state that no dose adjustment is necessary on concurrent use with moderate CYP3A4 inhibitors, such as erythromycin.

Macrolides + Tolterodine

Potent CYP3A4 inhibitors (such as clarithromycin and telithromycin) might increase the exposure to tolterodine, but possibly only in those who are poor metabolisers of CYP2D6. Erythromycin, a moderate CYP3A4 inhibitor, is also expected to increase the exposure to tolterodine, but to a lesser extent. Note that tolterodine might increase the risk of QT prolongation, and this effect can be additive with the QT-prolonging effects of some macrolides, see Drugs that prolong the QT interval, page 352 for further information.

Based on the interactions of other CYP3A4 inhibitors with tolterodine it would be prudent to monitor for tolterodine adverse effects in any patient (note that metaboliser status is rarely known), and to bear in mind the possibility of an interaction if antimuscarinic effects (dry mouth, constipation, drowsiness) are increased. However, note that the UK manufacturers advise avoiding concurrent use with potent CYP3A4 inhibitors, whereas the US manufacturers suggest reducing the tolterodine dose to 1 mg twice daily.

Macrolides + Toremifene

Based on theoretical considerations, the manufacturers advise care when toremifene is given with inhibitors of CYP3A such as the macrolides (they specifically name erythromycin, see macrolides, page 474, for more detail) as toremifene concentrations might be raised.

Although the clinical relevance of these interactions has not been established, note that CYP3A *inducers*, such as rifampicin (rifampin), page 574 have been found to interact, so a pharmacokinetic interaction with CYP3A inhibitors would be expected. It would seem prudent to monitor for toremifene adverse effects (e.g. hot flushes, uterine bleeding, fatigue, nausea, dizziness) on concurrent use with the macrolides. Note that the manufacturers suggest that toremifene is associated with a high risk of QT prolongation and life-threatening arrhythmias. For general information on QT prolongation see drugs that prolong the QT interval, page 352.

M

Macrolides + **Trazodone**

Clarithromycin impaired the clearance of trazodone and enhanced its sedative effects in a study in healthy subjects.

> The UK manufacturer of trazodone recommends that a lower dose of trazodone should be considered if it is given with a CYP3A4 inhibitor such as clarithromycin or erythromycin, but that concurrent use should be avoided where possible. Note that other macrolides might also interact, see macrolides, page 474. Note that trazodone and some macrolides might prolong the QT interval, see Drugs that prolong the QT interval, page 352 for further information.

Macrolides + **Triptans**

Almotriptan

Potent CYP3A4 inhibitors, such as clarithromycin and telithromycin, are predicted to increase the exposure to almotriptan.

> The US manufacturer of almotriptan recommends an almotriptan starting dose of 6.25 mg in the presence of potent CYP3A4 inhibitors, and this would be expected to include clarithromycin and telithromycin.

Eletriptan

Erythromycin moderately increases the exposure to eletriptan about 3.6-fold.

> The US manufacturer specifically recommends that eletriptan should not be given within 72 hours of potent CYP3A4 inhibitors, and they specifically name clarithromycin. The UK manufacturer suggests that concurrent use of erythromycin and other inhibitors of CYP3A4 (such as clarithromycin and telithromycin) should be avoided. Other macrolides seem less likely to interact, see macrolides, page 474.

Macrolides + **Ulipristal**

Erythromycin appears to moderately increase the exposure to ulipristal.

> The UK manufacturer of low-dose ulipristal for the symptomatic management of fibroids does not recommend its concurrent use with moderate and potent CYP3A4 inhibitors (which would include clarithromycin, erythromycin, and telithromycin). If low-dose ulipristal is given with one of these macrolides, monitor for an increase in the adverse effects of ulipristal (such as nausea, abdominal pain, and breast tenderness) or any unexpected outcome occurring during concurrent use. The UK manufacturer of ulipristal for emergency contraception states that CYP3A4 inhibitors are unlikely to have any clinically relevant effects.

Macrolides + **Warfarin and related oral anticoagulants**

Most controlled studies suggest that macrolides do not cause clinically relevant changes in the pharmacokinetics or anticoagulant effects of warfarin. There is less information about other anticoagulants, but two retrospective studies of acenocoumarol and phenprocoumon have variously shown an increased risk (azithromycin, clarithromycin), a non-significant increased risk (erythromycin) or no increased risk of bleeding (clarithromycin, erythromycin, roxithromycin). Furthermore, a number of case reports describe marked increases in INRs and/or bleeding in patients taking coumarins and macrolides.

> The available evidence suggests that, occasionally and unpredictably the effects of warfarin, acenocoumarol or phenprocoumon may be markedly increased by the macrolides. It would therefore be prudent to increase monitoring in all patients when they are first given any macrolide. There is some evidence that this may be particularly important in those who clear warfarin and other anticoagulants slowly and who therefore only need low doses. The elderly in particular would seem to fall into this higher risk category.

Macrolides + Zafirlukast

Erythromycin reduces the mean plasma concentration of zafirlukast by about 40%, which might reduce its anti-asthma effects.

> If these drugs are given concurrently, be alert for a reduced response; however, note that the manufacturers do not suggest that an alteration in the zafirlukast dose is necessary.

MAO-B inhibitors

MAO-B inhibitors + MAOIs

Severe orthostatic hypotension has been seen in patients given selegiline with MAOIs. Rasagiline would be expected to interact similarly.

> Avoid concurrent use wherever possible. If both drugs are used, monitor initial doses very carefully so hypotension can be rapidly managed. The manufacturers of selegiline contraindicate concurrent use and suggest that at least 14 days should elapse between stopping selegiline and starting an MAOI. The manufacturers of rasagiline contraindicate concurrent use, presumably because of the way selegiline interacts. At least 14 days should elapse between stopping rasagiline and starting an MAOI.

MAO-B inhibitors + Maprotiline

Cases of serotonin syndrome, page 580 have been reported on the concurrent use of selegiline or rasagiline with other drugs with serotonergic effects, such as the *SSRIs* and *tricyclics*. Maprotiline might interact similarly.

> Some manufacturers of selegiline advise avoiding the concurrent use of *tricyclics*: it may be prudent to consider this advice with maprotiline. Note that the US manufacturer of rasagiline advises avoiding the concurrent use of a tetracyclic antidepressant, during and for 14 days after stopping rasagiline. If the combination is used, the outcome should be well monitored for signs and symptoms of serotonin syndrome (such as flushing, ataxia, tremor, hyperthermia, agitation and confusion).

M

MAO-B inhibitors + **Mianserin**

Cases of serotonin syndrome, page 580 have been reported on the concurrent use of selegiline or rasagiline with other drugs with serotonergic effects, such as the *SSRIs* and *tricyclics*. Mianserin might interact similarly.

Some manufacturers of selegiline advise avoiding the concurrent use of *tricyclics*: it may be prudent to consider this advice with mianserin. Note that the US manufacturer of rasagiline advises avoiding the concurrent use of a tetracyclic antidepressant, during and for 14 days after stopping rasagiline. If the combination is used, the outcome should be well monitored for signs and symptoms of serotonin syndrome (such as flushing, ataxia, tremor, hyperthermia, agitation and confusion).

MAO-B inhibitors + **Mirtazapine**

Cases of serotonin syndrome, page 580 have been reported on the concurrent use of selegiline or rasagiline with other drugs with serotonergic effects, such as the *SSRIs* and *tricyclics*. Mirtazapine might interact similarly.

Some manufacturers of selegiline advise avoiding the concurrent use of *tricyclics*: it may be prudent to consider this advice with mirtazapine. Note that one US manufacturer of selegiline contraindicates concurrent use. If the combination is used, the outcome should be well monitored for signs and symptoms of serotonin syndrome (such as flushing, ataxia, tremor, hyperthermia, agitation and confusion).

MAO-B inhibitors + **Moclobemide**

The combination of an MAO-A inhibitor (moclobemide) with an MAO-B inhibitor (selegiline or rasagiline) causes MAO inhibition similar to that seen with the non-selective MAOIs.

Some manufacturers contraindicate concurrent use. If both drugs are given, patients should be given the same dietary restrictions for tyramine-rich foods and drinks (cheese, some wines and beers, etc.), which relate to the non-selective MAOIs. See food, page 389. It is suggested that if selegiline is replaced by moclobemide, the dietary restrictions can be relaxed after a wash-out period of about 2 weeks. If switching from moclobemide to selegiline, a wash-out period of 1 to 2 days is sufficient. Similar advice would seem prudent with rasagiline. Note that all of the interactions of the non-selective MAOIs, are likely to apply to patients taking this combination.

MAO-B inhibitors + **Nasal decongestants**

An isolated report describes a hypertensive crisis, which was attributed to an interaction between selegiline, ephedrine, and maprotiline. Rasagiline is expected to interact like selegiline.

In general, if selegiline is used at recommended doses it is selective for MAO-B and no restrictions are required. Nevertheless, this report suggests that, rarely, interactions are still possible, and some consider that patients taking selegiline should try to avoid pseudoephedrine. The manufacturers of rasagiline recommend against concurrent use of nasal decongestants that are indirectly-acting sympathomimetics, such as ephedrine and pseudoephedrine, due to the risk of hypertensive crises.

MAO-B inhibitors + Opioids

A case report describes a patient who fluctuated between stupor and agitation, and developed muscle rigidity, sweating and a raised temperature when given pethidine (meperidine) with selegiline. Rasagiline is expected to interact similarly. Some manufacturers of selegiline consider other opioids may interact similarly.

On the basis of this evidence the manufacturers of selegiline and rasagiline contraindicate pethidine (meperidine) and also suggest that pethidine should be avoided in the 14 days after rasagiline has been stopped. Some manufacturers of selegiline contraindicate concurrent use with all opioids, which is probably unnecessary, based on the evidence with non-selective MAOIs, page 489.

MAO-B inhibitors + Quinolones

Ciprofloxacin increases the AUC of rasagiline by 83%.

The clinical relevance of this pharmacokinetic interaction has not been assessed but it may be prudent to be alert for rasagiline adverse effects (e.g. headache, dyspepsia). Some other quinolones may also interact, see quinolones, page 564.

MAO-B inhibitors + SSRIs

Rasagiline with Fluoxetine or Fluvoxamine

The concurrent use of rasagiline and fluvoxamine should be avoided because of an increased risk of serotonin syndrome, page 580. In addition, fluvoxamine is predicted to inhibit the metabolism of rasagiline by CYP1A2, which may further increase the risk of adverse effects.

The manufacturers of rasagiline recommend avoiding the concurrent use of fluvoxamine or fluoxetine. Rasagiline should not be started for 5 weeks after stopping fluoxetine or 2 weeks after starting fluvoxamine, and fluoxetine should not be started for 2 weeks after stopping rasagiline.

Rasagiline with other SSRIs

The manufacturers of rasagiline report that, although in clinical studies no cases of serotonin syndrome were reported when some SSRIs (citalopram, paroxetine and sertraline) were given to patients also given rasagiline, cases of serotonergic adverse effects have been reported on concurrent use.

The UK manufacturer advises caution on the concurrent use of rasagiline with these SSRIs. Patients should be monitored for signs of serotonin syndrome, page 580, such as flushing, ataxia, tremor, and hyperthermia. Note that the US manufacturer states that the possibility of an interaction cannot be ruled out and they therefore recommend avoiding the concurrent use of rasagiline with an antidepressant, including these SSRIs, during and for 14 days after stopping rasagiline.

M

Selegiline with SSRIs

Although the safe concurrent use of selegiline and SSRIs has been reported in a number of patients, there are also documented cases of serotonin syndrome, page 580.

> The manufacturers of selegiline contraindicate the concurrent use of SSRIs. In addition, selegiline should not be started for 5 weeks after stopping fluoxetine, 2 weeks after stopping sertraline, and one week after stopping other SSRIs. SSRIs should not be started for 2 weeks after stopping selegiline.

MAO-B inhibitors + Tricyclics

In a clinical study in patients taking amitriptyline and given rasagiline, no symptoms or signs of serotonin syndrome were reported. However, rare cases of serotonin syndrome, page 580, and other CNS disturbances have been seen when selegiline or rasagiline have been given with a tricyclic.

> If the combination is used the outcome should be well monitored, but the likelihood of problems seems to be small. Nevertheless, some manufacturers of selegiline advise avoiding the concurrent use of tricyclics. The UK manufacturer of rasagiline advises similar caution if it is given with antidepressants, whereas the US manufacturer states that the possibility of an interaction cannot be ruled out, and they therefore recommend avoiding the concurrent use of rasagiline with an antidepressant, including the tricyclics, during and for 14 days after stopping rasagiline.

MAO-B inhibitors + Triptans

The UK manufacturer of selegiline contraindicates the concurrent use of serotonin agonists (and they name the triptans as an example). This is presumably because of the theoretical risk of the serotonin syndrome, page 580.

> Avoid concurrent use. The UK manufacturer states that at least 14 days should lapse between stopping selegiline and starting a triptan.

MAO-B inhibitors + Venlafaxine

Rasagiline

Cases of serotonin syndrome, page 580 have been reported when rasagiline was given with antidepressants (such as venlafaxine).

> The UK manufacturer of rasagiline advises caution, whereas the US manufacturer advises against the concurrent use of antidepressants, including the SNRIs, and for 14 days after stopping rasagiline. Patients should be monitored for signs and symptoms of serotonin syndrome (such as flushing, ataxia, tremor, hyperthermia, agitation and confusion).

Selegiline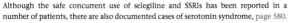

Serotonin syndrome, page 580 has been reported when selegiline was given with venlafaxine. This is in line with the manufacturers' prediction and the way that other serotonergic drugs behave with selegiline.

> The manufacturers of selegiline contraindicate the concurrent use of

M

venlafaxine. A 2-week washout period would seem appropriate when switching from one of these drugs to the other.

MAOIs

This section covers the non-selective MAOIs. Other drugs with MAO-inhibitory properties, such as linezolid, moclobemide, and the MAO-B inhibitors, selegiline and rasagiline, are discussed in their own sections.

MAOIs + Maprotiline ⊗

Toxic and sometimes fatal reactions (similar to or the same as serotonin syndrome, page 580) have very occasionally occurred in patients taking both MAOIs and *tricyclic antidepressants*. Maprotiline would be expected to interact similarly.

Avoid concurrent use. Maprotiline should not be started for 2 to 3 weeks after treatment with MAOIs has been stopped and an MAOI should not be started until at least 7 to 14 days after maprotiline has been stopped. If concurrent use is thought necessary it has been suggested that it should only be undertaken by specialists well aware of the problems and who can undertake adequate supervision.

MAOIs + Methyldopa ⊗

Theoretically hypertension may occur when non-selective MAOIs are taken with methyldopa, although additive blood-pressure lowering effects are also a possibility. The concurrent use of antidepressant MAOIs and methyldopa may not be desirable because methyldopa can sometimes cause depression.

It would seem prudent to avoid the combination wherever possible. Some manufacturers contraindicate concurrent use.

MAOIs + Methylphenidate ⊗

The concurrent use of non-selective MAOIs with methylphenidate can result in hypertensive crisis and/or serotonin syndrome. Dexmethylphenidate is predicted to interact similarly.

Methylphenidate and dexmethylphenidate should not be taken either with or within 14 days of an MAOI.

MAOIs + Mianserin ⊗

Toxic and sometimes fatal reactions (similar to or the same as serotonin syndrome, page 580) have very occasionally occurred in patients taking both MAOIs and *tricyclic antidepressants*. Case reports suggest that mianserin can interact similarly.

Avoid concurrent use. Mianserin should not be started for 2 to 3 weeks after treatment with MAOIs has been stopped and an MAOI should not be started until at least 7 to 14 days after mianserin has been stopped. If concurrent use is thought

M

necessary it has been suggested that it should only be undertaken by specialists well aware of the problems and who can undertake adequate supervision.

MAOIs + Mirtazapine

No data seem to be available about the concurrent use of mirtazapine with MAOIs.

The manufacturers say that the concurrent use of mirtazapine and the MAOIs should be avoided both during and within 2 weeks of stopping treatment. This is a general warning about the concurrent use of MAOIs that most of the manufacturers of antidepressants issue.

MAOIs + Nasal decongestants

The concurrent use of a number of nasal decongestants with indirect sympathomimetic actions, such as ephedrine, phenylpropanolamine, and pseudoephedrine, and non-selective MAOIs can result in a potentially fatal hypertensive crisis.

Avoid concurrent use both during and for 2 weeks after stopping the MAOI. These drugs are found in many proprietary cough, cold and influenza preparations, or are used as appetite suppressants. Counsel patients accordingly.

MAOIs + Nefopam

Nefopam has sympathomimetic activity, which theoretically might cause severe hypertension in those taking MAOIs.

The manufacturer of nefopam contraindicates concurrent use. With other drugs that interact in the manner predicted, it is usually advised that concurrent use should also be avoided for 2 weeks after the MAOI has been stopped.

MAOIs + Opioids

The concurrent use of pethidine (meperidine) and an MAOI has resulted in a serious and potentially life-threatening reaction in several patients. Excitement, muscle rigidity, hyperpyrexia, flushing, sweating and unconsciousness can occur very rapidly. Respiratory depression and hypertension or hypotension have also been seen. Similar interactions have been seen if tramadol is taken with MAOIs. Isolated cases of adverse reactions (e.g. hypertension, hypotension, hyperthermia and tachycardia) have been reported after fentanyl or morphine were given to patients taking MAOIs.

The interaction with pethidine (meperidine) is serious and potentially fatal, but the incidence is probably quite low. It may therefore be an idiosyncratic reaction. Nevertheless, it would be imprudent to give pethidine to any patient taking an MAOI. Bear in mind that the non-selective MAOIs are all essentially irreversible so that an interaction is possible for many days after their withdrawal (at least 2 weeks is the official advice). The manufacturers of tramadol contraindicate its use with MAOIs because of the risks of this reaction. Evidence for an interaction between other opioids and MAOIs is limited, and some of the cases appear to represent a different type of reaction to that seen with pethidine. Indeed, with some opioids there is evidence of safe concurrent use. Nevertheless, the manufacturers of many opioids contraindicate concurrent use both with and within 14 days of the use of an MAOI. These include alfentanil, buprenorphine, codeine,

M

dextropropoxyphene (propoxyphene), diamorphine, dipipanone, fentanyl, hydromorphone, methadone, morphine and oxycodone.

MAOIs + Oxcarbazepine ⊗

The use of *tricyclics*, page 491 and MAOIs results in a serious potentially fatal adverse reaction. Oxcarbazepine is structurally related to the tricyclics and may therefore interact similarly.

Avoid concurrent use. It is usual to wait until 2 weeks after an MAOI is stopped before starting a potentially interacting drug.

MAOIs + Phenobarbital ❓

Although the MAOIs can enhance and prolong the activity of barbiturates in *animals*, only a few isolated cases of adverse responses (profound sedation) attributed to an interaction have been described.

There is no well-documented evidence showing that concurrent use should be avoided, although some caution is clearly appropriate because of the case reports.

MAOIs + Reboxetine ⊗

No data seem to be available about the concurrent use of reboxetine with MAOIs. However, the manufacturers predict that a hypertensive reaction is possible.

Concurrent use should be avoided. With other drugs that interact in the manner predicted it is usually advised that concurrent use should also be avoided for 2 weeks after the MAOI has been stopped.

MAOIs + Salbutamol (Albuterol) and related bronchodilators ❓

An isolated case of tachycardia and apprehension has been described after a patient with asthma taking phenelzine also took salbutamol (albuterol).

This appears to be an isolated case, and is probably not of general importance as the reaction is not in line with the expected pharmacological effects of concurrent use. Nevertheless, on the basis of interactions with other sympathomimetic drugs, one manufacturer of fenoterol (with ipratropium) advises caution if MAOIs are also given.

MAOIs + SSRIs ⊗

A number of case reports describe serotonin syndrome, page 580, in patients given SSRIs with MAOIs: some have been fatal.

Direct information about the interaction between MAOIs and SSRIs is limited, and given that concurrent use is contraindicated, further reports seem unlikely. The manufacturers say that the SSRIs should not be given within 14 days of discontinuing an irreversible MAOI. Moreover, the manufacturers of each SSRI give guidance on the appropriate intervals that should be left between stopping the SSRI and starting an MAOI; that is, 7 days for sertraline, citalopram, escitalopram, fluvoxamine or paroxetine (14 days in the US for citalopram, escitalopram, sertraline and paroxetine) and at least 5 weeks for fluoxetine, with an even longer interval if long-term or high-dose fluoxetine has been used.

MAOIs + Trazodone ⊗

Toxic and sometimes fatal reactions (similar to or the same as serotonin syndrome, page 580) have very occasionally occurred in patients taking both MAOIs and *tricyclic antidepressants*. A case report suggests that trazodone may interact similarly; however, a small number of reports describe the successful use of low-dose trazodone with phenelzine for depression and insomnia.

Trazodone should not be started for 2 weeks after treatment with MAOIs has been stopped, and an MAOI should not be started until 1 week after trazodone has been stopped. If concurrent use is thought necessary it has been suggested that it should only be undertaken by specialists well aware of the problems and who can undertake adequate supervision.

MAOIs + Tricyclics ⊗

Occasionally very toxic and sometimes fatal reactions (similar to or the same as serotonin syndrome, page 580) have occurred in patients taking both MAOIs and tricyclic antidepressants.

Concurrent use is contraindicated. Tricyclic antidepressants should not be started for 2 weeks after treatment with MAOIs has been stopped (3 weeks if starting clomipramine or imipramine), and an MAOI should not be started until at least 7 to 14 days after a tricyclic or related antidepressant has been stopped (3 weeks in the case of clomipramine or imipramine). If concurrent use is thought necessary it has been suggested that it should only be undertaken by specialists well aware of the problems and who can undertake adequate supervision.

MAOIs + Triptans ⊗

Some have suggested that there might be a pharmacodynamic interaction between MAOIs (both selective and non-selective) and triptans, which could result in serotonin syndrome, page 580.

The manufacturers of rizatriptan and sumatriptan contraindicate their use both during, and for 2 weeks after stopping, treatment with a non-selective MAOI. The US manufacturer contraindicates the use of zolmitriptan both during, and for 2 weeks after, the use of *moclobemide*, whereas the UK manufacturer restricts the dose of zolmitriptan to 5 mg in 24 hours. In the absence of any direct information it would seem prudent to apply these warnings to the use of non-selective MAOIs. It would seem prudent to monitor for signs of serotonin syndrome (such as weakness, hyperreflexia, and incoordination) on concurrent use of other triptans and non-selective MAOIs.

MAOIs + Tryptophan ⚠

Although the concurrent use of MAOIs and tryptophan can be both safe and effective, a number of patients have developed severe behavioural and neurological signs of

M

toxicity (some similar to serotonin syndrome, page 580) after taking MAOIs with tryptophan, and fatalities have occurred.

> It has been recommended that patients taking MAOIs should start treatment with a low dose of tryptophan (500 mg). This should be gradually increased while monitoring the patient for changes suggesting hypomania, and neurological changes, including ocular oscillations and upper motor neurone signs.

MAOIs + Venlafaxine

Serious and potentially life-threatening reactions (serotonin syndrome, page 580) can develop if venlafaxine and non-selective, irreversible MAOIs are given concurrently, or even sequentially if insufficient time is left in between.

> Concurrent use is contraindicated. The manufacturers of venlafaxine recommend that at least one week should elapse between stopping the venlafaxine and starting an MAOI, and 2 weeks between stopping an MAOI and starting venlafaxine.

Maprotiline

Maprotiline + Moclobemide

One study did not find a serious hypertensive reaction, like that seen with the tricyclics and the MAOIs, when maprotiline was given with moclobemide. Nevertheless, such a reaction is thought possible.

> Concurrent use should be avoided. Moclobemide has a short duration of action so no treatment free period is required before starting a tricyclic or related antidepressant. However, some recommend waiting 24 hours. Moclobemide should not be started until at least one week after a tricyclic or related antidepressant has been stopped.

Maraviroc

Maraviroc + Phenobarbital

Phenobarbital is predicted to reduce the exposure to maraviroc. It might also be prudent to consider an interaction with primidone, which is metabolised to phenobarbital.

> The US HIV guidelines do not recommend concurrent use. However, if concurrent use is necessary, the UK and US manufacturers of maraviroc, and the US HIV guidelines, recommend increasing the maraviroc dose to 600 mg twice daily if phenobarbital is also given.

M

Maraviroc + Phenytoin

Phenytoin is predicted to reduce the exposure to maraviroc. It might also be prudent to consider an interaction with fosphenytoin, a prodrug of phenytoin.

The US HIV guidelines do not recommend concurrent use. However, if concurrent use is necessary, the UK and US manufacturers of maraviroc, and the US HIV guidelines, recommend increasing the maraviroc dose to 600 mg twice daily if phenytoin is also given.

Maraviroc + Rifabutin

Rifabutin is predicted to reduce the exposure to maraviroc.

Monitor for a reduction in maraviroc efficacy. The US HIV guidelines recommend a dose of maraviroc of 300 mg twice daily for use with rifabutin, which is the usual dose for use with non-interacting drugs.

Maraviroc + Rifampicin (Rifampin)

Rifampicin moderately reduces the exposure to maraviroc. This could result in a decrease in therapeutic efficacy and the development of viral resistance. Doubling the maraviroc dose negated the effects of this interaction.

The US HIV guidelines do not recommend concurrent use. If concurrent use is necessary, The UK and US manufacturers of maraviroc, and the US HIV guidelines, recommend increasing the dose of maraviroc to 600 mg twice daily. Note that the UK manufacturer of maraviroc does not recommend the concurrent use of maraviroc in patients taking both rifampicin and efavirenz, because the effect of two enzyme inducers has not been studied.

Mebendazole

Mebendazole + Phenobarbital

Carbamazepine and *phenytoin* lower mebendazole concentrations. Phenobarbital and primidone are expected to interact similarly.

When treating systemic worm infections it might be necessary to increase the mebendazole dose in patients taking phenobarbital or primidone. Monitor the outcome of concurrent use. This interaction is of no importance when mebendazole is used for intestinal worm infections where its action is a local effect on the worms in the gut.

Mebendazole + Phenytoin

Phenytoin lowers mebendazole concentrations. Fosphenytoin is expected to interact similarly.

When treating systemic worm infections it might be necessary to increase the

M

mebendazole dose in patients taking phenytoin or fosphenytoin. Monitor the outcome of concurrent use. This interaction is of no importance when mebendazole is used for intestinal worm infections where its action is a local effect on the worms in the gut.

Medroxyprogesterone

For the interactions of medroxyprogesterone used as a progestogen-only contraceptive, consider contraceptives, page 288.

Medroxyprogesterone + Warfarin and related oral anticoagulants ⚠

High-dose medroxyprogesterone acetate (1 g daily) increases the half-life and reduces the clearance of warfarin by about 70% and 35%, respectively.

Monitor the effect of concurrent use on the anticoagulant response and adjust the warfarin dose as necessary.

Mefloquine

Mefloquine + Quinidine ❓

The UK and US manufacturers of mefloquine warn that, in theory, there is an increased risk of convulsions if mefloquine is given with quinidine.

Caution is advised on concurrent use.

Mefloquine + Quinine ⚠

The plasma concentration of mefloquine might be increased by quinine. In theory there is an increased risk of convulsions. The manufacturers warn that, in theory, concurrent use might increase the risk of QT prolongation. See Drugs that prolong the QT interval, page 352 for more information on this effect.

It has been suggested that treatment with mefloquine should be delayed until 12 hours after the last dose of intravenous quinine.

Mefloquine + Rifampicin (Rifampin)

Rifampicin moderately reduces the exposure to mefloquine.

The clinical relevance of this is uncertain, but some suggest that simultaneous use should be avoided to prevent treatment failure and the risk of *Plasmodium falciparum* resistance to mefloquine. Until more is known, this would seem a sensible precaution.

Mefloquine + **Warfarin and related oral anticoagulants**

The effects of warfarin and an unnamed coumarin were increased in two patients who took mefloquine.

Patients taking mefloquine should have their warfarin effects checked before travel to allow for monitoring of any changes in anticoagulant effects.

Melatonin

Melatonin + **Quinolones**

In a study, *fluvoxamine* raised melatonin levels 12-fold probably by inhibiting CYP1A2. All subjects reported marked drowsiness after melatonin intake that was even more pronounced when *fluvoxamine* was also given. The manufacturer predicts that the quinolones, page 564 will interact similarly, but note that they differ in their ability to inhibit this isoenzyme.

Be aware that excessive drowsiness and related adverse effects may occur on concurrent use.

Melatonin + **SSRIs** ✕

In a study, fluvoxamine raised melatonin levels 12-fold. All subjects reported marked drowsiness after melatonin intake that was even more pronounced when fluvoxamine was also given.

The manufacturers advise avoiding concurrent use.

Melatonin + **Warfarin and related oral anticoagulants** ❓

Case reports suggest that melatonin may raise or lower the INR in response to warfarin.

Until more is known, bear these cases in mind in the event of an unexpected change in coagulation status in patients also taking melatonin.

Meropenem

Meropenem + **Probenecid**

Probenecid increases the AUC of meropenem by about 50%.

The manufacturers say that because the potency and duration of meropenem are adequate without probenecid, they do not recommend concurrent use.

M

Meropenem + **Valproate**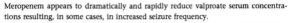

Meropenem appears to dramatically and rapidly reduce valproate serum concentrations resulting, in some cases, in increased seizure frequency.

Avoid concurrent use if possible. If it is essential, consider using intravenous valproate (which has been successfully substituted in some cases) and monitor valproate serum concentrations closely, adjusting the valproate dose if necessary. Consider using another antibacterial, or an alternative to valproate; limited evidence suggests that carbamazepine and phenytoin are not affected.

Methotrexate

Methotrexate + **Neomycin** ?

The gastrointestinal absorption of methotrexate can be reduced by neomycin.

The significance of this interaction is unclear, but bear it in mind in case of an unexpected response to treatment.

Methotrexate + **NSAIDs**

Increased methotrexate toxicity, sometimes life-threatening, has been seen in a few patients also taking an NSAID, whereas other patients have taken NSAIDs with methotrexate uneventfully. The mechanism of this interaction suggests that all NSAIDs have the potential to interact similarly. The pharmacokinetics of methotrexate (reduced clearance) can also be changed by some NSAIDs.

Concurrent use need not be avoided but close monitoring is necessary. Tell patients to report symptoms such as sore throat, dyspnoea or cough. If high-dose methotrexate is given with an NSAID, monitor methotrexate levels and increase routine methotrexate monitoring (e.g. full blood count, liver function tests). The risk appears to be lowest in those taking low-dose methotrexate for psoriasis or rheumatoid arthritis, with normal renal function. Patients must be counselled regarding non-prescription NSAIDs.

Methotrexate + **Penicillins**

Reduced clearance and acute methotrexate toxicity has been attributed to the concurrent use of various penicillins (amoxicillin, benzylpenicillin, carbenicillin, dicloxacillin, flucloxacillin, mezlocillin, oxacillin, phenoxymethylpenicillin, piperacillin, and ticarcillin) in a small number of case reports.

Serious interactions between methotrexate and penicillins are uncommon. Risk factors are as yet unknown and even patients taking low doses of methotrexate have been affected. Given the current evidence monitoring is advisable. Full blood count should be routinely monitored with methotrexate alone: consider twice-weekly platelet and white cell counts for 2 weeks initially, with the measurement of methotrexate levels if toxicity is suspected.

M

Methotrexate + **Probenecid**

Probenecid markedly increases methotrexate levels (3- to 4-fold).

A marked increase in both the therapeutic and toxic effects of methotrexate can occur, apparently even with low doses if other risk factors are present (e.g. renal impairment, concurrent NSAIDs). Anticipate the need to reduce the dose of methotrexate and monitor the effects well if probenecid is also taken. If this is not possible, avoid the combination.

Methotrexate + **Proton pump inhibitors**

The excretion of methotrexate is reported to have been reduced in patients given proton pump inhibitors. However, similar elevations in methotrexate concentrations in another patient taking omeprazole were independent of omeprazole use. One patient had myalgia and elevated 7-hydroxymethotrexate concentrations when given methotrexate and pantoprazole.

The general significance of this interaction is unclear but the risk seems greatest with high-dose methotrexate. Routine methotrexate monitoring should be adequate to detect any toxicity. If toxicity develops, consider the proton pump inhibitor as a possible cause. Some advise against concurrent use and suggest that omeprazole should be stopped 5 days before starting methotrexate.

Methotrexate + **Pyrimethamine**

Serious pancytopenia and megaloblastic anaemia may occur in patients given pyrimethamine (with or without sulfonamides) with other drugs that inhibit folate metabolism, such as methotrexate.

If the concurrent use of pyrimethamine and a drug that inhibits folate metabolism cannot be avoided, consider the use of a folate supplement, preferably folinic acid. This is recommended for all patients with toxoplasmosis taking high-dose pyrimethamine.

Methotrexate + **Quinolones**

A report describes methotrexate toxicity in 2 patients also taking ciprofloxacin.

Full blood count should be monitored when methotrexate is used. If any abnormalities arise, consider this interaction as a possible cause.

Methotrexate + **Retinoids**

Methotrexate concentrations might be increased by etretinate, and cases of severe liver toxicity have been reported. Acitretin (a metabolite of etretinate, which has a shorter half-life), might interact similarly.

Although methotrexate and etretinate have been used together with success for psoriasis, the risk of severe drug-induced hepatitis seems to be very considerably increased. If the concurrent use of methotrexate with either etretinate or acitretin is necessary, it would be prudent to increase the frequency of monitoring of liver

M

function tests. The UK and US manufacturers of acitretin advise avoiding concurrent use.

Methotrexate + Tetracyclines

Two case reports describe the development of methotrexate toxicity in patients also taking tetracycline or doxycycline.

The general significance of this interaction is unclear, but bear it in mind in case of an unexpected response to treatment.

Methotrexate + Theophylline

In one study theophylline clearance was reduced by 19% after 6 weeks of treatment with intramuscular methotrexate 15 mg weekly. A few patients complained of nausea and the theophylline dose had to be reduced in one. It seems possible that aminophylline could be similarly affected.

The clinical importance of this change is unclear; however bear it in mind should increased theophylline adverse effects (such as nausea and vomiting) occur with concurrent use. Note that one UK manufacturer of low-dose methotrexate recommends monitoring theophylline levels.

Methotrexate + Trimethoprim

The concurrent use of low-dose methotrexate and trimethoprim or trimethoprim with sulfamethoxazole has resulted in several cases of severe bone marrow depression, some of which were fatal.

Full blood count should be monitored when methotrexate is used. If any abnormalities arise, consider this interaction as a possible cause. Note that trimethoprim (as co-trimoxazole) is commonly used in some cytotoxic regimens.

Methotrexate + Vaccines

The immune response of the body is suppressed by cytotoxic antineoplastics. The effectiveness of vaccines may be poor and generalised infection may occur in patients immunised with live vaccines. In one study the antibody response to pneumococcal vaccination was reduced by 60% in patients receiving antineoplastics, and suboptimal responses to influenza and measles vaccines have been reported.

Live vaccines should not be given to patients who are receiving cytotoxics or other immunosuppressant antineoplastics. In the UK, it is recommended that live vaccines should not be given during or within at least 6 months of such treatment. Monitor the immune response to other types of vaccine. Consider whether vaccination can be carried out before or after methotrexate use.

M

Methylphenidate

Dexmethylphenidate is the *d*-isomer of methylphenidate, and therefore has the potential to interact similarly.

Methylphenidate + **Phenytoin**

Raised phenytoin levels and phenytoin toxicity have been seen in a few patients also given methylphenidate, but it is an uncommon reaction and studies suggest that most patients do not experience an interaction. It seems possible that dexmethylphenidate, the d-isomer of methylphenidate, and fosphenytoin, a prodrug of phenytoin, could interact similarly.

> This interaction is unlikely to be generally significant, but bear it in mind in case of an unexpected response to treatment. Indicators of phenytoin toxicity include blurred vision, nystagmus, ataxia or drowsiness.

Methylphenidate + **SSRIs**

Isolated reports describe delirium in one patient and a seizure in another when methylphenidate was taken with sertraline.

> The general significance of these cases is likely to be small, especially when set in the context of beneficial concurrent use with SSRIs (fluoxetine, paroxetine, sertraline). However, if adverse CNS effects become troublesome, it may be worth considering this interaction as a possible cause: in both cases the adverse effects resolved when one of the drugs was withdrawn.

Methylphenidate + **Tricyclics**

Methylphenidate can increase the plasma concentration and rate of response to imipramine and other tricyclic antidepressants. This has led to both increased beneficial and adverse effects. Dexmethylphenidate, the d-isomer of methylphenidate, would be expected to interact similarly.

> The combination of methylphenidate and tricyclic antidepressants might be beneficial, but might result in an increase in tricyclic adverse effects. If concurrent use is necessary it would seem prudent to monitor for adverse tricyclic effects (e.g. dry mouth, blurred vision, urinary retention) and adjust the dose of the tricyclic as necessary.

Methylphenidate + **Warfarin and related oral anticoagulants**

One study found that methylphenidate increased the half-life of the coumarin *ethyl biscoumacetate*, whereas another better-controlled study found that no interaction occurred. There seems to be no data regarding an interaction between other coumarins and methylphenidate; however, the manufacturers of methylphenidate and its d-isomer, dexmethylphenidate, predict that they will inhibit the metabolism of the coumarins.

> Although the findings of these studies are at odds with each other, the better-

controlled study and the lack of reports of problems in the literature suggest that an interaction between methylphenidate and coumarin anticoagulants is unlikely. However, the manufacturers suggest that patients taking coumarins should have their INR monitored if methylphenidate is started or stopped. This seems over-cautious; nevertheless, until more is known, it may be prudent to follow the same precautions with dexmethylphenidate.

Metoclopramide

Metoclopramide + Paracetamol (Acetaminophen)

Metoclopramide increases the rate of absorption of paracetamol and raises its maximum plasma levels.

As the total amount of paracetamol absorbed was unchanged this interaction is unlikely to be clinically significant, although a more rapid onset of action may be advantageous.

Metoclopramide + SSRIs

Case reports describe serotonin syndrome, page 580, in patients taking sertraline with metoclopramide. Extrapyramidal symptoms have occurred in patients given fluox-etine, fluvoxamine, paroxetine, or sertraline with metoclopramide.

Information seems to be limited to these reports, but they highlight the fact that care should be taken if two drugs with the potential to cause the same adverse effects are used together. Some monitoring for increased adverse effects would be advisable if an SSRI is taken with metoclopramide.

Metronidazole

Metronidazole + Mycophenolate

Metronidazole has no clinically relevant effect on the bioavailability of mycopheno-late mofetil. However, the combination of metronidazole and norfloxacin may reduce the exposure to mycophenolate by about 30%.

The US manufacturer of mycophenolate mofetil advises against the concurrent use of mycophenolate, metronidazole and norfloxacin. This seems particularly cautious as the reduction in exposure was slight. If both these antibacterials are given, consider monitoring for signs of reduced mycophenolate efficacy.

Metronidazole + Phenobarbital

Phenobarbital markedly increases the metabolism of metronidazole, and treatment failure as a result of this interaction has been reported in both adults and children.

Primidone is metabolised to phenobarbital and would be expected to interact similarly. Other barbiturates are also expected to interact.

Monitor the effects of concurrent use and anticipate the need to increase the metronidazole dose by 2- to 3-fold.

Metronidazole + Phenytoin

One study found that the half-life of intravenous phenytoin was modestly prolonged by metronidazole, whereas another found that metronidazole did not affect the pharmacokinetics of oral phenytoin. An anecdotal report describes a few patients who developed toxic phenytoin levels when given metronidazole. Fosphenytoin, a prodrug of phenytoin, may interact similarly.

This interaction is unlikely to be generally significant, but bear it in mind in case of an unexpected response to treatment. Indicators of phenytoin toxicity include blurred vision, nystagmus, ataxia or drowsiness.

Metronidazole + Warfarin and related oral anticoagulants

The anticoagulant effects of warfarin can be markedly increased by metronidazole and bleeding has been seen. Tinidazole may interact similarly.

Monitor the INR if either metronidazole or tinidazole is given with warfarin and adjust the warfarin dose accordingly. Nothing seems to be documented about other anticoagulants but it would be prudent to expect the coumarins to behave similarly.

Mexiletine

Mexiletine + NNRTIs

The manufacturers predict that etravirine may decrease the levels of mexiletine. However, note that mexiletine is more usually affected by CYP2D6 inhibitors or inducers, effects that etravirine does not appear to have.

The manufacturers recommend caution on concurrent use and state that mexiletine levels should be monitored, if this is possible.

Mexiletine + Opioids

The absorption of mexiletine is reduced in patients following a myocardial infarction, and further reduced and delayed if opioids (diamorphine or morphine) are given concurrently. Other opioids might interact similarly.

The delay and reduction in the absorption would seem to limit the value of oral mexiletine during the first few hours after a myocardial infarction, particularly if opioid analgesics are used. Mexiletine is no longer widely available, but the UK manufacturer previously suggested that a higher loading dose of oral mexiletine

M

might be preferable in this situation. Alternatively, an intravenous dose of mexiletine may be given.

Mexiletine + **Phenytoin**

Mexiletine exposure is moderately reduced by phenytoin. Fosphenytoin, a prodrug of phenytoin, might interact similarly.

It seems likely that the fall in mexiletine exposure will be clinically important in at least some individuals. Monitor for mexiletine efficacy, and where possible monitor mexiletine concentrations. Increase the dose if necessary.

Mexiletine + **Rifampicin (Rifampin)**

Rifampicin slightly reduces the exposure to mexiletine.

It seems likely that the reduction in mexiletine exposure will be clinically important in some individuals. Monitor for mexiletine efficacy and, where possible, monitor mexiletine concentrations. Increase the dose if necessary.

Mexiletine + **SSRIs**

Fluvoxamine slightly increases the exposure to mexiletine by inhibiting its metabolism by CYP1A2. Fluoxetine and paroxetine might also be expected to interact, by inhibiting mexiletine metabolism by CYP2D6.

There appear to be no reported interactions with fluoxetine or paroxetine, but given the way they interact with other CYP2D6 substrates some interaction seems possible. However, note that other CYP2D6 inhibitors have only modest effects on mexiletine metabolism. Nevertheless, until more is known it would be prudent to be alert for mexiletine adverse effects (e.g. nausea, tremor, hypotension) in patients given fluoxetine or paroxetine. If they develop, consider an interaction as a possible cause. Similar caution seems warranted with fluvoxamine.

Mexiletine + **Terbinafine**

In vitro studies suggest that terbinafine is an inhibitor of CYP2D6. It might therefore be expected to increase the plasma concentration of other drugs that are substrates of this isoenzyme, such as mexiletine.

Until more is known it would seem wise to be aware of the possibility of an increase in mexiletine adverse effects (e.g. nausea, tremor, hypotension) if mexiletine is given with terbinafine. Consider a dose reduction if necessary.

Mexiletine + **Theophylline**

Theophylline concentrations are increased by mexiletine (up to threefold in some cases) and toxicity might occur. Aminophylline would be expected to interact similarly.

Monitor the theophylline concentration on concurrent use and reduce the theophylline dose as necessary. It has been suggested that 50% dose reductions may be required.

M

Mexiletine + Tizanidine

Mexiletine moderately increases tizanidine exposure, which increases the hypotensive and sedative effects of tizanidine.

A clinical response or adverse effect with tizanidine might occur at lower doses of tizanidine in patients taking mexiletine, therefore if concurrent use is necessary, consider reducing the dose of tizanidine or use the lowest possible starting dose titrated to effect. Monitor closely for adverse effects such as bradycardia, hypotension, and drowsiness.

Mianserin

Mianserin + Moclobemide

A number of studies suggest that no interaction, or only a moderate non-significant rise in *tricyclic antidepressant* levels occurs when they are given with moclobemide. However, several case reports describe serotonin syndrome, page 580, in patients receiving the combination. There is little evidence regarding mianserin, but it seems likely that it could interact similarly.

Concurrent use should be avoided. Moclobemide has a short duration of action so no treatment free period is required before starting a tricyclic or related antidepressant. However, some recommend waiting 24 hours. Moclobemide should not be started until at least one week after a tricyclic or related antidepressant has been stopped.

Mianserin + Phenobarbital

Mianserin levels can be markedly reduced by phenobarbital. Note that primidone is metabolised to phenobarbital and therefore may interact similarly.

Monitor the response to mianserin and increase the dose as necessary. Note that mianserin lowers the convulsive threshold and may therefore be inappropriate for patients with epilepsy.

Mianserin + Phenytoin

Mianserin levels can be markedly reduced by phenytoin. Fosphenytoin, a prodrug of phenytoin, may interact similarly.

Monitor the response to mianserin and increase the dose as necessary. Note that mianserin lowers the convulsive threshold and may therefore be inappropriate for patients with epilepsy.

Mianserin + Warfarin and related oral anticoagulants

Mianserin increased the response to warfarin in one patient. A case of decreased acenocoumarol efficacy has also been reported with mianserin. However on the whole concurrent use seems uneventful.

The general significance of the case reports is unknown, but bear it in mind in case of an excessive response to anticoagulant treatment.

Mifepristone

Mifepristone + NSAIDs

Theoretically NSAIDs might reduce the efficacy of mifepristone, and combined use is often not recommended. However, evidence from two studies with naproxen and diclofenac suggests no reduction in mifepristone efficacy.

Because of theoretical concerns of antagonistic effects, NSAID analgesics have been avoided in protocols for medical abortion. However, the limited available evidence suggests that this might not be necessary. Nevertheless, some NSAID manufacturers continue to advise that NSAIDs should not be used for 8 to 12 days after mifepristone.

Mirtazapine

Mirtazapine + Phenobarbital

Phenytoin decreases the AUC and maximum levels of mirtazapine by 47% and 33%, respectively. Phenobarbital (and therefore primidone) would be expected to interact similarly.

The mirtazapine dose may need to be increased in the presence of phenobarbital or primidone. Monitor concurrent use to ensure mirtazapine is effective. Note that mirtazapine can lower the seizure threshold, and therefore its use should be carefully considered in patients given barbiturates for epilepsy.

Mirtazapine + Phenytoin

Phenytoin decreases the AUC and maximum levels of mirtazapine by 47% and 33%, respectively. Fosphenytoin, a prodrug of phenytoin, may interact similarly.

The mirtazapine dose may need to be increased in the presence of phenytoin or fosphenytoin. Monitor concurrent use to ensure mirtazapine is effective. Note that, mirtazapine can lower the seizure threshold, and therefore its use should be carefully considered in patients with epilepsy.

Mirtazapine + Rifampicin (Rifampin)

Rifampicin is predicted to lower mirtazapine levels. Other enzyme inducers (e.g. phenytoin) have been shown to have this effect.

The mirtazapine dose may need to be increased during concurrent use. Monitor to ensure that mirtazapine is effective.

Mirtazapine + SSRIs ❓

There are a couple of isolated cases of possible serotonin syndrome, page 580, when mirtazapine was used with fluoxetine and fluvoxamine, and there is a report of hypomania associated with the concurrent use of sertraline. Restless legs syndrome occurred with fluoxetine and mirtazapine. Fluvoxamine markedly increased plasma levels of mirtazapine in two cases.

> Caution is warranted on concurrent use. Monitor for adverse effects (most commonly sedation, fatigue, headache) and be aware that CNS excitation may occur. Extra caution might be appropriate with fluvoxamine, as the limited evidence suggests that this might markedly raise mirtazapine levels. However, this needs confirming.

Mirtazapine + Warfarin and related oral anticoagulants ❓

Mirtazapine may cause small, clinically insignificant increases in INR in patients taking warfarin.

> No action needed. One UK manufacturer of mirtazapine very cautiously advises that the prothrombin time should be controlled if mirtazapine is given with warfarin; however, another manufacturer does not consider monitoring to be necessary.

Moclobemide

Moclobemide + Nasal decongestants ✖

The concurrent use of ephedrine and moclobemide raises blood pressure, and this has resulted in palpitations and headache. Other related drugs (e.g. pseudoephedrine) would be expected to interact with the MAOIs similarly.

> The manufacturers of moclobemide advise avoiding drugs such as ephedrine, pseudoephedrine and phenylpropanolamine. Patients taking MAOIs should be strongly warned not to take any of these drugs either with or for 2 weeks after stopping their MAOI.

Moclobemide + Opioids ✖

Animal studies suggest that moclobemide may potentiate the effects of the opioids. A report of suspected serotonin syndrome in a patient given pethidine (meperidine) in addition to her usual treatment with moclobemide, nortriptyline and lithium, adds some weight to this suggestion. Similar predictions have been made for tramadol, and serotonin syndrome, page 580, has been seen in a patient given tramadol with moclobemide and clomipramine.

> Concurrent use should be avoided or undertaken with great caution. One manufacturer of moclobemide suggests that opioid dose adjustments may be

M

needed. Note that the concurrent use of pethidine (meperidine) with moclobemide is contraindicated.

Moclobemide + SSRIs ⊗

Some studies suggest that moclobemide may not interact with the SSRIs, but there have been case reports of serotonin syndrome, page 580 in patients taking the combination.

Concurrent use is contraindicated. Because the effects of moclobemide are readily reversible, only one day need elapse between stopping moclobemide and starting an SSRI. However, if stopping an SSRI and starting moclobemide the same intervals as for the irreversible MAOIs, page 490 are required.

Moclobemide + Trazodone ⊗

Isolated cases of serotonin syndrome, page 580 have been reported in patients receiving trazodone and moclobemide. A small number of reports describe the successful use of low-dose trazodone with moclobemide for depression and insomnia.

The balance of the evidence suggests that concurrent use is favourable if the dose of trazodone is low (200 mg daily or less). No specific advice appears to have been given for moclobemide with higher doses, but, because of its half-life, a 24-hour washout is usually considered appropriate when starting potentially interacting drugs in patients who have been taking moclobemide.

Moclobemide + Tricyclics ⊗

A number of studies suggest that no interaction, or only a moderate non-significant rise in tricyclic antidepressant levels occurs when they are given with moclobemide. However, several case reports describe serotonin syndrome, page 580 in patients receiving the combination.

Concurrent use should be avoided. Moclobemide has a short duration of action so no treatment free period is required before starting a tricyclic antidepressant. However, some recommend waiting 24 hours. Moclobemide should not be started until at least one week after a tricyclic antidepressant has been stopped.

Moclobemide + Triptans ⊗

Moclobemide moderately increases the exposure to rizatriptan and sumatriptan, and slightly increases the exposure to zolmitriptan. Note that there is a potential risk of serotonin syndrome, page 580 if triptans are given with moclobemide.

The manufacturers contraindicate the use of moclobemide with rizatriptan or sumatriptan. In the UK, a maximum intake of 5 mg of zolmitriptan in 24 hours is recommended by the manufacturers, whereas in the US the combination is contraindicated.

M

Moclobemide + **Venlafaxine**

The concurrent use of moclobemide and venlafaxine has led to the potentially fatal serotonin syndrome, page 580.

Concurrent use is contraindicated. The UK manufacturer of venlafaxine states that a withdrawal period shorter than 14 days may be used before starting venlafaxine (with other similar interactions with moclobemide 24 to 48 hours has been said to be adequate). At least 7 days should elapse between stopping venlafaxine and starting moclobemide.

Modafinil

Armodafinil is the *R*-isomer of modafinil and would be expected to interact in a similar way to modafinil.

Modafinil + **Phenytoin**

Modafinil may inhibit the metabolism of phenytoin. The manufacturers predict that phenytoin may reduce the levels of modafinil. Fosphenytoin, a prodrug of phenytoin, may interact similarly.

Monitor for evidence of increased phenytoin effects and toxicity (blurred vision, nystagmus, ataxia or drowsiness). An effect on modafinil seems unlikely as it has multiple routes of metabolism; nevertheless it may be prudent to monitor for modafinil efficacy.

Modafinil + **Sodium oxybate**

No pharmacokinetic interaction is expected between modafinil and sodium oxybate; however, case reports describe anxiety and depression in patients taking modafinil when sodium oxybate was added. Armodafinil, the *R*-isomer of modafinil, would be expected to behave in the same way.

Concurrent use is common, but consider the possibility of an interaction if psychiatric adverse effects develop on concurrent use. Withdrawal of either drug should stop these symptoms.

Modafinil + **Tricyclics**

The blood concentration of clomipramine was reported to be increased by modafinil in one patient. However, a study found that the concurrent use of modafinil and clomipramine did not affect the pharmacokinetics of either drug. Clomipramine is metabolised by CYP2D6 and possibly CYP2C19. It was suggested that the patient was a poor metaboliser of CYP2D6 (that is, she had low activity of this isoenzyme), so that CYP2C19 might play a greater role in clomipramine metabolism. Modafinil is a weak inhibitor of CYP2C19 and, in poor metabolisers of CYP2D6, additional inhibition of CYP2C19 by modafinil might result in an increase in clomipramine concentrations. Armodafinil, the *R*-isomer of modafinil, would be expected to interact similarly.

M

Information about other tricyclic antidepressants is lacking, but the UK and US manufacturers of modafinil state that CYP2D6 poor metabolisers (about 7 to 10% of the Caucasian population) might possibly also show increased tricyclic antidepressant exposure in the presence of modafinil. However, note that not all tricyclic antidepressants are metabolised in the same way, and only those that are also metabolised by CYP2C19 (such as amitriptyline, clomipramine, and imipramine) would be expected to be affected.

> As metaboliser status is not usually known in clinical practice, it would be prudent to monitor the concurrent use of these tricyclics with modafinil for an increase in tricyclic adverse effects (such as dry mouth and urinary retention).

Modafinil + Ulipristal △

The UK and US manufacturers of ulipristal predict that CYP3A4 inducers might reduce the plasma concentration of ulipristal and reduce its efficacy. Modafinil and armodafinil, the *R*-isomer of modafinil, would be expected to interact in this way.

> The US manufacturer of ulipristal gives no specific advice about how to manage this potential interaction, whereas the UK manufacturer advises that ulipristal should not be used for emergency contraception in women taking CYP3A4 inducers (such as modafinil), or who have stopped taking an enzyme inducer within the last 2 to 3 weeks. Until more is known, this advice seems prudent.

Modafinil + Warfarin and related oral anticoagulants △

In a controlled study, modafinil did not affect the pharmacokinetics or anticoagulant effect of a single dose of warfarin.

> A pharmacokinetic interaction seems unlikely; however, the manufacturers cautiously advise that the effects of warfarin should be monitored more frequently, particularly over the first 2 months of concurrent use. Similarly, the manufacturer of armodafinil, the *R*-isomer of modafinil, states that a pharmaco-dynamic interaction cannot be ruled out and advises more frequent monitoring of the prothrombin time or INR on concurrent use.

Montelukast

Montelukast + Phenobarbital

Phenobarbital slightly reduces the exposure to montelukast. Note that primidone is metabolised to phenobarbital and therefore might interact similarly.

> The UK manufacturer of montelukast advises caution on concurrent use, especially in children. Monitor for a reduction in montelukast efficacy but note that dose adjustments seem unlikely to be needed.

Montelukast + Phenytoin

Phenytoin (and therefore possibly fosphenytoin) is predicted to reduce the exposure to montelukast.

> The UK manufacturer of montelukast advises caution on concurrent use, especially in children. Monitor for a reduction in montelukast efficacy but note that dose adjustments seem unlikely to be needed.

Montelukast + Rifampicin (Rifampin)

Rifampicin is predicted to reduce the exposure to montelukast.

> The UK manufacturer of montelukast advises caution on concurrent use, especially in children. Monitor for a reduction in montelukast efficacy but note that dose adjustments seem unlikely to be needed.

Moxonidine

Moxonidine + Tricyclics

Tricyclic antidepressants may antagonise the blood-pressure lowering effects of clonidine, page 271. As moxonidine is related to clonidine it is expected to interact similarly. Tricyclics can also cause postural hypotension, which could potentially be additive with the effects of moxonidine.

> The manufacturers of moxonidine advise avoiding tricyclic antidepressants, because of the lack of clinical experience of concurrent use. If the combination is used, it would be prudent to carefully monitor blood pressure.

Mycophenolate

Mycophenolate + Nystatin

A selective bowel decontamination regimen of nystatin (with tobramycin and cefuroxime) appears to modestly reduce mycophenolate bioavailability, although the clinical relevance of this reduction has not been assessed.

> Until further information is available, it would seem prudent to monitor the outcome of concurrent use, and for a short period after stopping the antibacterial, to ensure that mycophenolate remains effective.

Mycophenolate + Penicillins

Amoxicillin (given with clavulanic acid) transiently reduces the trough levels of mycophenolate mofetil by about 50% in renal transplant patients, although the clinical relevance of this reduction has not been assessed.

> The UK manufacturer of mycophenolate considers that a change in the dose of

M

mycophenolate should not normally be necessary, in the absence of clinical evidence of graft dysfunction, if amoxicillin with clavulanic acid is also given. However, close clinical monitoring is advisable during the concurrent use of the antibacterial, and shortly after it is stopped.

Mycophenolate + **Proton pump inhibitors**

Lansoprazole, omeprazole and pantoprazole appear to modestly reduce mycophenolic acid concentrations from mycophenolate mofetil. Other proton pump inhibitors would be expected to interact similarly, although one study found that low doses of rabeprazole did not affect mycophenolic acid concentrations. Limited evidence suggests that mycophenolate sodium *enteric-coated tablets* may not interact in the same way, but this needs confirmation.

The clinical relevance of this interaction is unclear, and the lack of effect of rabeprazole might have been due to the low dose used. Until more is known, it would seem prudent to be aware of the possibility of reduced mycophenolic acid exposure with any proton pump inhibitor.

Mycophenolate + **Quinolones**

Ciprofloxacin taken for 7 days reduced mycophenolate trough levels by about 40% in renal transplant patients. The magnitude of the interaction was smaller with a longer course of ciprofloxacin (17% reduction in AUC at 14 days). The concurrent use of norfloxacin has no clinically relevant effect on the bioavailability of mycophenolate; however, the concurrent use of norfloxacin, metronidazole and mycophenolate reduces the bioavailability of mycophenolate by about 30%.

Although the effects are small, and monitoring is not considered necessary by some, others suggest that, as antibacterials can affect the gut bacteria that are involved in mycophenolate metabolism, monitoring for mycophenolate efficacy may be prudent. Note that the US manufacturer of mycophenolate mofetil advises against the concurrent use of mycophenolate, metronidazole and norfloxacin.

Mycophenolate + **Rifampicin (Rifampin)**

Rifampicin reduces the concentrations of mycophenolic acid (the active metabolite of mycophenolate) and increases the concentrations of the metabolite associated with mycophenolate adverse effects. An isolated case describes increased mycophenolate dose requirements in a patient taking rifampicin.

Mycophenolate should be closely monitored for both reduced efficacy and increased adverse effects if rifampicin is given, and the dose adjusted as required, both on starting and stopping rifampicin. Some suggest avoiding concurrent use.

Mycophenolate + **Sevelamer**

Sevelamer reduces the AUC of mycophenolate by 25%.

The clinical significance of this interaction is unclear, but it would seem prudent to monitor mycophenolate levels in any patient given sevelamer. One UK manufacturer of mycophenolate mofetil recommends that drugs for which a

M

reduction in bioavailability could be clinically important should be taken at least 1 hour before or three 3 hours after taking sevelamer. One US manufacturer advises taking mycophenolate 2 hours before sevelamer.

Mycophenolate + Vaccines

The body's immune response is suppressed by mycophenolate. The antibody response to vaccines may be reduced. The use of live attenuated vaccines may result in generalised infection.

For many inactivated vaccines even the reduced response seen is considered clinically useful and, in the case of renal transplant patients, influenza vaccination is actively recommended. If a vaccine is given, it may be prudent to monitor the response, so that alternative prophylactic measures can be considered where the response is inadequate. Note that even where effective antibody titres are produced, these may not persist as long as in healthy subjects, and more frequent booster doses may be required. The use of live vaccines is generally considered to be contraindicated. Ideally vaccines should take place before immunosuppressive treatment is started, and live vaccines should not be given for up to 6 months after treatment has stopped.

M

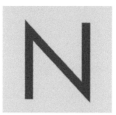

Nasal decongestants

Nasal decongestants + Theophylline

There is some information suggesting an increased frequency of adverse effects when ephedrine is used with theophylline. Aminophylline would be expected to interact similarly.

> Note that ephedrine is still an ingredient of a number of cough and cold remedies. It may be prudent to use an alternative. Patients taking theophylline or aminophylline and requiring ephedrine should be advised to report any adverse effects.

Neomycin

Neomycin + Penicillins

The serum levels of oral phenoxymethylpenicillin can be halved by oral neomycin.

> The clinical significance of this interaction is unclear. Monitor concurrent use to ensure phenoxymethylpenicillin is effective.

Neomycin + Vitamin A

Neomycin can markedly reduce the absorption of vitamin A (retinol). The extent to which chronic treatment with neomycin would impair the treatment of vitamin A deficiency has not been determined.

> The general importance of this interaction is unknown, but bear it in mind in case of an unexpected response to treatment.

Neomycin + Warfarin and related oral anticoagulants

Normally no interaction occurs, but in rare cases neomycin can cause a malabsorption syndrome, which may reduce vitamin K absorption and lead to over-anticoagulation.

This interaction seems rare, and only likely to occur in those with totally inadequate diets, starvation or some other condition in which the intake of vitamin K is very limited and who are given long-term antibacterial treatment.

Nicorandil

Nicorandil + Phosphodiesterase type-5 inhibitors

When avanafil, sildenafil, tadalafil, or vardenafil are given with *nitrates* potentially serious hypotension can occur, and myocardial infarction may be precipitated. A number of fatalities have occurred, possibly as a result of this interaction. Nicorandil is expected to interact in the same way as the nitrates.

The concurrent use of these phosphodiesterase inhibitors and nicorandil is contraindicated. Sildenafil should not be used within 24 hours of a *nitrate*, and some evidence suggests this is also a suitable separation for vardenafil. *Nitrates* should not be given for at least 48 hours after the last dose of tadalafil. Similar cautions would seem to apply to nicorandil.

Nicorandil + Riociguat

Nicorandil and riociguat both stimulate guanylate cyclase leading to vasodilation. Hence, concurrent use might lead to hypotension.

The UK and US manufacturer contraindicate concurrent use.

Nicotinic acid (Niacin)

Nicotinic acid (Niacin) + Statins

The risk of muscle toxicity, such as rhabdomyolysis, might be increased in patients taking a statin with nicotinic acid. In particular, a higher than expected incidence of myopathy has been reported in Chinese patients given simvastatin and nicotinic acid.

This interaction has been disputed; however, the latest data suggest that the risk of myopathy with simvastatin and nicotinic acid might be increased in Chinese patients. If the decision is made to use nicotinic acid with a statin the outcome should be closely monitored. All patients should be advised to report promptly any unexplained muscle aches, tenderness, cramps, stiffness, or weakness. The UK and US manufacturers of simvastatin recommend avoiding the 80 mg daily dose in Chinese patients taking nicotinic acid in daily doses of 1 g or more, whereas the US manufacturer of nicotinic acid recommends a maximum dose of simvastatin of 40 mg daily with a maximum daily dose of nicotinic acid of 2 g in all patients. The US manufacturer of lovastatin recommends a maximum dose of 20 mg daily in patients taking nicotinic acid in doses of 1 g or more daily, whereas the US manufacturer of nicotinic acid recommends a maximum daily dose of lovastatin of

40 mg with a maximum daily dose of nicotinic acid of 2 g. The US manufacturers of atorvastatin, pitavastatin, and rosuvastatin suggest that the lowest statin dose should be used or a statin dose reduction considered.

Nicotinic acid (Niacin) + Warfarin and related oral anticoagulants

The US manufacturer states that nicotinic acid has been associated with a small (4%) increase in the prothrombin time, which could be additive with the effects of anticoagulants. Nicotinic acid has also been associated with an 11% reduction in the platelet count.

> The US manufacturer advises caution on the concurrent use of anticoagulants and nicotinic acid, and states that the prothrombin time and platelet counts should be monitored.

Nilutamide

Nilutamide + Warfarin and related oral anticoagulants

The manufacturer notes that, *in vitro*, nilutamide has been shown to inhibit cytochrome P450 isoenzymes (specific isoenzymes not stated). Because of this, they suggest that nilutamide might decrease the metabolism of drugs with a narrow therapeutic range such as the vitamin K antagonists (i.e. coumarins and indanediones).

> Despite the lack of evidence for an interaction, the manufacturer of nilutamide recommends that the prothrombin time be carefully monitored in patients also taking vitamin K antagonists, and the coumarin or indanedione dose reduced if necessary.

Nitrates

Nitrates + Phosphodiesterase type-5 inhibitors

If avanafil, sildenafil, tadalafil, or vardenafil are given with organic nitrates (e.g. glyceryl trinitrate (nitroglycerin), isosorbide dinitrate, isosorbide mononitrate) potentially serious hypotension can occur, and myocardial infarction might be precipitated. A number of fatalities have occurred, possibly as a result of this interaction.

> The concurrent use of these phosphodiesterase type-5 inhibitors and all organic nitrates is contraindicated. Sildenafil should not be used within 24 hours of a nitrate, and some evidence suggests this is also a suitable separation for vardenafil. Nitrates should not be given for at least 48 hours after the last dose of tadalafil. The

US manufacturer of avanafil suggests that at least 12 hours should elapse after the last dose of avanafil before nitrates are given.

Nitrates + Riociguat

The concurrent use of riociguat with nitrates (e.g. isosorbide mononitrate, isosorbide dinitrate, and glyceryl trinitrate) can lead to hypotension.

Both the UK and US manufacturer contraindicates the concurrent use of riociguat and nitrates.

NNRTIs

The NNRTIs are extensively metabolised by cytochrome P450, particularly by CYP3A4. They are also inducers (nevirapine, efavirenz, and etravirine to a lesser degree) or inhibitors (delavirdine) of CYP3A4. The NNRTIs therefore have the potential to interact with drugs metabolised by CYP3A4, and may also be affected by CYP3A4 inhibitors and inducers. Delavirdine, efavirenz and etravirine may also inhibit some other cytochrome P450 isoenzymes and therefore the interaction profile varies between members of this drug group.

NNRTIs + Opioids

Alfentanil

Efavirenz decreases the exposure to oral and intravenous alfentanil.

Monitor concurrent use for reduced alfentanil effects: an increased alfentanil dose is likely to be needed.

Buprenorphine

Delavirdine moderately increases buprenorphine exposure, and efavirenz decreases buprenorphine exposure.

Monitor for buprenorphine adverse effects (such as drowsiness, respiratory depression) and consider adjusting the buprenorphine dose if necessary. One manufacturer states that the starting dose of sublingual buprenorphine (when used as a substitute for opioid dependence) should be halved; however, other manufacturers state that concurrent use should be avoided when buprenorphine is given parenterally or sublingually as a strong analgesic. One manufacturer states that no precaution is necessary in patients using transdermal buprenorphine. Be aware that buprenorphine might be less effective in patients also taking efavirenz.

Methadone

Methadone plasma concentrations can be greatly reduced by efavirenz or nevirapine, and methadone withdrawal symptoms have been seen.

If efavirenz or nevirapine are added to established treatment with methadone, be alert for evidence of opiate withdrawal, and raise the methadone dose accordingly. Some patients might require an increase in the methadone dose frequency to twice daily. In patients who subsequently discontinue the NNRTI, the methadone dose should be gradually reduced over 1 to 2 weeks.

NNRTIs + Orlistat

Orlistat might reduce the absorption of antiretroviral drugs, such as the NNRTIs, resulting in reduced efficacy.

> Monitoring of antiretroviral drug concentrations, if concurrent use is considered essential, would seem sensible. Further, the MHRA in the UK advises that orlistat should only be started after careful consideration of the possible impact it might have on the efficacy of antiretroviral medicines.

NNRTIs + Phenobarbital

Carbamazepine reduces the concentrations of delavirdine, efavirenz, and nevirapine, and is predicted to reduce the concentrations of etravirine and rilpivirine. This would be expected to lead to treatment failure. Phenobarbital and primidone would be expected to interact similarly, and this suggestion is supported by a study with delavirdine and phenobarbital, which found that delavirdine concentrations were greatly reduced by concurrent use.

> The UK and US manufacturers state that when efavirenz is given with phenobarbital, there is a potential for reduction or increase in the concentrations of each drug: they therefore recommend periodic therapeutic drug monitoring. Note that efavirenz can cause seizures and caution is recommended in patients with a history of convulsions. Although evidence for an interaction with nevirapine is lacking, it would seem prudent to follow the monitoring suggested for efavirenz. The UK and US manufacturers of delavirdine, etravirine, and rilpivirine advise against their concurrent use with phenobarbital.

NNRTIs + Phenytoin

Phenytoin reduces the concentrations of delavirdine and nevirapine, and is predicted to reduce the concentrations of efavirenz, etravirine, and rilpivirine. This suggestion is supported by cases of low or undetectable efavirenz concentrations in patients taking phenytoin. Treatment failure might result from these interactions. Fosphenytoin, a prodrug of phenytoin, might interact similarly.

> The UK and US manufacturers state that when efavirenz is given with phenytoin, there is a potential for a reduction or an increase in the concentrations of each drug: they therefore recommend periodic therapeutic drug monitoring of both drugs. Note that efavirenz can cause seizures and caution is recommended in patients with a history of convulsions. Although evidence for nevirapine is sparse it may be prudent to follow the same precautions given for efavirenz. The UK and US manufacturers of delavirdine, etravirine, and rilpivirine advise against the concurrent use of phenytoin.

NNRTIs + **Phosphodiesterase type-5 inhibitors**

Delavirdine

Delavirdine is predicted to increase sildenafil exposure. Vardenafil and tadalafil are likely to be similarly affected.

> Monitor the outcome of concurrent use, and decrease the dose of the phosphodiesterase type-5 inhibitor if adverse effects become troublesome. It would seem prudent to consider a lower starting dose of sildenafil, tadalafil, or vardenafil in patients taking delavirdine. The manufacturer of delavirdine recommends a maximum dose of sildenafil of 25 mg in 24 hours.

Other NNRTIs

Etravirine moderately reduces sildenafil exposure; nevirapine and efavirenz might interact similarly. Vardenafil and tadalafil are likely to be similarly affected.

> If these phosphodiesterase type-5 inhibitors are not effective in patients taking efavirenz, etravirine, or nevirapine, it would seem sensible to try a higher dose with close monitoring.

NNRTIs + **Prasugrel** ❓

Prasugrel may slightly inhibit the metabolism of *bupropion* by CYP2B6 and decrease the levels of its metabolite by 23%. The manufacturers suggest that the metabolism of other substrates of CYP2B6 with a narrow therapeutic margin, such as efavirenz, may also be affected.

> A clinically significant interaction would seem unlikely. Consider an interaction if efavirenz adverse effects (such as rash, dizziness and headache) are troublesome.

NNRTIs + **Propafenone** ⚠

The manufacturers predict that etravirine may decrease the levels of propafenone. However, note that propafenone is more usually affected by CYP2D6 inhibitors or inducers, effects that etravirine does not appear to have.

> The manufacturers recommend caution on concurrent use and state that propafenone levels should be monitored, if this is possible.

NNRTIs + **Proton pump inhibitors**

Delavirdine ⚠

Proton pump inhibitors are predicted to reduce delavirdine exposure.

> The long-term concurrent use of delavirdine and a proton pump inhibitor is not recommended.

Rilpivirine ✖

Omeprazole slightly reduces rilpivirine exposure. Other proton pump inhibitors might interact similarly.

> Concurrent use is contraindicated.

NNRTIs + Quinidine ⚠

The manufacturers predict that etravirine may decrease the levels of quinidine.

> The manufacturers recommend caution on concurrent use and state that quinidine levels should be monitored, if this is possible.

NNRTIs + Quinine ⚠

The exposure to quinine is decreased, and the plasma concentration of 3-hydroxyquinine, the major metabolite of quinine, is increased, by nevirapine.

> The clinical importance of this interaction is unclear, but it could lead to reduced quinine efficacy and possibly increased toxicity due to raised 3-hydroxyquinine concentrations. Monitor for an increase in quinine adverse effects (such as tinnitus, headache, vomiting, vertigo, or cardiac disorders) and efficacy, increasing the dose of quinine, if appropriate.

NNRTIs + Raltegravir ❓

Efavirenz slightly reduces raltegravir exposure, and nevirapine is predicted to interact similarly. Altered raltegravir plasma concentrations have been reported in patients taking etravirine.

> Consider monitoring virological efficacy more closely on the concurrent use of raltegravir and these NNRTIs.

NNRTIs + Rifabutin

Delavirdine ❌

Rifabutin causes a large reduction in delavirdine plasma concentrations. Rifabutin exposure was increased when the delavirdine dose was increased to compensate for this.

> The US manufacturer of delavirdine, and the Center for Disease Control (CDC) in the US, recommend that rifabutin should not be used with delavirdine.

Efavirenz ⚠

Rifabutin does not affect efavirenz pharmacokinetics, but efavirenz can decrease rifabutin concentrations: a case of treatment failure has been reported.

> US guidelines state that the combination is probably clinically useful, and they suggest increasing the dose of rifabutin to 450 mg or 600 mg (taken daily or intermittently). The British HIV Association (BHIVA) also recommend increasing the rifabutin dose to 450 mg daily in patients taking efavirenz. Monitor the outcome of concurrent use carefully.

Etravirine or Nevirapine ⚠

Only slight increases in nevirapine exposure seem to occur with rifabutin; however, some patients may be more susceptible to adverse effects due to raised rifabutin concentrations. Rifabutin slightly reduces etravirine exposure, but etravirine has little effect on rifabutin concentrations.

With both etravirine and nevirapine caution is recommended if rifabutin is also given due to the possibility of increased rifabutin exposure and the possibility of decreased etravirine efficacy.

Rilpivirine

Rilpivirine has little effect on rifabutin concentrations, and rifabutin halves rilpivirine exposure.

The UK manufacturer and the BHIVA guidelines recommend doubling the rilpivirine dose, whereas the US manufacturer contraindicates concurrent use. If concurrent use is essential, it should be well-monitored, bearing in mind that the dose of rilpivirine is likely to need increasing.

NNRTIs + Rifampicin (Rifampin)

Efavirenz and Nevirapine

Neither efavirenz nor nevirapine affect rifampicin concentrations, but rifampicin modestly reduces the concentrations of these NNRTIs.

There is a general lack of consensus regarding an appropriate dose of efavirenz to use in patients taking rifampicin. US guidelines suggest using the standard efavirenz dose while monitoring for virologic response, although they note that some clinicians suggest increasing the efavirenz dose to 800 mg daily in patients weighing more than 60 kg. Others suggest this dose increase regardless of weight. Until more is known, monitor for virological efficacy and efavirenz adverse effects, with therapeutic drug monitoring as necessary, adjusting the efavirenz dose accordingly. The UK manufacturers, US manufacturers and US guidelines suggest that the concurrent use of rifampicin with nevirapine is not recommended In the UK, the BHIVA guidelines state that if there are no alternatives to using nevirapine with rifampicin, then standard doses should be used with monitoring of nevirapine concentrations.

Other NNRTIs

Rifampicin greatly reduces delavirdine and rilpivirine plasma concentrations, and is predicted to reduce etravirine concentrations.

The concurrent use of these NNRTIs and rifampicin is generally considered to be contraindicated.

NNRTIs + Sirolimus

The UK manufacturer of etravirine predicts that it will induce the metabolism of sirolimus (by CYP3A4) and thus reduce sirolimus concentrations. However, note that etravirine is only a weak inducer of this isoenzyme.

The UK manufacturer of etravirine advises caution on concurrent use. Sirolimus concentrations and/or effects (e.g. on renal function) should usually be monitored as a matter of routine, but until more is known, it might be prudent to increase monitoring if etravirine is started or stopped, and adjust the dose if necessary.

NNRTIs + SSRIs

A case of serotonin syndrome, page 580, occurred in a woman taking fluoxetine when efavirenz was added; this resolved when the dose of fluoxetine was halved. Efavirenz decreases sertraline levels, and nevirapine decreases fluoxetine levels, whereas fluvoxamine modestly increases nevirapine levels.

> Monitor for fluoxetine efficacy if nevirapine is given, and sertraline efficacy if efavirenz is given: adjust the SSRI dose as required. Monitor for signs of nevirapine adverse effects in patients also taking fluvoxamine. Bear the case of serotonin syndrome in mind if efavirenz and fluoxetine are both given.

NNRTIs + Statins

Delavirdine

Delavirdine is expected to increase the exposure to atorvastatin, fluvastatin, simvastatin, and lovastatin. This expectation is supported by a case of rhabdomyolysis, which developed in a patient taking atorvastatin and delavirdine.

> The US manufacturer of delavirdine advises against the concurrent use of either simvastatin or lovastatin. Caution is advised with concurrent use of atorvastatin or fluvastatin, and the lowest possible statin dose should be used. Patients should be made aware of the risks of myopathy and rhabdomyolysis, and advised to report promptly muscle pain, tenderness, or weakness, especially if accompanied by malaise, fever, or dark urine.

Efavirenz, Etravirine or Nevirapine

Efavirenz (and possibly nevirapine) slightly to moderately reduces the exposure to atorvastatin, simvastatin, and pravastatin. Etravirine slightly reduces the exposure to atorvastatin and its active metabolites, and is predicted to have a similar effect on lovastatin and simvastatin. Etravirine is also predicted to *increase* fluvastatin concentrations.

> It would seem prudent to monitor the lipid profile of patients taking efavirenz, nevirapine, or etravirine and any of these statins, adjusting the dose as necessary, although bear in mind that if the NNRTI is part of a regimen containing HIV-protease inhibitors, page 436, these dramatically *increase* the concentrations of some statins.

NNRTIs + Tacrolimus

Limited evidence suggests that efavirenz may increase the clearance of tacrolimus resulting in reduced levels. Nevirapine and etravirine may interact similarly. Delavirdine is predicted to increase the levels of tacrolimus.

> Tacrolimus levels should be monitored as a matter of routine but it would seem prudent to increase monitoring if any of these NNRTIs is started, adjusting the tacrolimus dose as necessary.

NNRTIs + Ulipristal

The UK and US manufacturers of ulipristal predict that CYP3A4 inducers, such as efavirenz and nevirapine, might reduce the plasma concentration of ulipristal and reduce its efficacy.

> The US manufacturer of ulipristal gives no specific advice about how to manage this potential interaction, whereas the UK manufacturer advises that ulipristal should not be used for emergency contraception in women taking CYP3A4 inducers (such as efavirenz and nevirapine), or who have stopped taking an enzyme inducer within the last 2 to 3 weeks. Until more is known, this advice seems prudent.

NNRTIs + Warfarin and related oral anticoagulants

Three cases suggest that warfarin requirements are approximately doubled by nevirapine. One case of an unusually low warfarin dose requirement has been reported in a patient taking an efavirenz-based regimen. Etravirine appears to increase the exposure to warfarin; delavirdine is predicted to interact similarly.

> Monitor the effect of concurrent use of these NNRTIs on the anticoagulant response and adjust the coumarin dose as necessary.

NRTIs

The NRTIs are prodrugs, which need to be activated by phosphorylation within cells. Drugs may therefore interact with NRTIs by increasing or decreasing intracellular activation. NRTIs are water soluble, and are mainly eliminated by the kidneys (didanosine, lamivudine, and stavudine) or undergo hepatic glucuronidation (abacavir, zidovudine). The few important interactions with these drugs primarily involve altered renal clearance. For zidovudine (and possibly abacavir) some interactions occur via altered glucuronidation, but the clinical relevance of these are less clear. Cytochrome P450-mediated interactions are not important for this class of drugs. Didanosine chewable tablets are formulated with antacid buffers that are intended to facilitate didanosine absorption by minimising acid-induced hydrolysis in the stomach. These preparations can therefore alter the absorption of other drugs that are affected by antacids (e.g. azoles, quinolones, tetracyclines). This interaction may be minimised by separating administration by at least 2 hours. Alternatively, the enteric-coated preparation of didanosine (gastro-resistant capsules) may be used.

NRTIs + NSAIDs

Cidofovir or Tenofovir

NSAIDs might precipitate renal failure in patients taking cidofovir or tenofovir, particularly these with pre-existing risk factors or mild renal impairment.

> Avoid concurrent use. If this is not possible, the manufacturers advise weekly

monitoring of renal function. Potentially nephrotoxic drugs should be stopped at least 7 days before starting cidofovir.

Zidovudine

NSAIDs are said to increased the risk of haematological toxicity with zidovudine, and that there is evidence of an increased risk of haemarthroses and haematoma in HIV-positive patients with haemophilia taking zidovudine and ibuprofen.

Be aware that concurrent use increases the risk of bleeding. It is unclear if this is restricted to this particular patient group.

NRTIs + Opioids ⚠

Case reports describe patients who needed methadone dose increases after starting zidovudine or abacavir. Didanosine, stavudine, tenofovir, and a single dose of zidovudine with lamivudine do not appear to affect methadone pharmacokinetics. Methadone can increase zidovudine concentrations, and reduce the concentrations of abacavir, stavudine; and didanosine from the tablet formulation.

The clinical relevance of the changes in methadone concentrations is unclear, but be alert for any increase in zidovudine adverse effects. The reduction in didanosine concentrations with methadone might be clinically relevant, and it would seem prudent to monitor virological response, adjusting the dose of the tablet formulation, or swapping to the enteric-coated preparation (which is not affected), if needed. The reduction in abacavir and stavudine concentrations with methadone is probably not clinically relevant, but this needs confirmation.

NRTIs + Orlistat ⚠

Orlistat might reduce the absorption of antiretroviral drugs, such as the NRTIs, resulting in reduced efficacy.

Monitoring of antiretroviral drug concentrations, if concurrent use is considered essential, would seem sensible. Further, the MHRA in the UK advises that orlistat should only be started after careful consideration of the possible impact it might have on the efficacy of antiretroviral medicines.

NRTIs + Pentamidine ⚠

Additive pancreatic toxicity is predicted to occur with the concurrent use of intravenous pentamidine and didanosine or stavudine, and possibly lamivudine. Didanosine, stavudine, and lamivudine alone have all been associated with pancreatitis, which has been fatal in some cases. The concurrent use of zidovudine and systemic pentamidine can theoretically lead to additive haematological toxicity. Limited data suggest that no additive haematological toxicity occurs with nebulised pentamidine. The concurrent use of tenofovir and pentamidine might have additive adverse effects on renal function.

The manufacturers of didanosine advise that if pentamidine is needed, didanosine should be stopped, although if concurrent use is unavoidable, patients should be closely monitored. Similar precautions are advised with lamivudine. Careful monitoring is also recommended if pentamidine is given with stavudine. Monitor full blood count in patients given systemic pentamidine with zidovudine. If pentamidine is given with tenofovir, increase the frequency of renal function monitoring (the manufacturers of tenofovir advise at least weekly).

NRTIs + Phenobarbital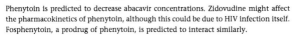

The UK manufacturer of abacavir predicts that phenobarbital (and therefore probably primidone) might slightly decrease abacavir concentrations.

The clinical significance of this prediction is unclear but it may be prudent to monitor to ensure abacavir is effective.

NRTIs + Phenytoin

Phenytoin is predicted to decrease abacavir concentrations. Zidovudine might affect the pharmacokinetics of phenytoin, although this could be due to HIV infection itself. Fosphenytoin, a prodrug of phenytoin, is predicted to interact similarly.

The clinical significance of these interactions is unclear. However, it would be prudent to monitor the concurrent use of these NRTIs with phenytoin, and adjust the NRTI or phenytoin dose as necessary.

NRTIs + Probenecid

Probenecid reduces the clearance of zidovudine, increasing its exposure. The incidence of adverse effects is reported to be very much increased by concurrent use.

Concurrent use need not be avoided, but monitor carefully for zidovudine toxicity. The effects of this interaction might be minimised by separating administration by 6 hours, but this needs confirmation.

NRTIs + Rifabutin

Studies suggest that rifabutin might slightly increase the clearance of zidovudine, whereas other studies have found no interaction.

The clinical implications of this interaction are unknown. Be alert for any evidence of a reduced response to zidovudine if rifabutin is given.

NRTIs + Rifampicin (Rifampin)

Several studies suggest that rifampicin more than doubles the clearance of zidovudine. In some subjects increased haematological toxicity was also seen. Rifampicin is predicted to interact similarly with abacavir.

Be alert for any evidence of a reduced response to these antivirals and monitor for haematological toxicity with zidovudine.

N

NRTIs + Tacrolimus

Tacrolimus-induced renal impairment might increase entecavir exposure.

Monitor renal function closely on concurrent use.

NRTIs + Valproate

Valproate increases zidovudine exposure. Cases of severe anaemia, liver toxicity, and respiratory failure have been attributed to this interaction.

It would seem prudent to monitor for zidovudine adverse effects and possible toxicity.

NSAIDs

NSAIDs + NSAIDs

The combined use of two or more NSAIDs increases the risk of gastrointestinal damage.

As there is no clear clinical rationale for the combined use of different NSAIDs, such use should be avoided.

NSAIDs + Opioids

NSAIDs, general ✅

On the whole the concurrent use of NSAIDs and opioids is successful and without incident; however, see the specific instances discussed below.

No action needed.

Diclofenac ❓

An isolated report describes grand mal seizures in a patient given diclofenac and pentazocine. Diclofenac did not alter morphine pharmacokinetics in one study. However, in another, diclofenac slightly increased respiratory depression despite a reduction in morphine use, possibly because of persistent levels of an active metabolite of morphine.

These interactions are not established and they seem unlikely to be of general significance, but be alert to the possibility of increased sedation, or, with pentazocine, use with caution in patients who are known to be seizure-prone.

Ketorolac ❓

A single case report describes marked respiratory depression in a man taking buprenorphine with ketorolac.

This seems unlikely to be of general significance but be alert to the possibility of increased sedation.

NSAIDs + Paracetamol (Acetaminophen)

On the whole the concurrent use of NSAIDs with paracetamol is beneficial and without serious adverse effects. One epidemiological study found that paracetamol alone, and particularly when given with an NSAID, was associated with an increased risk of gastrointestinal bleeding, but other studies have not found such an effect. Diflunisal raises paracetamol levels by 50% but does not alter its total bioavailability.

> The interaction with diflunisal has not been shown to be clinically significant but the manufacturers advise caution because of the risks of increased paracetamol levels. Paracetamol is not usually considered to increase the risk of upper gastrointestinal adverse effects and there is insufficient evidence to suggest that the concurrent use of paracetamol and any NSAID should be avoided.

NSAIDs + Penicillamine

Indometacin has been found to increase the peak levels of penicillamine by about 22%. The manufacturers warn that the concurrent use of NSAIDs and penicillamine may increase the risk of nephrotoxicity.

> The US manufacturer specifically recommends avoiding oxyphenbutazone or phenylbutazone because these drugs are also associated with serious haematological and renal effects. There seems to be no reason to avoid other NSAIDs and penicillamine, but if problems occur bear the possibility of a drug interaction in mind.

NSAIDs + Pentoxifylline

A review of bleeding events associated with the use of postoperative ketorolac revealed that a small number of patients were also taking pentoxifylline.

> The UK manufacturer of ketorolac, rather cautiously, contraindicates concurrent use, whereas the US manufacturer makes no mention of an interaction. There seems to be no evidence regarding this interaction with other NSAIDs; however, as both pentoxifylline and the non-selective NSAIDs may cause bleeding it would be prudent to be alert for this possible interaction.

NSAIDs + Phenytoin

Phenytoin concentrations can be increased by azapropazone, and toxicity can develop rapidly. A similar interaction has been seen with phenylbutazone, and it seems likely that oxyphenbutazone will interact similarly. Fosphenytoin, a prodrug of phenytoin, might interact similarly with these NSAIDs.

> Warn the patient to monitor for indicators of phenytoin toxicity (blurred vision, nystagmus, ataxia, or drowsiness), and reduce the phenytoin dose as necessary. Some manufacturers contraindicate concurrent use.

NSAIDs + Prasugrel

NSAIDs alone increase the risk of bleeding. The concurrent use of an antiplatelet drug (such as prasugrel) would be expected to further increase this risk.

> If concurrent use is necessary, patients should be monitored for signs of excessive

bleeding and advised to report any unusual bleeding. Consider giving additional gastrointestinal prophylaxis (e.g. an H_2-receptor antagonists or a proton pump inhibitor) in patients at risk of gastrointestinal ulceration and bleeding. Note that the need for any NSAID should be very carefully considered as NSAIDs (particularly coxibs and diclofenac, but also other non-selective NSAIDs) are associated with an increased thrombotic/cardiovascular risk, particularly when used at high doses and for long-term treatment. Therefore coxibs and diclofenac are contra-indicated, and other NSAIDs should generally be avoided, in those with ischaemic heart disease, cerebrovascular disease, or peripheral artery disease. Diclofenac is also contraindicated in those with congestive heart failure.

NSAIDs + Probenecid

Probenecid reduces the clearance of dexketoprofen, diflunisal, ketoprofen, ketorolac, indometacin, meclofenamate, naproxen, tenoxicam and tiaprofenic acid, and raises their levels. Increased clinical effects have been seen for indometacin, but indometacin toxicity has also occurred.

Increased levels do occur, which could reasonably be expected to result in increased beneficial and adverse effects. However, the clinical outcome of this interaction is uncertain and so action (e.g. dose adjustments) should be based on the response of the patient. Reduce the NSAID dose if necessary. Note that probenecid is specifically contraindicated by the manufacturers of ketorolac.

NSAIDs + Propafenone

Because valdecoxib (the metabolite of parecoxib) increases *dextromethorphan* levels about 3-fold and celecoxib increases *dextromethorphan* levels about 2.4-fold, the manufacturers predict that the levels of flecainide (which is similarly metabolised) will also be raised by these coxibs.

The general importance of this interaction is unclear. Monitor concurrent use for adverse effects, and consider reducing the dose of the antiarrhythmic if these become troublesome.

NSAIDs + Quinolones

Convulsions have been seen in patients given fenbufen with enoxacin, and several NSAIDs with ofloxacin or ciprofloxacin. The CSM in the UK warns that this interaction could occur with any combination of an NSAID and a quinolone.

Convulsions are rare, so in the majority of patients concurrent use should be without problem. Patients with epilepsy, or those predisposed to convulsions, seem to be at greater risk, so avoid concurrent use in these patients or monitor very closely.

NSAIDs + Rifampicin (Rifampin)

The levels of celecoxib, diclofenac, and etoricoxib are reduced by rifampicin.

The clinical relevance of these interactions is unclear, but it seems likely that the efficacy of these NSAIDs will be reduced by rifampicin. Concurrent use should be well monitored, and the NSAID dose increased if necessary.

NSAIDs + Rivaroxaban ❓

Naproxen does not affect the pharmacokinetics of rivaroxaban, or cause a clinically relevant change in the anticoagulant effects of rivaroxaban. However, the bleeding time during concurrent use might be slightly prolonged. Note that all NSAIDs increase the risk of bleeding, and concurrent use with rivaroxaban might possibly increase this risk.

Advise patients to be aware of increased bruising or prolonged bleeding, and to seek medical advice if this occurs.

NSAIDs + SSRIs ❓

SSRIs might increase the risk of gastrointestinal bleeding (especially upper gastrointestinal bleeding), and the risk appears to be further increased by the concurrent use of NSAIDs.

In general, the concurrent use of NSAIDs should be undertaken with caution. Alternatives such as paracetamol (acetaminophen) or less gastrotoxic NSAIDs such as ibuprofen should be considered, but if the combination of an SSRI and NSAID cannot be avoided, prescribing of gastroprotective drugs such as proton pump inhibitors, or H_2-receptor antagonists should be considered, especially in elderly patients or those with a history of gastrointestinal bleeding.

NSAIDs + Tacrolimus ⚠️

The UK manufacturers of tacrolimus suggest that all NSAIDs may have additive nephrotoxic effects with tacrolimus. Cases of renal failure have been reported in patients receiving the combination. However, a study in rheumatoid arthritis patients found no increased risk.

Tacrolimus levels and/or effects (e.g. on renal function) should be monitored as a matter of routine, but it may be prudent to increase monitoring if NSAIDs are started.

NSAIDs + Ticagrelor ❓

The manufacturer of ticagrelor states that the concurrent use of NSAIDs within 24 hours of taking ticagrelor might theoretically increase the risk of bleeding.

Advise patients to report signs of excessive bleeding. Consider gastroprotection if other risk factors for gastrointestinal bleeding are present. Note that giving NSAIDs to patients with ischaemic heart disease might increase the risk of thrombotic events.

NSAIDs + Ticlopidine ❓

NSAIDs alone increase the risk of bleeding. The concurrent use of an antiplatelet drug (such as ticlopidine) would be expected to further increase this risk.

If concurrent use is necessary, patients should be monitored for signs of excessive bleeding and advised to report any unusual bleeding. Consider giving additional gastrointestinal prophylaxis such as a proton pump inhibitor in patients at risk of gastrointestinal ulceration and bleeding. Note that the need for any NSAID should be very carefully considered as some NSAIDs (particularly coxibs and diclofenac, but also other non-selective NSAIDs) are associated with an increased thrombotic/cardiovascular risk, particularly when used at high doses and for long-term treatment. Therefore coxibs and diclofenac are contraindicated, and other NSAIDs should generally be avoided, in those with ischaemic heart disease, cerebrovascular disease, and peripheral artery disease. Diclofenac is also contraindicated in those with congestive heart failure.

NSAIDs + Tricyclics ⚠

The manufacturers of celecoxib (a CYP2D6 inhibitor) predict that it will raise the levels of the tricyclics (CYP2D6 substrates). The levels of other CYP2D6 substrates have been more than doubled by celecoxib.

Monitor concurrent use for tricyclic adverse effects (such as nausea, dry mouth, palpitations), and consider reducing the dose if these become troublesome.

NSAIDs + Vancomycin ⚠

Indometacin reduces the renal clearance of vancomycin in premature neonates. This interaction appears not to have been studied in adults.

The effect in adults is unclear, but in neonates be prepared to reduce the dose of vancomycin in the presence of indometacin.

NSAIDs + Warfarin and related oral anticoagulants

Azapropazone, Ketorolac, Oxyphenbutazone, Phenylbutazone ✗

The anticoagulant effects of warfarin are markedly increased by azapropazone, ketorolac, oxyphenbutazone and phenylbutazone. Bleeding has been reported in patients taking phenindione or phenprocoumon when given phenylbutazone.

Concurrent use is contraindicated.

Coxibs ❓

There is some evidence to suggest that celecoxib and parecoxib do not normally interact with warfarin. However, raised INRs accompanied by bleeding, particularly in the elderly, have been attributed to the use of warfarin and celecoxib. Etoricoxib causes a small increase in INR when it is taken with warfarin.

Monitor the anticoagulant effect if these NSAIDs are added to or withdrawn from the treatment of patients taking anticoagulants.

Other NSAIDs ❓

Case reports suggest that most NSAIDs can occasionally enhance the effects of warfarin and other coumarins (acenocoumarol, phenprocoumon), resulting in increased anticoagulant effects and sometimes severe bleeding events.

Monitor the anticoagulant effect if NSAIDs are added to or withdrawn from the treatment of patients taking anticoagulants. Note that since NSAIDs reduce platelet aggregation and cause gastrointestinal irritation they can prolong and worsen any bleeding events.

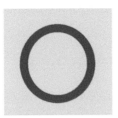

Opioids

Opioids with mixed agonist/antagonist properties (e.g. buprenorphine, butorphanol, nalbuphine, pentazocine) may precipitate opioid withdrawal symptoms in patients taking pure opioid agonists such as fentanyl, methadone, morphine and tramadol.

Opioids + Phenobarbital

Opioids, general 🚫

The concurrent use of opioids (including weak opioids such as codeine) and barbiturates appears to increase sedation and respiratory depression.

> Concurrent use need not be avoided, but be aware of the potential for respiratory depression, especially in patients with a restricted respiratory capacity. Note that tramadol should be avoided if possible as it might increase the risk of seizures. Counsel patients against driving or undertaking other skilled tasks if sedation occurs.

Buprenorphine, Fentanyl, Methadone, or Pethidine (Meperidine) ⚠

Phenobarbital and primidone appear to increase fentanyl and methadone requirements, and methadone withdrawal reactions have been seen. The analgesic effects of pethidine can be reduced by barbiturates, but in one study, increased sedation was seen with phenobarbital. The manufacturers predict that phenobarbital and primidone will reduce buprenorphine concentrations.

> Anticipate the need to increase the dose of these opioids in patients taking phenobarbital or primidone. Monitor concurrent use to ensure the opioid effects are adequate. It might be necessary to give the methadone twice daily, remembering to reduce the methadone dose if phenobarbital is stopped.

Tapentadol 🚫

The UK manufacturer of tapentadol states that caution is necessary if a strong enzyme inducer, such as phenobarbital or primidone, is started or stopped in a patient taking tapentadol, as this might lead to decreased efficacy or an increased risk of adverse

0

effects; however, the mechanism of this proposed interaction is unclear, and further study is required.

Until more is known, be aware that the dose of tapentadol might need to be adjusted in patients taking phenobarbital.

Opioids + Phenytoin ⚠

Phenytoin appears to increase fentanyl and methadone requirements and methadone withdrawal reactions have been seen. The manufacturers of buprenorphine predict that phenytoin will decrease its concentrations. Phenytoin increases the production of the toxic metabolite of pethidine (meperidine), which resulted in pethidine toxicity in one case. Fosphenytoin, a prodrug of phenytoin, might interact similarly with these opioids.

Anticipate the need to increase the dose of these opioids in patients taking phenytoin, and monitor concurrent use to ensure the opioid effects are adequate. It might be necessary to give the methadone twice daily. Remember to reduce the opioid dose if phenytoin is stopped.

Opioids + Pregabalin ❓

The manufacturer of pregabalin notes that there was no clinically relevant pharmacokinetic interaction between pregabalin and oxycodone, and that there was no clinically important effect on respiration. However, pregabalin appeared to cause an additive impairment in cognitive and gross motor function when given with oxycodone. It seems possible that all opioids may have this effect.

The degree of impairment will depend on the individual patient. However, warn all patients of the potential effects, and counsel against driving or undertaking other skilled tasks.

Opioids + Quinidine ⚠

The analgesic effects of codeine, and probably also hydrocodone, appear to be reduced or abolished by quinidine. Quinidine appears to increase the oral absorption and effects of fentanyl, methadone, and morphine, and might slightly increase the exposure to tramadol. Cardiac conduction might be affected with high-dose methadone is given with quinidine.

Monitor for analgesic efficacy and consider using an alternative to codeine or hydrocodone in the case of reduced efficacy. Monitor for increased opioid effects after the oral administration of fentanyl, methadone, and morphine. Bear the possibility of an interaction in mind should a patient taking both drugs develop an increase in tramadol adverse effects. Note that quinidine and high-dose methadone might prolong the QT interval, see drugs that prolong the QT interval, page 352.

Opioids + Quinolones ❓

It has been suggested that opioids decrease oral ciprofloxacin concentrations, but good evidence for this appears to be lacking.

Based on this rather slim evidence, some have suggested that the concurrent use of opioids and ciprofloxacin as pre-medication should be avoided. Note that both high-dose methadone and some quinolones might prolong the QT interval, see drugs that prolong the QT interval, page 352 for further information.

Opioids + Rifampicin (Rifampin)

Rifampicin (rifampin) appears to cause large reductions in the plasma concentrations of methadone and withdrawal symptoms have occurred in some patients. Similarly, rifampicin increases the metabolism of alfentanil, codeine, fentanyl, morphine and oral oxycodone, and reduces their effects. Rifampicin is predicted to induce the metabolism of tapentadol; however the mechanism of this interaction is unclear.

Monitor concurrent use for reduced opioid effects and adjust the dose accordingly.

Opioids + Sodium oxybate

Opioids are expected to have additive CNS depressant effects with sodium oxybate.

Concurrent use is contraindicated by the UK manufacturer of sodium oxybate. If both drugs are given be alert for CNS depression. Warn all patients of the potential effects, and counsel against driving or undertaking other skilled tasks.

Opioids + SSRIs

Tramadol

Several case reports describe the development of serotonin syndrome, page 580, in patients taking citalopram, fluoxetine, paroxetine, or sertraline with tramadol. Another patient developed hallucinations when taking tramadol with paroxetine. Tramadol analgesia might possibly be altered by paroxetine and potentially by fluoxetine

There would seem to be little reason for totally avoiding the concurrent use of the SSRIs and tramadol but it would clearly be prudent to use the combination cautiously and monitor the outcome closely. Bear the potential for an interaction in mind should a patient taking paroxetine or fluoxetine have a reduced response to tramadol, and adjust the dose of tramadol as necessary. Tramadol should be used with caution with SSRIs because of the possible increased risk of seizures.

Other opioids

In isolated cases the concurrent use of SSRIs and opioids (including fentanyl, hydromorphone, oxycodone, pentazocine, pethidine (meperidine), and possibly morphine) has resulted in the serotonin syndrome. Methadone plasma concentrations might be increased by fluvoxamine. Sertraline, paroxetine, and possibly fluoxetine, might also modestly increase methadone concentrations. The analgesic effects of codeine, and probably also hydrocodone, are predicted to be reduced or abolished by fluoxetine and paroxetine.

Serotonin syndrome, page 580, seems to be a rare occurrence, but the possibility should be borne in mind if an SSRI is given with one of these opioids. Be aware that the use of fluvoxamine, paroxetine, sertraline, or fluoxetine might alter the response to methadone. Monitor the outcome of concurrent use for methadone adverse effects. Monitor for analgesic efficacy and consider using an alternative to

0

codeine or hydrocodone in the case of reduced efficacy. Note that some SSRIs and methadone can prolong the QT interval, see Drugs that prolong the QT interval, page 352 for further information.

Opioids + Terbinafine ⚠

The analgesic effects of codeine, and probably also hydrocodone, are predicted to be reduced or abolished by terbinafine.

Monitor for analgesic efficacy and consider using an alternative to codeine or hydrocodone in the case of reduced efficacy.

Opioids + Tricyclics

Opioids, general ❓

In general, the concurrent use of most opioids and tricyclics is uneventful, although lethargy, sedation, and respiratory depression have been reported. In addition, the incidence of myoclonus (muscle twitching or spasm) in patients on high doses of morphine appeared to be increased by tricyclic antidepressants in one study.

Serious adverse interactions seem rare and concurrent use may be beneficial in pain management. Be alert for any evidence of increased CNS depression and warn patients that sedation can occur. Respiratory depression is more likely to be of significance in those who already have respiratory impairment. Note that some tricyclics and high-dose methadone may prolong the QT interval, see drugs that prolong the QT interval, page 352.

Tapentadol ⚠

The US manufacturer of tapentadol warns of an increased risk of serotonin syndrome, page 580 when tapentadol is given with a tricyclic antidepressant.

Be aware of the possibility that in rare cases patients may develop serotonin syndrome when taking tapentadol with a tricyclic.

Tramadol ⚠

The CSM in the UK recommends caution if tramadol is used with a tricyclic antidepressant as both drugs may reduce the seizure threshold. There have been reports of seizures on concurrent use. In addition, concurrent use may lead to the development of serotonin syndrome, page 580.

Consider an alternative analgesic or antidepressant if possible, or use with caution, particularly in epileptic patients or those taking other drugs that affect serotonin.

Opioids + Triptans ⚠

Sumatriptan given by injection does not appear to interact with butorphanol nasal spray, but if both drugs are given by nasal spray a slight reduction in butorphanol absorption may occur.

When butorphanol was given 30 minutes after sumatriptan no significant pharmacokinetic interaction was noted. It would therefore seem prudent to separate administration to ensure the full effects of butorphanol are achieved.

Opioids + **Warfarin and related oral anticoagulants**

Tramadol has been reported to increase the anticoagulant effects of acenocoumarol, fluindione, warfarin and phenprocoumon in a few patients and a retrospective cohort study also found an increased risk of bleeding when acenocoumarol or phenprocoumon was given with tramadol. Several patients taking warfarin have shown a marked increase in prothrombin times and/or bleeding when given co-proxamol (which contains dextropropoxyphene (propoxyphene)), but the interaction seems to be uncommon.

It would be prudent to consider monitoring prothrombin times in any patient taking anticoagulants when tramadol is first added, being alert for the need to reduce the anticoagulant dose. An interaction with dextropropoxyphene seems rare, but bear it in mind in case of an excessive response to anticoagulant treatment.

Orlistat

Orlistat + **Oxcarbazepine**

The MHRA in the UK suggests that the absorption of antiepileptics might be decreased by orlistat, leading to a loss of seizure control.

Although an interaction has not been established, the MHRA advises that patients should be monitored for changes in the severity or frequency of convulsions, and consideration given to separating the administration of orlistat and the antiepileptic.

Orlistat + **Perampanel**

The MHRA in the UK suggests that the absorption of antiepileptics might be decreased by orlistat, leading to a loss of seizure control.

Although an interaction has not been established, the MHRA advises that patients should be monitored for changes in the severity or frequency of convulsions, and consideration given to separating the administration of orlistat and the antiepileptic.

Orlistat + **Phenobarbital**

The MHRA in the UK suggests that absorption of antiepileptics, such as phenobarbital, might be decreased by orlistat, leading to a loss of seizure control. Primidone, a prodrug of phenobarbital, is predicted to interact similarly.

Although an interaction has not been established, the MHRA advises that patients should be monitored for changes in the severity or frequency of convulsions, and consideration given to separating the administration of orlistat and the antiepileptic.

Orlistat + Phenytoin ⚠

Orlistat does not appear to alter the pharmacokinetics of phenytoin. However, the MHRA in the UK suggests that the absorption of antiepileptics might be decreased by orlistat, leading to a loss of seizure control. Fosphenytoin, a prodrug of phenytoin, is predicted to interact similarly.

Although an interaction has not been established, the MHRA advises that patients should be monitored for changes in the severity or frequency of convulsions, and consideration given to separating the administration of orlistat and the antiepileptic.

Orlistat + Pregabalin ⚠

The MHRA in the UK suggests that the absorption of antiepileptics might be decreased by orlistat, leading to a loss of seizure control.

Although an interaction has not been established, the MHRA advises that patients should be monitored for changes in the severity or frequency of convulsions, and consideration given to separating the administration of orlistat and the antiepileptic.

Orlistat + Raltegravir ⚠

Orlistat might reduce the absorption of antiretroviral drugs, such as raltegravir, resulting in reduced efficacy.

Monitoring of antiretroviral drug concentrations, if concurrent use is considered essential, would seem sensible. Further, the MHRA in the UK advises that orlistat should only be started after careful consideration of the possible impact it might have on the efficacy of antiretroviral medicines.

Orlistat + Retigabine (Ezogabine) ⚠

The MHRA in the UK suggests that the absorption of antiepileptics might be decreased by orlistat, leading to a loss of seizure control.

Although an interaction has not been established, the MHRA advises that patients should be monitored for changes in the severity or frequency of convulsions, and consideration given to separating the administration of orlistat and the antiepileptic.

Orlistat + Tiagabine ⚠

The MHRA in the UK suggests that the absorption of antiepileptics might be decreased by orlistat, leading to a loss of seizure control.

Although an interaction has not been established, the MHRA advises that patients should be monitored for changes in the severity or frequency of convulsions, and consideration given to separating the administration of orlistat and the antiepileptic.

Orlistat + Topiramate

The MHRA in the UK suggests that the absorption of antiepileptics might be decreased by orlistat, leading to a loss of seizure control.

Although an interaction has not been established, the MHRA advises that patients should be monitored for changes in the severity or frequency of convulsions, and consideration given to separating the administration of orlistat and the antiepileptic.

Orlistat + Valproate

The manufacturers report that convulsions have been noted in patients taking valproate with orlistat. The MHRA in the UK suggests that the absorption of antiepileptics might be decreased by orlistat, leading to a loss of seizure control.

Although an interaction has not been established, the MHRA advises that patients should be monitored for changes in the severity or frequency of convulsions, and consideration given to separating the administration of orlistat and the antiepileptic.

Orlistat + Vigabatrin

The MHRA in the UK suggests that the absorption of antiepileptics might be decreased by orlistat, leading to a loss of seizure control.

Although an interaction has not been established, the MHRA advises that patients should be monitored for changes in the severity or frequency of convulsions, and consideration given to separating the administration of orlistat and the antiepileptic.

Orlistat + Vitamins

Orlistat decreases the absorption of supplemental betacarotene and vitamin E. There is some evidence to suggest that some patients may have low vitamin D levels while taking orlistat, even if they are also taking multivitamins.

It is recommended that multivitamin preparations should be taken at least 2 hours after orlistat, such as at bedtime. The US manufacturers suggest that patients taking orlistat should be advised to take multivitamins, because of the possibility of reduced vitamin levels. Note that it has been suggested that monitoring of vitamin D may be required, even if multivitamins are given.

Orlistat + Warfarin and related oral anticoagulants

Orlistat does not appear to affect the pharmacokinetics of warfarin, however it reduces fat absorption, and might therefore reduce vitamin K absorption and affect coagulation. Several cases of increased INR have been reported in patients taking either warfarin or acenocoumarol after also taking orlistat.

> Close monitoring for changes in coagulation parameters is recommended in patients taking orlistat with a coumarin or indanedione. As changes in diet are known to affect anticoagulant effects this seems prudent.

Oxcarbazepine

Oxcarbazepine is a derivative of carbamazepine and is an inducer of CYP3A4, with effects similar to carbamazepine in some cases. Oxcarbazepine can also act as an inhibitor of CYP2C19.

Oxcarbazepine + Perampanel

Oxcarbazepine decreases perampanel concentrations.

> Monitor for perampanel efficacy and increase the perampanel dose if necessary.

Oxcarbazepine + Phenobarbital

Oxcarbazepine concentrations, and those of its active metabolite, monohydroxyoxcarbazepine, are reduced by phenobarbital. Oxcarbazepine caused a minor increase in the concentrations of phenobarbital in one study. Primidone is expected to act similarly to phenobarbital.

> The increase in phenobarbital concentrations seems unlikely to be clinically important. However, the decrease in monohydroxyoxcarbazepine concentrations might reduce the antiepileptic activity of oxcarbazepine. More study is needed but it might be prudent to monitor concurrent use for antiplatelet efficacy, and adjust the oxcarbazepine dose if required.

Oxcarbazepine + Phenytoin

Oxcarbazepine has been shown to have no effect on phenytoin pharmacokinetics in one study, and to increase the concentration of phenytoin at higher doses in another study. Exposure to the active metabolite of oxcarbazepine is reduced by phenytoin, but the pharmacokinetics of oxcarbazepine were unaffected by phenytoin. Fosphenytoin, a prodrug of phenytoin, might interact similarly.

> A decrease in the phenytoin dose might be required when the oxcarbazepine dose is greater than 1200 mg daily. Consider monitoring phenytoin concentrations; decreasing the dose as necessary. Indicators of phenytoin toxicity include blurred vision, nystagmus, ataxia, or drowsiness.

Oxcarbazepine + Statins

Oxcarbazepine is predicted to reduce atorvastatin, lovastatin, and simvastatin exposure.

Monitor concurrent use to ensure the statin is effective, increasing the dose if needed.

Oxcarbazepine + Tacrolimus

Oxcarbazepine might decrease tacrolimus concentrations.

Monitor tacrolimus concentrations more frequently to ensure it remains effective, adjusting the dose as necessary.

Oxcarbazepine + Ulipristal

The UK and US manufacturers of ulipristal predict that CYP3A4 inducers such as oxcarbazepine might reduce the plasma concentration of ulipristal and reduce its efficacy.

The US manufacturer of ulipristal gives no specific advice about how to manage this potential interaction, whereas the UK manufacturer advises that ulipristal should not be used for emergency contraception in women taking CYP3A4 inducers (such as oxcarbazepine), or who have stopped taking an enzyme inducer within the last 2 to 3 weeks. Until more is known, this advice seems prudent.

Oxcarbazepine + Warfarin and related oral anticoagulants

A small study suggests that oxcarbazepine might not interact with warfarin; however, it did reduce the anticoagulant effects of warfarin in one case, although there were other complicating factors.

Oxcarbazepine might interact with warfarin, but not to the same extent as carbamazepine. Be aware that it might have an important effect in poor metabolisers and warfarin dose adjustments might be necessary.

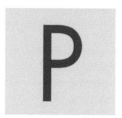

Paracetamol (Acetaminophen)

Paracetamol (Acetaminophen) + Rifampicin (Rifampin) ❓

Rifampicin induces the glucuronidation of paracetamol and increases its clearance, but does not increase the formation of hepatotoxic metabolites of paracetamol.

The clinical importance of these findings awaits further study.

Paracetamol (Acetaminophen) + Warfarin and related oral anticoagulants ❓

An equal number of randomised studies have found a modest increase in the anticoagulant effect (e.g. an increase in INR of 1) of coumarins as have reported no effect. Other cohort studies found no evidence of a change in anticoagulant effect. There are isolated case reports of an increase in anticoagulant effects in patients taking warfarin, acenocoumarol or fluindione and paracetamol.

On the basis of the available data, it is not possible to firmly recommend increased monitoring, or dismiss its advisability. Further study is clearly needed. Note that paracetamol is still considered to be safer than aspirin or NSAIDs as an analgesic in the presence of an anticoagulant because it does not affect platelets or cause gastric bleeding.

Penicillins

Penicillins + Probenecid ❓

Probenecid reduces the excretion of the penicillins, and usually raises their levels.

This is generally considered to be a beneficial interaction, but bear in mind that, in some cases, such as in patients with renal impairment, the increase in penicillin levels may be undesirably large.

Penicillins + **Warfarin and related oral anticoagulants**

Isolated cases of increased prothrombin times and/or bleeding in patients taking coumarins have been seen in patients given amoxicillin (with or without clavulanic acid) or intravenous benzylpenicillin. There is also some evidence that phenoxymethylpenicillin (penicillin V) does not increase the risk of bleeding in patients taking coumarins. In contrast, dicloxacillin might cause a modest reduction in warfarin effects, and an isolated case of thrombosis has been reported.

> For dicloxacillin, increase monitoring of the INR and anticipate the need to increase the warfarin dose on concurrent use. For the other penicillins, even though the general picture is of no interaction, factors associated with infection, such as fever, can also affect anticoagulant response. Therefore, if a patient is unwell enough to require an antibacterial, it would be prudent to increase monitoring of coagulation status. Monitor within 3 days of starting the antibacterial.

Pentamidine

Pentamidine + **Proton pump inhibitors**

Proton pump inhibitors can cause hypomagnesaemia, which might be additive with the magnesium-lowering effects of pentamidine.

> Hypomagnesaemia can develop after more than one year of concurrent use, so consider monitoring magnesium concentrations before and annually during proton pump inhibitor use, or in response to symptoms of hypomagnesaemia (e.g. muscle twitching or cramps, tremors, vomiting, tiredness, or loss of appetite). In those patients who develop hypomagnesaemia, oral and parenteral magnesium supplements might not be as effective as anticipated. Stopping the proton pump inhibitor (where possible) might be necessary.

Pentoxifylline

Pentoxifylline + **Quinolones**

Evidence from one study suggests that ciprofloxacin increases the peak serum levels of pentoxifylline by 60%, and may increase the incidence of adverse effects. In some clinical studies ciprofloxacin has been used to boost the levels of pentoxifylline.

> It has been suggested that the dose of pentoxifylline should be halved if ciprofloxacin is also given, which may be a sensible precaution. Alternatively, it may be sufficient to recommend a reduction in pentoxifylline dose only in those who experience adverse effects (e.g. nausea, headache). Note that other quinolones may also interact, see quinolones, page 564.

Pentoxifylline + Theophylline ⚠

Pentoxifylline appears to increase serum theophylline concentrations. Aminophylline is expected to be similarly affected.

Patients should be well monitored for theophylline adverse effects (such as headache, nausea, and tremor). If an interaction is suspected, monitor the theophylline concentration and adjust the theophylline or aminophylline dose, as necessary. Note that one UK manufacturer of intravenous aminophylline contra-indicates concurrent use.

Pentoxifylline + Warfarin and related oral anticoagulants ⚠

Some studies have found that pentoxifylline does not alter the anticoagulant effects of phenprocoumon or acenocoumarol; however, one study suggests that there might be an increased risk of serious bleeding if pentoxifylline is given with acenocoumarol. Pentoxifylline alone has rarely been associated with bleeding.

It may be prudent to increase the frequency of INR monitoring on the concurrent use of pentoxifylline and warfarin. This would seem sensible with any coumarin or indanedione.

Perampanel

Perampanel + Phenobarbital ⚠

Population data suggests that there is no clinically relevant pharmacokinetic interaction between perampanel and phenobarbital (an enzyme-inducing antiepileptic). However, other known enzyme-inducing antiepileptics have been seen to decrease perampanel concentrations. Primidone is metabolised to phenobarbital, and might interact similarly.

Until more is known, monitor perampanel efficacy and increase the dose if necessary.

Perampanel + Phenytoin ⚠

Phenytoin decreases perampanel concentrations. Fosphenytoin, a prodrug of phenytoin, is predicted to interact similarly.

Monitor perampanel efficacy and increase the dose if necessary.

Perampanel + Rifampicin (Rifampin) ⚠

Rifampicin is predicted to decrease perampanel exposure.

Monitor for perampanel efficacy and increase the perampanel dose if necessary.

Phenobarbital

Studies in man and *animals* clearly show that the barbiturates are potent liver enzyme inducers. The most commonly used barbiturate is phenobarbital, which is known to induce CYP3A4, amongst other isoenzymes. Most of the interaction information concerns phenobarbital, but all barbiturates would be expected to share its interactions to a greater or lesser extent. Note that primidone is metabolised to phenobarbital, and so would therefore also be expected to share many of its interactions.

Phenobarbital + Phenytoin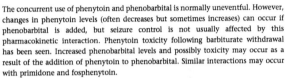

The concurrent use of phenytoin and phenobarbital is normally uneventful. However, changes in phenytoin levels (often decreases but sometimes increases) can occur if phenobarbital is added, but seizure control is not usually affected by this pharmacokinetic interaction. Phenytoin toxicity following barbiturate withdrawal has been seen. Increased phenobarbital levels and possibly toxicity may occur as a result of the addition of phenytoin to phenobarbital. Similar interactions may occur with primidone and fosphenytoin.

> Given the unpredictable outcome of concurrent use it would seem prudent to monitor levels if one drug is added to the other or if a dose is changed. Indicators of phenobarbital toxicity include drowsiness, ataxia or dysarthria.

Phenobarbital + Phosphodiesterase type-5 inhibitors

Phenobarbital (and therefore probably primidone) are expected to reduce the exposure of phosphodiesterase type-5 inhibitors, because other inducers of CYP3A4 have been shown to do so.

> It might be prudent to follow the same advice for rifampicin: if standard doses of these phosphodiesterase type-5 inhibitors are not effective for erectile dysfunction in patients taking phenobarbital or primidone, it would seem sensible to try a higher dose with close monitoring. For pulmonary hypertension, the UK manufacturer of sildenafil states that sildenafil efficacy should be closely monitored, with the sildenafil dose increased as necessary, whereas the manufacturers of tadalafil for pulmonary hypertension do not recommend the concurrent use of phenobarbital (and therefore, probably primidone). The UK and US manufacturers of avanafil contraindicate concurrent use with all CYP3A4 inducers.

Phenobarbital + Praziquantel

Phenobarbital (and therefore probably primidone) markedly reduces praziquantel exposure, but whether this results in neurocysticercosis treatment failures is unclear.

> When treating systemic worm infections such as neurocysticercosis some authors have advised increasing the praziquantel dose from 25 to 50 mg/kg if phenobarbital is being used; however, note that the recommended dose of praziquantel for neurocysticercosis is 50 mg/kg daily in three divided doses. The interaction with

antiepileptics is of no importance when praziquantel is used for intestinal worm infections (where its action is a local effect on the worms in the gut).

Phenobarbital + Propafenone ⚠

Phenobarbital increases the metabolism of propafenone and reduces its exposure. Other barbiturates might interact similarly. Primidone is metabolised to phenobarbital and might therefore interact similarly.

> The clinical importance of this interaction awaits assessment but check that propafenone remains effective if phenobarbital is added, and that toxicity does not occur if it is stopped.

Phenobarbital + Pyridoxine ⚠

Daily doses of pyridoxine 200 mg can cause reductions of 40 to 50% in phenobarbital levels in some patients. Primidone is metabolised to phenobarbital and may therefore be affected similarly, although this does not appear to have been studied.

> Concurrent use should be monitored if large doses of pyridoxine are used, being alert for the need to increase the phenobarbital dose. It seems unlikely that small doses (as in multivitamin preparations) will interact to any great extent.

Phenobarbital + Pyrimethamine ❓

Serious pancytopenia and megaloblastic anaemia may occur in patients given pyrimethamine (with or without sulfonamides) with other drugs that inhibit folate metabolism, such as phenobarbital or primidone.

> If the concurrent use of pyrimethamine and a drug that inhibits folate metabolism cannot be avoided, consider the use of a folate supplement, preferably folinic acid. This is recommended for all patients with toxoplasmosis taking high-dose pyrimethamine.

Phenobarbital + Quinidine ⚠

Quinidine levels can be reduced by the concurrent use of phenobarbital or primidone. Loss of arrhythmia control is possible if the quinidine dose is not increased.

> Concurrent use need not be avoided, but be alert for the need to increase the quinidine dose. If phenobarbital or primidone are withdrawn the quinidine dose may need to be reduced to avoid quinidine toxicity. Quinidine levels should be monitored if possible.

Phenobarbital + Ranolazine ⚠

Rifampicin (rifampin) reduces ranolazine levels by 95%, and loss of efficacy is expected. Phenobarbital (and therefore probably primidone, which is metabolised to phenobarbital) are predicted to interact in the same way as rifampicin.

> The manufacturers recommend avoiding concurrent use. In the absence of any

information on the magnitude of the effect of phenobarbital on ranolazine levels, this seems prudent.

Phenobarbital + Rifampicin (Rifampin)

Phenobarbital possibly modestly increases the clearance of rifampicin (up to a 40% reduction in rifampicin levels in one study). The effect of rifampicin on phenobarbital levels is unknown, but note that rifampicin markedly increases the clearance of hexobarbital. Primidone is metabolised to phenobarbital and may therefore interact similarly with rifampicin.

The outcome of concurrent use is unclear but a reduction in the levels of both rifampicin and the barbiturate seems possible. Concurrent use need not be avoided, but be alert for a reduced response to both drugs.

Phenobarbital + Rivaroxaban

Phenobarbital and primidone are predicted to decrease the exposure to rivaroxaban, and therefore decrease its anticoagulant effects.

Given the likely clinical risk of reduced rivaroxaban efficacy, it would seem prudent to consider using an alternative drug; however, if this is not possible, consider closely monitoring the prothrombin time to ensure the anticoagulant effect of rivaroxaban is maintained in patients given these drugs.

Phenobarbital + Roflumilast

Rifampicin (rifampin) increases the metabolism of roflumilast to its active metabolite, roflumilast *N*-oxide, but decreases the overall bioavailability of roflumilast *N*-oxide, resulting in a decrease in its phosphodiesterase inhibitory effects. Phenobarbital and primidone (which is metabolised to phenobarbital) might interact similarly.

Monitor concurrent use to ensure that roflumilast is effective, and consider increasing the dose of roflumilast, according to clinical need.

Phenobarbital + Rufinamide

Phenobarbital and primidone may modestly increase the clearance of rufinamide. Rufinamide does not appear to affect trough phenobarbital or primidone levels.

Until more is known it would seem prudent to monitor the plasma levels and clinical effects of rufinamide when it is started or stopped in patients taking phenobarbital or primidone.

Phenobarbital + Sirolimus

Phenobarbital (and therefore probably primidone) is predicted to reduce sirolimus concentrations.

It would seem prudent to increase the frequency of monitoring of sirolimus concentrations during concurrent use, and adjust the dose as necessary. The UK and US manufacturers of sirolimus state that concurrent use should be avoided.

Phenobarbital + Sodium oxybate

Barbiturates, such as phenobarbital or primidone, are expected to have additive CNS depressant effect with sodium oxybate.

Concurrent use is contraindicated. If both drugs are given be alert for CNS depression. Warn all patients of the potential effects, and counsel against driving or undertaking other skilled tasks.

Phenobarbital + Solifenacin

The manufacturers predict that potent CYP3A4 inducers, such as phenobarbital, will decrease solifenacin levels. Primidone, which is metabolised to phenobarbital, would be expected to interact similarly.

Monitor the outcome of concurrent use to ensure that solifenacin is effective and adjust the dose if necessary.

Phenobarbital + SSRIs

In one study in 6 subjects phenobarbital caused reductions of 10 to 86% in the AUC of paroxetine, but the mean values were not altered to a statistically significant extent. One subject showed an *increase* of about 60% in their AUC. Primidone is metabolised to phenobarbital and may therefore interact similarly with paroxetine.

Although there seems to be little correlation between plasma paroxetine levels and its efficacy, be alert for the need to increase its dose if phenobarbital is given. Note that SSRIs can decrease the seizure threshold and so they should be used with caution in patients given barbiturates for epilepsy.

Phenobarbital + Tacrolimus

Phenobarbital (and therefore probably primidone) decrease tacrolimus concentrations.

Monitor the concentrations and effects of tacrolimus (e.g. on renal function) more frequently if phenobarbital or primidone are given, adjusting the tacrolimus dose as necessary.

Phenobarbital + Tetracyclines

The serum levels of doxycycline are reduced and may fall below the accepted minimum inhibitory concentration in patients receiving long-term treatment with barbiturates.

It has been suggested that the doxycycline dose could be doubled to overcome this reaction. Alternatively, tetracycline, oxytetracycline, and chlortetracycline appear not to interact and may therefore be suitable alternatives.

Phenobarbital + Theophylline

Theophylline clearance is increased (by roughly one-third) by phenobarbital or pentobarbital. A single report describes a similar interaction with secobarbital, and an interaction would be expected to occur with other barbiturates. Aminophylline would be expected to interact similarly.

It would be prudent to monitor theophylline concentrations if a barbiturate is used concurrently to ensure theophylline remains effective, and adjust the theophylline or aminophylline dose if necessary.

Phenobarbital + Tiagabine

Tiagabine levels may be reduced 1.5- to 3-fold by both phenobarbital and primidone.

The manufacturers recommend that tiagabine 30 to 45 mg (in divided doses) should be given to patients taking enzyme-inducing antiepileptics.

Phenobarbital + Ticagrelor

Phenobarbital is predicted to decrease ticagrelor exposure. Primidone, a prodrug of phenobarbital, is predicted to interact similarly.

If concurrent use is unavoidable, be alert for reduced ticagrelor efficacy.

Phenobarbital + Topiramate

Phenobarbital and primidone can reduce topiramate levels by about 30%.

When topiramate is given with phenobarbital or primidone, its dose should be titrated to effect. If phenobarbital or primidone are added or withdrawn be aware that the dose of topiramate may be need adjustment.

Phenobarbital + Toremifene

Phenobarbital can reduce toremifene exposure. Primidone is metabolised to phenobarbital and might therefore interact similarly.

Monitor concurrent use to ensure toremifene remains effective. The UK manufacturer of toremifene suggests that the toremifene dose might need to be doubled in the presence of phenobarbital (and therefore probably primidone).

Phenobarbital + Tricyclics

Barbiturates reduce the levels of the tricyclic antidepressants, which has been associated with the re-emergence of depression. Although not all combinations have been studied, they would all be expected to interact similarly.

Monitor the outcome of concurrent use anticipating reduced tricyclic antidepressant effects. Consider an alternative to the barbiturate, or raise the tricyclic dose if problems occur. Note that tricyclics lower the seizure threshold and so they should be used with caution in patients given barbiturates for epilepsy.

Phenobarbital + Ulipristal

The UK and US manufacturers of ulipristal predict that CYP3A4 inducers such as phenobarbital might reduce the plasma concentrations of ulipristal and reduce its efficacy. Primidone is metabolised to phenobarbital and would be expected to interact similarly.

The US manufacturer of ulipristal gives no specific advice about how to manage this potential interaction, whereas the UK manufacturer advises that ulipristal should not be used for emergency contraception in women taking CYP3A4 inducers (such as phenobarbital), or who have stopped taking an enzyme inducer within the last 2 to 3 weeks. Until more is known, this advice seems prudent.

Phenobarbital + Vaccines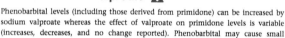

Influenza vaccine can cause a transient moderate (30%) rise in phenobarbital levels. Primidone is metabolised to phenobarbital and may therefore interact similarly.

Warn the patient to monitor for indicators of phenobarbital toxicity (drowsiness, ataxia or dysarthria), and take levels if necessary. Levels may still be moderately raised after 28 days. However, most patients seem unlikely to require dose adjustments.

Phenobarbital + Valproate

Phenobarbital levels (including those derived from primidone) can be increased by sodium valproate whereas the effect of valproate on primidone levels is variable (increases, decreases, and no change reported). Phenobarbital may cause small reductions in sodium valproate. The concurrent use of phenobarbital and valproate may cause an increase in serum liver enzymes.

Use of this combination may result in excessive sedation and lethargy. To control this interaction the dose of phenobarbital has been reduced by up to about 50%, without loss of seizure control. Indicators of phenobarbital toxicity include drowsiness, ataxia or dysarthria. Monitor levels as necessary. Valproate has been associated with serious hepatotoxicity, especially in children aged less than 3 years, and this has been more common in those receiving other antiepileptics. Valproate monotherapy is to be preferred in this group.

Phenobarbital + Vigabatrin

Vigabatrin causes a small decrease in phenobarbital and primidone levels. There is some evidence that phenobarbital may reduce the efficacy of vigabatrin in infantile spasms.

Generally no action seems necessary, but bear the possibility of reduced efficacy in mind.

Phenobarbital + Vitamin D

The long-term use of phenobarbital can disturb vitamin D and calcium metabolism, which may result in osteomalacia. There are a few reports of patients taking vitamin D supplements as replacement therapy who responded poorly while taking phenobarbital or primidone.

Monitor the outcome of concurrent use. Larger doses of vitamin D may be needed.

Phenobarbital + Warfarin and related oral anticoagulants

The effects of the coumarins (acenocoumarol, phenprocoumon and warfarin) are reduced by the barbiturates.

Reduced anticoagulant effects may occur within 2 to 4 days (maximum effect after about 3 weeks). Monitor the INR closely until stable and be aware that dose increases of 30 to 60% are likely to be needed. Also monitor if the barbiturate is stopped (note that the interaction may persist for up to several weeks after concurrent use is stopped). The benzodiazepines do not usually interact with anticoagulants, and may therefore be a suitable alternative in some circumstances.

Phenobarbital + Zonisamide

Phenobarbital (and therefore probably primidone) can cause a small to moderate reduction in zonisamide levels, but zonisamide appears not to affect phenobarbital or primidone levels.

The clinical importance of this interaction is unknown, but bear the possibility of reduced zonisamide levels in mind if either of these barbiturates is given.

Phenytoin

Phenytoin is extensively metabolised by hydroxylation, principally by CYP2C9, although CYP2C19 also plays a role. These isoenzymes show genetic polymorphism, and CYP2C19 may assume a greater role in individuals who have a poor metaboliser phenotype of CYP2C9. The concurrent use of inhibitors of CYP2C9, and sometimes also CYP2C19, can lead to phenytoin toxicity. In addition, phenytoin metabolism is saturable (it shows nonlinear pharmacokinetics), therefore, small changes in metabolism or phenytoin dose can result in marked changes in plasma levels. Fosphenytoin is a prodrug of phenytoin, which is rapidly and completely hydrolysed to phenytoin in the body. It is predicted to interact with other drugs in the same way as phenytoin. No drugs are known to interfere with the conversion of fosphenytoin to phenytoin.

Phenytoin + Phosphodiesterase type-5 inhibitors

Phenytoin (and therefore probably fosphenytoin) is predicted to reduce the exposure of phosphodiesterase type-5 inhibitors, because other inducers of CYP3A4 have been shown to do so.

It might be prudent to follow the same advice for rifampicin: if standard doses of these phosphodiesterase type-5 inhibitors are not effective for erectile dysfunction in patients taking phenytoin or fosphenytoin, it would seem sensible to try a higher dose with close monitoring. For pulmonary hypertension, the UK manufacturer of sildenafil states that sildenafil efficacy should be closely monitored, with the sildenafil dose increased as necessary, whereas the manufacturers of tadalafil do not recommend the concurrent use of phenytoin (and therefore probably fosphenytoin). The UK and US manufacturers of avanafil contraindicate concurrent use with all CYP3A4 inducers.

Phenytoin + Praziquantel

Phenytoin markedly reduces praziquantel exposure, but whether this results in neurocysticercosis treatment failures is unclear. Fosphenytoin, a prodrug of phenytoin, might interact similarly.

> When treating systemic worm infections such as neurocysticercosis some authors have advised increasing the praziquantel dose from 25 to 50 mg/kg if phenytoin is being used, but in one case this dose was not effective. Furthermore, note that the recommended dose for praziquantel for neurocysticercosis is 50 mg/kg daily in 3 divided doses. The interaction with antiepileptics is of no importance when praziquantel is used for intestinal worm infections (where its action is a local effect on the worms in the gut).

Phenytoin + Proton pump inhibitors

A study found that omeprazole 20 mg daily did not affect phenytoin levels, whereas earlier studies suggested that phenytoin levels might be modestly raised by omeprazole 40 mg daily. A study with esomeprazole also suggests that it may cause a minor rise in phenytoin levels. Lansoprazole does not normally interact with phenytoin, but an isolated case report of toxicity is tentatively attributed to an interaction. Fosphenytoin, a prodrug of phenytoin, may interact similarly with these proton pump inhibitors.

> This interaction is unlikely to be generally significant, but bear it in mind in case of an unexpected response to treatment. Indicators of phenytoin toxicity include blurred vision, nystagmus, ataxia or drowsiness. However, note that the manufacturers of esomeprazole recommend monitoring phenytoin levels.

Phenytoin + Pyridoxine

Daily doses of pyridoxine 80 to 400 mg can cause reductions of about 35% in phenytoin levels in some patients. The effect on fosphenytoin, a prodrug of phenytoin, does not appear to have been studied, but it may be prudent to assume it may interact similarly.

> Concurrent use should be monitored if large doses of pyridoxine are used, being alert for the need to increase the phenytoin dose. It seems unlikely that small doses (as in multivitamin preparations) will interact to any great extent.

Phenytoin + Pyrimethamine

Serious pancytopenia and megaloblastic anaemia may occur in patients given pyrimethamine (with or without sulfonamides) with other drugs that inhibit folate metabolism, such as phenytoin or fosphenytoin.

If the concurrent use of pyrimethamine and a drug that inhibits folate metabolism cannot be avoided, consider the use of a folate supplement, preferably folinic acid. This is recommended for all patients with toxoplasmosis taking high-dose pyrimethamine.

Phenytoin + Quinidine

Quinidine levels can be reduced by phenytoin. Loss of arrhythmia control is possible if the quinidine dose is not increased. Fosphenytoin, a prodrug of phenytoin, may interact similarly.

Concurrent use need not be avoided, but be alert for the need to increase the quinidine dose. If phenytoin is withdrawn the quinidine dose may need to be reduced to avoid quinidine toxicity. Quinidine levels should be monitored if possible.

Phenytoin + Quinolones

Studies suggest that ciprofloxacin does not usually have a clinically significant effect on phenytoin concentrations. However, case reports describe changes (both increases and decreases) in phenytoin concentrations in patients given ciprofloxacin. Fosphenytoin, a prodrug of phenytoin, might interact similarly.

It has been suggested that it would be prudent to consider monitoring phenytoin concentrations in those given ciprofloxacin. Quinolones alone very occasionally cause convulsions, therefore they should be used with caution in patients with epilepsy.

Phenytoin + Ranolazine

Rifampicin (rifampin) reduces ranolazine levels by 95%, and loss of efficacy is expected. Phenytoin (and therefore probably its prodrug, fosphenytoin) are predicted to interact in the same way as rifampicin.

The manufacturers recommend avoiding concurrent use. In the absence of any information on the magnitude of the effect of phenytoin on ranolazine levels, this seems prudent.

Phenytoin + Retigabine (Ezogabine)

Retigabine clearance is increased by phenytoin but retigabine does not affect phenytoin pharmacokinetics.

The clinical importance of this interaction is unknown, but bear it in mind in the case of an unexpected response to treatment.

Phenytoin + Rifampicin (Rifampin)

Phenytoin levels can be markedly reduced by rifampicin (clearance doubled in one study). If rifampicin is given with isoniazid, phenytoin levels may fall in patients who are fast acetylators of isoniazid, but may occasionally rise in those who are slow acetylators. Fosphenytoin, a prodrug of phenytoin, may interact similarly.

> It is unlikely that the acetylator status of the patient will be known. Therefore monitor phenytoin levels and adjust the dose accordingly.

P

Phenytoin + Rivaroxaban

Phenytoin and fosphenytoin are predicted to decrease the exposure to rivaroxaban, and therefore decrease its anticoagulant effects.

> Given the likely clinical risk of reduced rivaroxaban efficacy, it would seem prudent to consider using an alternative drug; however, if this is not possible, consider closely monitoring the prothrombin time to ensure the anticoagulant effect of rivaroxaban. The US manufacturer of rivaroxaban advises avoiding concurrent use.

Phenytoin + Roflumilast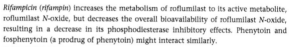

Rifampicin (rifampin) increases the metabolism of roflumilast to its active metabolite, roflumilast *N*-oxide, but decreases the overall bioavailability of roflumilast *N*-oxide, resulting in a decrease in its phosphodiesterase inhibitory effects. Phenytoin and fosphenytoin (a prodrug of phenytoin) might interact similarly.

> Monitor concurrent use to ensure that roflumilast is effective, and consider increasing the dose of roflumilast, according to clinical need.

Phenytoin + Rufinamide

Phenytoin may modestly increase the clearance of rufinamide. Rufinamide does not appear to affect trough phenytoin levels; however, the manufacturer of rufinamide suggests that the plasma levels of phenytoin may be increased. It may be prudent to expect fosphenytoin to behave similarly.

> The manufacturer of rufinamide suggests that the dose of phenytoin may need to be reduced. Until more is known it would seem prudent to monitor the clinical effects of rufinamide. Monitor for phenytoin and fosphenytoin adverse effects (e.g. blurred vision, nystagmus, ataxia or drowsiness) and consider taking levels if these occur.

Phenytoin + Sirolimus

Phenytoin (and therefore possibly fosphenytoin) is predicted to reduce sirolimus plasma concentrations: two cases of increased sirolimus requirements with phenytoin have been reported.

> It would seem prudent to increase the frequency of monitoring sirolimus concentrations, both during concurrent use and also if phenytoin is withdrawn.

The UK and US manufacturers of sirolimus state that concurrent use should be avoided.

Phenytoin + **Sodium oxybate** ⚠

The UK manufacturer of sodium oxybate predicts that phenytoin might affect its metabolism, however there are no clinical studies to confirm this prediction. Fosphenytoin, a prodrug of phenytoin, would be expected to interact similarly.

Monitor concurrent use, and adjust the dose of sodium oxybate as needed.

Phenytoin + **Solifenacin** ⚠

The manufacturers predict that potent CYP3A4 inducers, such as phenytoin, will decrease solifenacin levels. Fosphenytoin, a prodrug of phenytoin, would be expected to interact similarly.

Monitor the outcome of concurrent use to ensure that solifenacin is effective and adjust the dose if necessary.

Phenytoin + **SSRIs** ❓

Phenytoin levels can be increased by fluoxetine and fluvoxamine in some patients and toxicity may occur. Phenytoin and sertraline do not normally interact, but 2 patients have had increased phenytoin levels while taking sertraline. Fosphenytoin, a prodrug of phenytoin, may interact similarly with these SSRIs.

Monitor patients for signs of phenytoin toxicity, such as blurred vision, nystagmus, ataxia or drowsiness. Consider monitoring phenytoin levels and adjust the dose accordingly. Note that SSRIs should be avoided in unstable epilepsy and used with care in patients with controlled epilepsy.

Phenytoin + **Statins** ❓

A number of isolated case reports describe a reduced cholesterol-lowering effect of simvastatin, fluvastatin, and atorvastatin in patients taking phenytoin. In a study, the concurrent use of phenytoin and fluvastatin increased the exposure to both drugs but the effect was only slight.

The increase in phenytoin and fluvastatin exposure seen on concurrent use seems unlikely to be clinically important. The general importance of a reduced cholesterol-lowering effect is unknown, but bear the interaction in mind if lipid-lowering targets are not satisfactorily met.

Phenytoin + **Sulfinpyrazone** ⚠

Some limited evidence indicates that phenytoin levels may be markedly increased by sulfinpyrazone. Fosphenytoin, a prodrug of phenytoin, may interact similarly.

Warn the patient to monitor for indicators of phenytoin toxicity (blurred vision, nystagmus, ataxia or drowsiness). It would seem advisable to monitor phenytoin levels and adjust the dose accordingly.

Phenytoin + Sulfonamides

Phenytoin concentrations can be increased by co-trimoxazole (which contains sulfamethoxazole), sulfamethizole, sulfamethoxazole, and sulfadiazine. Phenytoin toxicity might develop in some cases. Fosphenytoin, a prodrug of phenytoin, might interact similarly.

> The risk of toxicity is small and is most likely in those with phenytoin concentrations at the top end of the range. Monitor phenytoin concentrations and adjust the dose accordingly. Indicators of phenytoin toxicity include blurred vision, nystagmus, ataxia, or drowsiness.

Phenytoin + Tacrolimus

An isolated report describes an increase in phenytoin concentrations attributed to the use of tacrolimus. Phenytoin decreased tacrolimus concentrations in several cases. Fosphenytoin, a prodrug of phenytoin, might interact similarly.

> Monitor tacrolimus concentrations and effects (e.g. on renal function) more frequently in patients given phenytoin. Similarly, based on the single case of phenytoin toxicity, it might also be advisable to monitor phenytoin concentrations.

Phenytoin + Tetracyclines

The serum levels of doxycycline are reduced and may fall below the accepted minimum inhibitory concentration in patients receiving long-term treatment with phenytoin. Fosphenytoin, a prodrug of phenytoin, may interact similarly.

> It has been suggested that the doxycycline dose could be doubled to overcome this interaction. Tetracycline, oxytetracycline and chlortetracycline appear not to interact and may therefore be suitable alternatives.

Phenytoin + Theophylline

Phenytoin increases the clearance of theophylline, but the magnitude of the effect reported varies widely. Limited evidence suggests that theophylline might also reduce phenytoin exposure. Fosphenytoin, a prodrug of phenytoin, would be expected to interact similarly to phenytoin, and aminophylline would be expected to interact similarly to theophylline.

> Theophylline concentrations should be monitored to ensure that they remain within the therapeutic range. Theophylline dose increases of up to 50% or more might be required. The effect of theophylline on phenytoin is not established, but it may be prudent to monitor phenytoin concentrations as well. Separating the oral dose by 1 to 2 hours appears to minimise the effects of theophylline on phenytoin.

Phenytoin + Tiagabine

Tiagabine levels may be reduced 1.5 to 3-fold by phenytoin. Fosphenytoin, a prodrug of phenytoin, may interact similarly.

> The manufacturers recommend that tiagabine 30 to 45 mg (in divided doses) should be given to patients taking enzyme-inducing antiepileptics.

Phenytoin + Ticagrelor

Phenytoin is predicted to decrease ticagrelor exposure. Fosphenytoin, a prodrug of phenytoin, is predicted to interact similarly.

> If concurrent use is unavoidable, be alert for reduced ticagrelor efficacy.

Phenytoin + Ticlopidine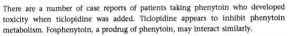

There are a number of case reports of patients taking phenytoin who developed toxicity when ticlopidine was added. Ticlopidine appears to inhibit phenytoin metabolism. Fosphenytoin, a prodrug of phenytoin, may interact similarly.

> It would be prudent to monitor phenytoin levels if ticlopidine is added. Warn the patient to monitor for indicators of phenytoin toxicity (blurred vision, nystagmus, ataxia or drowsiness).

Phenytoin + Topiramate

Phenytoin increases the clearance of topiramate 2- to 3-fold, which appears to result in topiramate levels that are up to 50% lower. Topiramate slightly increases the phenytoin AUC by up to about 55% but this is said not to be clinically significant based on several other analyses showing no interaction. Fosphenytoin, a prodrug of phenytoin, may interact similarly.

> Topiramate dose adjustments may be required if phenytoin is added or discontinued. Be aware that a few patients may have increased phenytoin levels, particularly at high topiramate doses. Warn the patient to monitor for indicators of phenytoin toxicity (blurred vision, nystagmus, ataxia or drowsiness). Consider monitoring phenytoin levels.

Phenytoin + Toremifene

Phenytoin might reduce toremifene exposure. Fosphenytoin, a prodrug of phenytoin, might interact similarly.

> Monitor concurrent use to ensure toremifene remains effective. The UK manufacturer of toremifene suggests that the toremifene dose may need to be doubled in the presence of phenytoin (and therefore probably fosphenytoin).

Phenytoin + Tricyclics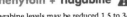

Some very limited evidence suggests that imipramine can raise phenytoin levels.

Phenytoin possibly reduces desipramine levels. Fosphenytoin, a prodrug of phenytoin, may interact similarly.

> None of these interactions is established. Note that the tricyclic antidepressants as a group lower the seizure threshold, which suggests that extra care should be taken if deciding to use them in patients with epilepsy.

Phenytoin + Trimethoprim ⚠

Phenytoin serum concentrations can be increased by trimethoprim. Fosphenytoin, a prodrug of phenytoin, might interact similarly.

> The risk of toxicity is small and is most likely in those with phenytoin concentrations at the top end of the range. Monitor phenytoin concentrations and adjust the dose accordingly. Indicators of phenytoin toxicity include blurred vision, nystagmus, ataxia, or drowsiness.

Phenytoin + Ulipristal ⚠

The UK and US manufacturers of ulipristal predict that CYP3A4 inducers such as phenytoin might reduce the plasma concentration of ulipristal and reduce its efficacy. Fosphenytoin, a prodrug of phenytoin, would be expected to interact similarly.

> The US manufacturer of ulipristal gives no specific advice about how to manage this potential interaction, whereas the UK manufacturer advises that ulipristal should not be used for emergency contraception in women taking CYP3A4 inducers (such as phenytoin), or who have stopped taking an enzyme inducer within the last 2 to 3 weeks. Until more is known, this advice seems prudent.

Phenytoin + Vaccines

Influenza vaccine is reported to increase, decrease or to have no effect on phenytoin levels. The efficacy of the vaccine is unaffected. Fosphenytoin, a prodrug of phenytoin, may interact similarly.

> Phenytoin levels appear to return to normal after about 14 days. Warn the patient to monitor for indicators of phenytoin toxicity (blurred vision, nystagmus, ataxia or drowsiness). However, be aware that any alteration in levels may take a couple of weeks to develop and usually resolves spontaneously.

Phenytoin + Valproate ⚠

The concurrent use of phenytoin and valproate is usually uneventful. Initially total phenytoin levels may fall by 20 to 50% but this is offset by a rise in the levels of free (and active) phenytoin, which may very occasionally cause some toxicity. After continued use total phenytoin levels rise once again. Phenytoin also reduces valproate levels. Fosphenytoin, a prodrug of phenytoin, may interact similarly.

> Monitor phenytoin levels and adjust the dose accordingly. When monitoring concurrent use it is important to understand fully the implications of changes in 'total', and 'free' or 'unbound' phenytoin levels. Where monitoring of free phenytoin levels is not available, various nomograms have been designed for

predicting unbound phenytoin levels during the use of sodium valproate. Consider monitoring valproate levels for an indication of toxicity if phenytoin is stopped.

Phenytoin + Vigabatrin ❓

Vigabatrin causes a small to moderate 20 to 30% reduction in phenytoin levels. Fosphenytoin, a prodrug of phenytoin, may interact similarly

Occasional patients may require a small adjustment in dose. Note that this interaction can take several weeks to develop.

Phenytoin + Vitamin D ⚠️

The long-term use of phenytoin can disturb vitamin D and calcium metabolism, which may result in osteomalacia. There are a few reports of patients taking vitamin D supplements for replacement therapy who responded poorly while taking phenytoin. Fosphenytoin, a prodrug of phenytoin, may interact similarly.

Monitor the outcome of concurrent use. Larger doses of vitamin D may be needed.

Phenytoin + Warfarin and related oral anticoagulants ⚠️

Phenytoin would be expected to reduce the anticoagulant effects of the coumarins and this has been seen with warfarin. However, cases where the effects of warfarin were *increased* have been reported, and one study found that the effects of phenprocoumon were generally unaltered by phenytoin. Limited evidence suggests that phenytoin levels may rise in patients taking phenprocoumon or, more rarely, warfarin. Fosphenytoin, a prodrug of phenytoin, may interact similarly.

None of these interactions have been extensively studied nor are they well established. Warn patients to monitor for indicators of phenytoin toxicity (blurred vision, nystagmus, ataxia or drowsiness) and to report any increased bruising or bleeding. Consider monitoring phenytoin levels and anticoagulant control if acenocoumarol, phenprocoumon or warfarin is given with phenytoin.

Phenytoin + Zonisamide ❓

Phenytoin can cause a small to moderate reduction in zonisamide levels. Zonisamide appears not to affect phenytoin levels in most studies, although two studies suggest a modest rise of about 20% may occur. Fosphenytoin, a prodrug of phenytoin, may interact similarly.

The general importance of this interaction is unknown although a serious interaction is unlikely. Consider the importance of a possible reduction in zonisamide levels. Bear the potential for a modest increase in phenytoin levels in mind should a patient taking zonisamide develop signs of phenytoin toxicity (blurred vision, nystagmus, ataxia or drowsiness).

Phosphodiesterase type-5 inhibitors

Phosphodiesterase type-5 inhibitors + **Rifampicin (Rifampin)**

Rifampicin markedly reduces the exposure to tadalafil by inducing CYP3A4. Rifampicin is predicted to reduce the exposure to avanafil, sildenafil, and vardenafil, which are also metabolised by CYP3A4.

> If standard doses of these phosphodiesterase type-5 inhibitors are not effective for erectile dysfunction in patients taking rifampicin, it would seem sensible to try a higher dose with close monitoring. For pulmonary hypertension, the UK manufacturer of sildenafil states that sildenafil efficacy should be closely monitored, with the sildenafil dose increased as necessary, whereas the manufacturers of tadalafil for pulmonary hypertension do not recommend its concurrent use with rifampicin. The UK and US manufacturers of avanafil contraindicate concurrent use with all CYP3A4 inducers.

Phosphodiesterase type-5 inhibitors + **Riociguat**

The concurrent use of riociguat and phosphodiesterase type-5 inhibitors (e.g. avanafil, sildenafil, tadalafil, and vardenafil) can lead to hypotension. However, riociguat does not affect the pharmacokinetics of sildenafil.

> Both the UK and US manufacturers of riociguat contraindicate the concurrent use with phosphodiesterase type-5 inhibitors.

Prasugrel

Prasugrel + **Rivaroxaban** ?

The concurrent use of rivaroxaban and prasugrel might increase the risk of bleeding.

> Advise patients to be aware of increased bruising or prolonged bleeding, and to seek medical advice if this occurs.

Prasugrel + **SSRIs** ?

The bleeding risk associated with antiplatelet drugs such as prasugrel might be further increased by the concurrent use of an SSRI, although the data appears to be conflicting.

> In general, the manufacturers of the SSRIs advise caution on the concurrent use of drugs that affect platelet function, such as prasugrel. Consider giving gastroprotective drugs to those at high risk of gastrointestinal bleeding (e.g. the elderly, those with a history of gastrointestinal bleeding, patients taking multiple antiplatelet drugs). Advise patients to report any signs of excessive bleeding.

Prasugrel + Ticagrelor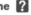

The concurrent use of prasugrel and ticagrelor might theoretically increase the risk of bleeding.

> Although combinations of antiplatelet drugs are commonly used and can be clinically beneficial in some indications, be aware of the increased risk of bleeding.

Prasugrel + Ticlopidine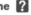

The concurrent use of prasugrel and ticlopidine might theoretically increase the risk of bleeding.

> Although combinations of antiplatelet drugs are commonly used and can be clinically beneficial in some indications, be aware of the increased risk of bleeding.

Prasugrel + Venlafaxine

The bleeding risk associated with antiplatelet drugs such as prasugrel might be further increased by the concurrent use of an SSRI, although the data appears to be conflicting. SNRIs (e.g. venlafaxine) are expected to interact similarly.

> The manufacturer of venlafaxine advises caution on concurrent use in patients taking antiplatelet drugs (such as prasugrel). Consider giving gastroprotective drugs to those at high risk of gastrointestinal bleeding (e.g. the elderly, those with a history of gastrointestinal bleeding, patients taking multiple antiplatelet drugs). Advise patients to report any signs of excessive bleeding.

Prasugrel + Warfarin and related oral anticoagulants ⚠

Prasugrel has no effect on the pharmacokinetics of warfarin. However, concurrent use may increase the risk of bleeding.

> If the concurrent use of prasugrel and a coumarin or indanedione is necessary, the patient should be monitored for signs of increased bleeding, and told to report any unexplained bruising or bleeding.

Praziquantel

Praziquantel + Rifampicin (Rifampin) ✖

Rifampicin reduces the plasma concentration of praziquantel.

> It is predicted that rifampicin will reduce the efficacy of praziquantel, and therefore the combination should be avoided.

Probenecid

Probenecid + Pyrazinamide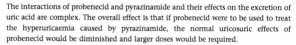

The interactions of probenecid and pyrazinamide and their effects on the excretion of uric acid are complex. The overall effect is that if probenecid were to be used to treat the hyperuricaemia caused by pyrazinamide, the normal uricosuric effects of probenecid would be diminished and larger doses would be required.

Note that pyrazinamide should be used with caution or is contraindicated in patients with a history of gout. If hyperuricaemia accompanied by gouty arthritis occurs, pyrazinamide should be stopped.

Probenecid + Quinolones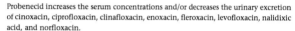

Probenecid increases the serum concentrations and/or decreases the urinary excretion of cinoxacin, ciprofloxacin, clinafloxacin, enoxacin, fleroxacin, levofloxacin, nalidixic acid, and norfloxacin.

This is unlikely to be of clinical significance unless other drugs that affect renal clearance (such as some penicillins or cephalosporins) are taken concurrently, or in the presence of renal impairment. Moxifloxacin, sparfloxacin, and probably ofloxacin, appear not to interact with probenecid.

Procainamide

Procainamide + Trimethoprim ⚠

Trimethoprim causes a marked increase in the plasma levels of procainamide and its active metabolite, *N*-acetylprocainamide.

The need to reduce the procainamide dose should be anticipated if trimethoprim is given to patients already taking stable doses of procainamide.

Proguanil

Proguanil + Pyrimethamine ❓

Serious pancytopenia and megaloblastic anaemia may occur in patients given pyrimethamine (with or without sulfonamides) with other drugs that inhibit folate metabolism, such as proguanil.

If the concurrent use of pyrimethamine and a drug that inhibits folate metabolism cannot be avoided, consider the use of a folate supplement, preferably folinic acid. This is recommended for all patients with toxoplasmosis taking high-dose pyrimethamine.

Proguanil + Warfarin and related oral anticoagulants

An isolated report describes bleeding in a patient taking warfarin after she took proguanil for about 5 weeks; however, factors related to travel (such as a changing diet and changing dose times in different time zones) may have had a part to play. The UK manufacturer speculates that proguanil possibly interferes with the metabolic pathway of warfarin and related anticoagulants; however, a pharmacokinetic interaction seems unlikely.

> The general importance of this isolated case is uncertain. Note that the UK manufacturer of proguanil advises caution on concurrent use; however a clinically relevant interaction seems unlikely.

P

Propafenone

Propafenone + Quinidine ⚠

Quinidine doubles the plasma concentrations of propafenone and halves the concentrations of its active metabolite in some patients, but the antiarrhythmic effects appear to be unaffected.

> Anticipate the need to reduce the propafenone dose (maybe by as much as half) if the combination is used. Monitor well for an increase in propafenone adverse effects (such as hypotension, bradycardia, dizziness, dry mouth), and adjust the propafenone dose as necessary.

Propafenone + Ranolazine

Ranolazine increases the levels of *metoprolol* by about 80% (by inhibiting CYP2D6). The manufacturers predict that propafenone will be similarly affected.

> Be aware of a possible interaction if propafenone adverse effects (such as hypotension, bradycardia, dizziness, dry mouth) occur. The manufacturer of ranolazine suggests a dose reduction of propafenone may be needed.

Propafenone + Rifampicin (Rifampin) ⚠

When given orally, propafenone serum concentrations and therapeutic effects can be reduced by rifampicin (bioavailability approximately halved). This has resulted in the re-emergence of arrhythmias in some cases. Limited evidence suggests that *intravenous* propafenone is not affected.

> The dose of oral propafenone will probably need increasing if rifampicin is given. Alternatively, if possible, it has been advised that another antibacterial be used because of the probable difficulty in adjusting the propafenone dose.

Propafenone + SSRIs

Fluoxetine markedly inhibits the metabolism (5-hydroxylation) of propafenone, and paroxetine would also be expected to behave similarly, but the clinical consequences of this are unknown. Fluvoxamine would be expected to inhibit the metabolism of propafenone by *N*-dealkylation, but in most patients this is only expected to have a small effect.

> Until more is known, it would be prudent to use caution when giving any of these SSRIs with propafenone, monitoring for an increase in propafenone adverse effects (e.g. hypotension, bradycardia, dizziness, dry mouth) and consider decreasing the dose of propafenone if these become troublesome.

P

Propafenone + Terbinafine

In vitro studies suggest that terbinafine is an inhibitor of CYP2D6. It might therefore be expected to increase the plasma concentration of other drugs that are substrates of this isoenzyme, such as propafenone.

> Until more is known it would seem wise to be aware of the possibility of an increase in propafenone adverse effects (e.g. hypotension, bradycardia, dizziness, dry mouth) if propafenone is given with terbinafine and consider a dose reduction if necessary.

Propafenone + Tizanidine

Propafenone is predicted to increase the exposure to tizanidine, increasing its hypotensive and sedative effects.

> The UK and US manufacturers suggest that concurrent use should be avoided. Until more is known be alert for adverse effects such as bradycardia, hypotension, and drowsiness.

Propafenone + Warfarin and related oral anticoagulants

The anticoagulant effects of warfarin are increased by propafenone. Case reports suggest that phenprocoumon and fluindione interact similarly.

> Monitor the anticoagulant effect if propafenone is added or withdrawn. This interaction appears to start in the first week of concurrent use.

Proton pump inhibitors

Proton pump inhibitors + Sirolimus ?

Proton pump inhibitors can cause hypomagnesaemia, and might be additive with the magnesium-lowering effects of sirolimus.

> Hypomagnesaemia can develop after more than one year of concurrent use, so consider monitoring magnesium concentrations before and annually during proton pump inhibitor use, or in response to symptoms of hypomagnesaemia (e.g. muscle twitching or cramps, tremors, vomiting, tiredness, or loss of appetite). In

those patients who develop hypomagnesaemia, oral and parenteral magnesium supplements might not be as effective as anticipated. Stopping the proton pump inhibitor (where possible) might be necessary.

Proton pump inhibitors + SSRIs

Fluvoxamine

Fluvoxamine inhibits the metabolism of lansoprazole, omeprazole and rabeprazole in most patients. Theoretically other proton pump inhibitors may be similarly affected.

> The proton pump inhibitors have a wide therapeutic margin and therefore the clinical significance of this interaction is unknown. Bear it in mind in case of increased proton pump inhibitors adverse effects (such as headache, diarrhoea or skin rashes) and consider reducing the dose if necessary.

Other SSRIs

Omeprazole (and therefore probably esomeprazole) increases escitalopram (and therefore probably citalopram) levels by 50%.

> Monitor concurrent use for SSRI adverse effects (such as nausea, diarrhoea, dry mouth, palpitations). The UK manufacturer of escitalopram suggests that dose adjustments may be necessary, but this would seem unlikely in most patients.

Proton pump inhibitors + Tacrolimus

Lansoprazole and omeprazole might increase tacrolimus concentrations, but the outcome of concurrent use, particularly with omeprazole, is variable. Case reports suggest that esomeprazole might interact with tacrolimus similarly. Both proton pump inhibitors and tacrolimus can cause hypomagnesaemia and these effects might be additive when they are used together.

> Until more is known, it might be prudent to be alert for the possibility of an interaction with any proton pump inhibitor, and consider increasing monitoring of tacrolimus concentrations. Some evidence suggest that rabeprazole is unlikely to interact and could be a suitable alternative, but this needs confirmation. Consider monitoring magnesium concentrations before, and annually during, proton pump inhibitor use, and if symptoms of hypomagnesaemia (e.g. muscle twitching or cramps, tremors, vomiting, tiredness, or loss of appetite) occur. In those patients who develop hypomagnesaemia, oral and parenteral magnesium supplements might not be as effective as anticipated. Stopping the proton pump inhibitor (where possible) might be necessary.

Proton pump inhibitors + Warfarin and related oral anticoagulants

Omeprazole causes a minor increase in the anticoagulant effect of warfarin. Conversely, in studies dexlansoprazole, lansoprazole, pantoprazole, and rabeprazole did not alter warfarin pharmacokinetics or its anticoagulant effect, although cases of an enhanced effect have been reported. Esomeprazole and lansoprazole appear to increase the risk of overanticoagulation with acenocoumarol, but omeprazole, pantoprazole and rabeprazole do not, although a case of an enhanced effect have been reported with acenocoumarol and omeprazole. Omeprazole and pantoprazole does not appear to alter the effects of phenprocoumon.

The very minor pharmacokinetic interaction between omeprazole and warfarin is probably of limited clinical relevance. It is possible that the isolated cases of interactions with proton pump inhibitors just represent idiosyncratic effects attributable to other factors, and not to any interaction with warfarin. Nevertheless, it would seem prudent to bear in mind that rarely bleeding can occur. Note that some manufacturers of the proton pump inhibitors recommend monitoring the INR in all patients taking a coumarin.

P

Pyrimethamine

Pyrimethamine + Sulfonamides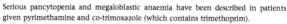

Serious pancytopenia and megaloblastic anaemia have been described in patients given pyrimethamine and either co-trimoxazole (which contains sulfamethoxazole) or other sulfonamides.

Pyrimethamine is usually given with a sulfonamide for toxoplasmosis and malaria. Nevertheless, caution should be used , especially in the presence of other drugs (e. g. methotrexate) or disease states that predispose to folate deficiency. When high-dose pyrimethamine is used for the treatment of toxoplasmosis, the manufacturer recommends that all patients should receive a folate supplement. Note that the US manufacturer of sulfadoxine with pyrimethamine recommended that the concurrent use of sulfonamides (including co-trimoxazole) should be avoided.

Pyrimethamine + Trimethoprim

Serious pancytopenia and megaloblastic anaemia have been described in patients given pyrimethamine and co-trimoxazole (which contains trimethoprim).

Caution should be used, especially in the presence of other drugs (e.g. methotrexate) or disease states that can predispose to folate deficiency. When high-dose pyrimethamine is used for the treatment of toxoplasmosis, the manufacturer recommends that all patients should receive a folate supplement. Note that the US manufacturer of sulfadoxine with pyrimethamine recommended that the concurrent use of trimethoprim should be avoided.

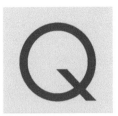

Quinidine

Quinidine + Rifabutin

The levels of quinidine and its therapeutic effects can be markedly reduced by *rifampicin*. In one case quinidine levels were reduced from 4 to 0.5 micrograms/mL. Rifabutin is predicted to interact similarly, but probably to a lesser extent.

> A quinidine dose increase may be necessary if rifabutin is given. Monitor concurrent use (including quinidine levels, where possible) and adjust the dose as necessary.

Quinidine + Rifampicin (Rifampin)

The levels of quinidine and its therapeutic effects can be markedly reduced by rifampicin. In one case quinidine levels were reduced from 4 to 0.5 micrograms/mL.

> The dose of quinidine will need to be increased (possibly more than doubled in some patients) if rifampicin is given concurrently. The quinidine dose will need to be reduced when the rifampicin is stopped. Monitor quinidine levels where possible.

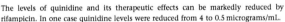

Quinidine + Tamoxifen

Paroxetine reduces the metabolism of tamoxifen to one of its active metabolites (by inhibiting CYP2D6): this might decrease the efficacy of tamoxifen and possibly increase the risk of breast cancer recurrence. The MHRA predicts that other CYP2D6 inhibitors (such as quinidine) might possibly interact similarly.

> The European Medicines Agency and the MHRA in the UK state that concurrent of CYP2D6 inhibitors use should be avoided whenever possible in patients taking tamoxifen, and they specifically name quinidine. Consider alternatives to tamoxifen in patients clearly benefiting from quinidine.

Quinidine + Ticagrelor

Quinidine might increase ticagrelor exposure.

> The UK manufacturer recommends that concurrent use is avoided, but if both drugs are given, monitor for increased ticagrelor effects (e.g. bleeding).

Quinidine + Tricyclics ⚠

Quinidine can significantly reduce the clearance of some tricyclics (desipramine, imipramine, nortriptyline and trimipramine), thereby increasing their levels, to varying degrees.

This interaction is expected to be clinically relevant with nortriptyline, and possibly desipramine, but probably not with imipramine. Monitor for signs of tricyclic adverse effects (dry mouth, urinary retention, constipation) on concurrent use. Additive QT-prolonging effects are also possible, see drugs that prolong the QT interval, page 352.

Quinidine + Warfarin and related oral anticoagulants ✓

Quinidine does not appear to alter the anticoagulant effect of warfarin. However, a few isolated cases of decreased anticoagulant effects and increased anticoagulant effects with bleeding have been reported.

No interaction would normally be anticipated.

Quinine

Quinine + Rifampicin (Rifampin) ⚠

Rifampicin increases the clearance of quinine.

It has been suggested that rifampicin should not be given with quinine for the treatment of malaria. Increased quinine doses should be considered if the concurrent use of rifampicin is essential: monitor concurrent use carefully to assess efficacy.

Quinine + Warfarin and related oral anticoagulants ❓

Normally no significant interaction occurs between warfarin and quinine but two women required warfarin dose reductions and one man taking phenprocoumon developed extensive haematuria after drinking large amounts of quinine-containing tonic water.

Any interaction seems rare, but bear it in mind in case of unexpected bleeding.

Quinolones

The quinolones are generally considered to be inhibitors of CYP1A2; however, it should be noted that they vary in the strength of this effect. Quinolones that are more potent inhibitors of CYP1A2 are likely to have greater effects on substrates of this isoenzyme, and therefore their use seems more likely to be associated with greater clinical consequences. Caffeine is used as a probe substrate for CYP1A2. Therefore the magnitude of the effect the quinolones have on caffeine can be used as a guide to the strength of their effect on CYP1A2. The interactions of the quinolones with caffeine suggests that enoxacin has the greatest effects, ciprofloxacin and pipemidic acid have moderate effects, while gatifloxacin, levofloxacin, lomefloxacin, moxifloxacin, nalidixic acid, norfloxacin, ofloxacin, pefloxacin, rufloxacin and sparfloxacin only inhibit CYP1A2 to a small or clinically irrelevant extent.

Quinolones + Roflumilast

Enoxacin increases the exposure to roflumilast and its active metabolite, roflumilast *N*-oxide, and also increases its phosphodiesterase type-4 inhibitory effect. Ciprofloxacin (and other quinolones that inhibit CYP1A2) might also interact, although to a lesser extent than enoxacin.

> Some patients might develop roflumilast adverse effects (such as nausea, diarrhoea, headache). Be alert for these and, if possible, adjust the roflumilast dose as necessary.

Quinolones + Sevelamer

Sevelamer reduced the bioavailability of ciprofloxacin by 48% in one study. It seems possible that other quinolones could be similarly affected.

> The manufacturers advise that ciprofloxacin should be taken at least one hour before or 3 hours after sevelamer. Until more is known, it would seem prudent to apply this advice to all quinolones.

Quinolones + Strontium

The manufacturer of strontium predicts that it will form a complex with quinolones, and therefore prevent their absorption.

> It is recommended that when treatment with a quinolone is required, strontium ranelate should be temporarily suspended.

Quinolones + Sucralfate

Sucralfate causes a marked reduction in the absorption of ciprofloxacin, enoxacin, gemifloxacin, lomefloxacin, moxifloxacin, ofloxacin, norfloxacin, and sparfloxacin, which may lead to therapeutic failure. It seems possible that other quinolones could be similarly affected.

> Separate the doses as much as possible, giving the quinolone first. The manufacturer advises that ciprofloxacin should be given 1 to 2 hours before or 4 hours after sucralfate. The UK manufacturer of moxifloxacin advises separating administration by 6 hours, whilst the US manufacturer recommends that moxifloxacin is taken at least 4 hours before or 8 hours after sucralfate. Proton pump inhibitors and H₂-receptor antagonists do not normally interact with the quinolones and may therefore be possible alternatives in some patients.

Quinolones + Theophylline

Theophylline concentrations can be moderately to markedly increased in most patients by enoxacin. Pipemidic acid is likely to interact similarly. Theophylline concentrations can also be increased in some patients by ciprofloxacin, and possibly by pefloxacin. Norfloxacin and ofloxacin normally cause a much smaller rise in theophylline concentrations, although serious toxicity has been seen in a few patients taking norfloxacin. Convulsions have been reported with theophylline and cipro-floxacin, norfloxacin, or pefloxacin. With some of these cases it is difficult to know if this was due to increased theophylline concentration, to patient predisposition, to potential additive effects on the seizure threshold, or to all three factors combined. Aminophylline would be expected to interact similarly.

Monitor the theophylline concentration closely. The theophylline dose should be modified based on the theophylline concentration on day 2 of quinolone use. Theophylline dose reductions of 50 to 75% have been suggested for enoxacin, and 30 to 50% for ciprofloxacin, although this is not always needed. It might be prudent to follow similar precautions with ofloxacin, pipemidic acid, and norfloxacin. Seizures resulting from concurrent use are relatively rare. Gatiflox-acin, levofloxacin, lomefloxacin, moxifloxacin, nalidixic acid, and sparfloxacin appear not to significantly affect the theophylline concentration and might therefore be suitable alternatives in some cases.

Quinolones + Tizanidine

Ciprofloxacin markedly increases tizanidine exposure, which increases the hypoten-sive and sedative effects of tizanidine. Other quinolones might also interact, see quinolones, page 564.

Concurrent use of ciprofloxacin with tizanidine is contraindicated, and the UK and US manufacturers state that concurrent use of enoxacin and norfloxacin should generally be avoided, or undertaken with caution. If concurrent use is necessary, anticipate the need to reduce the tizanidine dose before starting ciprofloxacin, and if starting tizanidine, start with the lowest dose, increasing gradually according to clinical response. Closely monitor for adverse effects such as marked hypotension, bradycardia, and sedation. Note that tizanidine and some quinolones have been associated with QT prolongation, see Drugs that prolong the QT interval, page 352 for more information.

Quinolones + Triptans

Quinolones are predicted to increase the plasma concentration of zolmitriptan.

The UK manufacturer recommends a dose reduction of zolmitriptan to a maximum of 5 mg in 24 hours in patients taking quinolones, such as ciproflox-acin. Other quinolones might interact to varying extents, see quinolones, page 564.

Quinolones + Warfarin and related oral anticoagulants

The quinolones do not normally alter the effects of the coumarins in most patients, but increased effects and even bleeding have been seen in some patients.

It would be prudent to monitor the effects of concurrent use. Monitor the INR within 3 to 5 days of starting the quinolone.

Quinolones + Zinc ⚠

Limited evidence suggests zinc interacts like iron, page 450 to reduce quinolone levels.

As the quinolones are rapidly absorbed, taking them 2 hours before the zinc should minimise the risk of admixture in the gut and largely avoid this interaction.

Q

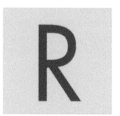

R

Raloxifene

Raloxifene + Warfarin and related oral anticoagulants ⚠

Raloxifene may cause a minor increase in warfarin levels. However, a 10% decrease in prothrombin time may also occur. The manufacturers report that modest changes in prothrombin times may occur over a period of several weeks. Other coumarins would be expected to be similarly affected.

The manufacturers recommend that prothrombin times should be monitored on the concurrent use of coumarin anticoagulants.

Raltegravir

Raltegravir + Rifampicin (Rifampin) ⚠

Rifampicin reduces raltegravir exposure and minimum concentrations; doubling the raltegravir dose does not minimise the effect on its minimum concentration.

If concurrent use cannot be avoided, the UK and US manufacturers of raltegravir suggest doubling the raltegravir dose; however, note that the raltegravir minimum concentration might still be low. Monitor the virological response closely.

Ranolazine

Ranolazine + Rifabutin ⚠

Rifampicin (rifampin) reduces ranolazine levels by 95%, and loss of efficacy is expected. Rifabutin is predicted to interact in the same way as rifampicin.

The manufacturers recommend avoiding concurrent use. In the absence of any information on the magnitude of the effect of rifabutin on ranolazine levels, this seems prudent.

Ranolazine + **Rifampicin (Rifampin)**

Rifampicin reduces ranolazine levels by 95%, and loss of efficacy is expected.

The manufacturers contraindicate concurrent use.

Ranolazine + **SSRIs**

Paroxetine increases ranolazine levels, but the effects are only slight.

No dose adjustments would be expected to be necessary on concurrent use. Note that ranolazine and some SSRIs can prolong the QT interval, see Drugs that prolong the QT interval, page 352 for further information.

R

Ranolazine + **Statins**

Ranolazine increases the exposure to simvastatin. Other statins that are similarly metabolised (lovastatin and to a lesser extent, atorvastatin) might also be affected. Cases of rhabdomyolysis have been reported for simvastatin in which ranolazine may have been a contributing factor.

The increased simvastatin exposure seen appears to be slight; however, it might be clinically relevant in some patients. The US manufacturer of simvastatin recommends a maximum dose of 20 mg daily in patients taking ranolazine. All patients taking statins should be warned about the symptoms of myopathy and advised to report muscle pain or weakness. It would be prudent to reinforce this advice if patients given simvastatin, lovastatin, and possibly atorvastatin, are also given ranolazine.

Ranolazine + **Tricyclics**

Ranolazine increases the levels of *metoprolol* by about 80% (by inhibiting CYP2D6). The manufacturers predict that the tricyclics, which are metabolised, at least in part, by CYP2D6 will be similarly affected.

Be aware of a possible interaction if tricyclic adverse effects (nausea, dry mouth, urinary retention) increase. The manufacturer of ranolazine suggests a dose reduction of the tricyclic may be needed. Note that ranolazine prolongs the QT interval, and effect that may be additive with some tricyclics, see drugs that prolong the QT interval, page 352.

Reboxetine

Reboxetine + SSRIs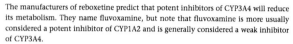

The manufacturers of reboxetine predict that potent inhibitors of CYP3A4 will reduce its metabolism. They name fluvoxamine, but note that fluvoxamine is more usually considered a potent inhibitor of CYP1A2 and is generally considered a weak inhibitor of CYP3A4.

> The manufacturers say that concurrent use of fluvoxamine should be avoided, although this appears to be over-cautious.

Retinoids

Retinoids + Tetracyclines ⊗

Additive increased intracranial pressure might occur on the concurrent use of tetracyclines and retinoids.

> Avoid concurrent use.

Retinoids + Vitamins ⚠

A condition similar to vitamin A (retinol) overdose may occur if oral retinoids such as acitretin, alitretinoin, isotretinoin or tretinoin are given with vitamin A.

> The UK and US manufacturers of acitretin advise avoiding the concurrent use of high-dose vitamin A: in the UK, they advise no more than 4000 to 5000 units of vitamin A daily, which is the recommended daily allowance, and in the US they advise doses of no more than the minimum recommended daily allowance. Similarly, the UK manufacturers of oral alitretinoin, and the UK and US manufacturers of isotretinoin and oral tretinoin state that vitamin A should be avoided.

Rifabutin

Rifabutin + Sirolimus ⚠

Rifabutin is predicted to reduce sirolimus concentrations.

> The UK and US manufacturers of sirolimus state that concurrent use is not recommended. If both drugs are given, monitor sirolimus concentrations closely and adjust the dose as necessary.

Rifabutin + Tacrolimus

Rifabutin is predicted to increase tacrolimus concentrations.

Tacrolimus concentrations and effects (e.g. on renal function) should be monitored as a matter of routine, but it is advisable to increase monitoring if rifabutin is started or stopped, adjusting the dose of tacrolimus as necessary.

Rifabutin + Ulipristal

The UK and US manufacturers of ulipristal predict that CYP3A4 inducers such as *rifampicin* might reduce the plasma concentrations of ulipristal and reduce its efficacy. Rifabutin would be expected to interact similarly, although to a lesser extent than rifampicin.

The US manufacturer of ulipristal gives no specific advice about how to manage this potential interaction, whereas the UK manufacturer advises that ulipristal should not be used for emergency contraception in women taking CYP3A4 inducers (such as rifabutin), or who have stopped taking an enzyme inducer within the last 2 to 3 weeks. Until more is known, this advice seems prudent.

Rifabutin + Warfarin and related oral anticoagulants

The anticoagulant effects of warfarin are markedly reduced by *rifampicin (rifampin)*. Other coumarins may be similarly affected. The manufacturers and the CSM in the UK therefore warn that rifabutin may reduce the effects of oral anticoagulants, although it is likely to interact to a lesser degree.

Expect any interaction to occur within 7 days of starting rifabutin. It may persist for several weeks after the rifabutin is stopped. Monitor the INR closely.

Rifampicin (Rifampin)

Of the rifamycins, rifampicin (rifampin) is the best studied; it is known to potently inhibit a number of cytochrome P450 isoenzymes. There is much less data available for rifapentine, but it is known to be a moderate enzyme inducer. Therefore some have predicted that it will interact with other drugs in the same way as rifampicin, although this is likely to be to a lesser extent.

Rifampicin (Rifampin) + Rivaroxaban

Rifampicin reduces rivaroxaban exposure and therefore decreases its anticoagulant effects.

Given the likely clinical risk of reduced rivaroxaban efficacy, it would seem prudent to consider using an alternative drug; however, if this is not possible, consider closely monitoring the prothrombin time to ensure the anticoagulant effect of rivaroxaban is maintained in patients given these drugs. The US manufacturer of rivaroxaban advises avoiding concurrent use.

Rifampicin (Rifampin) + Roflumilast

Rifampicin increases the metabolism of roflumilast to its active metabolite, roflumilast N-oxide, but decreases the overall bioavailability of roflumilast N-oxide, resulting in a decrease in its phosphodiesterase inhibitory effects.

Monitor concurrent use to ensure that roflumilast is effective, and consider increasing the dose of roflumilast according to clinical need.

Rifampicin (Rifampin) + Sirolimus

Rifampicin greatly decreases sirolimus concentrations.

The UK and US manufacturers of sirolimus state that concurrent use is not recommended. If both drugs are given, monitor sirolimus concentrations closely and adjust the dose as necessary.

Rifampicin (Rifampin) + Solifenacin

The manufacturers predict that CYP3A4 inducers, such as rifampicin, will reduce solifenacin levels.

Monitor the outcome of concurrent use to ensure that solifenacin is effective and adjust the dose if necessary.

Rifampicin (Rifampin) + SSRIs

In two cases rifampicin decreased the efficacy of citalopram and sertraline. In theory rifampicin could similarly affect other SSRIs but there appear to be no reports of this.

Information is limited. The dose adjustment of any SSRI on starting or stopping rifampicin should be guided by clinical effect. Be alert for evidence of SSRI withdrawal symptoms of loss of effect.

Rifampicin (Rifampin) + Statins

In studies where the administration of the statin and rifampicin (at steady state) were separated, rifampicin markedly to very markedly reduced the exposure to atorvastatin and simvastatin. However, when rifampicin (at steady state) and atorvastatin are given simultaneously the exposure to atorvastatin is slightly *increased*. Steady-state rifampicin appears to slightly to moderately reduce fluvastatin exposure, and slightly increase steady-state pitavastatin exposure.

The UK and US manufacturers of atorvastatin recommend that, if concurrent use cannot be avoided, the atorvastatin should be taken at the same time as rifampicin. This advice seems prudent when rifampicin is at steady state. However, as *single-dose* rifampicin given simultaneously with atorvastatin increases atorvastatin exposure, some caution might be appropriate for the first few days of concurrent use, or when short courses of single doses of rifampicin are given. In this situation, separating administration might be prudent. The increase in pitavastatin exposure would not be expected to be clinically relevant. Nevertheless, the manufacturer limits the maximum pitavastatin dose to 2 mg daily when taken with rifampicin. If simvastatin is given separately to steady-state rifampicin, it would be likely that a simvastatin dose increase would be required to maintain efficacy: the effects of simultaneous dosing do not appear to have been studied. Until more is known about the other statins, it would seem prudent to monitor the concurrent use of rifampicin, keeping the dose interval constant, and adjusting the statin dose according to clinical response.

Rifampicin (Rifampin) + Sulfonamides

Rifampicin modestly reduces the AUC of sulfamethoxazole (given as co-trimoxazole) by 28% in HIV-positive subjects.

> This would not be expected to be clinically relevant with sulfamethoxazole alone; however, a greater effect is seen on trimethoprim levels, which may affect the efficacy when sulfamethoxazole is given as co-trimoxazole, see co-trimoxazole, page 311. The effect of rifampicin on other sulfonamides does not appear to have been studied.

Rifampicin (Rifampin) + Tacrolimus

Rifampicin decreases the exposure to tacrolimus after oral and intravenous administration.

> Anticipate the need to increase the dose of tacrolimus, sometimes greatly, if rifampicin is given to any patient taking tacrolimus concurrently. Tacrolimus concentrations and effects (e.g. on renal function) should be monitored as a matter of routine, but it is essential to increase monitoring if rifampicin is started or stopped in order to avoid the risk of transplant rejection.

Rifampicin (Rifampin) + Tamoxifen

Rifampicin increased the metabolism of tamoxifen in one study (in men). The efficacy of tamoxifen would be expected to be reduced, however this does not appear to have been studied.

> Further study is needed to assess the clinical impact of the long-term concurrent use of these drugs. Until more is known, it would be prudent to be cautious with the use of rifampicin in women taking tamoxifen.

Rifampicin (Rifampin) + Terbinafine

The exposure to terbinafine is reduced by rifampicin.

> Terbinafine seems likely to be less effective in the presence of rifampicin. Monitor carefully and consider increasing the terbinafine dose if necessary.

Rifampicin (Rifampin) + Tetracyclines

Rifampicin may cause a marked reduction in doxycycline exposure (AUC reported to be reduced by 60% in one study), which has led to treatment failures in some cases.

Monitor the effects of concurrent use and increase the doxycycline dose as necessary.

Rifampicin (Rifampin) + Theophylline

Rifampicin increases the clearance of theophylline (given either as aminophylline or theophylline) by up to about 85%. In one study rifampicin (with isoniazid) increased theophylline clearance during the initial few days of treatment, but another study suggested that these antimycobacterials decreased theophylline clearance within 4 weeks.

Monitor the theophylline concentration. An effect has been seen within 36 hours of starting rifampicin. Expect to need to increase the aminophylline or theophylline dose. The picture is less clear when isoniazid is also taken. In this situation it would seem prudent to monitor the theophylline concentration closely for the first month of treatment.

Rifampicin (Rifampin) + Ticagrelor

Rifampicin decreases ticagrelor exposure.

If concurrent use is unavoidable, be alert for reduced ticagrelor efficacy.

Rifampicin (Rifampin) + Toremifene

Rifampicin decreases toremifene exposure, and might be expected to reduce its efficacy.

Monitor the outcome of concurrent use to ensure toremifene remains effective. The UK manufacturer of toremifene suggests that the toremifene dose might need to be doubled.

Rifampicin (Rifampin) + Trimethoprim

Rifampicin reduces the AUC of trimethoprim (given as co-trimoxazole) by 56% in HIV-positive subjects, but apparently has no effect on trimethoprim alone in healthy subjects.

The interaction between rifampicin and trimethoprim seems unlikely to be relevant in subjects who are not infected with HIV. Consider also co-trimoxazole, page 311.

Rifampicin (Rifampin) + Ulipristal

The UK manufacturers of ulipristal briefly note that, in a study in healthy subjects, rifampicin decreased the plasma concentrations of ulipristal and reduced its efficacy.

The US manufacturer of ulipristal gives no specific advice about how to manage this potential interaction, whereas the UK manufacturer advises that ulipristal should not be used for emergency contraception or the symptomatic management of fibroids in women taking CYP3A4 inducers (such as rifampicin), or who have stopped taking an enzyme inducer within the last 2 to 3 weeks. Until more is known, this advice seems prudent.

Rifampicin (Rifampin) + Warfarin and related oral anticoagulants ⚠

The anticoagulant effects of acenocoumarol, phenprocoumon and warfarin are markedly reduced by rifampicin.

A marked reduction occurs within 5 to 7 days of starting rifampicin, persisting for up to 5 weeks after the rifampicin is stopped. Monitor the INR closely. The warfarin dose may need to be markedly increased (2- to 5-fold) over a number of weeks. Remember to re-adjust the coumarin dose when rifampicin is stopped.

R

Riociguat

Riociguat + Theophylline

The US manufacturer predicts that the concurrent use of riociguat and theophylline will lead to hypotension. Aminophylline is expected to interact similarly.

Avoid concurrent use

Rivaroxaban

Rivaroxaban + Sulfinpyrazone ⚠

The concurrent use of antiplatelet drugs with rivaroxaban might theoretically increase the risk of bleeding.

If both drugs are essential, patients should be closely monitored for signs and symptoms of bleeding.

Rivaroxaban + Ticagrelor

The concurrent use of rivaroxaban and ticagrelor might increase the risk of bleeding.

It would be prudent to advise patients to be aware of increased bruising or prolonged bleeding, and to seek medical advice if this occurs.

Rivaroxaban + Ticlopidine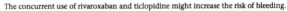

The concurrent use of rivaroxaban and ticlopidine might increase the risk of bleeding.

Advise patients to be aware of increased bruising or prolonged bleeding, and to seek medical advice if this occurs.

Rivaroxaban + Warfarin and related oral anticoagulants ⚠

The concurrent use of rivaroxaban and anticoagulants increases the risk of bleeding.

Monitor for signs of bleeding on concurrent use. The US manufacturer advises avoiding rivaroxaban for prophylaxis of deep vein thrombosis in patients taking anticoagulants. The UK manufacturer of rivaroxaban contraindicates concurrent use unless switching between anticoagulants.

Roflumilast

Roflumilast + SSRIs ❓

The exposure to roflumilast and its active metabolite, roflumilast N-oxide, is increased by fluvoxamine, resulting in an overall increase in its total phosphodiesterase inhibitory effects.

Some patients might develop roflumilast adverse effects (such as nausea, diarrhoea, headache). Be alert for these and if possible, adjust the roflumilast dose as necessary. Note that roflumilast is associated with an increased risk of depression, and its use in those requiring antidepressants should be carefully considered.

Roflumilast + Theophylline ❓

Theophylline has been reported to slightly increase the exposure to roflumilast, but this does not affect its overall pharmacodynamic effect to a clinically relevant extent. Aminophylline would be expected to interact similarly.

Because of the lack of clinical efficacy data, the UK manufacturer suggests that concurrent use should be avoided.

Rufinamide

Rufinamide + Ulipristal ⚠

The UK and US manufacturers of ulipristal predict that CYP3A4 inducers (such as *phenytoin* and *carbamazepine*) might reduce the plasma concentration of ulipristal and reduce its efficacy. Rufinamide might interact similarly.

The US manufacturer of ulipristal gives no specific advice about how to manage this potential interaction, whereas the UK manufacturer advises that ulipristal should not be used for emergency contraception in women taking CYP3A4 inducers (such as rufinamide), or who have stopped taking an enzyme inducer within the last 2 to 3 weeks. Until more is known, this advice seems prudent.

Rufinamide + Valproate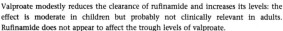

Valproate modestly reduces the clearance of rufinamide and increases its levels: the effect is moderate in children but probably not clinically relevant in adults. Rufinamide does not appear to affect the trough levels of valproate.

No dose adjustment is recommended for patients weighing more than 30 kg. In patients weighing less than 30 kg, the manufacturer advises starting rufinamide at 200 mg daily, and increasing the dose by no more than 200 mg every 2 days (according to clinical response and efficacy) until a maximum dose of 600 mg daily is achieved.

R

Rufinamide + Warfarin and related oral anticoagulants ⚠

The manufacturers of rufinamide predict that it may interact with warfarin by inducing CYP3A4. However, warfarin is only metabolised to a limited extent by this isoenzyme, and moderate CYP3A4 *inhibitors* do not generally interact with warfarin, although cases of bleeding may occur.

The manufacturers recommend monitoring for 2 weeks after starting, stopping, or changing the dose of rufinamide, and making dose adjustments as appropriate.

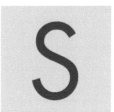

S

Salbutamol (Albuterol) and related bronchodilators

Salbutamol (Albuterol) and related bronchodilators + Theophylline ❓

The concurrent use of theophylline and beta$_2$ agonist bronchodilators, such as salbutamol, is a useful option in the management of asthma and chronic obstructive pulmonary disease, but potentiation of some adverse reactions can occur. The most serious of these are hypokalaemia and tachycardia, particularly with high-dose theophylline. Some patients might have a decrease in their theophylline concentration if given oral or intravenous salbutamol or intravenous isoprenaline (isoproterenol).

> Potassium should be monitored, particularly in acutely unwell patients receiving high-dose intravenous beta$_2$ agonists. The CSM in the UK particularly recommends monitoring potassium concentrations in those with severe asthma as the hypokalaemic effects of beta$_2$ agonists can be potentiated by concurrent use of theophylline, corticosteroids, and diuretics and by hypoxia.

Sevelamer

Sevelamer + Tacrolimus ⚠

Sevelamer reduced the absorption of tacrolimus in one patient (AUC *increased* 2.4-fold when sevelamer *stopped*).

> Tacrolimus levels should be closely monitored as a matter of routine; however, it may be prudent to increase monitoring when sevelamer is started or stopped, adjusting the tacrolimus dose as needed. The manufacturers advise that tacrolimus should be taken at least 1 hour before or 3 hours after sevelamer.

Sevelamer + Vitamin D

Sevelamer carbonate reduces the exposure to calcitriol.

Give calcitriol at least one hour before or 3 hours after sevelamer carbonate. Routine monitoring of the effect of calcitriol should determine if this sufficiently manages the interaction.

Sirolimus

Sirolimus + Vaccines

The body's immune response is suppressed by sirolimus. The antibody response to vaccines may be reduced and the use of live attenuated vaccines may result in generalised infection.

For many inactivated vaccines even the reduced response seen is considered clinically useful and, in the case of renal transplant patients, influenza vaccination is actively recommended. If a vaccine is given, it may be prudent to monitor the response, so that alternative prophylactic measures can be considered where the response is inadequate. Note that even where effective antibody titres are produced, these may not persist as long as in healthy subjects, and more frequent booster doses may be required. The use of live vaccines is generally considered to be contraindicated. Ideally vaccines should take place before immunosuppressive treatment is started, and live vaccines should not be given for up to 6 months after treatment has stopped.

Sodium oxybate

Sodium oxybate + Tricyclics

The UK manufacturer of sodium oxybate states that the rate of adverse events was increased when it was given with tricyclic antidepressants.

Concurrent use need not be avoided, but consider the interaction if adverse effects become troublesome.

Sodium oxybate + Valproate

The UK manufacturer of sodium oxybate predicts that valproate might affect its metabolism, however there are no clinical studies to confirm this prediction.

Monitor concurrent use, and adjust the dose of sodium oxybate as needed.

SSRIs

Although the SSRIs are likely to share pharmacodynamic interactions (for example development of serotonin syndrome with other serotonergic drugs) they do have differing effects on cytochrome P450, which leads to different metabolic actions. Fluvoxamine is a potent inhibitor of CYP1A2, whereas fluoxetine and paroxetine have

S

moderate inhibitory effects on CYP2D6. Citalopram (and therefore probably escitalopram) and sertraline only weakly inhibit this isoenzyme.

Serotonin syndrome

Serotonin syndrome is thought to result from the over-stimulation of the $5-HT_{1A}$ and $5-HT_{2A}$ receptors and possibly other serotonin receptors in the central nervous system. It can, exceptionally, occur with the use of one drug, but much more usually it develops when two or more drugs with serotonergic actions are given together. The characteristic symptoms fall into three main areas, namely altered mental status (agitation, confusion, mania), autonomic dysfunction (diaphoresis, diarrhoea, fever, shivering) and neuromuscular abnormalities (hyperreflexia, incoordination, myoclonus, tremor). Serotonin syndrome usually resolves within about 24 hours if the offending drugs are withdrawn and supportive measures given. Most patients recover uneventfully, but there have been a few fatalities. Many drugs have serotonergic actions, but the advice on concurrent use of these drugs varies greatly between manufacturers. The SSRIs are amongst the most commonly implicated drugs, and it is generally advised that the concurrent use of serotonergic drugs with SSRIs should be undertaken with caution. The most practical approach therefore seems to be to monitor for potential symptoms, and to seek medical advice should they occur.

SSRIs + Tacrine ⚠

Fluvoxamine can increase the AUC of tacrine by up to 8-fold. Tacrine adverse effects (nausea, vomiting, diarrhoea, sweating) are increased.

> It is likely that standard tacrine doses will be poorly tolerated and a decrease in the tacrine dose will probably be needed. Other SSRIs such as fluoxetine, paroxetine, or sertraline, may theoretically be suitable alternatives, as these are unlikely to inhibit tacrine metabolism.

SSRIs + Tamoxifen ✖

Paroxetine, a CYP2D6 inhibitor, reduces the metabolism of tamoxifen to one of its active metabolites and it has been suggested that this might decrease the efficacy of tamoxifen. Several case-control studies and one retrospective cohort study investigating the effects of SSRIs on tamoxifen have not found an increase in breast cancer recurrence, although one case-control study with CYP2D6 inhibitors did suggest an increased recurrence. In addition, one retrospective cohort study reported an increased risk of breast cancer recurrence in patients taking paroxetine with tamoxifen.

> Many commentators suggest that paroxetine (and therefore probably fluoxetine, which has similar CYP2D6 inhibitory potential) should be avoided. Given that alternatives to these SSRIs are available, and given the potential seriousness of the proposed interaction, until the risks are established, it would seem prudent to use an alternative SSRI (such as citalopram) or perhaps the SNRI, venlafaxine, which have a low potential for affecting CYP2D6.

SSRIs + Terbinafine ❓

Terbinafine modestly increased paroxetine levels in one study. Other SSRIs may interact similarly.

> The clinical relevance of this interaction is unclear; increases of the magnitude

seen would seem likely to increase adverse effects, although this was not seen in one study. Nevertheless be alert for an increase in SSRI adverse effects, and consider reducing the dose if these become troublesome.

SSRIs + Theophylline ⚠️

Exposure to theophylline (given as aminophylline or theophylline) can be rapidly increased (to almost 3-fold in one study) by the concurrent use of fluvoxamine. Toxicity has occurred.

Ideally concurrent use should be avoided. If this is not possible, reduce the theophylline (or aminophylline) dose by half when fluvoxamine is added, and monitor the outcome of concurrent use on the theophylline concentration carefully. Citalopram (and therefore probably escitalopram), fluoxetine, paroxetine, and sertraline are not expected to interact, and might therefore be suitable alternatives.

SSRIs + Ticagrelor ❓

The bleeding risk associated with antiplatelet drugs such as ticlopidine might be further increased by the concurrent use of an SSRI, although the data appears to be conflicting.

In general, the manufacturers of the SSRIs advise caution on the concurrent use of drugs that affect platelet function, such as ticagrelor. Consider giving gastro-protective drugs to those at high risk of gastrointestinal bleeding (e.g. the elderly, those with a history of gastrointestinal bleeding, patients taking multiple antiplatelet drugs). Advise patients to report any signs of excessive bleeding.

SSRIs + Ticlopidine ❓

The bleeding risk associated with antiplatelet drugs such as ticlopidine might be further increased by the concurrent use of an SSRI, although the data appears to be conflicting.

In general, the manufacturers of the SSRIs advise caution on the concurrent use of drugs that affect platelet function, such as ticlopidine. Consider giving gastro-protective drugs to those at high risk of gastrointestinal bleeding (e.g. the elderly, those with a history of gastrointestinal bleeding, patients taking multiple antiplatelet drugs). Advise patients to report any signs of excessive bleeding.

SSRIs + Tizanidine ❌

Fluvoxamine causes a very marked increase in tizanidine exposure with a consequent increase in its adverse effects such as hypotension, bradycardia, and sedation.

Concurrent use is contraindicated. Consider changing fluvoxamine to another SSRI, as they are not expected to affect tizanidine metabolism to a clinically relevant extent. Note that tizanidine and some SSRIs can prolong the QT interval, see Drugs that prolong the QT interval, page 352 for further information.

SSRIs + Trazodone ⚠

Trazodone and fluoxetine have been used concurrently with advantage, although fluoxetine might modestly increase trazodone concentrations, and some patients have developed increased adverse effects. Additive adverse effects such as sedation are predicted to possibly occur with other SSRIs.

> It would be prudent to monitor for an increase in adverse effects (such as dysarthria, tremor and sedation) when trazodone is used with any SSRI. Note that trazodone and some SSRIs (escitalopram and citalopram) have been associated with QT prolongation, see Drugs that prolong the QT interval, page 352 for more information.

SSRIs + Tricyclics ⚠

The concentrations of the tricyclic antidepressants can be increased by the SSRIs, but the extent varies greatly, from 20% to 10-fold: fluvoxamine, fluoxetine, and paroxetine appear to cause the greatest increase. Tricyclic toxicity has been seen in a number of cases. Tricyclics can increase the concentrations of citalopram and possibly fluvoxamine, but the significance of this is unclear. There are several case reports of serotonin syndrome, page 580, following concurrent and even sequential use of the SSRIs and tricyclics.

> The increased tricyclic antidepressant concentrations can be beneficial. However, it has been suggested that patients given fluoxetine should have their tricyclic dose reduced to one quarter. Similar recommendations have been made with fluvoxamine (reduction in tricyclic dose to one-third) and sertraline. It would also seem prudent to consider a dose reduction of the tricyclic if paroxetine is added. Some suggest that a small initial dose of the SSRI should also be used. Patients taking any combination of tricyclic and SSRI should be monitored for adverse effects (e.g. dry mouth, sedation, confusion) with tricyclic concentrations monitored where possible. Note that the active metabolite of fluoxetine has a half-life of 7 to 15 days, and so any interaction can persist for some time after the fluoxetine is withdrawn, and might therefore occur on sequential use. The UK manufacturer of clomipramine advises a washout period of 2 to 3 weeks before and after treatment with fluoxetine. Serotonin syndrome seems to occur rarely, but patients and prescribers should be aware of the symptoms so that prompt action can be taken if problems occur. Note that some tricyclics and some SSRIs can prolong the QT interval, see Drugs that prolong the QT interval, page 352 for further information.

SSRIs + Triptans ⚠

The concurrent use of a triptan and an SSRI is normally uneventful, but adverse reactions (such as serotonin syndrome, page 580, reported with sumatriptan and some SSRIs) do occasionally occur. Fluvoxamine has been shown to inhibit the metabolism of frovatriptan, and is predicted to inhibit the metabolism of zolmitriptan.

> The combination need not be avoided, but monitor carefully for signs of serotonin syndrome (such as weakness, hyperreflexia, and incoordination), especially during treatment initiation and dose increases, and if other serotonergic drugs are also used. Because of the elevated triptan concentrations, reactions seem more likely on concurrent use of fluvoxamine with zolmitriptan or frovatriptan. The manufacturers of zolmitriptan recommend a dose reduction to a maximum of 5 mg in 24 hours in the presence of fluvoxamine. Caution and strict adherence to the recommended dose is also advised with frovatriptan.

SSRIs + Tryptophan

Central and peripheral toxicity developed in a number of patients taking fluoxetine with tryptophan and adverse effects (headache, nausea, sweating, and dizziness) have been reported with concurrent use of paroxetine. On theoretical grounds, an adverse reaction (such as serotonin syndrome, page 580) seems possible between any SSRI and tryptophan.

> The combination is probably best avoided; however, if tryptophan is given with an SSRI, the SSRI should be started at a low dose and tryptophan gradually introduced, starting with a low dose. Patients should be closely monitored for adverse effects.

SSRIs + Venlafaxine

The manufacturer of venlafaxine cautions its use with SSRIs because of the potential risks of serotonin syndrome. Cases of this reaction have been reported. Additive antimuscarinic effects have also been seen.

> Monitor concurrent use carefully. Patients should told to report any symptoms of serotonin syndrome, page 580 and antimuscarinic adverse effects (such as dry mouth, blurred vision and urinary retention).

SSRIs + Warfarin and related oral anticoagulants

Fluvoxamine

Warfarin concentrations can be increased by fluvoxamine. Increased INRs have been seen in several cases when fluvoxamine was given with coumarins or indanediones.

> It might be prudent to monitor the INR when fluvoxamine is first added, being alert for the need to decrease the anticoagulant dose.

Other SSRIs

Isolated reports describe raised INRs and/or haemorrhage in patients taking SSRIs with coumarins or indanediones, although no pharmacokinetic interaction appears to occur. SSRIs alone have, rarely, been associated with bleeding.

As SSRIs alone can rarely cause bleeding, caution is advised with the concurrent use of oral anticoagulants and SSRIs; consider monitoring with other SSRIs, but note only a few patients appear to have demonstrated this interaction.

Statins

Lovastatin and simvastatin are extensively metabolised by CYP3A4 so that drugs that moderately or potently inhibit this enzyme can cause marked rises in statin levels. Atorvastatin is also metabolised by CYP3A4, but to a lesser extent than lovastatin or simvastatin. Fluvastatin is metabolised primarily by CYP2C9, rosuvastatin by CYP2C9 and CYP2C19, while the cytochrome P450 system does not appear to be involved in the metabolism of pravastatin. Therefore the statins tend to interact differently. In order to reduce the risk of myopathy the CSM in the UK advises that statins should be used with care in patients who are at increased risk of this adverse effect, such as those taking interacting drugs. They also recommend that patients should be made aware of the risks of myopathy and rhabdomyolysis, and asked to promptly report muscle pain, tenderness or weakness, especially if accompanied by malaise, fever or dark urine.

Statins + Ticagrelor

Ticagrelor increases the exposure to simvastatin, and is predicted to have a similar effect on lovastatin.

> Use a maximum dose of simvastatin 40 mg daily and a maximum dose of lovastatin 40 mg daily in patients taking ticagrelor. If both drugs are given, advise patients to report any unexplained muscle pain, tenderness, or weakness.

Statins + Warfarin and related oral anticoagulants

Fluvastatin and Rosuvastatin

Studies and case reports have suggested that fluvastatin can increase warfarin levels and/or effects. Rosuvastatin can increase the anticoagulant effects of warfarin but does not alter warfarin levels. Not all patients are affected.

> Increased monitoring is required when starting or stopping fluvastatin or rosuvastatin, or changing the statin dose.

Other statins

Studies with atorvastatin, lovastatin, pravastatin, and simvastatin suggest that they do not usually significantly alter the effects of warfarin, although cases of bleeding have been seen when these statins were given with coumarins and fluindione.

> It has been suggested that it would be prudent to monitor the early stages of concurrent use of statins and anticoagulants in all patients, or if the dose of statin is changed, being alert for the need to adjust the anticoagulant dose, and many manufacturers recommend this. However, this interaction has only been clinically significant in a handful of patients, so monitoring every patient may be over-cautious. Note that pitavastatin does not appear to interact with warfarin, but the US manufacturer nevertheless advises that INR and prothrombin time should be monitored on concurrent use.

Strontium

Strontium + Tetracyclines

The manufacturer of strontium ranelate predicts that it will complex with tetracyclines, and therefore prevent their absorption.

> It is recommended that when treatment with a tetracycline is required, strontium ranelate should be temporarily suspended.

Sucralfate

Sucralfate + Tetracyclines

On theoretical grounds the absorption of tetracycline may possibly be reduced by sucralfate, but clinical confirmation of this appears to be lacking.

The manufacturers suggest that they should be given 2 hours apart to minimise their admixture in the gut.

Sucralfate + Theophylline

Two studies found that sucralfate caused only negligible changes in theophylline pharmacokinetics, but another suggests that the absorption of sustained-release theophylline is reduced by sucralfate.

Be alert for any evidence of a reduced response to theophylline on concurrent use. Give sucralfate 2 hours before or after a dose of aminophylline or theophylline.

Sucralfate + Warfarin and related oral anticoagulants ?

Case reports describe a marked reduction in the effects of warfarin in patients given sucralfate. Other evidence suggests that this interaction is uncommon.

Concurrent use need not be avoided but bear this interaction in mind if a patient has a reduced anticoagulant response to warfarin. Information about other anticoagulants is lacking, but be aware that a similar interaction is possible.

Sulfinpyrazone

Sulfinpyrazone + Theophylline

Sulfinpyrazone causes a small 22% increase in the clearance of theophylline.

This small reduction is unlikely to be clinically relevant.

Sulfinpyrazone + Warfarin and related oral anticoagulants ⚠

The anticoagulant effects of warfarin and acenocoumarol are increased by sulfinpyrazone and serious bleeding has occurred.

The INR should be well monitored and suitable anticoagulant dose reductions made. Halving the dose of warfarin and reducing the acenocoumarol dose by 20% has proven to be adequate in some patients. Bear in mind that the antiplatelet effects of sulfinpyrazone might increase the risk of bleeding with oral antic-oagulants.

Sulfonamides

Sulfonamides + Warfarin and related oral anticoagulants ⚠

The anticoagulant effects of warfarin, acenocoumarol, and phenprocoumon are increased by co-trimoxazole (sulfamethoxazole with trimethoprim). Bleeding may occur if the anticoagulant dose is not reduced appropriately. There is also evidence that sulfaphenazole, sulfafurazole (sulfisoxazole), and sulfamethizole might interact like co-trimoxazole. Anecdotal evidence suggests that phenindione might not interact with co-trimoxazole, but sulfaphenazole has been reported to increase the effects of phenindione.

The incidence of the interaction between coumarins and co-trimoxazole appears to be high. If bleeding is to be avoided the INR should be well monitored and the coumarin dose should be reduced. Some suggest avoiding concurrent use because of the difficulties with re-establishing anticoagulation. Phenindione is said not to interact; however, bear the case report of an interaction with sulfaphenazole in mind. The other interactions are poorly documented. However, it would seem prudent to follow the precautions suggested for co-trimoxazole if any sulfonamide is given with a coumarin or indanedione.

S

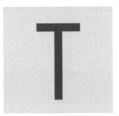

Tacrine

Tacrine + Theophylline

Limited evidence suggests that tacrine reduces the clearance of theophylline by about 50%. Aminophylline would be expected to be similarly affected.

Be alert for theophylline adverse effects (such as headache, nausea, and tremor) on concurrent use, and if indicated, monitor theophylline concentrations, reducing the theophylline or aminophylline dose accordingly.

Tacrine + Tizanidine

Tacrine is predicted to increase the exposure to tizanidine, increasing its hypotensive and sedative effects.

The UK and US manufacturers suggest that concurrent use should be avoided. Until more is known be alert for adverse effects such as bradycardia, hypotension, and drowsiness.

Tacrolimus

Tacrolimus + Vaccines

The body's immune response is suppressed by tacrolimus. The antibody response to vaccines may be reduced and the use of live attenuated vaccines may result in generalised infection.

For many inactivated vaccines even the reduced response seen is considered clinically useful and, in the case of renal transplant patients, influenza vaccination is actively recommended. If a vaccine is given, it may be prudent to monitor the response, so that alternative prophylactic measures can be considered where the response is inadequate. Note that even where effective antibody titres are produced, these may not persist as long as in healthy subjects, and more frequent booster doses may be required. The use of live vaccines is generally considered to be contraindicated. Ideally vaccines should take place before immunosuppressive treatment is started, and live vaccines should not be given for up to 6 months after treatment has stopped.

Tamoxifen

Tamoxifen + Tibolone ⊗

Tibolone increases the risk of recurrent breast cancer in women including those taking tamoxifen.

Concurrent use should be avoided.

Tamoxifen + Warfarin and related oral anticoagulants ⚠

Tamoxifen appears to increase the effects of warfarin and cases of serious bleeding, in one case fatal, have been reported. A case report describes a similar effect with acenocoumarol.

Monitor the effects closely if tamoxifen is given to patients taking warfarin or acenocoumarol, and reduce the dose as necessary. Reports indicate that, generally, a reduction of between one-half to two-thirds might be needed for warfarin. Consider also that, from a disease perspective, when treating venous thromboembolic disease in patients with cancer, warfarin is generally inferior (higher risk of major bleeds and recurrent thrombosis) to low-molecular-weight heparins.

Terbinafine

Terbinafine + Tricyclics ⚠

Terbinafine moderately increases the exposure to desipramine. Case reports describe increases in the serum concentrations of amitriptyline, desipramine, imipramine, and nortriptyline, with associated toxicity, in patients given oral terbinafine.

Monitor for any increase in the adverse effects of the tricyclic (e.g. dry mouth, blurred vision, constipation), and be aware that the dose may need to be decreased, sometimes substantially. Note that due to the long half-life of terbinafine, clinically significant interactions might occur if these tricyclics are given within 3 months of stopping terbinafine.

Terbinafine + Venlafaxine ?

The metabolism of venlafaxine to its active metabolite O-desmethylvenlafaxine is reduced in the presence of terbinafine. However, the combined AUC of venlafaxine and its metabolite is only raised by a modest 22%.

Until more is known, it may be prudent to be alert for any indication of increased venlafaxine adverse effects (e.g. nausea, insomnia, dry mouth) in patients also taking terbinafine.

Testosterone

Testosterone + Warfarin and related oral anticoagulants ⚠

A woman showed a 78% and a 65% increase in prothrombin times on two occasions when using a 2% testosterone propionate vaginal ointment twice daily concomitantly with warfarin. A 25% reduction in her warfarin dose was needed. Acenocoumarol and phenindione might interact similarly.

Until more is known it would seem prudent to increase the frequency of INR monitoring if testosterone is given with coumarins or indanediones.

Tetracyclines

Tetracyclines + Warfarin and related oral anticoagulants ⚠

Isolated cases suggest that doxycycline and tetracycline can increase the effects of coumarins. Similarly, some small studies (none controlled) suggest that chlortetracycline (alone or with oxytetracycline), doxycycline, or the tetracyclines as a class may increase the risks of over-anticoagulation.

The clinical importance of this interaction is unknown, but bear it in mind in case of an excessive response to anticoagulant treatment. If a patient is unwell enough to require an antibacterial, it may be prudent to increase monitoring of coagulation status even if no specific drug interaction is expected. Monitor within 3 days of starting the antibacterial.

Tetracyclines + Zinc ⚠

The absorption of tetracycline is reduced by up to 50% by zinc. All tetracyclines (with perhaps the exception of doxycycline) are expected to interact similarly.

Separate administration. In the case of *iron*, which interacts by the same mechanism, 2 to 3 hours is sufficient. Doxycycline may be a useful non-interacting alternative.

Theophylline

Theophylline is metabolised by cytochrome P450 in the liver, principally by CYP1A2. Many drugs interact with theophylline by inhibition or potentiation of its metabolism. Theophylline has a narrow therapeutic range, and small increases in serum concentrations can result in toxicity. Moreover, symptoms of serious toxicity such as convulsions and arrhythmias can occur before minor symptoms suggestive of toxicity. Furthermore, age, cigarette smoking, chronic obstructive airways disease, congestive heart failure, and liver disease (cirrhosis, acute hepatitis) can also affect theophylline clearance. Within the context of interactions, aminophylline is expected to behave like theophylline, because it is a complex of theophylline with ethylenediamine.

Theophylline + Ticlopidine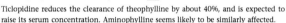

Ticlopidine reduces the clearance of theophylline by about 40%, and is expected to raise its serum concentration. Aminophylline seems likely to be similarly affected.

> Monitor concurrent use for theophylline toxicity (such as headache, nausea, palpitations), particularly in situations where the metabolism of the theophylline might already be reduced (other drugs or diseases), and monitor theophylline concentrations accordingly.

Theophylline + Vaccines

BCG vaccine might reduce the clearance of theophylline. Normally influenza vaccines (whole-virion, split-virion, and surface antigen) do not interact with theophylline, but raised theophylline concentrations and toxicity have been seen in occasional cases.

> No action is needed as any interaction with BCG vaccine seems likely to resolve spontaneously. Problems with influenza vaccines are very unlikely to arise now that purer vaccines are available; however, bear these interactions in mind in case of an unexpected response to treatment.

Theophylline + Zafirlukast

Zafirlukast has no effect on theophylline concentrations, although isolated cases of an increase in theophylline concentration have been reported on concurrent use. Zafirlukast concentrations are modestly reduced by theophylline, but this does not appear to be clinically important. Aminophylline would be expected to interact similarly.

> No adverse interaction would normally seem to occur with zafirlukast and theophylline.

Theophylline + Zileuton

Zileuton increases the exposure to theophylline and increases the incidence of adverse effects. Aminophylline would be expected to interact similarly.

> Be alert for theophylline adverse effects (headache, nausea, tremor) and, if required, monitor the effect of concurrent use on theophylline concentrations and

reduce the dose as needed. The US manufacturer of zileuton recommends reducing the theophylline dose by 50%. Similarly, the initial dose of theophylline should be reduced if it is given to a patient already taking zileuton, and adjusted according to theophylline concentrations.

Tibolone

Tibolone + Toremifene

Tibolone appears to increase the risk of recurrent breast cancer in women taking anti-oestrogenic drugs, such as tamoxifen and the aromatase inhibitors. Toremifene would be expected to interact similarly.

Until more is known it would seem prudent to avoid concurrent use.

Ticagrelor

Ticagrelor + Ticlopidine

The concurrent use of ticagrelor and ticlopidine might theoretically increase the risk of bleeding.

Although combinations of antiplatelet drugs are commonly used and can be clinically beneficial in some indications, be aware of the increased risk of bleeding.

Ticagrelor + Venlafaxine

The bleeding risk associated with antiplatelet drugs such as ticagrelor might be further increased by the concurrent use of an SNRI.

The manufacturer of venlafaxine advises caution on concurrent use in patients taking antiplatelet drugs (such as ticagrelor). Consider giving gastroprotective drugs to those at high risk of gastrointestinal bleeding (e.g. the elderly, those with a history of gastrointestinal bleeding, patients taking multiple antiplatelet drugs). Advise patients to report any signs of excessive bleeding.

Ticagrelor + Warfarin and related oral anticoagulants

The UK manufacturer of ticagrelor states that the concurrent use of oral anticoagulants within 24 hours of taking ticagrelor might theoretically increase the risk of bleeding.

Be aware that the risk of bleeding might be increased.

Ticlopidine

Ticlopidine + Tizanidine ⚠

Ciprofloxacin, a CYP1A2 inhibitor, markedly increases tizanidine exposure, which increases the hypotensive and sedative effects of tizanidine. Other CYP1A2 inhibitors (the UK and US manufacturers name ticlopidine) are expected to interact similarly.

The effects of ticlopidine on CYP1A2 appear to be less potent than those of ciprofloxacin, nevertheless the manufacturers suggest that concurrent use should be avoided. Until more is known be alert for tizanidine adverse effects such as bradycardia, hypotension, and drowsiness.

Ticlopidine + Venlafaxine ❓

The bleeding risk associated with antiplatelet drugs such as ticlopidine might be further increased by the concurrent use of an SSRI, although the data appears to be conflicting. SNRIs (e.g. venlafaxine) are expected to interact similarly.

The manufacturer of venlafaxine advises caution on concurrent use in patients taking antiplatelet drugs (such as ticlopidine). Consider giving gastroprotective drugs to those at high risk of gastrointestinal bleeding (e.g. the elderly, those with a history of gastrointestinal bleeding, patients taking multiple antiplatelet drugs). Advise patients to report any signs of excessive bleeding.

Ticlopidine + Warfarin and related oral anticoagulants ⚠

The anticoagulant effects of acenocoumarol may be modestly reduced by ticlopidine. However, the anticoagulant effects of warfarin are unchanged by ticlopidine. As with other antiplatelet drugs, concurrent use with coumarins might possibly increase bleeding risk. Cholestatic hepatitis has been reported in some patients given warfarin and ticlopidine.

The US manufacturer recommends that if a patient is switched from an anticoagulant to ticlopidine, the anticoagulant should be stopped before ticlopidine is started. As with other antiplatelet drugs, an increased risk of bleeding is anticipated if coumarins or indanediones are also given.

Tizanidine

Tizanidine + Zileuton ⚠

Zileuton is predicted to increase the exposure to tizanidine, increasing its hypotensive and sedative effects.

The UK and US manufacturers suggest that concurrent use should be avoided.

Until more is known be alert for adverse effects such as bradycardia, hypotension, and drowsiness.

Topiramate

Topiramate + Ulipristal

The UK and US manufacturers of ulipristal predict that CYP3A4 inducers might reduce the plasma concentration of ulipristal and reduce its efficacy. High-dose topiramate might interact in this way.

The US manufacturer of ulipristal gives no specific advice about how to manage this potential interaction, whereas the UK manufacturer advises that ulipristal should not be used for emergency contraception in women taking CYP3A4 inducers (such as high-dose topiramate), or who have stopped taking an enzyme inducer within the last 2 to 3 weeks. Until more is known, this advice seems prudent.

Toremifene

Toremifene + Warfarin and related oral anticoagulants

The anticoagulant effects of acenocoumarol and warfarin are predicted to be increased by toremifene, increasing the risk of bleeding.

Monitor the anticoagulant response closely if toremifene is added to treatment with any coumarin, and reduce the dose as necessary. Note that the UK manufacturer of toremifene recommends avoiding the concurrent use of coumarins. Consider also that, from a disease perspective, when treating venous thromboembolic disease in patients with cancer, warfarin is generally inferior (higher risk of major bleeds and recurrent thrombosis) to low-molecular-weight heparins.

Trazodone

Trazodone + Venlafaxine

Isolated cases of serotonin syndrome have been reported in patients taking venlafaxine with trazodone.

Concurrent use should be monitored carefully. For more information, see serotonin syndrome, page 580.

Trazodone + **Warfarin and related oral anticoagulants** ⚠️

A handful of case reports describe a moderate reduction in the anticoagulant effects of warfarin caused by trazodone, and another case report describes a rise in INR.

> It might be prudent to monitor the INR in all patients taking warfarin if trazodone is started or stopped, adjusting the warfarin dose if necessary.

Tricyclics

Tricyclics + **Valproate** ❓

Amitriptyline and nortriptyline plasma levels can be increased by sodium valproate and valpromide. Status epilepticus, tremulousness and/or sleep disturbances have been attributed to elevated clomipramine or nortriptyline levels in patients taking valproate or valproic acid.

> It would seem prudent to monitor for tricyclic adverse effects (such as dry mouth, blurred vision and urinary retention) and reduce the dose of the tricyclic if necessary. Tricyclics can lower the convulsive threshold and should therefore be used with caution in patients with epilepsy.

Tricyclics + **Venlafaxine** ⚠️

The use of venlafaxine with the tricyclics is expected to increase the risk of serotonin syndrome, page 580, and cases have been seen. Increased antimuscarinic adverse effects, movement disorders and seizures have also been reported. Venlafaxine appears to increase the levels of desipramine or its 2-hydroxydesipramine metabolite. Other tricyclics are expected to interact similarly.

> Be alert for any evidence of increased antimuscarinic adverse effects. Although there appears to be only one report, the possibility of an increased risk of seizures with concurrent use should be borne in mind, especially in those already at risk of seizures. It may be necessary to withdraw one or both of the drugs. The reports of serotonin syndrome highlight the need for caution when one or more serotonergic drugs are given.

Tricyclics + **Warfarin and related oral anticoagulants** ❓

Limited evidence suggests that amitriptyline and possibly other tricyclics can cause unpredictable increases or decreases in prothrombin times in patients taking coumarins, which can make stable anticoagulation difficult.

> There is insufficient evidence to recommend an increased frequency of INR monitoring, but it would at least seem prudent to bear this interaction in mind when prescribing a coumarin and a tricyclic.

Triptans

Triptans + Venlafaxine

Concurrent use of venlafaxine and a triptan (e.g. sumatriptan) might lead to serotonin syndrome, page 580: cases have been reported to the FDA in the US.

> The combination need not be avoided, but monitor concurrent use carefully for signs of serotonin syndrome (such as weakness, hyperreflexia, and incoordination), especially during treatment initiation and dose increases, and if other serotonergic drugs are used.

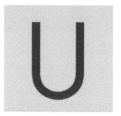

No interactions monographs have been included for drugs beginning with the letter U.

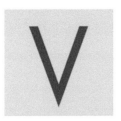

Vaccines

Vaccines + **Warfarin and related oral anticoagulants** ❓

The concurrent use of warfarin and influenza vaccine is usually safe and uneventful, but there are reports of bleeding in a handful of patients (life-threatening in one case) attributed to an interaction. Acenocoumarol also does not normally interact.

This interaction seems rare, but bear it in mind in case of unexpected bleeding. Note that, because of the theoretical risk of local muscle haematoma, it may be preferable to give influenza vaccines by deep subcutaneous injection in patients taking coumarins and related anticoagulants.

Venlafaxine

Venlafaxine + **Warfarin and related oral anticoagulants** ❓

Unpublished cases of bleeding and raised prothrombin times have been reported with venlafaxine and warfarin. Note that venlafaxine alone has, rarely, been associated with bleeding, and there is the theoretical possibility that the risk might be increased when used with warfarin and related drugs.

The general significance of these case reports is unclear. Consider increasing INR monitoring if venlafaxine is added or withdrawn from treatment with warfarin or any coumarin. Also bear in mind the possibility of increased bleeding risk in the absence of alterations in INR.

Vitamins

Vitamins + **Warfarin and related oral anticoagulants** ⚠

The effects of coumarins and indanediones can be reduced or abolished by vitamin K. This effect can be used to manage overdose, but unintentional and unwanted antagonism has occurred in patients after taking some proprietary chilblain preparations, health foods, food supplements, enteral feeds or exceptionally large amounts of some green vegetables, seaweed, or green tea, which can contain significant amounts of vitamin K. Giving 10 to 50 micrograms of vitamin K_1 (phytomenadione) generally will not significantly affect the INR in response to warfarin; however, patients with poor vitamin K status, even low vitamin K doses of 25 micrograms daily may have an important effect.

> The drug intake and diet of any patient who shows warfarin resistance' should be investigated for the possibility of this interaction. It can be accommodated either by increasing the anticoagulant dose, or by reducing the intake of vitamin K. However, patients taking vitamin K-rich diets should not change their eating habits without at the same time reducing the anticoagulant dose, because excessive anticoagulation and bleeding may occur.

V

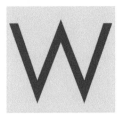

Warfarin and related oral anticoagulants

Warfarin, phenprocoumon, and acenocoumarol are racemic mixtures of *S*- and *R*-enantiomers. The *S*-enantiomers of these coumarins have several times more anticoagulant activity than the *R*-enantiomers. The *S*-enantiomer of warfarin is metabolised primarily by CYP2C9. The metabolism of *R*-warfarin is more complex but this enantiomer is primarily metabolised by CYP1A2, CYP3A4, CYP2C19, and CYP2C8. There is much more known about the metabolism of warfarin compared to other anticoagulants but it is established that *S*-phenprocoumon and *S*-acenocoumarol are also substrates for CYP2C9. Whilst the metabolism of the coumarins, especially warfarin, is well known, the numerous interaction pathways and the variability in patient responses makes the clinical consequences of alterations in metabolism difficult to predict.

Warfarin and related oral anticoagulants +
Zafirlukast

Zafirlukast increases the anticoagulant effects of warfarin and bleeding has been seen. Other coumarins might be similarly affected.

> If zafirlukast is given to patients stable taking a coumarin, monitor prothrombin times closely and be alert for the need to reduce the coumarin dose to avoid over-anticoagulation.

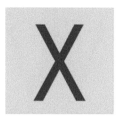

No interactions monographs have been included for drugs beginning with the letter X.

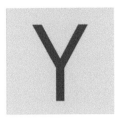

No interactions monographs have been included for drugs beginning with the letter Y.

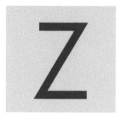

No interactions monographs have been included for drugs beginning with the letter Z.

Index

Index

Index

Index